Lippincott's Review for

NCLEX-PN

SEVENTH EDITION

Lippincott's Review for
NCLEX-PN
SEVENTH EDITION

Barbara Kuhn Timby, RN, BC, BSN, MA
Nursing Professor
Glen Oaks Community College
Centerville, Mich.

Ann Carmack, RN, BSN
Director of Educational Services
Baptist-Lutheran Medical Center
Kansas City, Mo.

Diana L. Rupert, RNC, MSN
Faculty
Registered Nursing Program
Conemaugh School of Nursing
Johnstown, Pa.

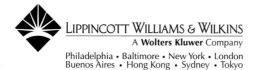

LIPPINCOTT WILLIAMS & WILKINS
A **Wolters Kluwer** Company
Philadelphia • Baltimore • New York • London
Buenos Aires • Hong Kong • Sydney • Tokyo

STAFF

Executive Publisher
Judith A. Schilling McCann, RN, MSN

Senior Acquisitions Editor
Elizabeth Nieginski

Editorial Director
David Moreau

Clinical Director
Joan M. Robinson, RN, MSN

Senior Art Director
Arlene Putterman

Editorial Project Manager
Coleen M.F. Stern

Clinical Project Manager
Beverly Ann Tscheschlog, RN, BS

Editor
Diane M. Labus

Copy Editors
Kimberly Bilotta (supervisor), Karen C. Comerford,
Amanda Bradford Cortright, Pamela Wingrod

Designers
Will Boehm (book design), E. Jane Spencer (project manager)

Digital Composition Services
Diane Paluba (manager), Joyce Rossi Biletz, Donna S. Morris

Manufacturing
Patricia K. Dorshaw (director), Beth J. Welsh

Editorial Assistants
Megan Aldinger, Karen J. Kirk, Linda Ruhf

The clinical treatments described and recommended in this publication are based on research and consultation with nursing, medical, and legal authorities. To the best of our knowledge, these procedures reflect currently accepted practice. Nevertheless, they can't be considered absolute and universal recommendations. For individual applications, all recommendations must be considered in light of the patient's clinical condition and, before administration of new or infrequently used drugs, in light of the latest package-insert information. The authors and publisher disclaim any responsibility for any adverse effects resulting from the suggested procedures, from any undetected errors, or from the reader's misunderstanding of the text.

LRNCLEXPN011205 – 030307

Library of Congress Cataloging-in-Publication Data

Timby, Barbara Kuhn.
  Lippincott's review for NCLEX-PN.—7th ed. / Barbara Kuhn Timby, Ann Carmack, Diana L. Rupert.
     p. ; cm.
  Includes bibliographical references.
  1. Practical nursing—Examinations, questions, etc. 2. National Council Licensure Examination for Practical/Vocational Nurses—Study guides. I. Carmack, Ann. II. Rupert, Diana L. III. Lippincott Williams & Wilkins. IV. Title.
  [DNLM: 1. Nursing, Practical—Examination Questions. WY 18.2 T583L 2006]
RT62.T56 2006
610.7306'93076—dc22
ISBN13: 978-1-58255-540-9
ISBN10: 1-58255-540-0 (alk. paper)   2005025758

Contents

CONTRIBUTORS   ix
PREFACE   x
ACKNOWLEDGMENTS   xii
FREQUENTLY ASKED QUESTIONS   xiii
HOW TO USE THIS BOOK   xxi

UNIT I
The Nursing Care of Adults with Medical-Surgical Disorders   **1**

TEST 1
The Nursing Care of Clients with Musculoskeletal Disorders   **2**

Nursing Care of Clients with Musculoskeletal Injuries   2
Nursing Care of Clients with Fractures   3
Nursing Care of Clients with Casts   5
Nursing Care of Clients with Traction   7
Nursing Care of Clients with Inflammatory Joint
    Disorders   8
Nursing Care of Clients with Degenerative Bone
    Disorders   12
Nursing Care of Clients with Amputations   12
Nursing Care of Clients with Skeletal Tumors   13
Nursing Care of Clients with a Herniated Intervertebral
    Disk   14
Correct Answers and Rationales   15

TEST 2
The Nursing Care of Clients with Neurologic System Disorders   **30**

Nursing Care of Clients with Infectious and
    Inflammatory Conditions   30
Nursing Care of Clients with Seizure Disorders   31
Nursing Care of Clients with Neurologic Trauma   32

Nursing Care of Clients with Degenerative Disorders   33
Nursing Care of Clients with Cerebrovascular Disorders   36
Nursing Care of Clients with Tumors of the Neurologic
    System   37
Nursing Care of Clients with Nerve Disorders   38
Correct Answers and Rationales   40

TEST 3
The Nursing Care of Clients with Disorders of Sensory Organs and the Integument   **51**

Nursing Care of Clients with Eye Disorders   51
Nursing Care of Clients with Disorders of Accessory
    Eye Structures   55
Nursing Care of Clients with Ear Disorders   56
Nursing Care of Clients with Nasal Disorders   59
Nursing Care of Clients with Disorders of the Skin and
    Related Structures   60
Correct Answers and Rationales   63

TEST 4
The Nursing Care of Clients with Endocrine Disorders   **77**

Nursing Care of Clients with Disorders of the Pituitary
    Gland   77
Nursing Care of Clients with Disorders of the Thyroid
    Gland   78
Nursing Care of Clients with Disorders of the
    Parathyroid Glands   80
Nursing Care of Clients with Disorders of the Adrenal
    Glands   80
Nursing Care of Clients with Pancreatic Endocrine
    Disorders   82
Correct Answers and Rationales   86

TEST 5
The Nursing Care of Clients with Cardiac Disorders 97

Nursing Care of Clients with Hypertensive Heart
    Disease 97
Nursing Care of Clients with Coronary Artery Disease 98
Nursing Care of Clients with Myocardial Infarction 102
Nursing Care of Clients with Congestive Heart Failure 104
Nursing Care of Clients with Conduction Disorders 106
Nursing Care of Clients with Valvular Disorders 106
Nursing Care of Clients with Infectious and
    Inflammatory Disorders of the Heart 108
Correct Answers and Rationales 109

TEST 6
The Nursing Care of Clients with Peripheral Vascular, Hematologic, and Lymphatic Disorders 124

Nursing Care of Clients with Venous Disorders 124
Nursing Care of Clients with Arterial Disorders 127
Nursing Care of Clients with Red Blood Cell Disorders 129
Nursing Care of Clients with White Blood Cell
    Disorders 131
Nursing Care of Clients with Bone Marrow Disorders 133
Nursing Care of Clients with Coagulation Disorders 135
Nursing Care of Clients with Inflammatory and
    Obstructive Lymphatic Disorders 135
Correct Answers and Rationales 136

TEST 7
The Nursing Care of Clients with Respiratory Disorders 152

Nursing Care of Clients with Upper Respiratory
    Infections 152
Nursing Care of Clients with Inflammatory and
    Allergic Disorders of the Upper Airways 153
Nursing Care of Clients with Cancer of the Larynx 154
Nursing Care of Clients with Inflammatory and
    Infectious Disorders of the Lower Airways 154
Nursing Care of Clients with Asthma 158
Nursing Care of Clients with Chronic Obstructive
    Pulmonary Disease 159
Nursing Care of Clients with Lung Cancer 160
Nursing Care of Clients with Chest Injuries 161
Nursing Care of Clients with Pulmonary Embolism 162
Nursing Care of Clients with a Tracheostomy 163
Nursing Care of Clients with a Sudden Airway
    Occlusion 163
Correct Answers and Rationales 164

TEST 8
The Nursing Care of Clients with Disorders of the Gastrointestinal System and Accessory Organs of Digestion 179

Nursing Care of Clients with Disorders of the Mouth 179
Nursing Care of Clients with Disorders of the
    Esophagus 180
Nursing Care of Clients with Disorders of the Stomach 182
Nursing Care of Clients with Disorders of the Small
    Intestine 185
Nursing Care of Clients with Disorders of the Large
    Intestine 186
Nursing Care of Clients with Disorders of the Rectum
    and Anus 190
Nursing Care of Clients with Disorders of the
    Gallbladder 191
Nursing Care of Clients with Disorders of the Liver 193
Nursing Care of Clients with Disorders of the Pancreas 195
Correct Answers and Rationales 196

TEST 9
The Nursing Care of Clients with Urologic Disorders 216

Nursing Care of Clients with Urinary Incontinence 216
Nursing Care of Clients with Infectious and
    Inflammatory Urologic Disorders 217
Nursing Care of Clients with Renal Failure 220
Nursing Care of Clients with Urologic Obstructions 222
Nursing Care of Clients with Urologic Tumors 224
Nursing Care of Clients with Urinary Diversions 224
Correct Answers and Rationales 225

TEST 10
The Nursing Care of Clients with Disorders of the Reproductive System 236

Nursing Care of Clients with Breast Disorders 236
Nursing Care of Clients with Disturbances in
    Menstruation 238
Nursing Care of Clients with Infectious and
    Inflammatory Disorders of the Female
    Reproductive System 239
Nursing Care of Clients with Benign and Malignant
    Disorders of the Uterus and Ovaries 240
Nursing Care of Clients with Miscellaneous Disorders
    of the Female Reproductive System 243
Nursing Care of Clients with Inflammatory Disorders
    of the Male Reproductive System 243
Nursing Care of Clients with Structural Disorders
    of the Male Reproductive System 244

Nursing Care of Clients with Benign and Malignant
  Disorders of the Male Reproductive System 244
Nursing Care of Clients with Sexually
  Transmitted Diseases 245
Nursing Care of Clients Practicing Family Planning 247
Correct Answers and Rationales 249

UNIT II
The Nursing Care of the Childbearing Family 265

TEST 11
The Nursing Care of Clients During the Antepartum Period 266

Anatomy and Physiology of the Male and Female
  Reproductive Systems 266
Signs and Symptoms of Pregnancy 267
Assessing the Pregnant Client 268
Nutritional Needs During Pregnancy 269
Teaching the Pregnant Client 271
Common Discomforts of Pregnancy 272
High-Risk Factors and Pregnancy 273
Complications of Pregnancy 274
Elective Abortion 277
Correct Answers and Rationales 278

TEST 12
The Nursing Care of Clients During the Intrapartum and Postpartum Periods 291

Admission of the Client to a Labor and Delivery
  Facility 291
Nursing Care of Clients During the First Stage of
  Labor 292
Nursing Care of Clients During the Second Stage of
  Labor 294
Nursing Care of Clients During the Third Stage of
  Labor 295
Nursing Care of Clients During the Fourth Stage of
  Labor 296
Nursing Care of Clients Having a Cesarean Birth 296
Nursing Care of Clients Having an Emergency Delivery 298
Nursing Care of Clients Having a Stillborn Baby 298
Nursing Care of Clients During the Postpartum Period 299
Nursing Care of the Newborn Client 301
Nursing Care of Newborns with Complications 304
Correct Answers and Rationales 306

UNIT III
The Nursing Care of Children 321

TEST 13
The Nursing Care of Infants, Toddlers, and Preschool Children 322

Normal Growth and Development of Infants, Toddlers,
  and Preschool Children 322
Nursing Care of an Infant with Myelomeningocele 324
Nursing Care of an Infant with Hydrocephalus 325
Nursing Care of an Infant with Cleft Lip 325
Nursing Care of an Infant with Pyloric Stenosis 326
Nursing Care of an Infant with Bilateral Clubfoot 326
Nursing Care of a Child with Otitis Media 327
Nursing Care of a Child with a Congenital Heart Defect 327
Nursing Care of a Child with an Infectious Disease 328
Nursing Care of a Child with Human
  Immunodeficiency Virus (HIV) Infection 328
Nursing Care of a Child with Atopic Dermatitis 329
Nursing Care of a Toddler with Sickle Cell Crisis 329
Nursing Care of a Toddler with Cystic Fibrosis 329
Nursing Care of a Toddler with Asthma 330
Nursing Care of a Toddler Who Has Swallowed a Toxic
  Substance 330
Nursing Care of a Toddler with Croup 331
Nursing Care of a Toddler with Pneumonia 332
Nursing Care of a Preschooler with Seizure Disorder 332
Nursing Care of a Preschooler with Leukemia 333
Nursing Care of a Preschooler with Strabismus 334
Nursing Care of a Preschooler Having a Tonsillectomy
  and Adenoidectomy 334
Correct Answers and Rationales 335

TEST 14
The Nursing Care of School-Age Children and Adolescents 350

Nursing Care of a Child with Rheumatic Fever 350
Nursing Care of a Child with Diabetes Mellitus 351
Nursing Care of a Child with Partial- and
  Full-Thickness Burns 353
Nursing Care of a Child with Juvenile Rheumatoid
  Arthritis 353
Nursing Care of a Child with an Injury 354
Nursing Care of a Child with a Head Injury 354
Nursing Care of a Child with a Brain Tumor 355
Nursing Care of a Child in Traction 356
Nursing Care of a Child with a Kidney Disorder 356
Nursing Care of a Child with a Blood Disorder 357

Nursing Care of a Child with a Communicable Disease 357
Nursing Care of a Child with a Nutritional Deficiency 357
Nursing Care of a Child with a Musculoskeletal
    Disability 358
Nursing Care of an Adolescent with Appendicitis 358
Nursing Care of an Adolescent with Dysmenorrhea 359
Nursing Care of an Adolescent Who Is Abusing Drugs 359
Nursing Care of an Adolescent with a Sexually
    Transmitted Disease 360
Nursing Care of an Adolescent with Scoliosis 362
Dosage Calculations for Children and Adolescents 362
Correct Answers and Rationales 363

UNIT IV
The Nursing Care of Clients with Mental Health Needs 375

TEST 15
The Nursing Care of Infants, Children, and Adolescents with Mental Health Needs 376

Mental Health Needs During Infancy 376
Mental Health Needs During Childhood 378
Mental Health Needs During Adolescence 383
Correct Answers and Rationales 388

TEST 16
The Nursing Care of Adult Clients with Mental Health Needs 401

Mental Health Needs During Young Adulthood 401
Mental Health Needs During Middle Age (35-65) 405
Mental Health Needs During Late Adulthood
    (Over 65) 409
Correct Answers and Rationales 413

UNIT V
Postreview Tests 427

Comprehensive Test 1 428
Correct Answers and Rationales 440

Comprehensive Test 2 456
Correct Answers and Rationales 468

BIBLIOGRAPHY 484

Contributors

Coauthor of Previous Editions

Jeanne C. Scherer, RN, BSN, MS
Formerly Assistant Director and Medical-Surgical Coordinator
Sisters School of Nursing
Buffalo, N.Y.

Contributor to Previous Editions

Bennita W. Vaughans, RN, MSN
Instructor
Practical Nursing Program
Councill Trenholm State Technical College
Montgomery, Ala.

Reviewers for this Edition

Barbara C. Anderson, RN, BSN, MED
Director
Virginia Beach City Public Schools,
Virginia Beach School of Practical
Nursing
Virginia Beach, Va.

Janice W. Chapman, RN, MSN
Site Coordinator, Instructor of Nursing
Health Careers Department
Reid State College
Atmore, Ala.

Diane J. Lane, RN, MSN
Instructor—Vocational Nursing
Maxine L. Silva Magnet High School for
Health Care Professions
El Paso, Tex.

Kendra S. Seiler, RN, MSN, CNOR
Nursing Instructor
Rio Hondo Community College
Whittier, Calif.

Preface

Lippincott's Review for NCLEX-PN, Seventh Edition, has been written to help the candidate prepare for the National Council Licensure Examination for Practical/Vocational Nurses (NCLEX-PN). Several features make this review book especially helpful.

First and foremost, the most recent NCLEX-PN Test Plan approved by the National Council of State Boards of Nursing (effective April 2005) was used as a guide for preparing this book. Consequently, the review questions presented here reflect the components in the Test Plan as well as current nursing practice. In addition, the substance of the questions is based entirely on information contained in textbooks that are widely used in practical nursing programs throughout the United States.

An effort has also been made to divide the book content into comprehensive yet manageable sections. To accomplish this goal, the topics for review are organized into four major units according to specialty areas of nursing practice:

• Unit I: The Nursing Care of Adults with Medical-Surgical Disorders
• Unit II: The Nursing Care of the Childbearing Family
• Unit III: The Nursing Care of Children
• Unit IV: The Nursing Care of Clients with Mental Health Needs.

The decision to arrange the content according to specific subject areas was made for several reasons. First, it helps you correlate your review with courses commonly taught in most practical nursing programs. Second, it allows you to focus your energy on reviewing a limited amount of information at any one time.

The four major units are further subdivided into a total of 16 separate review tests. The first unit, which pertains to the nursing care of clients with medical-surgical disorders, contains 10 review tests. The remaining three units each contain two review tests. This distribution is appropriate because medical-surgical nursing is the most common clinical area where new practical nurses are employed. In addition, the Test Plan is based on a job survey of newly employed practical nurses 6 months following their graduation; therefore, it is logical to assume that a majority of the licensing examination questions will reflect items of a medical-surgical nature.

All the questions in the review tests are integrated in the same manner as the licensing examination. This means that each test question—whether it is one that concerns a medical-surgical, obstetric, pediatric, or mental health situation—reflects a specific category and subcategory of client need. Both of these test components are discussed further in *Frequently Asked Questions,* page xiii.

Another helpful feature of this review book is the fifth unit, which consists of a two-part comprehensive examination that follows the 16 review tests. The examination, beginning on page 428, is as much like the national licensing examination as possible. Like the NCLEX-PN, the questions in the comprehensive examination are a mix of all nursing content areas and the Test Plan components.

Each part of the comprehensive examination contains 130 items, for a total of 260 items. The number of questions in each part is slightly higher than the average number of items answered by candidates on the NCLEX-PN (115 items in 2000 [National Council of State Boards of Nursing, 2001]). Taken in total, the comprehensive examination provides practice with more than the maximum of 205 questions asked on the NCLEX-PN, and it offers you a rough estimate of how long it might take to answer all the potential NCLEX-PN items, should that possibility occur.

In addition to the review tests and two-part comprehensive examination in the text, the accompanying CD-ROM provides a way to realistically simulate the computerized method for taking the NCLEX-PN. You can use the CD-ROM to test yourself in a number of ways: by general content area; by number of questions; or by time. This functionality allows you to tailor your studying to the specific areas in which you need practice or to the time you have available in a study session, while simulating the NCLEX-PN as closely as possible.

Other advantages to using this book include the sections containing the *Correct Answers and Rationales,* which follow each review test and comprehensive examination. These sections provide the best answer to each test question, the rationale for the correct answer, and reasons why the other answer choices are incorrect. Reading the rationales is an excellent technique for reviewing the domain of practical nursing.

In summary, there are more than 1,800 items in the 16 review tests and 260 items in the two-part comprehensive examination, for a total of more than 2,000 items. The items that compose the 16 review tests are found on the CD-ROM as well. Although it is unreasonable to believe that any item in this book will be identical to one in the national examination, it is reasonable to expect that the NCLEX-PN will test the same kinds of content, knowledge, and skills. Although no review book or licensing examination can cover all aspects of nursing, this book serves as a resource for a comprehensive review and realistic simulation of the NCLEX-PN process.

As a candidate for the NCLEX-PN, you are further urged to read the section titled *Frequently Asked Questions,* which begins on page xiii. This section provides information about the NCLEX-PN testing process, how the test is designed, and suggestions on how to prepare for the examination. The National Council of State Boards of Nursing Web site (www.ncsbn.org) provides the most up-to-date information on the Test Plan and testing process. The *How to Use This Book* section, which begins on page xxi, introduces you to the testing format used in this review book.

Although this book's primary purpose is to help practical nurses prepare for the national licensing examination, it can serve other purposes as well. For example, it can be used to study for various types of achievement tests in nursing. Inactive practical nurses who wish to return to nursing will also find the book useful for review and self-appraisal, as will others who seek course credit by taking challenge examinations for advanced placement. And, finally, faculty may find the book helpful for developing expertise in test construction. However, regardless of the purpose for which this book is used, its ultimate goal is to help prepare practicing nurses to provide safe, effective nursing care.

Acknowledgments

Many thanks to Ann Carmack and Diana Rupert, coauthors of this edition, for their efforts in updating and revising test items as well as generating new material. The authors express sincere thanks for the contributions of Bennita Vaughans, RN, MSN, contributor to the previous edition, and Jeanne C. Scherer, RN, BSN, MS, coauthor of the 4th edition, whose previous work made this revision easier.

Finally, recognition is due for the conscientious assistance from the editors and staff who have helped develop this book through its various stages of production. Among that legion, the authors wish to thank Elizabeth Nieginski, Acquisitions Editor.

Barbara Kuhn Timby, RN, BC, BSN, MA

Frequently Asked Questions

The following are frequently asked questions concerning the NCLEX-PN and the most current information that is available about the testing process.

What is the NCLEX-PN?

The abbreviation *NCLEX-PN* stands for the National Council Licensure Examination for Practical/Vocational Nurses. In short, the NCLEX-PN is a computerized test developed by the National Council of State Boards of Nursing. The test is used to regulate the licensing of practical and vocational nurses in each of its member states.

MEMBERS OF THE NATIONAL COUNCIL OF STATE BOARDS OF NURSING

Members include representatives from:
- all 50 United States
- District of Columbia
- Puerto Rico
- Guam
- American Samoa
- Virgin Islands
- Mariana Islands.

What is the purpose of the NCLEX-PN?

All National Council member states and territories currently use the NCLEX-PN as the standard for licensing practical and vocational nurses. *Practical nurse* and *vocational nurse* are regional terms; they differ in name only. Whether referred to as practical or vocational, each nurse completes similar educational programs, and graduates from both take the NCLEX-PN. The terms *practical nurse* and *practical nursing* are used in this book to refer to both.

Licensing serves to assure the public that a graduate practical nurse is a competent practitioner. Passing the NCLEX-PN demonstrates that a graduate of a practical nursing program can perform entry-level nursing skills that meet the needs of clients with common health problems, have predictable outcomes, and demonstrate at least a minimum level of competency.

Can foreign-educated nurses take the NCLEX-PN?

Foreign-educated nurses can take the NCLEX-PN. However, before taking the test, they must first meet eligibility requirements in the state where they wish to practice. In most states, foreign-educated nurses are asked to present credentials describing their course of study in the country where they were schooled.

How is the NCLEX-PN developed?

Before the examination is administered, it goes through several stages of development.

STEPS IN THE NCLEX-PN TEST DEVELOPMENT

- Survey newly licensed practical nurses every 3 years
- Analyze practical nurse job responsibilities
- Formulate a test plan based on the data
- Select and approve item writers
- Submit questions to item reviewers
- Implement trial testing of items
- Give state boards of nursing an opportunity to review items
- Obtain approval of NCLEX-PN test items
- Maintain two alternating NCLEX-PN test pools

What is the NCLEX-PN Test Plan?

The Test Plan, which changes from time to time, serves as the framework for the content that is included in the NCLEX-PN. The current Test Plan, which was implemented in April 2005, is based on the results of a study called the *Report of Findings from the 2003 LPN/LVN Practical Analysis: Linking the NCLEX-PN ® Examination to Practice* (Smith and Crawford, 2003). This study sampled data from newly licensed practical nurses who provided information on how often they performed each of the studied nursing activities, the impact of the nursing activities on their clients' well-being, and the setting in which the activities were performed.

The tabulated results of the job analysis study influence the subject matter tested and the percentage of questions asked in particular NCLEX-PN test categories. The test categories on the current NCLEX-PN Test Plan follow the framework of Client Needs Categories and Client Needs Subcategories. (See illustration below.)

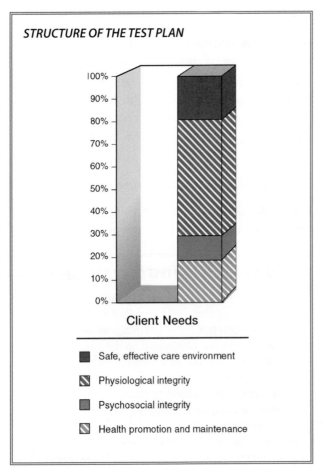

The distribution of NCLEX-PN test items in the Client Needs Categories and Subcategories is as follows:
- Physiological integrity
  - Basic care and comfort 11%-17%
  - Pharmacological therapies 9%-15%
  - Reduction of risk potential 10%-16%
  - Physiological adaptation 12%-18%
- Safe, effective care environment
  - Coordinated care 11%-17%
  - Safety and infection control 8%-14%
- Health promotion and maintenance 7%-13%
- Psychosocial integrity 8%-14%

Client Needs Categories and Subcategories

Of the four Client Needs Categories, the emphasis is on physiological integrity. The remaining categories (in descending order) are safe, effective care environment; health promotion and maintenance; and psychosocial integrity.

PHYSIOLOGICAL INTEGRITY

This category tests the candidates's knowledge in the following areas:
- **Basic care and comfort** (11%-17%)—providing comfort and assistance in performance of activities of daily living
- **Pharmacological therapies** (9%-15%)—providing care related to administration of medications and monitoring clients receiving parenteral therapies
- **Reduction of risk potential** (10%-16%)—reducing the possibility of developing complications or additional health problems related to treatments, procedures, or existing conditions
- **Physiological adaptation** (12%-18%)—providing care during acute and chronic phases of health disorders, including emergency situations.

SAFE, EFFECTIVE CARE ENVIRONMENT

This category covers questions concerning:
- **Coordinated care** (11%-17%)—providing care and collaborating with health team members to coordinate client care, including legal and ethical issues
- **Safety and infection control** (8%-14%)—protecting clients and health care personnel from injury.

HEALTH PROMOTION AND MAINTENANCE

This category tests the candidate's ability to answer questions about the expected stages of growth and development and the prevention or early detection of health problems.

PSYCHOSOCIAL INTEGRITY

This category covers questions concerning the promotion and support of the emotional, mental, and social well-being of clients.

Integrated processes

Phases of the nursing process are integrated throughout the Client Needs Categories and Subcategories. This review book codes all questions according to the Client Needs Categories and Subcategories. Other integrated processes—caring, communication and documentation, teaching, and learning—are represented as well.

What is the style of questions asked on the NCLEX-PN?

The NCLEX-PN is composed primarily of multiple-choice questions. A multiple-choice question, also called an *item*, has two main parts: the *stem* and the *options*.

The stem

The *stem* presents the problem or situation that requires a solution. The stem of an NCLEX-PN multiple-choice question is stated as a complete sentence. If all the essential information for answering the question is contained in the stem, it is called a *stand-alone item*. Sometimes the stem is preceded by a *case scenario*, which gives background information that is pertinent to the item.

The options

The *options* are the choices from which an answer is selected. There are four options in multiple-choice questions. The options on the NCLEX-PN are labeled *1, 2, 3, 4*. In this type of question, there is one correct answer among the choices given. The three incorrect options, called distractors, are intended to appear as good answers; they may even be partially correct. But an option is incorrect if it is not the best answer to the question.

Alternate-format questions

Besides the traditional four-option multiple-choice questions, the NCLEX-PN also includes alternate-format questions. These are as follows:

- multiple-response multiple-choice questions that provide up to six options (1, 2, 3, 4, 5, 6) from which the candidate must select all applicable answers.
- fill-in-the-blank questions, which require the candidate to use calculations to solve dosage problems or make conversions.
- hot-spot questions, which require the candidate to use the computer mouse to click onto an appropriate area on a graphic image appearing on the computer screen.
- drag-and-drop questions, which require the candidate to order all the options sequentially or chronologically by clicking and dragging the items using the computer mouse.
- chart/exhibit questions, which require the candidate to arrive at the correct answer by reviewing information presented in a chart, table, or graph.

Most of the questions on the NCLEX-PN, however, are of the traditional variety—multiple-choice questions with four options—and these standard questions make up the bulk of this review book. Regardless of the style, any question may include a chart, table, or graphic image.

STANDARD MULTIPLE-CHOICE STEM AND OPTIONS

Which assessment finding best justifies withholding the continued I.M. administration of penicillin (Bicillin) until consulting with the prescribing physician?
[ ] 1. The client states that the injection sites are painful.
[ ] 2. The client shows the nurse a red, itchy rash.*
[ ] 3. The client's oral body temperature is 100° F (37.8° C).
[ ] 4. The client has been having two stools a day.

*Correct answer

How is the NCLEX-PN administered?

The NCLEX-PN is an adaptive computerized test. The term *adaptive* means that the computer creates a unique test for each candidate. (See "How does the computer select test questions?" for more information.)

The computerized method of testing offers several advantages over the earlier way of taking the NCLEX-PN. For example, it:

- facilitates year-round testing.
- offers convenient scheduling choices.
- personalizes the test for each candidate.
- shortens the length of the examination.
- expedites notification of test results.

A candidate may request any testing site regardless of the state in which he or she wishes to be licensed. Since the test is adapted to each candidate, it can be completed in 5 hours or less; the average time is just over 2 hours (National Council of State Boards of Nursing, 2001). Also, because scoring is computerized, examination results are available more rapidly than in the past.

What is the testing site like?

Each of more than 200 testing sites is able to accommodate up to 15 candidates at the same time. A sample of the basic floor plan of a test site is shown in Figure 2. Each candidate is assigned to a separate testing cubicle that contains a table with computer equipment, a desk lamp, and scratch paper. Personal articles can be placed in secured storage or lockers outside the test room.

Persons with special physical needs, or those requesting modifications in the testing process or environment, must make that information known to the board of nursing at the time of application. A letter from a professional (usually the director of the nursing program) confirming the candidate's disability is also required. If the board of nursing approves the applicant's request, special accommodations are made if they do not jeopardize the security of the test or give the candidate an unfair advantage.

Precautions are taken to ensure that the candidate who is registered for the NCLEX-PN and the person at the test site are one and the same.

Once the examination commences, test security is maintained in two ways. All candidates are observed directly and continuously by a proctor who can view the testing cubicles without entering the room. In addition, candidates are monitored by video and audio equipment that has taping capability.

> **TEST SITE SECURITY POLICIES**
>
> Before the test, each person must:
> - possess an Authorization to Test (ATT) affidavit.*
> - present two forms of signature identification.
>   - One must contain a recent photograph.
>   - The name on the photograph identification must match exactly the name on the ATT.
> - be photographed and thumbprinted.
>
> *See "How do I register for the NCLEX-PN?" on page xviii.

Will I be given a chance to practice using the computer?

Regardless of the candidates' computer skills, each is given an opportunity to practice before the actual test begins. If necessary, computer assistance is also available during the examination. Thus far, candidates with computer experience have not demonstrated any advantage in test performance.

How does the computer select test questions?

The NCLEX-PN questions vary in their level of difficulty. When the test begins, the first questions are generally at a moderately difficult level. If the candidate answers such a question incorrectly, the computer selects an easier question next. Conversely, if the candidate answers a moderately difficult item correctly, the next question is more difficult. Passing the examination depends on both the number of correctly answered questions and their level of difficulty.

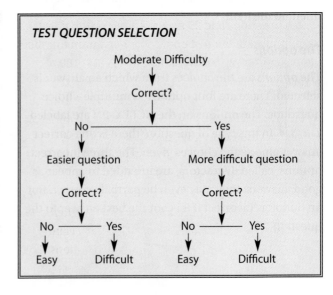

TEST QUESTION SELECTION

How do I indicate my answers to the NCLEX-PN questions?

Answers are selected by using the keyboard or mouse. The only two working keys are the *space bar* and the *enter key*. The space bar moves the cursor to highlight a choice. The enter key is pressed to record the highlighted choice. A description of the two keys, along with a written explanation on how to use them, is included at each computer terminal. A mouse interface and drop-down calculator are also provided. The CD-ROM included with this book also features a drop-down calculator.

How long do the questions remain on the screen?

Each question remains on the screen until an answer is recorded. Candidates are *not* able to:

- skip a question.
- review previous questions.
- change answers.

The underlying reason is that the difficulty of each test question is based on the candidate's answer to preceding test questions.

How many questions are asked on the NCLEX-PN?

Each candidate's test is unique. The test is made up of a comparatively small number of items from among the vast quantity stored in the memory of the computerized test pool. However, each candidate must answer a minimum of 85 questions. Of these questions, 60 are scored questions and 25 are tryout items that may be used in subsequent test pools. The maximum number of questions given to any candidate is 205—180 of which are scored.

There is no way for a candidate to determine which questions are tryout items. The tryout items are *not* calculated in the final NCLEX-PN score, regardless of whether the candidate answers the questions correctly.

On average, approximately 50% of NCLEX-PN candidates answer the minimum number of test items. Fewer than one-third, or 33%, of NCLEX-PN candidates answer the maximum number of questions. The latter group usually consists of those whose test performances are on the borderline between passing and failing. The remaining test candidates answer between 85 and 205 items.

NCLEX-PN TESTING PARAMETERS	
Minimum number of questions	85
Maximum number if questions	205
Minimum testing time	None
Maximum testing time	5 hours
Mandatory break	After 2½ hours
Optional break	After 4 hours

How long does the NCLEX-PN take?

Since each test is tailor-made for the candidate, there is no minimum amount of time for the test. The maximum length of time allowed for the NCLEX-PN is 5 hours; however, most candidates finish much sooner. The examination time varies depending on how speedily the candidate reads and answers each test item and how well or poorly the questions are answered.

The test is terminated when the computer has sufficient data to determine with 95% confidence whether the candidate has demonstrated sufficient knowledge to pass the examination. The test ends automatically when the candidate:

- answers at least a minimum number of 85 questions correctly.
- answers 85 to 205 questions at or below the passing standard.
- answers 205 questions without enough certainty to determine a passing or failing score.
- is still testing when the 5-hour time limit expires.

Who decides the pass/fail score for the NCLEX-PN?

The National Council's Board of Directors ultimately establishes the official minimum passing standard for the NCLEX-PN. The Board of Directors' decision is made after receiving recommendations from a panel of nine judges. The panel, which represents diverse geographic regions and areas of clinical practice, determines what portion of minimally competent practical nurses would correctly answer each test question in a sample test.

The passing standard for the NCLEX-PN is reevaluated whenever the Test Plan changes or at 3-year intervals, whichever comes first. Each state has the authority to set the minimum passing score in its own jurisdiction. However, most states use the same minimum passing score proposed by the National Council of State Boards of Nursing.

How do I register for the NCLEX-PN?

There are several basic steps that all candidates must complete before taking the NCLEX-PN.

NCLEX-PN applications may be obtained on request from the state board of nursing, or they may be available from the candidate's school of nursing. After receiving an application, the state board of nursing determines if the applicant meets licensure eligibility requirements.

Once the candidate's eligibility is confirmed, NCLEX-PN registration with Pearson VUE, an electronic testing service, can go forward. Pearson VUE offers three different methods of registration: via its Web site (www.pearsonvue.com), by contacting a Pearson VUE agent, or by contacting the test center directly. Forms and information on registering for the NCLEX-PN can be obtained by requesting the *NCLEX Candidate Bulletin* from the National Council of State Boards of Nursing (available at www.ncsbn.org). Fee payment of $225 is required at the time of direct registration.

After registration with Pearson VUE is processed, the candidate is sent a publication titled *Scheduling and Taking Your NCLEX*, along with a printed form called an Authorization to Test (ATT). There are three pieces of important information on the ATT: a candidate examination number, an authorization number, and an expiration date.

STEPS FOR NCLEX-PN REGISTRATION

1. Apply to the board of nursing in the state from which licensure is sought.
2. Request that the nursing program provide the board with proof of eligibility to take the NCLEX-PN.
3. Register with Pearson VUE.
4. Pay a fee of $225.

When and how do I arrange to take the NCLEX-PN?

After receiving an ATT, candidates can schedule a test date by phone with the test site of their choice or online at Pearson VUE's Web site before the expiration date that appears on the ATT. The locations and phone numbers of all available test sites are provided in the scheduling brochure and can also be found online by using the Test Center Locator function of the Pearson VUE Web site.

After contacting the test site, first-time candidates are offered a test date within 30 days; repeating candidates may be scheduled within a 45-day period. Either type of candidate can request a date beyond the 30 or 45 days as long as the date occurs prior to the expiration date on the ATT.

If the candidate wishes to cancel or reschedule a testing date, it must be done within 3 business days of the original appointment; otherwise, all fees are forfeited and the ATT is revoked. The same policy applies if a candidate is more than 30 minutes late on the date of the test.

How will I be informed of my NCLEX-PN results?

Test results, either Pass or Fail, are reported by mail from the state board of nursing where the candidate desires licensure. Although each candidate's score is electronically transmitted from the testing service to the respective board of nursing within 48 hours following an examination, the interim for informing the candidate varies from state to state. Generally, most candidates receive their test results 1 month after taking the examination.

A candidate who fails the NCLEX-PN is provided with a testing analysis in the form of a printed diagnostic profile. The profile gives data on how close the candidate came to the minimum passing score, how many items were answered, and performance achieved in each of the Test Plan categories. The statistical data are offered to assist failing candidates to improve their potential for success when retaking the NCLEX-PN. Weak areas suggest where an unsuccessful candidate might concentrate his or her review.

What if I feel my test result is incorrect?

Some (but not all) states provide a process for reviewing and challenging NCLEX-PN results. If a failed candidate feels that his or her test performance measurement is invalid, or wants the opportunity to dispute the answer to missed items, arrangements can be made to examine the questions that were answered in error. The review and challenge involves a fee and is limited to no more than 2 1/2 hours.

When can I retake the NCLEX-PN if I fail?

Presently, a repeating candidate may retake the examination up to four times a year, but no more frequently than every 91 days. This allows for a variation in items within the existing test pool. When, and if, the test pool of items increases, the frequency for retesting may be amended.

What are some strategies for NCLEX-PN success?

There are certain strategies that promote success on the NCLEX-PN. Some are more appropriate for long-term planning, while others are more pertinent as the test date nears.

STRATEGIC PLAN FOR NCLEX-PN PREPARATION

- Develop a time schedule for a comprehensive review.
- Divide the review topics into manageable amounts.
- Refresh your knowledge of topics in nursing courses.
- Reread sections in nursing textbooks, classroom notes, and written assignments.
- Reexamine tests from previous nursing courses.
- Concentrate on information that is necessary for self-care.
- Use this review book to assess your areas of competence.
- Identify weak areas, and restudy or clarify information.

Long-term strategies

Long-term strategies are best implemented as early as possible after completion of a nursing program. In fact, some nursing programs include standardized comprehensive examinations for graduating nurses to help predict how well the potential graduate will perform on the NCLEX-PN. But most new graduates are left to their own initiative when it comes to preparing for the licensing examination. Whatever approaches are used, it is best to begin preparing for the NCLEX-PN well in advance.

A systematic and comprehensive review is more effective than last-minute cramming. Cramming contributes to disorganized thinking; facts and concepts are likely to be confused. Also, with cramming there is always an underlying fear of being unprepared, which only heightens test anxiety.

One method of continued learning and retention of learned material is to focus on the review of subjects recently covered in the classroom. For example, after a focused review of the nursing care of clients with disorders of the cardiovascular system, it is advantageous to take the corresponding review test in this book. This is considered a practical approach because, although the NCLEX-PN basically tests the four categories in the

---

LONG-TERM REVIEW STRATEGIES

- Give priority attention to your weaker subjects first.
- Review key concepts in nursing textbooks.
- Summarize information identified in chapter objectives.
- Process critical-thinking questions in nursing books.
- Concentrate on how each Client Needs Category and Subcategory applies to the specific review topic.
- Organize or join a study group preparing for the NCLEX-PN.
- Select an environment that is conducive to concentration.
- Choose to review when you are most energetic and focused.
- Keep review periods short, regular, and on task.
- Take an NCLEX-PN review course if your motivation weakens.
- Invest in NCLEX-PN computerized testing programs.

SHORT-TERM STRATEGIES FOR ENSURING SUCCESS

- Correct vision or hearing problems prior to the test date.
- Make a trial run to the test site location.
- Obtain hotel or motel reservations if the test site is distant.
- Plan some leisure activity the day before the test.
- Get an adequate amount of sleep the night before the test.
- Awaken early.
- Eat sensibly.
- Avoid taking any mind- or mood-altering drugs.
- Take required admission papers and identification.
- Bring a snack or beverage for scheduled breaks.
- Distance yourself from anyone who looks frantic; anxiety is contagious.
- Locate the restroom, and use it shortly before the test.
- Use relaxation techniques.
- Make positive statements to yourself about your ability.

Test Plan, the test questions are asked from a medical, surgical, obstetric, pediatric, or mental health perspective.

Above all, it is best to include review strategies that have been successful in the past.

Short-term strategies

Some strategies are more appropriate as the testing date draws near.

If you use several of the suggested long- and short-term strategies, you can approach the NCLEX-PN with a feeling of confidence and a positive mental attitude. You will be off to a good start by continuing to work your way through this review book.

How to Use This Book

Lippincott's Review for NCLEX-PN, Seventh Edition, contains a series of tests covering a wide variety of health-related problems that can be used as a helpful adjunct for preparing for the NCLEX-PN. Although one of its objectives is to simulate the NCLEX-PN as much as possible, this book's primary purpose is to provide graduate nurses with an effective resource for reviewing nursing content. By answering the majority of questions correctly, you will not only have a solid foundation for taking the national licensure examination, but also a keen understanding of how to manage client situations in real-life clinical settings.

Reading the book's *Preface* and the section on *Frequently Asked Questions* will provide you with a thorough overview of the latest NCLEX Test Plan and address your concerns about the number and types of questions you may be asked on the actual examination. You will also learn valuable information about how to register for testing, what to expect at the test site facility, and helpful review strategies to ensure a successful test-taking experience.

In the sections below, you will learn how this book is organized, practical tips for choosing correct responses to test questions, and important information about the book's answers and rationales, classification of test items, and comprehensive examinations.

How the book is organized

This review book is divided into five units. The first four units are devoted to specific specialty areas of clinical practice—including adult medical-surgical disorders, care of the childbearing family, care of children, and mental health needs. These units are further subdivided into two or more review tests that concentrate on particular types of clients, health problems, and nursing care.

The last unit—a two-part printed comprehensive examination—and a CD-ROM containing all the questions from the 16 tests in the book serve as a final resource for your NCLEX-PN review.

DIVISIONS FOR REVIEW

- Unit I: The Nursing Care of Adults with Medical-Surgical Disorders
- Unit II: The Nursing Care of the Childbearing Family
- Unit III: The Nursing Care of Children
- Unit IV: The Nursing Care of Clients with Mental Health Needs
- Unit V: Comprehensive Test Parts 1 and 2

Editorial policies

Throughout the book, the word *client* is used when referring to the person receiving nursing services. Although the word *patient* is more familiar to some, *client* is the term that is used throughout the NCLEX-PN.

Clients are identified generically by age, gender, and medical information. No personal names are given, as you might have experienced on other examinations. The same principle is followed on the NCLEX-PN.

An effort has also been made to avoid using feminine pronouns when referring to the nurse because more and more men are joining their female colleagues in nursing practice. A similar decision was made regarding the use of only masculine pronouns when referring to physicians. In most cases, they are identified as the *nurse* or the *physician*. You can assume that the nurse to which the question refers is a practical nurse; if not, that information is identified.

Last, in multiple-choice questions involving drugs, both the generic and a brand name are provided wherever possible. The generic name is given first; a common brand or trade name follows in parentheses.

Testing format

Just like the latest NCLEX-PN examination, this review book primarily includes traditional multiple-choice questions consisting of a stem and four answer choices (options). However, a small percentage of alternate-format questions—such as multiple-response multiple-choice (typically, six-option questions), fill-in-the-blank (generally, a calculation), hot spot (graphically illustrated), drag-and-drop (including up to six options which the test-taker must place in chronological order), and chart/exhibit (information presented in a chart, table, or graph)—are also included in each test, reflecting the most recent changes to the NCLEX Test Plan.

In some cases, test questions are preceded by a case scenario that contains descriptive information about a client's condition or circumstances that are pertinent to answering the question. Such descriptions are italicized and appear above the stem, as shown below.

Sample case scenario

The nurse is caring for a 49-year-old man who is short of breath, has a heart rate of 110 beats/minute, and has moist breath sounds.

1. Which position is best for promoting ventilation in this client?　　**<stem**

[ ] **1.** Supine　　**<distractor**

[ ] **2.** Fowler's　　**<correct answer**

[ ] **3.** Prone　　**<distractor**

[ ] **4.** Sims'　　**<distractor**

Choosing answers

There are several necessary steps in choosing an answer. They include analyzing the information, looking for key words or terms, selecting an option, and making your choice.

ANALYZING THE INFORMATION

It is always best to read each case scenario and stem carefully. Focus on the information that makes the situation unique. Arriving at a correct answer involves integrating the pertinent facts within the context of the question. For example, if you are informed that a client is 3 years old, the answer to the question might be different than if the client is 65 years old, based on variations in the life cycle.

LOOKING FOR KEY TERMS

Key terms are words and their modifiers that help call attention to the critical information in the question. Identifying key terms can help you select the answer that fits the intent of the question.

EXAMPLES OF KEY WORDS AND MODIFIERS

Key words

Best	Least
Most	Except
Next	Earliest
At this time	Essential
Immediately	Initially

Key words and modifiers

Best response	Most important
Best evidence	Most appropriate
Best measure	Most accurate
Best answer	Most indicative
Best explanation	Most suggestive

SELECTING AN OPTION

When selecting an option, make sure you have read each one carefully because there may only be subtle differences between them. It is always helpful to narrow your options by using the process of elimination, being aware of distractor choices. Remember, the process of selecting an option may be different when answering alternate-format questions. For example, with multiple-response multiple-choice questions, more than one option is correct.

MAKING YOUR CHOICE

Once you have decided which option is best, you can record your answer by blackening the space in front of that option in the review test. If you are answering alternate-format questions: blacken the spaces in front of the options you think are correct for multiple-response multiple-choice questions; write your answer on the blank line provided for fill-in-the-blank questions; draw an "X" over the appropriate place on the illustration for hot spot questions; place the options in the correct order by writing them in the boxes provided for drag-and-drop questions; and blacken the space in front of the option you think is correct after reviewing the chart, table, or graph provided for chart/exhibit questions. See the electronic help file that accompanies the CD-ROM for directions on how to mark your choices while taking a test or conducting a review on the computer.

A word of warning: As in the actual NCLEX-PN, the correct answers are *randomized;* that is, they do not follow any particular pattern. It is therefore foolhardy to choose an answer by trying to predict some planned sequence in the numbered choices.

Correct answers and rationales

Refer to the sections titled *Correct Answers and Rationales* after completing each test and the comprehensive examinations. Compare your answers with those identified as the correct answers. Remember to place a check mark next to any items you answered incorrectly.

Study the rationale for each item regardless of whether you answered it correctly or incorrectly. The rationales often contain additional information that will enhance your NCLEX-PN review.

Next, analyze the reason you chose an incorrect answer. If you answered incorrectly because you did not read the item carefully or because you blackened the wrong space, plan to concentrate more on reading and marking the answers more accurately. If you made an error because you lacked the knowledge required to answer the question correctly, make a point of restudying that specific health-related problem.

Comprehensive examinations

Once you have taken all the individual tests and completed your review, you'll be ready to take the two-part comprehensive examination in the book or the examination on CD-ROM, or both. Whatever your decision, take these examinations as seriously as if you were taking the actual licensing examination.

Both of these practice examinations are intended to simulate the NCLEX-PN. The printed version contains a few more items than the maximum number asked on the NCLEX-PN. Because of its length, it provides the greatest opportunity for practice in answering a mix of questions from all the review test material.

The CD-ROM can generate mixes of questions that relate to topics in each of the four review test units, so you can practice by time or number of questions. In addition, the computerized version simulates the same testing process candidates are required to use when taking the NCLEX-PN.

When all the components of this book and CD-ROM are utilized along with recommended areas for further review, most candidates can acquire the self-confidence that will make passing the NCLEX-PN that much easier.

UNIT 1

The Nursing Care of Adults with Medical-Surgical Disorders

The Nursing Care of Clients with Musculoskeletal Disorders

⇨ **Nursing Care of Clients with Musculoskeletal Injuries**
⇨ **Nursing Care of Clients with Fractures**
⇨ **Nursing Care of Clients with Casts**
⇨ **Nursing Care of Clients with Traction**
⇨ **Nursing Care of Clients with Inflammatory Joint Disorders**
⇨ **Nursing Care of Clients with Degenerative Bone Disorders**
⇨ **Nursing Care of Clients with Amputations**
⇨ **Nursing Care of Clients with Skeletal Tumors**
⇨ **Nursing Care of Clients with a Herniated Intervertebral Disk**
⇨ **Correct Answers and Rationales**

Directions: With a pencil, blacken the space in front of the option you have chosen for your correct answer.

Nursing Care of Clients with Musculoskeletal Injuries

A male client who golfs at least three times a week has been experiencing wrist pain aggravated by movement. The physician diagnoses his condition as tenosynovitis and recommends temporarily avoiding repetitive wrist motion.

1. Which client statement provides the best evidence that he understands the therapeutic plan?
[ ] **1.** "I should keep my hand as still as possible."
[ ] **2.** "I should stop playing golf for the time being."
[ ] **3.** "I can substitute playing miniature golf."
[ ] **4.** "I can wear a tight leather glove when golfing."

The nurse examines a female client who slipped and fell while climbing stairs and now has ankle swelling and pain on movement.

2. The nurse reports to the physician that the client's ankle is *ecchymotic*. When the client asks what this means, which response by the nurse accurately describes the ankle's appearance?
[ ] **1.** Freckled
[ ] **2.** Mottled
[ ] **3.** Bruised
[ ] **4.** Blanched

3. While the client is waiting for her ankle to be X–rayed, which nursing measure is most helpful for relieving the soft-tissue swelling?
[ ] **1.** Place a heating pad on the ankle.
[ ] **2.** Apply ice to the ankle.
[ ] **3.** Exercise the client's foot.
[ ] **4.** Immobilize the client's foot.

The ankle X-ray reveals that the bones are not fractured. The physician tells the client that she has a severely sprained ankle.

4. The physician directs the nurse to wrap the client's lower extremity with an elastic bandage. Where should the nurse begin applying the bandage?
[ ] **1.** Below the knee
[ ] **2.** Above the ankle
[ ] **3.** Across the phalanges
[ ] **4.** At the metatarsals

5. Which technique is best to use when applying the elastic bandage?
[ ] **1.** Making figure-eight turns with the bandage
[ ] **2.** Making spiral-reverse turns with the bandage
[ ] **3.** Making recurrent turns with the bandage
[ ] **4.** Making spica turns with the bandage

Before the client is discharged from the emergency department, the nurse provides her with instructions on how to care for her sprained ankle at home.

6. The nurse advises the client that, besides routinely removing and reapplying the elastic bandage, it is essential for someone with a sprained ankle to rewrap the bandage following which situation?

[ ] **1.** After she sits for a long time
[ ] **2.** When the ankle feels painful
[ ] **3.** If her toes look swollen
[ ] **4.** When she wears tennis shoes

A male client arrives in the emergency department with a shoulder injury after falling from a stepladder.

7. When the nurse assesses the client, which finding best indicates that he has dislocated his shoulder?

[ ] **1.** The client is experiencing intense pain.
[ ] **2.** There is obvious swelling about the joint.
[ ] **3.** The client is hesitant to move his arm.
[ ] **4.** The affected arm is longer than the other.

The physician informs the client of plans to correct his shoulder dislocation by manipulation.

8. When the client asks the nurse what is meant by the term *manipulation,* which explanation is most accurate?

[ ] **1.** Manipulation involves making an incision to realign the bones.
[ ] **2.** Manipulation involves the insertion of a pin or wire into the joint.
[ ] **3.** Manipulation repositions the bone ends manually.
[ ] **4.** Manipulation strengthens the joint with exercise.

After learning that the client is uninsured and cannot afford to purchase a commercial canvas sling, the nurse teaches a family member how to apply a triangular sling made from muslin.

9. Which statement made by the family member indicates the need for further teaching?

[ ] **1.** "His hand should be elevated higher than his elbow."
[ ] **2.** "The knot should be tied at the back of the neck."
[ ] **3.** "His elbow should be flexed within the sling."
[ ] **4.** "The sling is used to elevate and support the arm."

Nursing Care of Clients with Fractures

While backpacking with a youth group, a 17-year-old boy sustains an injury to his lower leg. A nurse who is accompanying the group suspects a fracture of the tibia.

10. To immobilize the suspected fracture, how should the nurse apply a splint?

[ ] **1.** Below the knee to above the hip
[ ] **2.** Above the knee to below the hip
[ ] **3.** Above the ankle to below the knee
[ ] **4.** Below the ankle to above the knee

An X-ray of the injured teenager's leg reveals a comminuted fracture of the distal tibia.

11. Which explanation by the nurse can best help this client to understand the pathophysiology of a comminuted fracture?

[ ] **1.** One bone end is driven into the other.
[ ] **2.** The bone is splintered into pieces.
[ ] **3.** There is no open break in the skin.
[ ] **4.** A portion of the bone is split away.

After consulting the attending physician, the nurse learns that the teenager will require surgery to realign the bones in his fractured tibia.

12. In this case, from whom is it most appropriate to obtain consent to perform the surgical procedure?

[ ] **1.** The client himself
[ ] **2.** The client's physician
[ ] **3.** The client's youth leader
[ ] **4.** The client's parent

13. The client is about to go to surgery but is still wearing his class ring. Which nursing action is appropriate regarding care of the client's valuables?

[ ] **1.** Put the ring in the bedside stand.
[ ] **2.** Tape the ring to the client's finger.
[ ] **3.** Give the ring to a security guard.
[ ] **4.** Take the ring to the hospital safe.

14. The nurse correctly recognizes which physical finding as an early clinical manifestation of a fat embolism?

[ ] **1.** Respiratory distress
[ ] **2.** Abdominal distention
[ ] **3.** Difficulty swallowing
[ ] **4.** Swelling at the incision site

15. The nurse knows that a client who sustains multiple fractures of long bones in a motor vehicle accident is at risk for developing fat embolism syndrome. Which findings suggest that the client is developing this complication? Select all that apply.

[ ] **1.** Bradycardia
[ ] **2.** Petechiae
[ ] **3.** Dyspnea
[ ] **4.** Mental changes
[ ] **5.** Hypertension
[ ] **6.** Hematuria

A nurse stops to assist a woman who was involved in a motor vehicle accident. The victim was not wearing her seat belt and was thrown from the car.

16. Of the following emergency measures, which one should the nurse perform first?
[ ] **1.** Check the victim's breathing.
[ ] **2.** Cover the victim with a blanket.
[ ] **3.** Move the victim to the curb.
[ ] **4.** Assess the victim for injuries.

The nurse suspects that the victim has sustained rib fractures.

17. Which assessment finding best indicates that the client is experiencing secondary complications from the fractured ribs?
[ ] **1.** Irregular pulse rate
[ ] **2.** Asymmetrical chest expansion
[ ] **3.** Expiratory wheezing on auscultation
[ ] **4.** Coughing up pink, frothy sputum

Besides the suspected rib fractures, the nurse sees a bone fragment protruding from the client's thigh as well as profuse bleeding from the wound.

18. Which technique is most appropriate to control the bleeding?
[ ] **1.** Place a tourniquet around the leg.
[ ] **2.** Apply direct pressure on the wound.
[ ] **3.** Compress the femoral artery.
[ ] **4.** Elevate the injured extremity.

The nurse suspects that the accident victim might also have a broken back.

19. Which position is most preferred when transporting a victim with a possible back injury?
[ ] **1.** Side-lying
[ ] **2.** Prone
[ ] **3.** Supine
[ ] **4.** Semi-Fowler's

An 80-year-old woman who sustained a fall at a long-term care facility is suspected of having a fractured right hip.

20. Which finding would the nurse expect to document while assessing a client with an intertrochanteric fracture of the hip?
[ ] **1.** Paralysis of the affected leg
[ ] **2.** Bruising of the affected leg
[ ] **3.** Lengthening of the affected leg
[ ] **4.** External rotation of the leg

21. Which statements support the nurse's belief that the client has a fractured hip? Select all that apply.

[ ] **1.** The client has pain near the distal femur.
[ ] **2.** The client cannot bear weight on the affected leg.
[ ] **3.** The client's affected leg is shorter than her unaffected leg.
[ ] **4.** The client's affected leg is adducted.
[ ] **5.** The client's affected leg is externally rotated.
[ ] **6.** The client prefers to sit rather than lie flat.

22. Which risk factor found in the client's medical record is most significant for sustaining a hip fracture?
[ ] **1.** The client is postmenopausal.
[ ] **2.** The client is somewhat obese.
[ ] **3.** The client walks several blocks each day.
[ ] **4.** The client is lactose intolerant.

23. The nurse uses a diagram of the hip to explain to the client and her family where an intertrochanteric fracture of the femur has occurred. Identify the anatomic location of the injury.

After the client's fractured hip is stabilized with an open reduction and internal fixation, the nurse teaches her to perform isometric quadriceps setting exercises with her unaffected leg.

24. Which exercise should the nurse reinforce must be done correctly?
[ ] **1.** Moving her toes toward and away from her head
[ ] **2.** Contracting and relaxing her thigh muscles
[ ] **3.** Lifting her lower leg up and down from the bed
[ ] **4.** Bending her knee and pulling her lower leg upward

After surgery, the client is instructed to wear knee-high antiembolism stockings.

25. Which statement provides the best explanation about the preventative nature of antiembolism stockings?

[ ] **1.** Antiembolism stockings prevent blood from pooling in the legs.

[ ] **2.** Antiembolism stockings reduce blood flow to the extremities.

[ ] **3.** Antiembolism stockings keep the blood pressure lower in the legs.

[ ] **4.** Antiembolism stockings keep the blood vessels constricted.

26. The nurse supervises a clinical assistant in applying the client's antiembolism stockings. Which is the correct technique for applying these stockings?

[ ] **1.** The nursing assistant applies the stockings before getting the client out of bed.

[ ] **2.** The nursing assistant applies the stockings just before helping the client do leg exercises.

[ ] **3.** The nursing assistant applies the stockings after noting that the client's legs are cool.

[ ] **4.** The nursing assistant applies the stockings at night prior to the client's bedtime.

27. Postoperatively, which intervention should be completed prior to turning the client onto her nonoperative side?

[ ] **1.** Placing pillows between the client's legs

[ ] **2.** Having the client point her toes downward

[ ] **3.** Flexing the client's knee on the affected side

[ ] **4.** Elevating the head of the client's bed

28. The physician orders chair rest for a client with a hip prosthesis. To facilitate client transfer, how should the nurse position the chair?

[ ] **1.** At the end of the bed

[ ] **2.** Perpendicular to the bed

[ ] **3.** Parallel with the bed

[ ] **4.** Against a side wall

A client with a hip prosthesis is allowed to ambulate with a walker using a three-point partial weight-bearing gait.

29. Which return demonstration completed by the client indicates that she understands the correct way to ambulate with this type of walker?

[ ] **1.** The client advances the walker and operative leg while putting most of her weight on the walker's handgrips.

[ ] **2.** The client advances the walker and operative leg while putting most of her weight on the back legs of the walker.

[ ] **3.** The client advances the walker and operative leg while putting most of her weight on the toes of her operative leg.

[ ] **4.** The client advances the walker and operative leg while putting most of her weight on the heel of her nonoperative leg.

30. Following a client's hip replacement surgery, which nursing actions are essential? Select all that apply.

[ ] **1.** Keeping the client's knees apart at all times

[ ] **2.** Avoiding flexing the client's hips more than 90 degrees

[ ] **3.** Having the client use a raised toilet seat

[ ] **4.** Raising the head of the client's bed 90 degrees

[ ] **5.** Placing two pillows beneath the client's knees

[ ] **6.** Keeping the client's legs internally rotated

Nursing Care of Clients with Casts

A plaster arm cast will be applied to an adult male client with a compound fracture of his radius.

31. When preparing the client for cast application, which statement by the nurse is most accurate?

[ ] **1.** "Your cast will feel tight as it's applied."

[ ] **2.** "Your arm will feel warm as the wet plaster sets."

[ ] **3.** "You can expect a foul odor until the cast is dry."

[ ] **4.** "You may feel itchy while the cast is wet."

32. How can the nurse best support the wet cast while the physician wraps the arm with rolls of wet plaster?

[ ] **1.** By using a soft mattress

[ ] **2.** By resting it on a firm surface

[ ] **3.** By using the tips of her fingers

[ ] **4.** By using the palms of her hand

33. After the arm cast has been applied, which observation made by the nurse best indicates that the client may be developing compartment syndrome?

[ ] **1.** The client experiences severe pain.

[ ] **2.** The client's hand becomes reddened.

[ ] **3.** The fingers develop muscle spasms.

[ ] **4.** The radial pulse feels bounding.

34. Which is the best material for the nurse to place under a wet cast immediately after application?

[ ] **1.** Synthetic sheepskin

[ ] **2.** A vinyl sheet

[ ] **3.** An absorbent pad

[ ] **4.** Several pillows

35. Which technique does the nurse commonly use for drying a wet plaster cast?

[ ] **1.** Leave the casted arm uncovered.

[ ] **2.** Apply a heating blanket to the cast.

[ ] **3.** Use a hair dryer to blow hot air onto the cast.

[ ] **4.** Place a heat lamp directly above the cast.

36. Which is the best method to assess circulation in the casted extremity?
[ ] **1.** Ask the client if he can wiggle his fingers.
[ ] **2.** Feel the cast to determine if it is unusually hot or cold.
[ ] **3.** Depress the client's nailbeds, and document the time it takes for the color to return.
[ ] **4.** See if there is enough room to insert a finger between the cast and the extremity.

While waiting for his cast to dry, the client asks the nurse about the differences between plaster casts and those made of synthetic materials such as fiberglass.

37. Which statement by the nurse about fiberglass casts is most accurate?
[ ] **1.** Fiberglass casts are less expensive.
[ ] **2.** Fiberglass casts are lightweight.
[ ] **3.** Fiberglass casts are flexible.
[ ] **4.** Fiberglass casts are less restrictive.

Before discharging the client, the nurse provides him with cast care instructions and information about signs and symptoms of complications. The client returns to the clinic several hours later with bloody drainage seeping through the cast.

38. After assessing the client's cast, what action should the nurse take next?
[ ] **1.** Document the finding in the medical record.
[ ] **2.** Call the physician and report the finding.
[ ] **3.** Circle the area on the cast with ink, then record the time in the client's chart.
[ ] **4.** Apply an ice bag over the drainage area.

A hip spica cast is applied to a 16-year-old boy who sustained a fractured femur in a motorcycle accident.

39. The client states to the nurse, "My father is furious with me. He does not want me to ride a motorcycle." Which response by the nurse is most appropriate?
[ ] **1.** "As they say, 'Father knows best.'"
[ ] **2.** "All parents want their children to be safe."
[ ] **3.** "It can be frustrating when a father and son disagree."
[ ] **4.** "I think you should obey your father's wishes."

40. Which developmental task should the nurse keep in mind while planning the client's care?
[ ] **1.** The client is searching for his sexual identity.
[ ] **2.** The client is testing his physical abilities.
[ ] **3.** The client is acquiring his own independence.
[ ] **4.** The client is learning to control his emotions.

41. Which equipment should the nurse anticipate needing to facilitate the client's bowel elimination?
[ ] **1.** Bedside commode
[ ] **2.** Fracture bedpan
[ ] **3.** Mechanical lift
[ ] **4.** Raised toilet seat

The client asks the nurse to explain the purpose of the bar running between the thighs on his hip spica cast.

42. Which statement by the nurse about the cast's bar is most accurate?
[ ] **1.** The bar facilitates lifting and turning clients.
[ ] **2.** The bar enhances physical exercise.
[ ] **3.** The bar strengthens the cast.
[ ] **4.** The bar maintains the proper position.

The client tells the nurse that his skin itches terribly beneath the cast.

43. Which nursing action is most appropriate at this time?
[ ] **1.** Collaborate with the physician on prescribing an antipruritic medication.
[ ] **2.** Provide powder for the client to sprinkle in the cast.
[ ] **3.** Bend a wire coat hanger so the client can scratch inside the cast.
[ ] **4.** Apply a commercially prepared ice bag to the outside of the cast.

After the client has had the hip spica cast for nearly 3 weeks, the nurse detects a foul odor coming from the cast.

44. Which rationale is most accurate regarding the cast's unpleasant odor?
[ ] **1.** The plaster has dried improperly.
[ ] **2.** There is bleeding under the cast.
[ ] **3.** The cast is disintegrating.
[ ] **4.** There is an infected wound.

The physician cuts a small window in the hip spica cast to inspect the underlying tissue.

45. Which nursing action is most appropriate after the piece of plaster is removed to create a window in the cast?
[ ] **1.** Dispose of the piece of plaster in a plastic biohazard bag.
[ ] **2.** Replace the piece of plaster in the cast hole with tape.
[ ] **3.** Put the piece of plaster in the client's bedside table.
[ ] **4.** Send the piece of plaster to the laboratory for culturing.

46. Which nursing action is most correct when the rough edges on the client's hip spica cast begin to threaten the integrity of the skin?
[ ]   **1.** Line the cast edge with adhesive petals of mole-skin.
[ ]   **2.** Apply a fresh strip of plaster to the cast edge.
[ ]   **3.** Trim the rough cast edge with a cast cutter.
[ ]   **4.** Cover the cast edge with a gauze dressing.

47. Which assessment finding suggests that the client in the hip spica cast may be developing a response to his confinement known as *cast syndrome?*
[ ]   **1.** The client becomes nauseated and vomits.
[ ]   **2.** The client becomes disoriented and confused.
[ ]   **3.** The client becomes feverish and hypotensive.
[ ]   **4.** The client becomes dyspneic and hyperventi-lates.

Nursing Care of Clients with Traction

Before undergoing surgery for a fractured hip, an older female client is placed in Buck's traction.

48. Which technique is best when planning to change the client's bed linens?
[ ]   **1.** Roll the client from one side of the bed to the other.
[ ]   **2.** Apply the linens from the foot to the top of the bed.
[ ]   **3.** Leave the bottom sheets in place until after surgery.
[ ]   **4.** Raise the client from the bed with a mechanical lift.

49. Which assessment finding warrants immediate action when a client is in Buck's traction?
[ ]   **1.** The traction weights are hanging above the floor.
[ ]   **2.** The leg is in line with the pull of the traction.
[ ]   **3.** The client's foot is touching the end of the bed.
[ ]   **4.** The rope is in the groove of the traction pulley.

50. Which technique is the best strategy for assessing circulation in the leg in Buck's traction?
[ ]   **1.** Observe whether the client can wiggle or move her toes.
[ ]   **2.** Palpate for pulsation of the dorsalis pedis artery.
[ ]   **3.** Take the client's blood pressure with a thigh cuff positioned on her affected leg.
[ ]   **4.** Determine whether the client can feel sharp and dull sensations.

An older male client is placed in Russell's traction while awaiting surgery.

51. To prevent skin breakdown while the client is in traction, the nurse must frequently inspect the skin in which area?
[ ]   **1.** Over the ischial spines
[ ]   **2.** In the popliteal space
[ ]   **3.** Near the iliac crests
[ ]   **4.** At the zygomatic arch

The nurse enters the client's room to assess the traction apparatus.

52. Which of the following might interfere with the effectiveness of the Russell's traction?
[ ]   **1.** The rope is strung tautly from pulley to pulley.
[ ]   **2.** The trapeze is hanging above the client's chest.
[ ]   **3.** The rope is knotted at the location of a pulley.
[ ]   **4.** The weight is hanging about 24″ (61 cm) from the floor.

On the day of surgery, the client in Russell's traction is transported to the operating room in his bed.

53. Which nursing action is appropriate while the client is being transported?
[ ]   **1.** The nurse leaves the traction as is.
[ ]   **2.** The nurse removes the weights during his transport.
[ ]   **3.** The nurse rests the weights on the end of the bed.
[ ]   **4.** The nurse takes the client's leg out of the traction.

A cervical halter type of skin traction is applied to a client who has experienced a whiplash injury in a motor vehicle accident.

54. When the nurse makes rounds at the beginning of the shift, which observation requires the nurse's immediate attention?
[ ]   **1.** The halter rests under the client's chin and occiput.
[ ]   **2.** The client's ears are clear of the traction ropes.
[ ]   **3.** The weight hangs between the headboard and wall.
[ ]   **4.** There is a soft pillow beneath the client's head.

A woman with acute low back pain is being treated with pelvic-belt traction intermittently throughout the day.

55. When applying pelvic-belt traction to the client, where should the nurse place the top of the belt?
[ ]   **1.** Just below her rib cage
[ ]   **2.** Even with her waistline
[ ]   **3.** Level with her iliac crest
[ ]   **4.** Where it is most comfortable

A client with a fractured femur is in skeletal traction with a pin through the distal femur. The affected leg is supported by balanced suspension.

56. Which material is best for covering the tips of the pin to prevent injuries while the client is in skeletal leg traction?
[ ] **1.** Gauze squares
[ ] **2.** Cotton balls
[ ] **3.** Cork blocks
[ ] **4.** Rubber tubes

57. Which assessment finding best indicates that the client has an infection at the pin site?
[ ] **1.** Serous drainage at the pin site
[ ] **2.** Bloody drainage at the pin site
[ ] **3.** Mucoid drainage at the pin site
[ ] **4.** Purulent drainage at the pin site

The physician orders antibiotic therapy for the client's infection.

58. If the client is allergic to penicillin, the nurse must question a medical order for which type of antibiotics?
[ ] **1.** Aminoglycosides such as gentamicin sulfate (Garamycin)
[ ] **2.** Cephalosporins such as cefaclor (Ceclor)
[ ] **3.** Tetracyclines such as doxycycline (Vibramycin)
[ ] **4.** Sulfonamides such as co-trimoxazole (Bactrim)

An adult male client with a fractured cervical vertebra is placed in halo-cervical traction, a type of skeletal traction consisting of pins inserted into the skull that are incorporated into a vest of plaster.

59. Which description by the nurse most accurately states the purpose of halo-cervical traction?
[ ] **1.** "It restricts neck movement but enables physical activity."
[ ] **2.** "It allows head movement while immobilizing the spine."
[ ] **3.** "It accelerates healing by facilitating physical therapy."
[ ] **4.** "It promotes faster bone repair within a shorter time span."

60. Which observation by the nurse provides the best indication that the halo traction device is applied appropriately?
[ ] **1.** The client has full range of motion in his neck.
[ ] **2.** The client's neck pain is within a tolerable level.
[ ] **3.** The client can speak and hear at preinjury levels.
[ ] **4.** The client reports the ability to see straight ahead.

61. Which assessment finding best indicates that the halo traction needs to be readjusted by the physician?

[ ] **1.** The client experiences orthostatic hypotension.
[ ] **2.** The client needs assistance with shaving.
[ ] **3.** The client cannot open his mouth widely.
[ ] **4.** The client complains about irritation in his axillae.

Nursing Care of Clients with Inflammatory Joint Disorders

An adult woman consults a physician about persistent joint pain and stiffness.

62. Which laboratory test, if elevated, is the best diagnostic indicator of rheumatoid arthritis?
[ ] **1.** Erythrocyte sedimentation rate (ESR)
[ ] **2.** Partial thromboplastin time (PTT)
[ ] **3.** Fasting blood sugar (FBS)
[ ] **4.** Blood urea nitrogen (BUN)

63. If the client is typical of most people with rheumatoid arthritis, when would the nurse expect the client's symptoms first developed?
[ ] **1.** In very early childhood
[ ] **2.** At the onset of puberty
[ ] **3.** During young adulthood
[ ] **4.** After menopause

The physician diagnoses rheumatoid arthritis and prescribes a total of 5 g of aspirin per day.

64. If each tablet contains 5 grains, how many tablets should the nurse make sure are stocked in the distributing system for the client in each 24-hour period?
[ ] **1.** 5
[ ] **2.** 10
[ ] **3.** 15
[ ] **4.** 20

The client says she is surprised the physician prescribed a common drug such as aspirin to treat her condition.

65. The nurse should plan to include which information related to the therapeutic benefits of aspirin in the teaching plan for this client?
[ ] **1.** Aspirin stimulates the immune system.
[ ] **2.** Aspirin relaxes skeletal muscles.
[ ] **3.** Aspirin reduces joint inflammation.
[ ] **4.** Aspirin interrupts nerve synapses.

The client tells the nurse that she gets an upset stomach when she takes aspirin.

66. Which modification in the client's care plan is most appropriate to relieve the client's stomach discomfort?

[ ] **1.** Give aspirin before meals only.
[ ] **2.** Give aspirin with cold water.
[ ] **3.** Give aspirin with hot tea.
[ ] **4.** Give aspirin with food or meals.

67. Because the client takes large amounts of aspirin daily, the nurse monitors her for signs and symptoms of aspirin toxicity. Which assessment finding best indicates aspirin toxicity?
[ ] **1.** Ringing in the ears
[ ] **2.** Dizziness
[ ] **3.** Metallic taste in the mouth
[ ] **4.** Proteinuria

The client tells the nurse that watching television helps decrease her discomfort.

68. Which conclusion made by the nurse is most accurate given the above information?
[ ] **1.** The client is improving due to electronic signals.
[ ] **2.** The client is having less pain than she thinks.
[ ] **3.** The client is experiencing a slight case of arthritis.
[ ] **4.** The client is being distracted from her pain.

69. Which finger joints would the nurse expect to be most affected by the client's rheumatoid arthritis?
[ ] **1.** Proximal finger joints
[ ] **2.** Medial finger joints
[ ] **3.** Distal finger joints
[ ] **4.** Lateral finger joints

The physician recommends applying heat to the client's hands to relieve some of her discomfort.

70. Which heat application method is best for the nurse to use with this client?
[ ] **1.** Hot water bottle
[ ] **2.** Warm moist compresses
[ ] **3.** Electric heating pad
[ ] **4.** Infrared heat lamp

71. While planning care for the client, when would the nurse expect her to need more time and assistance with activities of daily living?
[ ] **1.** In the early morning
[ ] **2.** At noon
[ ] **3.** In the late afternoon
[ ] **4.** Before bed

72. Which nursing recommendation has the greatest potential for helping the client maintain her ability to care for herself?
[ ] **1.** Move to a warm climate.
[ ] **2.** Buy clothes that are easy to pull or slip on.
[ ] **3.** Enroll in an aerobic exercise class.
[ ] **4.** Sleep on a waterbed.

During an acute episode of rheumatoid arthritis, the physician asks the nurse to apply a splint to each of the client's hands.

73. Which explanation most accurately explains to the client the primary purpose of the splints?
[ ] **1.** To rest the affected joints
[ ] **2.** To cure her joint disease
[ ] **3.** To improve her hand strength
[ ] **4.** To increase her range of motion

The client has not responded to the usual drug therapy and now takes the corticosteroid prednisone (Deltasone) daily.

74. Which of the following should the nurse monitor closely while the client is receiving prednisone (Deltasone)?
[ ] **1.** Daily weight
[ ] **2.** Pulse rate
[ ] **3.** Red blood cell count
[ ] **4.** Skin integrity

75. Which statement made by the client indicates that further instruction regarding corticosteroid therapy is necessary?
[ ] **1.** "I'm susceptible to getting infections."
[ ] **2.** "I should never stop taking my medication abruptly."
[ ] **3.** "I may become very depressed and perhaps suicidal."
[ ] **4.** "I may develop low blood sugar and need glucose."

In addition to prednisone (Deltasone), the client is prescribed methotrexate (Rheumatrex), a drug commonly used to treat clients with cancer.

76. Which assessment finding would the nurse consider a likely adverse effect of the client's methotrexate (Rheumatrex) therapy?
[ ] **1.** Constipation
[ ] **2.** Polyuria
[ ] **3.** Mouth sores
[ ] **4.** Chest pain

A 75-year-old man with osteoarthritis in his left hip has been told by his physician to apply a heating pad to the area several times a day.

77. Which instruction about heating pads is essential to include in the client's teaching plan?
[ ] **1.** Keep the heating pad on the low setting.
[ ] **2.** Place the heating pad directly next to the skin for maximal effect.
[ ] **3.** Cover the heating pad with plastic during use.
[ ] **4.** Apply the heating pad for 2 hours at a time.

78. Which nursing instruction is most beneficial to minimize stress on the client's painful joints?
[ ] **1.** Maintain a normal weight.
[ ] **2.** Apply a topical analgesic cream.
[ ] **3.** Use restrictive assistive devices.
[ ] **4.** Become more physically active.

79. The client uses a cane when ambulating. When the nurse observes him walking, which assessment finding indicates that he needs more instruction regarding the use of his cane?
[ ] **1.** The tip of the cane is covered with a rubber cap.
[ ] **2.** The client wears athletic shoes with nonskid soles.
[ ] **3.** The client uses the cane on his painful side.
[ ] **4.** The client holds his head up and looks straight ahead.

The client tells the nurse that he usually takes 400 mg of ibuprofen (Motrin) four times a day at home.

80. Which question best helps the nurse determine whether the client is experiencing an adverse effect from taking nonsteroidal anti-inflammatory drugs (NSAIDs) such as ibuprofen (Motrin)?
[ ] **1.** "Have you noticed any hand tremors?"
[ ] **2.** "Are you urinating more frequently?"
[ ] **3.** "Has your interest in food changed?"
[ ] **4.** "What color are your stools?"

A total hip replacement (hip arthroplasty) is planned for a 70-year-old man with osteoarthritis. The physician instructs the client to stop taking his enteric-coated aspirin (Ecotrin) 1 week prior to surgery.

81. Which statement by the nurse best explains the rationale for the physician's instructions?
[ ] **1.** "Aspirin can increase your risk of wound infection."
[ ] **2.** "Aspirin impairs your ability to control bleeding."
[ ] **3.** "Aspirin can make it difficult to assess your pain."
[ ] **4.** "Aspirin interferes with your ability to heal."

Before the total hip replacement, the nurse teaches the client how to use an incentive spirometer.

82. Which statement indicates that the client understands how to use the incentive spirometer correctly?
[ ] **1.** "I should position the mouthpiece and inhale deeply."
[ ] **2.** "I should position the mouthpiece and exhale forcefully."
[ ] **3.** "I should position the mouthpiece and cough effectively."
[ ] **4.** "I should position the mouthpiece and breathe naturally."

Just before the total hip replacement, the nurse prepares a large area of the client's skin for surgery.

83. Which technique is most appropriate for the nurse to use when preparing the operative site?
[ ] **1.** Washing the area with soap and water
[ ] **2.** Pressing the razor deeply into the skin while shaving
[ ] **3.** Clipping the hair around the intended incisional area
[ ] **4.** Shaving in the direction of hair growth

84. After the client undergoes a total hip replacement, how should the nurse position the affected hip?
[ ] **1.** Adduct the hip
[ ] **2.** Abduct the hip
[ ] **3.** Flex the hip
[ ] **4.** Extend the hip

85. Which equipment is most helpful to have on hand when caring for the client postoperatively?
[ ] **1.** A bed cradle
[ ] **2.** A bed board
[ ] **3.** An overhead trapeze
[ ] **4.** Power side rails

86. Which equipment best prevents external rotation of the operative leg when caring for a client with a total hip replacement?
[ ] **1.** A footboard
[ ] **2.** A trochanter roll
[ ] **3.** A turning sheet
[ ] **4.** A foam mattress

Following the client's total hip replacement, the nurse provides discharge instructions regarding positions he must temporarily avoid.

87. Which statement indicates that the client understands the restrictions he must follow?
[ ] **1.** "I shouldn't cross my legs."
[ ] **2.** "I should avoid pointing my toes."
[ ] **3.** "I shouldn't lie flat in bed."
[ ] **4.** "I shouldn't stand upright."

88. When planning the client's discharge, the nurse must help the client obtain which essential piece of equipment for his home care?
[ ] **1.** A wheelchair
[ ] **2.** A hospital bed
[ ] **3.** A raised toilet seat
[ ] **4.** A mechanical lift

89. Which area of health teaching is essential to include in the discharge instructions for a client who has undergone a total hip replacement?

[ ] **1.** Modifying ways of donning clothing
[ ] **2.** Using special equipment for bathing
[ ] **3.** Taking vigorous daily walks
[ ] **4.** Receiving a daily stool softener

A 36-year-old male client undergoes an arthroscopy of his right knee for diagnosing and treating chronic joint pain.

90. Which information is most appropriate to teach the client before the arthroscopy procedure?
[ ] **1.** Signs and symptoms of arthritis
[ ] **2.** Technique for using crutches
[ ] **3.** Adverse effects of drug therapy
[ ] **4.** Need to balance rest and exercise

A 60-year-old man with osteoarthritis is scheduled to undergo knee arthroplasty in which an artificial joint will replace his natural knee joint. A continuous passive motion (CPM) machine will be used postoperatively.

91. What should the nurse explain is the purpose of the CPM machine while teaching the client?
[ ] **1.** To strengthen the leg muscles
[ ] **2.** To relieve foot swelling
[ ] **3.** To reduce surgical pain
[ ] **4.** To restore joint function

92. When documenting the client's progress while using a CPM machine, which assessment data are essential to include?
[ ] **1.** Degree of flexion, number of cycles, and condition of the sutures around the incision
[ ] **2.** Degree of flexion, number of cycles, and amount of time the client used the machine
[ ] **3.** Degree of flexion, number of cycles, and characteristics of drainage from the wound
[ ] **4.** Degree of flexion, number of cycles, and presence and quality of arterial pulses

93. Which evidence best indicates that the client who had a knee arthroplasty can discontinue wearing a resting knee extension splint (immobilizer)?
[ ] **1.** The client has minimal pain when ambulating.
[ ] **2.** The client can flex the operative knee 90 degrees.
[ ] **3.** The client can perform straight-leg raising.
[ ] **4.** The client's surgical wound is approximated.

A 54-year-old man is being treated for gout.

94. When the nurse examines the client, which body part is usually affected by gout?
[ ] **1.** Great toe
[ ] **2.** Index finger
[ ] **3.** Sacrococcygeal vertebrae
[ ] **4.** Temporomandibular joint

95. The nurse knows that elevated levels of which laboratory test typically validates a diagnosis of gout?
[ ] **1.** Creatinine clearance
[ ] **2.** Blood urea nitrogen
[ ] **3.** Serum uric acid
[ ] **4.** Serum calcium

96. Which equipment can best promote comfort during the client's acute gout attack?
[ ] **1.** A bed cradle
[ ] **2.** An electric fan
[ ] **3.** A foam mattress
[ ] **4.** A fracture bedpan

After the physician orders a low-purine diet for the client, the nurse assesses the client's dietary needs and his knowledge of appropriate foods.

97. The nurse would be correct to consult a dietitian if the client chooses a meal that includes which food?
[ ] **1.** Beets
[ ] **2.** Milk
[ ] **3.** Eggs
[ ] **4.** Liver

The client suffers an acute attack of gout. The physician prescribes colchicine (Colgout) to be given every hour until the client's pain is relieved.

98. Which finding indicates that the drug should be discontinued even if the client's pain is unrelieved?
[ ] **1.** Vomiting
[ ] **2.** Dizziness
[ ] **3.** Drowsiness
[ ] **4.** Headache

To reduce the client's risk of forming urinary stones, the nursing care plan includes administering 3,000 mL of fluid daily.

99. When implementing the care plan, the nurse would encourage the major intake of fluids at which time of the day?
[ ] **1.** Before bedtime
[ ] **2.** Early evening
[ ] **3.** In the morning
[ ] **4.** Mid-afternoon

The nurse advises the client to continue consuming a high intake of fluid following discharge.

100. The nurse correctly instructs the client that he should avoid which type of fluid?
[ ] **1.** Coffee
[ ] **2.** Alcohol
[ ] **3.** Cranberry juice
[ ] **4.** Carbonated drinks

Nursing Care of Clients with Degenerative Bone Disorders

101. The physician orders passive range-of-motion (ROM) exercises for an elderly client on bed rest. Which statement regarding the appropriate method of ROM exercises is correct?
[ ] **1.** ROM exercises should be completed independently with verbal cues from the nurse.
[ ] **2.** Force may be needed during ROM exercises to achieve maximum benefit.
[ ] **3.** Support should be maintained to the proximal and distal areas of the joint during ROM exercise.
[ ] **4.** ROM exercises should be performed until the client verbalizes discomfort.

A middle-aged woman asks the nurse about methods for preventing or delaying the onset of osteoporosis.

102. Which assessment finding most likely indicates that a client has osteoporosis?
[ ] **1.** Swollen joints
[ ] **2.** Discomfort when sitting
[ ] **3.** Spinal deformity
[ ] **4.** Diminished energy level

103. A client diagnosed with osteoporosis receives nursing instructions on methods to reduce disease progression. Which substances should the nurse advise her to avoid?
[ ] **1.** Aspirin and carbonated beverages
[ ] **2.** Nicotine and sources of caffeine
[ ] **3.** Sodium and substances containing alcohol
[ ] **4.** Calcium and dairy products

104. The nurse is caring for a client who was just diagnosed with osteoporosis. In this lateral view of the spine, identify the area where an abnormality will most likely be observed.

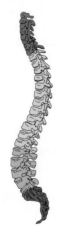

A 55-year-old man has developed bone necrosis as a result of chronic osteomyelitis in the tibia of his left leg.

105. Which nursing intervention is most appropriate for preventing a pathological fracture?
[ ] **1.** Encouraging a high fluid intake
[ ] **2.** Providing a nutritional diet
[ ] **3.** Supporting the limb during movement
[ ] **4.** Relieving pressure on bony prominences

A 68-year-old Mexican American man immigrated to the United States 3 months ago. The client comes to the emergency department with complaints of severe shoulder, elbow, and knee pain. The physician diagnoses bursitis.

106. Based on the nurse's knowledge of the client's culture and beliefs, which statement regarding his health-seeking behavior is probably most accurate?
[ ] **1.** Home remedies have been unsuccessful, and the client's condition threatens his role expectations.
[ ] **2.** The power to cure comes from physicians and is based on advances in medical technology.
[ ] **3.** The client has lost faith in prayer, supernatural forces, and his curandero.
[ ] **4.** The client's condition is the result of the mal de ojo (evil eye).

A client diagnosed with osteomalacia has been told that his condition may improve with the addition of vitamin D.

107. Besides recommending the consumption of foods fortified with vitamin D, which suggestion by the nurse is most appropriate?
[ ] **1.** Obtain more direct exposure to sunlight.
[ ] **2.** Eat meat from growth-stimulated cattle.
[ ] **3.** Consume bright orange vegetables.
[ ] **4.** Purchase organically grown produce.

Nursing Care of Clients with Amputations

During a farming accident, a 50-year-old man's arm was caught in a grain elevator. His lower left arm and hand have been crushed.

108. If the client is in shock, how should the nurse position his body while continuing to assess and care for him?
[ ] **1.** Prone
[ ] **2.** Supine
[ ] **3.** On his back with his legs elevated
[ ] **4.** On his side with his neck extended

The client is rushed to surgery where his arm is amputated above the elbow.

109. Postoperatively, the client screams obscenities at the nurse when he realizes that his forearm is missing. Which nursing action is most appropriate at this time?
[ ] **1.** Leave until the client works through his anger.
[ ] **2.** Stay quietly with the client at his bedside.
[ ] **3.** Tell the client to get control of himself.
[ ] **4.** Call the physician and request a sedative.

Later the client says, "I know my arm isn't there, but I feel it throbbing."

110. Which response by the nurse would be most accurate?
[ ] **1.** "You may be experiencing referred pain from an adjacent muscle."
[ ] **2.** "You may be experiencing phantom pain from the amputated site."
[ ] **3.** "You may be experiencing psychogenic pain from emotional distress."
[ ] **4.** "You may be experiencing intractable pain that can best be treated with opioids."

The physician orders transcutaneous electric nerve stimulation (TENS) in the location of the discomfort on the arm opposite the amputation.

111. Which statement reflects the most widely recognized theory for TENS use?
[ ] **1.** The sensation created by the TENS unit blocks the brain's perception of pain impulses.
[ ] **2.** The sensation created by the TENS unit travels to the nerve root of the amputated arm.
[ ] **3.** The sensation created by the TENS unit destroys the brain's pain center.
[ ] **4.** The sensation created by the TENS unit weakens the arm's sensory nerves.

An older diabetic woman is admitted with vascular problems. The nurse notes that some toes on her left foot are black. She is scheduled for a below-the-knee amputation.

112. When planning the client's postoperative care, the nurse knows to avoid placing the client in which least desirable position?
[ ] **1.** Lying prone
[ ] **2.** Lying supine
[ ] **3.** Sitting in a chair
[ ] **4.** Standing to shower

The nursing team meets to develop a plan for strengthening the client's muscles to prepare her for ambulating with crutches following surgery.

113. Which activity is best to begin implementing immediately after the client's surgery?
[ ] **1.** Standing at the side of the bed
[ ] **2.** Balancing between parallel bars
[ ] **3.** Lifting herself with the trapeze
[ ] **4.** Transferring from the bed to a chair

The client asks the nurse why her stump is rewrapped with elastic bandages several times a day.

114. While teaching the client, what does the nurse explain is the purpose of stump bandaging?
[ ] **1.** It lengthens and tones muscles.
[ ] **2.** It shrinks and shapes the stump.
[ ] **3.** It maintains joint flexibility.
[ ] **4.** It absorbs blood and drainage.

115. When caring for a client with a below-the-knee amputation, the nurse promotes the client's potential use of a prosthesis. To ensure optimum rehabilitation, what nursing actions are appropriate? Select all that apply.
[ ] **1.** Encourage the client to sit in a chair for at least 2 hours at a time.
[ ] **2.** Instruct the client to place a pillow under the thigh of her amputated limb while in bed.
[ ] **3.** Teach her to wrap the stump distally to proximally with an elastic roller bandage.
[ ] **4.** Have the client tighten her thigh muscles and press her knee into the bed several times a day.
[ ] **5.** Have her remove and replace the stump bandage every other day.

Nursing Care of Clients with Skeletal Tumors

Just before his 18th birthday, a male client is diagnosed with a cancerous bone tumor (osteogenic sarcoma) in his femur. An above-the-knee amputation is performed.

116. Which equipment should be kept at the client's bedside during the immediate postoperative period?
[ ] **1.** Gauze dressings
[ ] **2.** Rubber tourniquet
[ ] **3.** Oropharyngeal airway
[ ] **4.** Oxygen equipment

A rigid plaster shell surrounds the client's stump. A pylon, or temporary prosthesis, allows the client to ambulate with crutches soon after surgery.

117. Which observation by the nurse best suggests that the client's crutches need further adjustment?
[ ] **1.** The client stands straight without bending forward.
[ ] **2.** The client's elbows are slightly flexed when he is standing in place.
[ ] **3.** The top bars of the crutches fit snugly into the axillae.
[ ] **4.** The client's wrists are hyperextended when he grasps the handgrips.

118. Due to the location of a malignant bone tumor like osteogenic sarcoma, the nurse knows to assess for which possible complication?
[ ] **1.** Bowel obstruction
[ ] **2.** Liver dysfunction
[ ] **3.** Mental status changes
[ ] **4.** Anemia

119. Which diagnostic test result should the nurse monitor when assessing for evidence of metastasis?
[ ] **1.** Lung scan
[ ] **2.** Urinalysis
[ ] **3.** Spinal tap
[ ] **4.** Blood glucose

Nursing Care of Clients with a Herniated Intervertebral Disk

A male construction worker has an acute onset of severe low back pain. The physician suspects that the client has a herniated intervertebral disk in the lumbar spine.

120. When assessing the characteristics of pain in a client with a herniated disk, the nurse would expect to document increased intensity of pain during which activity?
[ ] **1.** Eating
[ ] **2.** Sneezing
[ ] **3.** Sleeping
[ ] **4.** Urinating

121. If the client is typical of others with a herniated disk, the nurse would expect him to report which additional symptom?
[ ] **1.** Pain radiating into the buttocks and leg
[ ] **2.** Tenderness over one or both iliac crests
[ ] **3.** Diminished sensation in one or both knees
[ ] **4.** Brief periods when his toes feel quite cold

The physician makes a tentative diagnosis of herniated intervertebral disk and prescribes 30 mg of cyclobenzaprine hydrochloride (Flexeril) orally b.i.d.

122. While teaching the client, what does the nurse explain is the purpose of prescribing this medication?
[ ] **1.** To reduce emotional depression
[ ] **2.** To relax skeletal muscles
[ ] **3.** To promote restful sleep
[ ] **4.** To relieve inflammation

The physician orders a myelogram with a water-soluble contrast dye to confirm the diagnosis of a herniated intervertebral disk.

123. Which nursing intervention is most important after the client returns from the myelogram?
[ ] **1.** Reducing glare from bright lights
[ ] **2.** Withholding food and fluids for 12 hours
[ ] **3.** Administering sedatives every 6 hours
[ ] **4.** Encouraging a high fluid intake

Conservative treatment does not relieve the client's symptoms and physical disability. The client consents to have a laminectomy and spinal fusion in the lumbar area of the spine.

124. Before turning the client postoperatively, which nursing instruction is especially important to prevent postoperative complications?
[ ] **1.** "Hold your breath as you are turning."
[ ] **2.** "Move your lower body first, then your chest."
[ ] **3.** "As you hold onto the trapeze, lift your hips off the bed."
[ ] **4.** "Let me roll you as if you were a log."

The nurse includes principles of good body mechanics in the discharge teaching for a client who has undergone spinal surgery. The client is from a foreign country and speaks very little English.

125. Which teaching method provides the best information regarding body mechanics when dealing with a non-English-speaking client?
[ ] **1.** Speak slowly while looking at the client.
[ ] **2.** Write the instructions on paper.
[ ] **3.** Use colorful pictures or diagrams.
[ ] **4.** Have the client watch a video.

126. The nurse correctly instructs the client to use which technique when picking something up?
[ ] **1.** Flex both his knees.
[ ] **2.** Keep his feet together.
[ ] **3.** Lift with his arms extended.
[ ] **4.** Bend from the waist.

Correct Answers and Rationales

Nursing Care of Clients with Musculoskeletal Injuries

1. 2. Temporarily eliminating the activity that has injured the tendons, in this case playing golf, is the best action to take at this time. Keeping the hand and wrist immobile is unnecessary. Playing miniature golf would continue to injure the tendon. Golfers wear gloves to prevent their skin from becoming blistered. Wearing a tight glove does not protect the joint from injury.
Client Needs Category—Health promotion and maintenance
Client Needs Subcategory—None

2. 3. Ecchymosis refers to a black and blue skin discoloration (bruise) caused by the rupture of small blood vessels bleeding into the skin. Freckled skin is evidenced as scattered small brown-pigmented spots on the skin. Mottled skin contains patchy areas of light- or blue-colored skin seen primarily in hypothermic infants and dying clients. Blanched skin appears pale.
Client Needs Category—Physiological integrity
Client Needs Subcategory—Physiological adaptation

3. 2. Applying ice and elevating a swollen extremity relieves swelling. Heat is not used immediately after the injury because it increases circulation to the injured part, causing more swelling. Exercise causes pain and further swelling in the early stage of an injury. Immobilization can help relieve pain and promote healing.
Client Needs Category—Physiological integrity
Client Needs Subcategory—Basic care and comfort

4. 4. When wrapping the lower extremity with an elastic bandage, bandaging starts at the metatarsal bones, which form the ball of the foot and instep. The toes, or phalanges, are left uncovered to assess circulation. To relieve swelling, the injured area is wrapped distally (from the metatarsals) to proximally (the calf). Wrapping from below the knee toward the foot would not relieve swelling.
Client Needs Category—Physiological integrity
Client Needs Subcategory—Basic care and comfort

5. 1. By overlapping the roller bandage in an alternately ascending and descending oblique pattern around a joint, the figure-eight turn is made. Each turn crosses the one preceding it so that it resembles the number eight. This method is used frequently for sprained ankles. A spiral reverse turn is used to bandage a cone-shaped body part, such as the thigh or leg. The recurrent turn is used to cover the tip of a body part, such as the stump of an amputated limb. A spica turn is an adaptation of the figure-eight wrap; it is used when the wrap goes around an adjacent body part, such as the thumb and hand or the thigh and hip.
Client Needs Category—Physiological integrity
Client Needs Subcategory—Basic care and comfort

6. 3. If the roller bandage is applied too tightly, venous blood and lymph may become trapped in the toes, producing a swollen appearance. The toes may also feel numb or look blue. Rewrapping the extremity may restore or improve circulation. Sitting will not disturb the application of the bandage. The injured area will not be pain-free until the swelling subsides and injured tissue heals. Wearing tennis shoes is not an indication for rewrapping the elastic bandage. It is unlikely that the client will be able to wear a shoe until after the swelling subsides.
Client Needs Category—Health promotion and maintenance
Client Needs Subcategory—None

7. 4. A dislocation is caused by the tearing of the ligaments that connect and hold two bone ends within a joint, resulting in temporary displacement of the bone from its normal position. When the nurse assesses the client's injury, the affected arm will look longer than the other one. Most traumatic musculoskeletal injuries, including sprains, strains, and fractures, are accompanied by pain, swelling, and compromised mobility. Consequently, these symptoms do not provide the best evidence of a dislocation.
Client Needs Category—Physiological integrity
Client Needs Subcategory—Physiological adaptation

8. 3. Restoring function for a dislocation involves repositioning two adjacent bones so that they are again in contact with one another. The physician manually does the repositioning, with or without anesthesia. A surgical incision is necessary when doing a procedure called an open reduction. Inserting a pin or wire is a type of internal fixation. To allow time for healing, exercise is prescribed only after a period of stabilization.
Client Needs Category—Physiological integrity
Client Needs Subcategory—Physiological adaptation

9. 2. When a triangular sling is used, the knot is tied at the side of the neck to avoid pressure on the cervical vertebrae. All other statements made by the family member indicate correct information concerning the application and use of a triangular sling.
Client Needs Category—Health promotion and maintenance
Client Needs Subcategory—None

Nursing Care of Clients with Fractures

10. 4. To immobilize a broken bone, a splint is applied to prevent movement of the joints above and below the injury. The tibia is between the knee and the ankle. Therefore, it is correct to apply the splint from below the ankle to above the knee. All other areas mentioned would not stabilize the injury correctly.

Client Needs Category—Physiological integrity
Client Needs Subcategory—Physiological adaptation

11. 2. A comminuted fracture means that there are pieces, fragments, or splinters of bone in the area where the bone was broken. An impacted fracture is one in which the bone ends are driven together. A simple or closed fracture is one in which there is no break in the skin. A greenstick fracture involves a longitudinal split that extends partially through one side of the bone.

Client Needs Category—Physiological integrity
Client Needs Subcategory—Basic care and comfort

12. 4. Hospital personnel should first attempt to obtain permission from a minor client's parent or guardian. Minors cannot give permission under most circumstances. If permission is obtained over the telephone, at least two people must hear the verbal consent and co-sign as witnesses to what they heard. The physician's role is to explain the procedure and the risk factors associated with the surgery. The nurse's responsibility is to witness the signing of the consent. The youth leader is not an appropriate person to give consent unless previous arrangements were made in case of emergency. The best choice is the parent or guardian.

Client Needs Category—Safe, effective care environment
Client Needs Subcategory—Coordinated care

13. 4. Jewelry is removed preoperatively, then itemized, identified, and locked in a secure area such as the hospital safe. The nurse is responsible for documenting in the client's record the items that were taken and how they are being kept secure. In some agencies, the client is given a receipt for his property. If a client asks that a wedding ring be left on, the nurse can secure it to the finger or hand with tape or a strip of gauze. Class rings, however, generally contain multiple grooves or crevices that trap and hold microorganisms. Therefore, to reduce the risk of infection, it is best to remove and safeguard the ring.

The ring is subject to theft if left in the bedside stand. Security guards usually are not responsible for the safekeeping of personal valuables. Another alternative is to give the client's valuables to a family member.

Client Needs Category—Safe, effective care environment
Client Needs Subcategory—Coordinated care

14. 1. A fat embolus can be seen in clients with fractures of the long bones or the pelvis and usually occurs more frequently in young men. When the bone is broken, fat globules are released into the bloodstream, where they combine with platelets. Most fat emboli travel to the pulmonary circulation. Once emboli partially or totally occlude blood flow through a pulmonary vessel, the client may experience dyspnea, rapid breathing and heart rate, cyanosis, chest pain, cough, blood-streaked sputum, and a feeling of doom. Emboli may also travel to the brain, causing confusion, agitation, and coma. Abdominal distention and difficulty swallowing are not associated with fat emboli. Swelling at the incision site is expected after surgery and does not relate to the formation of fat emboli.

Client Needs Category—Physiological integrity
Client Needs Subcategory—Reduction of risk potential

15. 2, 3, 4. During the first 72 hours following a traumatic injury, especially to long bones, the nurse should suspect fat embolism syndrome if the client manifests the following cluster of signs and symptoms: chest pain, dyspnea, tachycardia, tachypnea, fever, disorientation, restlessness, and petechiae over the chest, axillary folds, conjunctiva, buccal membrane, and hard palate.

Client Needs Category—Health promotion and maintenance
Client Needs Subcategory—None

16. 1. The first step a rescuer should take is to see that the victim is breathing because maintaining ventilation is essential for sustaining life—one of the ABCs (airway, breathing, and circulation) that are a nurse's highest priority. The nurse should be careful about moving the client until spinal cord injuries are confirmed or ruled out. Observing for injuries and covering the client with a blanket are important, but only after breathing has been assessed.

Client Needs Category—Physiological integrity
Client Needs Subcategory—Physiological adaptation

17. 2. The ribs enclose the lungs. This makes injuries to the pulmonary system the prime complication associated with fractured ribs. Broken ribs may puncture the pleura and collapse a lung. One classic sign of a flail chest injury is asymmetrical or paradoxical chest expansion, which results in dyspnea. Although the heart is also in the thorax, it is somewhat better protected in the center of the chest. Tachycardia and a weak, thready pulse (rather than an irregular pulse rate) are more likely to indicate damage to major blood vessels. Expiratory wheezing is generally associated

with asthma; pink, frothy sputum is commonly found with heart failure.
> ***Client Needs Category***—*Physiological integrity*
> ***Client Needs Subcategory***—*Reduction of risk potential*

18. 3. The best method to control bleeding in the case of a compound fracture is to compress the major artery above the injury site. Direct pressure on the wound may cause additional injuries to the soft tissue surrounding the fracture. A tourniquet is only used if all other efforts to control bleeding are unsuccessful. When used, a tourniquet is periodically released to allow oxygenated blood to the distal tissue. Elevating the extremity is helpful after applying pressure on the artery, but should be done with caution to prevent further damage to the bone and soft tissue.
> ***Client Needs Category***—*Physiological integrity*
> ***Client Needs Subcategory***—*Physiological adaptation*

19. 3. The neck and back of any accident victim with a suspected spinal injury should be immobilized before transport. The victim is typically positioned flat on her back (supine) and secured to a rigid stretcher before being moved and transported. Rescuers need to keep the head and spine extended and straight. Placing the client in a side-lying, face-lying (prone), or semisitting (semi-Fowler's) position may cause more injury to the vertebrae or the spinal cord because of the flexion and extra movement.
> ***Client Needs Category***—*Physiological integrity*
> ***Client Needs Subcategory***—*Physiological adaptation*

20. 4. Typical signs of a fractured hip include external rotation and shortening of the affected leg. Bruising may or may not be present, depending on the circumstances of the fracture. Sensation is usually intact. Movement results in increased pain.
> ***Client Needs Category***—*Physiological integrity*
> ***Client Needs Subcategory***—*Physiological adaptation*

21. 2, 3, 5. A client with a fractured hip develops pain in the injured area—the joint between the proximal end of the femur and the acetabulum of the pelvis—and weight-bearing is difficult. The fracture results in shortening and external rotation of the affected leg because of discontinuity of the femur. Also, the client typically has muscle spasms involving the iliopsoas muscle attached to the lesser trochanter of the femur, and the abductor and rotator muscles that are inserted on the greater trochanter of the femur. Therefore, the client's affected leg is not drawn toward the midline in an adducted position. The client would probably be too uncomfortable in an adducted position or when sitting or lying.

> ***Client Needs Category***—*Health promotion and maintenance*
> ***Client Needs Subcategory***—*None*

22. 1. Estrogen deficiency, which occurs postmenopausally, is linked to loss of calcium from the bones. Decreased bone mass weakens the skeletal system, increasing a person's susceptibility for fractures. Being overweight exerts more stress on the skeletal system; however, as long as bone integrity remains intact, the risk of fractures is the same as that for the general population. The bones and joints can be kept strong by walking and exercising daily. Lactose intolerance is not necessarily a risk factor as long as the client gets calcium from other sources such as vegetables.
> ***Client Needs Category***—*Physiological integrity*
> ***Client Needs Subcategory***—*Reduction of risk potential*

23.

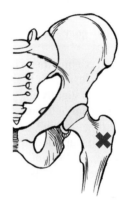

An intertrochanteric fracture refers to a break in the continuity of the femur between the greater and lesser trochanters, the bony prominences that lie outside the joint capsule. An intertrochanteric fracture is also referred to as an extracapsular fracture. The head and neck of the proximal femur are within the acetabulum. A fracture below the head of the femur (subcapital) or across the neck of the femur (transcervical) is referred to as an intracapsular fracture.
> ***Client Needs Category***—*Physiological integrity*
> ***Client Needs Subcategory***—*Physiological adaptation*

24. 2. To perform isometric exercises, a client tenses and releases muscles. These exercises do not involve any appreciable movement of a joint. The quadriceps muscles are on the anterior aspect of the thigh. All other options describe isotonic exercises that involve joint movement.
> ***Client Needs Category***—*Health promotion and maintenance*
> ***Client Needs Subcategory***—*None*

25. 1. Elastic stockings, known as antiembolism or thromboembolic disease hose, support the valves within veins. The supported valves keep the blood flowing upward, toward the heart. When blood moves, rather than pools, in the lower extremities, it is less likely to clot. Properly fitted antiembolism stockings should neither restrict arterial blood from flowing into the lower extremities nor affect blood pressure. Even though they are tight fitting, antiembolism stockings do not constrict the blood vessels.

Client Needs Category—Health promotion and maintenance
Client Needs Subcategory—None

26. **1.** To prevent trapping venous blood in the lower extremities, elastic stockings are applied while the client is in a nondependent position. The best time to apply these stockings is in the morning, before getting out of bed or after elevating the legs a short time. Elastic stockings are worn almost continuously. They are removed once per shift or once per day to assess the skin.

Client Needs Category—Safe, effective care environment
Client Needs Subcategory—Coordinated care

27. **1.** A client who has a prosthesis inserted to repair a fractured hip is turned using sufficient pillows so that the operative leg remains slightly abducted. Hip abduction prevents displacement of the fixation device. Pointing the toes, flexing the knee, or elevating the head will not promote hip abduction.

Client Needs Category—Physiological integrity
Client Needs Subcategory—Physiological adaptation

28. **3.** When helping the client transfer from the bed to a chair, it is best to place the chair parallel to and near the head of the bed on the client's stronger side. The distance between the bed and chair should be as short as possible because the client is weak and at risk for losing her balance. Transferring to a chair at the end of the bed or against a side wall requires much more physical effort and poses safety hazards. Placing the chair perpendicularly interferes with assisting the client.

Client Needs Category—Safe, effective care environment
Client Needs Subcategory—Safety and infection control

29. **1.** In a three-point partial weight-bearing gait, the weaker leg and walker are advanced together. The hands support most of the weight while the stronger leg is lifted and advanced. In the other options, the weight distribution is incorrect.

Client Needs Category—Health promotion and maintenance
Client Needs Subcategory—None

30. **1, 2, 3.** Until healing occurs, the client's legs must be spread outward (abducted) from the body. Adduction of the hip or flexion greater than 90 degrees may

dislocate the prosthesis from the joint. Postoperative nursing care also requires using a foam wedge splint between the legs while the client is in bed, using a raised toilet seat for elimination, keeping the knees lower than the hips when sitting, and reminding the client to avoid bending forward when dressing. Raising the head of the bed 90 degrees creates excessive hip flexion and can dislocate the hip. The knees should always be lower than the hips, and the leg should be in neutral position following hip replacement surgery.

Client Needs Category—Physiological integrity
Client Needs Subcategory—Reduction of risk potential

Nursing Care of Clients with Casts

31. **2.** When plaster combines with water, a chemical reaction takes place. Energy is given off in the form of heat. Therefore, it is appropriate to warn the client that his arm may feel quite warm temporarily. Steam or heat waves may even be seen rising from the surface of the wet cast. The cast supports the broken bone, but it should not constrict the underlying tissue or feel tight. Wet plaster does not produce a disagreeable odor. The client should not feel itchy when the cast is applied.

Client Needs Category—Health promotion and maintenance
Client Needs Subcategory—None

32. **4.** A wet cast is held and supported with the palms of the hands. Using the fingers is likely to cause indentations in the cast, which may create pressure areas on the underlying tissue. After the cast is applied, it is dried while supported on a soft surface. A wet cast on a hard surface can become flattened.

Client Needs Category—Physiological integrity
Client Needs Subcategory—Physiological adaptation

33. **1.** Sharp pain is the first symptom of compartment syndrome. Ischemia, the impairment of arterial blood flow that is caused by swelling of the surrounding muscle within the inelastic fascia, causes pain. Paralysis and sensory loss follow as nerves become damaged by compression and lack of blood supply. Muscle spasms do not typically occur. The hand may appear pale or white, not reddened, and feel cold because of inadequate arterial blood. If the radial artery is assessed, the nurse typically finds that it is weak or absent.

Client Needs Category—Physiological integrity
Client Needs Subcategory—Reduction of risk potential

34. **4.** A wet cast is supported along its entire length with soft pillows as it dries. This soft support distributes the weight of the cast over a greater surface and pre-

vents flattening of the underlying portion. Using pillows also elevates the extremity, which relieves temporary swelling. A synthetic sheepskin or vinyl sheet interferes with water evaporation from the wet plaster. An absorbent pad does not sufficiently cushion the weight of the cast.
***Client Needs Category**—Physiological integrity*
***Client Needs Subcategory**—Physiological adaptation*

35. 1. Natural evaporation is the best way to dry a plaster cast. This process takes 24 to 48 hours. It involves leaving the casted area uncovered and turning the client at frequent intervals so that the entire cast circumference is exposed to the air. Intense heat, such as with a heating blanket, hair dryer, or heat lamp, may burn the client or just dry the superficial surface of the cast.
***Client Needs Category**—Physiological integrity*
***Client Needs Subcategory**—Basic care and comfort*

36. 3. The nurse assesses circulation in an extremity by performing the blanching test to determine capillary refill time. After releasing pressure on the nailbed, the color normally returns within 2 to 3 seconds. This assessment is also performed on the opposite extremity. If the capillary refill time is similar in both extremities, the cast or tissue swelling is not a factor. Asking the client whether the cast feels heavy and palpating it to feel the cast temperature are inappropriate techniques for assessing circulation. Determining that there is space between the cast and the skin is not totally reliable. If circulation is impaired due to compartment syndrome, there may still be room to insert a finger at the cast margins.
***Client Needs Category**—Physiological integrity*
***Client Needs Subcategory**—Physiological adaptation*

37. 2. Casts made of fiberglass or other synthetic materials have several advantages, one of which is that they are lighter weight than plaster casts. A synthetic cast dries more quickly, is more durable, and is unlikely to soften if it becomes wet. Fiberglass casts are no less flexible or less restrictive than plaster ones. The major disadvantage is that they are more expensive than traditional plaster casts.
***Client Needs Category**—Physiological integrity*
***Client Needs Subcategory**—Physiological adaptation*

38. 3. Marking the outer margin of the drainage on the cast helps the nurse evaluate the status of the bleeding. The nurse needs to return soon for another assessment. By comparing the subsequent size of the bloody spot, the nurse evaluates the seriousness of the bleeding. It is important to monitor vital signs each time the drainage is assessed. All information is documented. If the bleeding is not controlled and vital signs indicate that the client's condition is changing, the physician must be notified immediately. An ice bag is generally used to control swelling postoperatively; it may also help decrease bleeding.
***Client Needs Category**—Physiological integrity*
***Client Needs Subcategory**—Physiological adaptation*

39. 3. When a client expresses a concern, it is best for the nurse to verbalize the feeling or message that the sender conveyed. This response shows understanding and a willingness to listen. Using clichés, agreeing with the client, stereotyping the family, or offering opinions are all nontherapeutic. They are of little help to a client who is struggling with a personal problem.
***Client Needs Category**—Psychosocial integrity*
***Client Needs Subcategory**—None*

40. 3. Most adolescents seek to become independent of their parents and develop relationships with nonrelatives. Developmental tasks concerned with self-identity, sexuality, testing the body's abilities, and learning to control emotional behavior occur more commonly just before young adulthood.
***Client Needs Category**—Health promotion and maintenance*
***Client Needs Subcategory**—None*

41. 2. A hip spica cast interferes with hip flexion and assuming a sitting position. A fracture bedpan elevates the buttocks just slightly enough for bowel elimination. Because this client cannot sit, a bedside commode, mechanical lift, and raised toilet seat are inappropriate.
***Client Needs Category**—Physiological integrity*
***Client Needs Subcategory**—Physiological adaptation*

42. 3. One of the weakest areas of a hip spica cast is at the groin. This area tends to crack because it is stressed when the client is turned and repositioned. The bar helps to strengthen the cast. The bar is never used for lifting, turning, or performing physical exercise. The bar will maintain proper alignment, but this is not its primary purpose.
***Client Needs Category**—Health promotion and maintenance*
***Client Needs Subcategory**—None*

43. 1. Obtaining a medical order for administering an antihistamine/antipruritic drug such as cyproheptadine (Periactin) chemically relieves the client's itching. Distraction may also be an alternative technique for relieving discomfort, but it takes commitment and repeated practice to be effective. The client should be cautioned against using a coat hanger or any method that scratches the skin. If the integrity of the skin is impaired, organisms may begin to grow in the warm, dark, moist environment.

Powder is inappropriate because it can cake under the cast, causing potential skin breakdown. Ice bags to the outside of the cast are ineffective in preventing itching.
> **Client Needs Category**—*Physiological integrity*
> **Client Needs Subcategory**—*Pharmacological therapies*

44. 4. The most common cause of an odor from a cast is an infected wound. Infected wounds produce purulent drainage, causing unpleasant odors as the pus accumulates. To confirm the suspicion that an infection exists, the nurse should monitor the client for a cluster of additional signs and symptoms, including elevated temperature, tachycardia, anorexia, and malaise. None of the other options provides reasons for foul-smelling odors.
> **Client Needs Category**—*Physiological integrity*
> **Client Needs Subcategory**—*Reduction of risk potential*

45. 2. The piece of plaster that is removed to make a window should be replaced in the opening and secured with tape or a roller bandage. Allowing the window to remain open may cause the tissue to bulge into the opening. This uneven pressure on the skin can cause it to break down. There is no need to dispose of the plaster piece or to send it to the laboratory.
> **Client Needs Category**—*Physiological integrity*
> **Client Needs Subcategory**—*Reduction of risk potential*

46. 1. Rough or crumbling edges of a plaster cast are smoothed or repaired by applying petals made from moleskin or adhesive tape. Petals, formed in rectangular or oval pieces, are inserted on the inside of the cast edge and then folded over the outside edge of the cast. The strips are made to overlap, resembling the appearance of flower petals. The physician usually applies more plaster strips or uses a cast cutter if needed. Trimming a cast does not usually stop it from crumbling. Fragments of plaster are likely to continue breaking off if the nurse uses gauze to cover the cast edge.
> **Client Needs Category**—*Physiological integrity*
> **Client Needs Subcategory**—*Physiological adaptation*

47. 1. Cast syndrome, also known as superior mesenteric syndrome, causes gastrointestinal symptoms, such as abdominal distention, bloating, nausea, vomiting, and abdominal pain. The symptoms are caused by a partial or total intestinal obstruction. Symptoms related to anxiety may also be present. The other options, if they develop, are more likely to be caused by complications other than cast syndrome.
> **Client Needs Category**—*Physiological integrity*
> **Client Needs Subcategory**—*Physiological adaptation*

Nursing Care of Clients with Traction

48. 2. The leg of the client in Buck's traction must remain in alignment with the pull of the traction. This means, rather than making the bed as usual from side to side, the nurse removes and applies linen at the top or bottom of the bed and pulls it underneath the client. A person in Buck's traction is not turned from side to side or raised with a mechanical lift. A client in traction, as any other hospitalized client, has bed linen changed whenever it is soiled, wet, or needs replacement.
> **Client Needs Category**—*Physiological integrity*
> **Client Needs Subcategory**—*Basic care and comfort*

49. 3. To maintain countertraction, the client's foot must never press against the foot of the bed. If this occurs, the nurse should help pull the client back up toward the head of the bed. The weights must always hang free, rather than rest on the floor or the bed. The body must be in alignment with the pull of the traction. The traction rope must move freely within the groove of the pulley.
> **Client Needs Category**—*Physiological integrity*
> **Client Needs Subcategory**—*Physiological adaptation*

50. 2. The best technique for assessing circulation among the options provided is to palpate the distal peripheral pulse such as the dorsalis pedis artery, which is on the top of the foot. Other pertinent circulatory assessments include checking the client's skin color, temperature, capillary refill time, and subjective complaints concerning pain. Checking movement and sensation are neurologic assessment techniques. Taking the blood pressure on the thigh rather than the arm is unnecessary.
> **Client Needs Category**—*Physiological integrity*
> **Client Needs Subcategory**—*Physiological adaptation*

51. 2. The popliteal space behind the knee is especially prone to pressure and irritation when Russell's traction is used. This area is suspended in a sling, which can become wrinkled. A piece of thick felt is sometimes used to line the sling to keep the surface smooth. The ischial spines are part of the inferior portion of the pelvic bones. The iliac crests are the upper flared portions of the bony pelvis. Neither of these areas is included in Russell's traction. The zygomatic arches are in the cheek.
> **Client Needs Category**—*Physiological integrity*
> **Client Needs Subcategory**—*Reduction of risk potential*

52. 3. Two pieces of rope are sometimes spliced together with a knot to provide sufficient length for traction. However, if the knot prevents free movement over and within a pulley, it interferes with the traction's effectiveness. Traction ropes are taut. Locating the trapeze above the client's chest facilitates its use. Traction weights must hang freely above the floor for effective use.

Client Needs Category—Physiological integrity
Client Needs Subcategory—Reduction of risk potential

53. 1. Preoperatively, the traction remains applied to the client at all times, even during transport to the operating room. Its purpose is to relieve muscle spasms and immobilize the fractured bone. If the nurse removes the traction or releases the weights, muscle spasms recur. Any realignment that may have been achieved with the use of traction is jeopardized.

Client Needs Category—Physiological integrity
Client Needs Subcategory—Physiological adaptation

54. 4. A pillow is usually contraindicated when a client is in cervical skin traction because it alters the direction of pull. If any kind of head support is necessary, it is usually provided with a cervical or neck pillow that fits under the nape of the neck. The other options are correct and do not require the nurse's attention.

Client Needs Category—Physiological integrity
Client Needs Subcategory—Reduction of risk potential

55. 3. The uppermost edge of a pelvic belt hugs the client's hips. The pelvic belt helps to relieve spasms and pain in the muscles in the lumbar area. Placing the belt below the rib cage or at the midabdomen does not promote maximum effective use. Though using pelvic-belt traction will promote comfort, the location for its application is not arbitrarily determined on that basis.

Client Needs Category—Physiological integrity
Client Needs Subcategory—Physiological adaptation

56. 3. The tips of the pin used for skeletal traction are skewered into a block of cork or a rubber ball similar to one used for playing jacks. Gauze and cotton are inadequate for preventing punctures and abrasions. The pin may also pierce rubber tubes, thus exposing the sharp tip.

Client Needs Category—Safe, effective care environment
Client Needs Subcategory—Safety and infection control

57. 4. Purulent drainage, sometimes referred to as pus, indicates an infection. Purulent drainage is a collection of fluid containing white blood cells and pathogens. The presence of white blood cells indicates that the body is attempting to destroy and remove infecting organisms. Serous drainage, which is clear, is

made up of plasma or serum. Bloody drainage indicates trauma. Mucoid drainage, which is released from mucous membranes, is sticky and transparent.

Client Needs Category—Physiological integrity
Client Needs Subcategory—Physiological adaptation

58. 2. There is a high probability that individuals who are allergic to penicillin will also exhibit a cross-sensitivity to cephalosporins. Both types of drugs are very similar in their structure. All clients with known drug sensitivity are closely observed when a new medication, especially an antibiotic, is administered. Individuals with a penicillin allergy seem to react more frequently to cephalosporins than to the other types of antibiotics mentioned.

Client Needs Category—Physiological integrity
Client Needs Subcategory—Pharmacological therapies

59. 1. Halo-cervical traction immobilizes the vertebrae in the neck while allowing clients to assume physical activity, such as standing, sitting, and walking. Halo-cervical traction, however, restricts head movement. Vertebral fractures proceed to heal at a standard rate regardless of whether halo traction or some other medical or surgical management is instituted. Physical therapy is not prescribed until the vertebral fracture is stabilized and the halo traction is removed.

Client Needs Category—Health promotion and maintenance
Client Needs Subcategory—None

60. 4. A client's ability to see straight ahead is the best sign that halo traction is keeping the neck immobilized in a neutral position. Clients should not be able to move the neck at will while in halo traction. Clients may experience mild neck discomfort even though halo traction is applied appropriately. The abilities to speak and to hear are unrelated to the use of halo traction.

Client Needs Category—Physiological integrity
Client Needs Subcategory—Physiological adaptation

61. 3. Signs that the metal rods in halo traction require readjustment include an inability to fully open the mouth and difficulty swallowing. Orthostatic hypotension, if it occurs, is not due to the malfunction of the halo traction. Men in halo traction typically need help with shaving because they cannot change their head position to see where to shave; the nurse should anticipate offering assistance. Irritation in the axilla is usually related to the plaster vest and does not indicate a need for readjustment. Nursing intervention, however, is needed to prevent further skin breakdown.

Client Needs Category—Physiological integrity
Client Needs Subcategory—Reduction of risk potential

Nursing Care of Clients with Inflammatory Joint Disorders

62. 1. The ESR is a nonspecific test that indicates the presence and progress of an inflammatory disease. It is elevated in a number of inflammatory conditions, including rheumatoid arthritis. A PTT helps determine a person's ability to clot blood; it is commonly ordered for clients receiving heparin therapy. A FBS is performed to diagnose and evaluate the treatment of diabetes mellitus. BUN levels are commonly checked to assess renal function.
> *Client Needs Category—Health promotion and maintenance*
> *Client Needs Subcategory—None*

63. 3. Although some people acquire juvenile arthritis, most experience the onset of rheumatoid arthritis early in adult life. The disease profoundly affects the ability to maintain employment during the productive years of life.
> *Client Needs Category—Health promotion and maintenance*
> *Client Needs Subcategory—None*

64. 3. Five grams of drug supplied in dosage strength of 5 grains per tablet requires 15 tablets in a 24-hour period. 1 g contains approximately 15 grains; 5 g contains 75 grains ($5 \times 15 = 75$). To solve the problem using the ratio and proportion method, use the following steps:

$$\frac{1 \text{ tablet}}{5 \text{ grains}} = \frac{X \text{ tablet}}{75 \text{ grains}}$$

$$5X = 75$$
$$X = 15 \text{ tablets}$$
> *Client Needs Category—Safe, effective care environment*
> *Client Needs Subcategory—Coordinated care*

65. 3. Aspirin has the ability to produce analgesic, anti-inflammatory, and antipyretic effects. Its analgesic and anti-inflammatory effects are probably achieved by inhibiting chemicals called prostaglandins, not by interrupting nerve synapses. Prostaglandins increase sensitivity of peripheral pain receptors. Aspirin does not relax skeletal muscles or stimulate the immune system.
> *Client Needs Category—Physiological integrity*
> *Client Needs Subcategory—Pharmacological therapies*

66. 4. Taking irritating drugs with food or at mealtimes helps to decrease gastric distress. Aspirin, especially in large doses, tends to irritate the stomach mucosa, resulting in bleeding. Giving aspirin on an empty stomach increases discomfort. Cold water and hot tea do not protect the stomach or alter aspirin's acidity. The caffeine in tea actually stimulates an increase in the production of stomach acid. Enteric-coated aspirin is needed for clients who take large doses of aspirin because the enteric coating protects the stomach.
> *Client Needs Category—Physiological integrity*
> *Client Needs Subcategory—Pharmacological therapies*

67. 1. Ringing in the ears, called tinnitus, is a sign of aspirin toxicity and is seen when clients take large amounts of salicylates on a daily basis. Clients may also report a buzzing, tinkling, or hissing sound. Diseases or conditions affecting the ear can also cause tinnitus. Dizziness, metallic tastes in the mouth, and proteinuria are not typically associated with aspirin toxicity.
> *Client Needs Category—Physiological integrity*
> *Client Needs Subcategory—Pharmacological therapies*

68. 4. Distraction is a legitimate and often very effective method for relieving discomfort. Watching television is one method of distraction. There are no reports that electronic television signals are an effective treatment for arthritis. If the client had only a slight case of arthritis, she would be likely to feel pain relief at times other than when watching television.
> *Client Needs Category—Physiological integrity*
> *Client Needs Subcategory—Physiological adaptation*

69. 1. The proximal finger joints are most commonly affected in clients with rheumatoid arthritis. In some cases, the joints are so affected that the fingers actually turn laterally. In osteoarthritis, the distal finger joints are more commonly deformed. Traumatic arthritis, which is associated with a specific injury, can affect any joint.
> *Client Needs Category—Physiological integrity*
> *Client Needs Subcategory—Physiological adaptation*

70. 2. Moist heat is more effective than forms of dry heat, such as a hot water bottle, an electric heating pad, or an infrared heat lamp. This phenomenon is attributed to the fact that water is a better conductor of heat than air. Whenever any form of heat is used, the nurse must take care to ensure that the client is not accidentally burned.
> *Client Needs Category—Physiological integrity*
> *Client Needs Subcategory—Physiological adaptation*

71. 1. People with rheumatoid arthritis are more stiff and uncomfortable in the early morning hours after being inactive during the hours of sleep. Therefore, it is best to allow extra time and distribute self-care activities over later hours of the day.
> *Client Needs Category—Physiological integrity*
> *Client Needs Subcategory—Basic care and comfort*

72. **2.** Hand deformities and muscle atrophy make it difficult for the client with rheumatoid arthritis to perform fine motor movement with the fingers. Purchasing clothes that can be easily pulled or slipped on enables the client to maintain a degree of independence. Although exercise is important to help maintain the client's joint mobility, aerobic exercise is unrealistic because it is likely to be too strenuous and tiring (clients with rheumatoid arthritis are often anemic and tire easily). Sleeping on a waterbed or moving to a warm climate will have little if any effect on the disease process.

Client Needs Category—*Health promotion and maintenance*
Client Needs Subcategory—*None*

73. **1.** During an acute attack, splints are used primarily to keep the inflamed joints somewhat inactive. Resting the affected joint in a splint limits the movement and alleviates additional stress on the diseased joints. The acute inflammation subsides with a combination of drug therapy and the body's natural healing processes. By limiting the damage during the acute attack, a certain amount of strength and joint flexibility is preserved, but these are not the primary purpose of splints. Splinting the affected fingers will not cure the disease.

Client Needs Category—*Health promotion and maintenance*
Client Needs Subcategory—*None*

74. **1.** Corticosteroid therapy causes sodium and water retention, which can lead to hypernatremia. Because this condition manifests as weight gain, the nurse needs to monitor the client's daily weight. This excess fluid can also cause the client's blood pressure to rise, so it is also closely monitored. The pulse rate is not likely to change appreciably; however, the pulse may feel bounding with an increase of fluid in the blood volume. The nurse should monitor the client's white blood cell count, not the red, because corticosteroids can mask the signs of infection. The skin of a person taking steroids undergoes various changes but generally remains intact. The nurse may observe that the skin becomes thin and bruises easily. The face may become edematous. Other possible changes include increased hair growth, petechiae, redistribution of body fat, and striae. If the skin does become impaired as a result of injury or surgery, wound healing is prolonged.

Client Needs Category—*Physiological integrity*
Client Needs Subcategory—*Pharmacological therapies*

75. **4.** Individuals receiving corticosteroids tend to have elevated blood glucose levels. Diabetics may need to increase their dosage of insulin or oral hypoglycemic agents. Nondiabetics should also be monitored for hyperglycemia and glycosuria. Because steroids depress the inflammatory response, they place the client at high risk for acquiring infections. To prevent acute adrenal insufficiency, steroids are tapered and withdrawn gradually if therapy is discontinued. Depression is common among individuals receiving corticosteroids.

Client Needs Category—*Physiological integrity*
Client Needs Subcategory—*Pharmacological therapies*

76. **3.** The mucosa of the mouth and entire gastrointestinal tract may become ulcerated as a consequence of taking methotrexate (Rheumatrex). Therefore, it is especially important to inspect the oral cavity. This drug also causes diarrhea and renal failure. Chest pain is not a usual adverse effect of methotrexate.

Client Needs Category—*Physiological integrity*
Client Needs Subcategory—*Pharmacological therapies*

77. **1.** To avoid burning the skin, a heating pad is always kept on a low setting. The client is cautioned not to turn the heat setting higher when becoming adapted to the sensation of warmth. Because of the client's age and changes in his skin and sensory functioning, the risk of burns is high if the heating pad is placed directly next to the skin. A heating pad is covered with fabric such as flannel. Heat is not applied for longer than 20 to 30 minutes at a time.

Client Needs Category—*Safe, effective care environment*
Client Needs Subcategory—*Safety and infection control*

78. **1.** Because obesity puts additional stress on weight-bearing joints and contributes to the discomfort of osteoarthritis, maintaining a desired weight will help to minimize stress and decrease pain. Applying a topical analgesic cream may improve joint mobility and help with sore muscles but does not directly relieve the joint stress related to arthritis. Restrictive devices may cause stiffness from joint disuse. Physical activity is likely to cause more discomfort to a person whose hips are affected by osteoarthritis.

Client Needs Category—*Health promotion and maintenance*
Client Needs Subcategory—*None*

79. **3.** A cane should always be held on the unaffected side. This allows the client to transfer or redistribute body weight from the painful joint to the hand with the cane when taking a step. Covering the tip with a rubber cap, wearing supportive shoes, and maintaining good posture are all appropriate techniques for using a cane.

Client Needs Category—*Health promotion and maintenance*
Client Needs Subcategory—*None*

80. 4. Gastrointestinal adverse effects and the potential for bleeding are common among clients who take nonsteroidal anti-inflammatory drugs (NSAIDs). By asking the client to identify the color of his stools, the nurse is assessing if the drug is causing gastrointestinal bleeding. NSAIDs are not known to cause increased urination or hand tremors. NSAIDs may or may not affect appetite, depending on the amount of GI upset.
>*Client Needs Category*—*Physiological integrity*
>*Client Needs Subcategory*—*Pharmacological therapies*

81. 2. Aspirin increases the possibility of postoperative bleeding. It interferes with the ability of platelets to clump together, one of the first mechanisms in clot formation. Aspirin does not increase the risk of wound infection or affect the body's ability to heal. Aspirin is not discontinued to facilitate assessing the client's pain. However, if the client takes aspirin for arthritis and is asked to stop it for a week, he may demonstrate signs of joint stiffness, tenderness, swelling, and immobility.
>*Client Needs Category*—*Physiological integrity*
>*Client Needs Subcategory*—*Pharmacological therapies*

82. 1. An incentive spirometer helps a client measure the effectiveness of deep inhalation. Postoperatively, it is important for the client to breathe deeply to open the airways and alveoli. This helps improve the oxygenation of blood, eliminate carbon dioxide, and prevent atelectasis and pneumonia. None of the other options indicate the correct use of an incentive spirometer.
>*Client Needs Category*—*Health promotion and maintenance*
>*Client Needs Subcategory*—*None*

83. 3. Clipping the hair around the intended incisional area is preferred over shaving to avoid microabrasions that support bacterial growth. Pressing the razor firmly or deeply onto the skin can cause cuts. Altering the integrity of the skin because of cuts and bleeding increases the risk of postoperative wound infections. Soap is used to decrease the numbers of transient skin organisms. For surgery, a stronger antiseptic such as Betadine is usually used.
>*Client Needs Category*—*Safe, effective care environment*
>*Client Needs Subcategory*—*Safety and infection control*

84. 2. The hip of a client who has undergone a total hip replacement (arthroplasty) is maintained in a position of abduction, or away from the midline. Adduction is positioned toward the midline, and flexion is a bent position. Extension is keeping the body part straight. If the client flexes his hip more than 90 degrees or adducts the hip, the prosthetic femoral head may become dislocated. A triangular foam wedge is generally kept between the client's legs while the client is in bed.
>*Client Needs Category*—*Physiological integrity*
>*Client Needs Subcategory*—*Physiological adaptation*

85. 3. A trapeze helps the client move and lift his body. Encouraging the client to participate actively helps maintain muscular strength and reduces the nurse's effort when moving and positioning a client. A bed cradle is used to keep bed linen off lower extremities. A bed board is used to support the client's spine. Lower side rails are appropriate when maintaining the safety of a confused client or one with a perceptual disorder.
>*Client Needs Category*—*Physiological integrity*
>*Client Needs Subcategory*—*Physiological adaptation*

86. 2. A trochanter roll is used to maintain the hip in a position of extension. Placing this positioning device at the trochanter helps keep the hip from rotating outward. A footboard is used to prevent plantar flexion and footdrop deformity. A turning sheet is used to reposition a client. A foam mattress helps relieve pressure from bony prominences.
>*Client Needs Category*—*Physiological integrity*
>*Client Needs Subcategory*—*Physiological adaptation*

87. 1. A client with a total hip replacement is instructed to avoid crossing his legs because this places the hip in a position of adduction and flexion. These two positions can displace the prosthetic device. Pointing the toes, as in plantar flexion or dorsiflexion, will not impair the surgical procedure. Laying flat and standing upright are not harmful.
>*Client Needs Category*—*Health promotion and maintenance*
>*Client Needs Subcategory*—*None*

88. 3. Postoperatively and for an extended time afterward, a client with a total hip replacement must avoid flexing the hip more than 90 degrees. This necessitates using a raised toilet seat. The client does not need a wheelchair and can ambulate using a walker. The client can continue to use his own bed at home. The nurse teaches the client the proper techniques for transferring from bed to a chair; therefore, a mechanical lift is unnecessary.
>*Client Needs Category*—*Health promotion and maintenance*
>*Client Needs Subcategory*—*None*

89. 1. The client with a total hip replacement must avoid bending over to put on or take off socks, pants, underwear, and shoes. Someone should help with these items of clothing, or assistive devices may be used. Another approach is to modify the clothing so that the client can slip items on without flexing the hip more than 90 degrees. No special equipment is needed for bathing; however, the client must be cautious when getting in and out of the shower and with the water temperature. Instructing the client about home safety is also important. Additional areas to cover include water and environmental temperatures, furniture placement, lighting, medication administration, burglary protection, and fire safety. Taking vigorous walks is inappropriate immediately after discharge because the client's activity level should be increased gradually. Stool softeners are not usually included in the client's discharge instructions.

Client Needs Category—Health promotion and maintenance
Client Needs Subcategory—None

90. 2. Most clients who undergo arthroscopy use crutches for a period of time following the procedure. Because postprocedural discomfort and recovery from anesthesia or light conscious sedation interfere with learning and practice, it is best to teach clients how to use crutches during their preoperative preparation. Most clients who undergo arthroscopy have already personally experienced the signs and symptoms of arthritis. Drug teaching is postponed until the physician writes postoperative orders. Balancing rest with exercise is important, but the physician indicates those specific orders after the procedure.

Client Needs Category—Health promotion and maintenance
Client Needs Subcategory—None

91. 4. A CPM machine is used primarily to restore full range of joint motion. Clients with knee joint replacement are often reluctant to exercise the operative knee actively because of pain. Discomfort usually accompanies use of the CPM machine. Exercise tones and strengthens muscles and relieves dependent swelling by promoting venous circulation; however, these are considered secondary benefits. It is appropriate for the nurse to administer a prescribed analgesic before the client uses a CPM machine.

Client Needs Category—Health promotion and maintenance
Client Needs Subcategory—None

92. 2. The length of time the client spends on the CPM machine helps determine his response to treatment following arthroplasty. Inspecting and documenting the wound's appearance and the drainage on the dressing, and checking presence and quality of arterial pulses are important data to record. However, this information is more pertinent to the client's general physical health, not his progress with treatment.

Client Needs Category—Physiological integrity
Client Needs Subcategory—Reduction of risk potential

93. 3. A resting knee extension splint (immobilizer) is worn on the operative leg until the client demonstrates enough quadriceps strength to independently perform straight leg raising. A decrease in pain, wound approximation, and increase in knee flexion are positive signs of healing and rehabilitation, but they are not criteria for discontinuing the immobilizer.

Client Needs Category—Physiological Integrity
Client Needs Subcategory—Physiological adaptation

94. 1. Gout is a metabolic disease caused by hyperuricemia as well as a form of acute arthritis. Marked by acute inflammation, gout can affect any joint; however, approximately 80% of those with the disease experience symptoms in their great toe, which makes ambulation painful.

Client Needs Category—Physiological integrity
Client Needs Subcategory—Physiological adaptation

95. 3. An elevated serum uric acid level is diagnostic among clients with gout. An elevated serum creatinine clearance and blood urea nitrogen level are indicative of renal failure. Serum calcium is elevated in hyperparathyroidism, primary cancers such as Hodgkin's disease or multiple myeloma, and bone metastasis.

Client Needs Category—Physiological integrity
Client Needs Subcategory—Physiological adaptation

96. 1. Acute gout attacks can be very painful. A bed cradle can help prevent the affected joints, particularly the toe joints, from being touched or otherwise bumped. An electric fan, foam mattress, or fracture bedpan will not promote comfort in this situation.

Client Needs Category—Physiological integrity
Client Needs Subcategory—Basic care and comfort

97. 4. Organ meats, such as liver, kidney, brain, and sweetbreads, are high in purines. Other sources of high purine levels include fish roe (eggs), sardines, and anchovies. Foods that are moderately high in purines are meats, seafood, dried beans, lentils, spinach, and peas. The other choices are not high in purines and may be included in the client's diet.

Client Needs Category—Safe, effective care environment
Client Needs Subcategory—Coordinated care

98. 1. Colchicine (Colgout) is an antigout agent used to treat acute attacks and to prevent recurrences of gout. The nurse would withhold this drug if the client manifests adverse gastrointestinal disturbances, such as nausea and vomiting, abdominal pain, or diarrhea. While the client is receiving the drug, the nurse should frequently assess the joints for pain, mobility, and edema. Dizziness, drowsiness, and headache are not signs of an adverse reaction to this drug.

Client Needs Category—Physiological integrity
Client Needs Subcategory—Pharmacological therapies

99. **3.** It is best to provide the greater share of fluid in the morning to compensate for the long period without oral fluids while sleeping. Frequent urination related to increased intake will most likely occur during the day. Providing a large volume of fluid after a meal contributes to gastrointestinal fullness or upset. Consuming large amounts of fluid during evening hours or before bedtime usually results in nocturia and interferes with sleep.

Client Needs Category—Physiological integrity
Client Needs Subcategory—Basic care and comfort

100. **2.** There is a correlation between the consumption of alcohol and the recurrence of gout symptoms. Therefore, it is best to instruct clients with gout to abstain from drinking alcohol. Coffee, cranberry juice, and carbonated beverages are safe to consume.

Client Needs Category—Health promotion and maintenance
Client Needs Subcategory—None

Nursing Care of Clients with Degenerative Bone Disorders

101. **3.** The nurse is correct to support the joint being exercised by holding areas proximal and distal to the joint. ROM exercises do not necessarily need to be completed independently. Force on a joint is not needed and can have serious consequences. Exercise should be stopped when discomfort occurs.

Client Needs Category—Health promotion and maintenance
Client Needs Subcategory—None

102. **3.** Clients with osteoporosis tend to present with spinal deformities, such as kyphosis (dowager's hump) or an inability to assume an erect posture. Although clients with osteoporosis experience swollen joints, discomfort in sitting, and diminished energy, these conditions are not uniquely associated with this disorder.

Client Needs Category—Physiological integrity
Client Needs Subcategory—Physiological adaptation

103. **2.** Smoking and caffeine consumption contribute to the severity of osteoporosis. Although aspirin, carbonated beverages, and sodium are best used in moderation, they are not considered pathologically related to osteoporosis. Alcohol is associated with loss of bone density. Currently, it is unclear whether chronic alcohol ingestion destroys bone-forming cells, interferes with calcium absorption, or contributes to osteoporosis simply because of its correlation with an inadequate nutritional intake. Supplemental calcium and consumption of dairy products are therapeutic measures for individuals who are at risk for or who have acquired osteoporosis.

Client Needs Category—Health promotion and maintenance
Client Needs Subcategory—None

104.

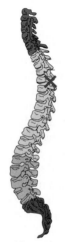

The client with osteoporosis typically develops progressive kyphosis, an exaggerated curvature of the thoracic spinal vertebrae. Kyphosis accompanies a loss of height. Osteoporosis of the spine can also cause back pain from spinal compression fractures.

Client Needs Category—Physiological integrity
Client Needs Subcategory—Physiological adaptation

105. **3.** Supporting the limb affected by osteomyelitis and handling it gently help reduce the risk of a pathological fracture. Meeting the client's needs for nutrition and fluids addresses the metabolic problems that accompany an infection that is often accompanied by a fever. Because the activity of a client with osteomyelitis is often limited, using pressure-relieving devices becomes imperative in maintaining skin integrity.

Client Needs Category—Physiological integrity
Client Needs Subcategory—Basic care and comfort

106. **1.** Health-seeking behaviors and illness beliefs vary among Mexican Americans. These behaviors and beliefs are influenced by geography, length of time spent in the United States, financial issues, age, and social standing. Because this client is an older adult and has just immigrated to the United States, the nurse may assume that his health-seeking behaviors are deeply rooted in traditional Mexican culture and health care practices.

In a traditional Mexican home, female members of the household provide medical care. Many clients will not go to the hospital or physician until all attempts at treating the illness with home remedies have been exhausted. Because Mexican American men are traditionally expected to be strong, the client's illness may be perceived as interfering with his ability to provide for his family.

Some Mexican Americans believe that medical technology assists the physician in curing illnesses; however, since the client has been in the United States for a short time, it is unlikely he would be aware of the medical advances in this country. A *curandero* is a faith healer. There is no evidence in this question to validate that the client no longer believes in curanderos. Some Mexican Americans believe that illness is caused by the "evil eye," which would be treated by spiritual ceremonies, candles, and prayer.

Client Needs Category—Psychosocial integrity
Client Needs Subcategory—None

107. 1. Vitamin D is necessary for calcium absorption. Exposure to sunlight helps to convert dehydrocholesterol in the skin and ergosterol, a plant precursor, to provitamins that eventually become vitamin D. The beneficial and harmful effects of eating cattle injected with bovine growth hormone have not been conclusively determined. Orange vegetables are good sources of beta carotene, a precursor of vitamin A. Organically grown produce does not provide any additional nutritional benefit over other produce; however, eliminating the ingestion of chemical fertilizers, herbicides, and pesticides may be beneficial.

Client Needs Category—Health promotion and maintenance
Client Needs Subcategory—None

Nursing Care of Clients with Amputations

108. 3. With very few exceptions, a person in shock is kept flat with the lower extremities slightly elevated. Gravity helps to maintain blood in the area of the vital organs. Keeping the client supine, in a back-lying position, does not provide the added benefit of elevating the legs. Keeping the client prone (in a face-lying position) or on his side would interfere with emergency assessment and care.

Client Needs Category—Physiological integrity
Client Needs Subcategory—Physiological adaptation

109. 2. Staying with a grief-stricken client provides emotional support and may help the client feel he can depend on the nurse to be available and respond to his future needs. Leaving an uncomfortable situation is one method health professionals use to cope with their own feelings of inadequacy; however, the client would probably interpret the desertion as a sign that the nurse is not a caring individual. Allowing the client to release his rage can be therapeutic as long as it does not endanger him or others. Feeling angry is one of the early steps in the grieving process. Calling the physician is inappropriate because it does not address the real problem of anger related to the missing limb.

Client Needs Category—Psychosocial integrity
Client Needs Subcategory—None

110. 2. Phantom pain or sensation is a phenomenon experienced by some people who have had a limb amputated. The person typically feels a physical sensation in the missing limb. The feelings range from a sense that the amputated part is still there to other sensations that cause discomfort, such as pain, cramping, burning, and itching. Referred pain is discomfort experienced in a location that is distant from the actual area of pathology. Psychogenic pain is discomfort that is emotional in origin. Intractable pain is severe and unrelenting and may require a combination of therapies.

Client Needs Category—Physiological integrity
Client Needs Subcategory—Physiological adaptation

111. 1. Most believe the TENS unit generates sensations that the brain perceives in place of the pain from the missing limb. The process is compared to a car waiting while a train crosses the highway. The impulses from the TENS unit are like the train. As long as the TENS impulses flood the brain, the pain impulses are blocked. Thus, the TENS unit does not travel to a nerve root, weaken sensory muscles, or destroy the brain's pain center.

Client Needs Category—Physiological integrity
Client Needs Subcategory—Physiological adaptation

112. 3. Sitting in a chair, especially frequently or for long periods, is undesirable because below-the-knee amputees are prone to knee flexion contractures. A knee flexion contracture interferes with wearing a prosthesis and being able to walk again. For this reason, the stump is kept in an extended or neutral position as much as possible. The prone, supine, and standing positions all allow for extension of the stump.

Client Needs Category—Physiological integrity
Client Needs Subcategory—Basic care and comfort

113. 3. Almost immediately after surgery, the client should begin to lift up using the trapeze to build up muscle strength in preparation for using crutches. The muscles that need the most strengthening are those in the arms, neck, shoulders, chest, and back. The client may also squeeze rubber balls and perform arm push-ups. Doing arm push-ups involves placing the palms flat on the bed and raising the buttocks. Some health care professionals provide the client with sawed-off crutches to use in bed to condition the same muscles needed during ambulation. Standing at the side of the bed and transferring from the bed to a chair should not be attempted without assistance because of the risk of falling. The client needs to get used to balancing with one leg; therefore, parallel bars are unnecessary.

Client Needs Category—Health promotion and maintenance
Client Needs Subcategory—None

114. 2. Wrapping the stump decreases stump edema, thereby shrinking and shaping the stump. A permanent prosthesis is not constructed until the stump is cone-shaped and no longer undergoing changes in size. An equal amount of compression is applied with each turn of the roller bandage. Isotonic and isometric exercises are used to tone muscles. Range-of-motion exercises help maintain joint flexibility. Gauze dressings absorb blood and drainage.

Client Needs Category—Physiological integrity
Client Needs Subcategory—Physiological adaptation

115. 3, 4. To ensure optimal rehabilitation, the client needs to wrap the stump to control edema and shrink it to its final shape and size before a permanent prosthesis can be made. Active isometric exercises, such as quadriceps and gluteal setting exercises, help strengthen the muscles required for ambulation. The client should be taught to tighten his thigh muscles and to press his knee into the bed several times a day. Flexion, abduction, and external rotation should be avoided. Therefore, the client must avoid sitting for long periods or putting a pillow under his thigh. He should be encouraged to keep his knee and leg in a neutral position. The stump bandage should be removed and reapplied at least two or three times a day, or whenever it becomes soiled or loose.

Client Needs Category—Physiological integrity
Client Needs Subcategory—Reduction of risk potential

Nursing Care of Clients with Skeletal Tumors

116. 2. A rubber tourniquet is usually kept at the bedside in case the client begins to hemorrhage and elevating the stump and applying direct pressure cannot control bleeding. An emergency supply of gauze dressings should not be necessary. If the airway becomes compromised, the nurse would maintain temporary patency by using the chin-lift/head-tilt maneuver. Most clients are transferred to the nursing unit from the recovery room with oxygen already in place.

Client Needs Category—Physiological integrity
Client Needs Subcategory—Physiological adaptation

117. 3. If crutches are measured and fitted appropriately, there should be enough room to fit at least two fingers between the axilla and the axillary bar of the crutch. Prolonged pressure under the arm can affect circulation or impair nerve function, resulting in permanent paralysis. All of the other options indicate that the crutch length and the handgrip position are correct.

Client Needs Category—Physiological integrity
Client Needs Subcategory—Physiological adaptation

118. 4. Malignant bone tumors cause secondary anemia if bone marrow function is disrupted. Although primary bone tumors can spread to any organ, the bowel and liver are not common metastatic sites. Mental status changes may occur, but they are not related to the location of a bone tumor.

Client Needs Category—Physiological integrity
Client Needs Subcategory—Physiological adaptation

119. 1. The most common site for bone tumor metastasis is the lungs; therefore, the nurse should monitor lung scan results. The other tests are unrelated to determining whether the primary tumor has metastasized.

Client Needs Category—Physiological integrity
Client Needs Subcategory—Reduction of risk potential

Nursing Care of Clients with a Herniated Intervertebral Disk

120. 2. Any activity that increases intraspinal pressure, such as sneezing, causes lower back pain to intensify. Other activities that can worsen back pain include coughing, lifting an object, and straining to have a bowel movement. Eating and urinating do not normally affect the intensity of pain. Resting and inactivity help relieve pain caused by a herniated intervertebral disk.

Client Needs Category—Physiological integrity
Client Needs Subcategory—Basic care and comfort

121. 1. Many clients feel pain radiate into their buttocks and down the leg where the herniating disk protrudes on the spinal nerve root. The sciatic nerve is commonly affected when the herniated disk occurs between lumbar vertebrae. The iliac crests, knees, and toes are not generally symptomatic.

Client Needs Category—Physiological integrity
Client Needs Subcategory—Physiological adaptation

122. 2. Cyclobenzaprine hydrochloride (Flexeril) is a central-acting skeletal muscle relaxant used to treat muscle spasms related to a herniated intervertebral disk. It does not reduce depression and should not be given with alcohol or other central nervous system depressants. NSAIDs are given to decrease inflammation, while sedatives and hypnotics are used to promote rest and sleep.

Client Needs Category*—Physiological integrity*
Client Needs Subcategory*—Pharmacological therapies*

123. **4.** Encouraging extra fluids and maintaining a quiet environment can help prevent headaches following a myelogram. Drinking fluid dilutes and hastens excretion of the contrast medium used during the procedure. Increasing oral fluid intake also helps replace cerebrospinal fluid withdrawn prior to or after the procedure. Keeping the room dim can help relieve a spinal headache once it manifests; however, this is not generally done as a standard of care following a myelogram. Food may be withheld if the client becomes nauseated, but this is not routinely done. Administering sedatives at scheduled intervals following a myelogram can mask early signs of central nervous system complications.

Client Needs Category*—Physiological integrity*
Client Needs Subcategory*—Physiological adaptation*

124. **4.** The client with a laminectomy and spinal fusion should be rolled from side to side without twisting the spine. This type of movement, called logrolling, prevents displacing bone grafts until they have become solidly fused. Holding one's breath increases discomfort when accompanied by bearing down. Because the client cannot twist his spine, moving his lower body and then the upper would be harmful. Likewise, raising his upper body and hips off of the bed would be contraindicated.

Client Needs Category*—Physiological integrity*
Client Needs Subcategory*—Reduction of risk potential*

125. **3.** Because the client has limited English-speaking ability, showing the client pictures and diagrams is the most appropriate teaching method in this situation. Demonstrating may also help to get the point across. Speaking slowly and looking at the client may or may not facilitate his understanding of the verbal instructions. Looking directly at a client in some cultures is considered offensive. Similarly, writing the instructions on paper or watching a video in English does not address the client's inability to understand or speak English.

Client Needs Category*—Health promotion and maintenance*
Client Needs Subcategory*—None*

126. **1.** Bending both knees and keeping the back straight makes best use of the longest and strongest muscles in the body. The feet are spread apart for a

broad base of support. Extending the arms strains the weaker muscles by placing the weight of the lifted object outside the body's center of gravity.

Client Needs Category*—Health promotion and maintenance*
Client Needs Subcategory*—None*

The Nursing Care of Clients with Neurologic System Disorders

⇨ *Nursing Care of Clients with Infectious and Inflammatory Conditions*
⇨ *Nursing Care of Clients with Seizure Disorders*
⇨ *Nursing Care of Clients with Neurologic Trauma*
⇨ *Nursing Care of Clients with Degenerative Disorders*
⇨ *Nursing Care of Clients with Cerebrovascular Disorders*
⇨ *Nursing Care of Clients with Tumors of the Neurologic System*
⇨ *Nursing Care of Clients with Nerve Disorders*
⇨ *Correct Answers and Rationales*

Directions: With a pencil, blacken the space in front of the option you have chosen for your correct answer.

Nursing Care of Clients with Infectious and Inflammatory Conditions

A 23-year-old man is brought to the hospital after efforts to relieve his fever are unsuccessful. The tentative diagnosis is meningitis.

1. If the diagnosis is accurate, which assessment finding is the nurse most likely to document?
[ ] **1.** Double vision
[ ] **2.** A stiff neck
[ ] **3.** Joint aches
[ ] **4.** Extreme thirst

The physician plans to do a lumbar puncture (spinal tap) to confirm the diagnosis of meningitis.

2. To facilitate performing the lumbar puncture, the nurse should place the client in which position?
[ ] **1.** Knee-chest (genupectoral) position
[ ] **2.** Sitting in an orthopneic position
[ ] **3.** Side-lying position with his neck flexed
[ ] **4.** Left lateral position with right knee flexed

3. Which intervention is most appropriate after the lumbar puncture has been performed?
[ ] **1.** Keep the client positioned on his side.
[ ] **2.** Ambulate the client around the room.
[ ] **3.** Withhold food and fluids for 1 hour.
[ ] **4.** Keep the client flat for several hours.

4. While awaiting the diagnostic test results of a client with possible meningitis, which transmission-based precautions are best to implement?

[ ] **1.** Droplet precautions
[ ] **2.** Airborne precautions
[ ] **3.** Contact precautions
[ ] **4.** Standard precautions

The physician orders a cooling blanket to reduce the fever of a client with meningitis.

5. When implementing the medical order, which nursing action is most appropriate?
[ ] **1.** Place the blanket on top of the client.
[ ] **2.** Enclose the blanket in a light cloth cover.
[ ] **3.** Add normal saline solution to the fluid chamber.
[ ] **4.** Replace crushed ice periodically as it melts.

6. To promote comfort and reduce the potential for seizures in a client with meningitis, how is it best for the nurse to keep the room?
[ ] **1.** Dark and quiet
[ ] **2.** Warm and sunny
[ ] **3.** Cool and well-ventilated
[ ] **4.** Warm and well-humidified

The care plan of a client with viral encephalitis indicates that the nurse should perform neurologic checks every 2 hours.

7. If the client had been unresponsive except to painful stimuli, which new assessment finding indicates that the client is improving?
[ ] **1.** Pupils are fixed when stimulated with light.
[ ] **2.** Pupils dilate when stimulated with light.
[ ] **3.** Eyes open when the client's name is called.
[ ] **4.** Cheek stroked with a swab causes swallowing.

The nursing team discusses the case of a new client who has Guillain-Barré syndrome.

8. When the medical history is reviewed, which fact is most likely related to the client's diagnosis?

[ ] **1.** The client had an immunization in the last week.

[ ] **2.** The client was bitten by a spider 2 days ago.

[ ] **3.** The client drinks fresh unpasteurized milk from his cows.

[ ] **4.** The client sprayed his garden with insecticide this week.

9. When the nursing team plans the care of a client with Guillain-Barré syndrome, which assessment can most accurately determine whether the client is developing ineffective breathing?

[ ] **1.** Pulse rate

[ ] **2.** Skin color

[ ] **3.** Red blood cell (RBC) count

[ ] **4.** Pulse oximetry

The client with Guillain-Barré syndrome begins to have difficulty swallowing food.

10. When the nurse is asked to recommend a technique for nourishing the client, which feeding method is most appropriate at this time?

[ ] **1.** Crystalloid I.V. fluid

[ ] **2.** Nasogastric (NG) tube feedings

[ ] **3.** Total parenteral nutrition (TPN)

[ ] **4.** Gastrostomy tube feedings

The nurse assigned to a client with postpolio syndrome reads the client's health history.

11. If the nurse finds the following information documented in the client's medical record, which item best explains how the client first contracted poliomyelitis?

[ ] **1.** The client was immunized with killed injectable polio vaccine as an infant.

[ ] **2.** The client was immunized with live oral polio vaccine (OPV) as an infant.

[ ] **3.** The client received his polio immunization before he was 9 months old.

[ ] **4.** The client received his polio and rubella immunization at the same time.

A hospice nurse makes a visit to the home of a client with acquired immunodeficiency syndrome (AIDS) dementia complex.

12. Which nursing instruction would be best if the client becomes confused?

[ ] **1.** Turn the television on so the client can hear human voices.

[ ] **2.** Play some of the client's favorite music when he is disturbed.

[ ] **3.** Tell the client where he is, who the caregiver is, and what is happening.

[ ] **4.** Look at and talk about pictures in a photo album of the client's life.

Nursing Care of Clients with Seizure Disorders

13. The nurse recognizes which of the following as an autonomic manifestation of a seizure?

[ ] **1.** Numbness and tingling

[ ] **2.** Changes in taste and speech

[ ] **3.** Increased epigastric secretions

[ ] **4.** A subjective aura or sensation

A 23-year-old woman who experienced a generalized seizure while at work is undergoing diagnostic tests.

14. When preparing the client for an EEG, which nursing action is most appropriate?

[ ] **1.** Administer a sedative 1 hour before the test.

[ ] **2.** Withhold food and water after midnight on the day of the test.

[ ] **3.** Assist the client with shampooing her hair.

[ ] **4.** Take the client's blood pressure while she is lying and sitting.

The nurse notes that seizure precautions have been included in the client's care plan.

15. When implementing seizure precautions, which nursing action is most appropriate?

[ ] **1.** Move the client to a room closer to the nursing station.

[ ] **2.** Serve the client's food in paper and plastic containers.

[ ] **3.** Leave the overhead light on at all times.

[ ] **4.** Make sure the side rails on the bed are padded.

16. If the client begins to have a seizure after her EEG, which action should the nurse take first?

[ ] **1.** Administer oxygen by nasal cannula.

[ ] **2.** Take her blood pressure and pulse.

[ ] **3.** Restrain her arms and upper body.

[ ] **4.** Place her in a side-lying position.

17. When documenting a seizure, which information is most important to include?

[ ] **1.** The time the seizure started

[ ] **2.** The duration of the seizure

[ ] **3.** The client's mood just before the seizure

[ ] **4.** The client's comments after the seizure

18. Which nursing actions are essential when finding a client experiencing a tonic-clonic seizure? Select all that apply.
[ ] **1.** Calling out the client's name
[ ] **2.** Holding the client's body during the seizure activity
[ ] **3.** Placing a belt buckle in the mouth to maintain the airway
[ ] **4.** Rolling the client's body to the side
[ ] **5.** Removing environmental hazards to protect the client
[ ] **6.** Activating the emergency response system

19. When a client is injured during a seizure, which fact is most important to document on the accident report to reduce the risk of liability?
[ ] **1.** The client was assigned to a licensed nurse.
[ ] **2.** The signal cord was within the client's reach.
[ ] **3.** The client's vital signs had been stable.
[ ] **4.** The client was last observed reading.

A client begins the postictal phase of a tonic-clonic (grand mal) seizure.

20. Which clinical manifestation will the nurse most likely observe first?
[ ] **1.** Frequent jerking in one extremity that gradually spreads to adjacent areas
[ ] **2.** Distant staring with a sense of aloofness to the surrounding environment
[ ] **3.** Loss of consciousness with body rigidity and violent muscle contractions
[ ] **4.** Drooling with loss of facial muscle control and frequent coughing episodes

21. What is the priority nursing intervention in the postictal phase of a seizure?
[ ] **1.** Assess the client's level of arousal.
[ ] **2.** Assess the client's breathing pattern.
[ ] **3.** Reorient the client to the surroundings.
[ ] **4.** Reposition the client on a hard surface.

The medical record of a client with epilepsy indicates that he has had two previous episodes of status epilepticus.

22. Which emergency drug should the nurse plan to have available in case the client has a similar episode?
[ ] **1.** Diazepam (Valium)
[ ] **2.** Phenytoin (Dilantin)
[ ] **3.** Carbamazepine (Tegretol)
[ ] **4.** Phenobarbital sodium (Luminal)

23. When a client takes phenytoin sodium (Dilantin), which hygiene measure is especially important to perform?

[ ] **1.** Shampooing hair
[ ] **2.** Trimming fingernails
[ ] **3.** Brushing teeth
[ ] **4.** Bathing

Nursing Care of Clients with Neurologic Trauma

A nurse who witnesses a motor vehicle accident stops to provide emergency assistance to the injured motorists.

24. When the nurse assesses a male victim who has been thrown from the vehicle, which assessment finding is most suggestive that he has a serious head injury?
[ ] **1.** The victim says he has a bad headache.
[ ] **2.** The victim asks the nurse, "What happened?"
[ ] **3.** The victim holds his head with his hands.
[ ] **4.** The victim has serous drainage from his ears.

25. Which nursing action is most important to do next?
[ ] **1.** Maintain the victim's present position.
[ ] **2.** Assist the victim to the shade of a tree.
[ ] **3.** Cover the victim with a light blanket.
[ ] **4.** Give the victim some water to drink.

26. To reduce the risk of liability, what is most appropriate for the nurse to do?
[ ] **1.** Avoid giving the accident victim any personal identification.
[ ] **2.** Remain with the accident victim until paramedics arrive.
[ ] **3.** Conceal the fact that she is a nurse.
[ ] **4.** Let others at the scene provide direct care.

The accident victim is taken to the emergency department, where he is evaluated.

27. While waiting for the physician to examine the client, how should the nurse position him?
[ ] **1.** Dorsal recumbent position with his legs elevated
[ ] **2.** Supine position with his head slightly elevated
[ ] **3.** Left lateral position with his knees flexed
[ ] **4.** Right lateral position with his neck flexed

The client is diagnosed with a head injury and is admitted after X-rays are taken of his head, neck, and spine.

28. When assessing the client with a head injury, which of the following should receive priority attention?
[ ] **1.** Lung sounds
[ ] **2.** Skin integrity
[ ] **3.** Urine characteristics
[ ] **4.** Pupillary responses

29. If the nurse obtains the following data, which one should be reported to the physician immediately?
[ ] **1.** The client rates his headache as 3 on a scale of 0 to 10.
[ ] **2.** The client leaves most of the food on his dietary tray.
[ ] **3.** The client is difficult to arouse.
[ ] **4.** The client says he feels exhausted.

30. When assessing the client's head injury, which assessment finding is most likely contributing to changes in his condition?
[ ] **1.** The client has been disturbed every hour.
[ ] **2.** The client has had very little fluid intake.
[ ] **3.** The client's neck is flexed toward his chest.
[ ] **4.** The client's bladder is becoming quite full.

The client is treated with mannitol (Osmitrol).

31. Which of the following is most important for the nurse to assess while the client is receiving mannitol (Osmitrol)?
[ ] **1.** Urine output
[ ] **2.** Respiratory rate
[ ] **3.** Level of pain
[ ] **4.** Skin condition

A 22-year-old man suffers a complete transection of his spinal cord at the level of the 5th thoracic (T5) vertebra at the time of a diving accident.

32. Which statement indicates that the client has an accurate understanding of his prognosis?
[ ] **1.** "After surgery, I can expect full function."
[ ] **2.** "My recovery depends on my rehabilitation efforts."
[ ] **3.** "I will retain functions above my chest."
[ ] **4.** "No one can predict my potential outcome at this time."

33. In this lateral view of the spine, identify the area on the thoracic vertebrae where the injury to the spinal cord has occurred.

After the client's condition stabilizes, he is transferred to a rehabilitation unit.

34. When the nursing team discusses the client's physical management, which plan has the highest priority?
[ ] **1.** Relieving the client's physical discomfort
[ ] **2.** Strengthening the client's upper body muscles
[ ] **3.** Confronting the client's denial of his condition
[ ] **4.** Letting the client verbalize his feelings

The client develops a severe headache and hypertension. Autonomic dysreflexia is suspected.

35. Besides helping the client to sit up, which other nursing action is most appropriate at this time?
[ ] **1.** Talking quietly to the client to relieve his anxiety
[ ] **2.** Inserting an oral airway in case he has a seizure
[ ] **3.** Compressing the client's abdomen with firm pressure
[ ] **4.** Checking to see if his urinary catheter is patent

36. When planning a bowel retraining program for a client with a spinal cord injury, which nursing intervention is most appropriate?
[ ] **1.** Administering a tap-water enema just before bedtime
[ ] **2.** Encouraging a high-fiber diet to increase stool bulk
[ ] **3.** Changing disposable undergarments when soiled
[ ] **4.** Padding the rim of the bedpan to prevent skin breakdown

37. Before discharge, which home care suggestion is best for promoting the mobility of the client with a spinal cord injury?
[ ] **1.** Rent or buy a conventional hospital bed.
[ ] **2.** Build a wheelchair ramp to the door.
[ ] **3.** Apply for a handicapped parking sticker.
[ ] **4.** Purchase a pair of supportive shoes.

Nursing Care of Clients with Degenerative Disorders

An older woman with Parkinson's disease is placed in a nursing home for basic nursing care.

38. Which assessment finding is most important to consider before developing the client's care plan?
[ ] **1.** The client's ability to perform activities of daily living (ADLs)
[ ] **2.** The client's preferences and dislikes of various foods
[ ] **3.** The client's family members and her network of social support
[ ] **4.** The client's feelings about giving up her independent living

39. Which clinical manifestation is the initial sign of Parkinson's disease?
[ ] **1.** Muscle rigidity
[ ] **2.** Muscle tremors
[ ] **3.** Muscle weakness
[ ] **4.** Muscle deterioration

The client with Parkinson's disease takes levodopa (Dopar) b.i.d.

40. When the nurse observes that the client has difficulty swallowing the capsule of medication, which action is best to take?
[ ] **1.** Soak the capsule in water until soft.
[ ] **2.** Tell her to chew the capsule.
[ ] **3.** Empty the capsule in the client's mouth.
[ ] **4.** Offer water before giving her the capsule.

The physician also prescribes a stool softener, a multivitamin, and a drug to counteract the client's osteoporosis.

41. Which nursing action is best when preparing to administer the prescribed medications?
[ ] **1.** Administer them all at the prescribed time.
[ ] **2.** Question the order for the multivitamin.
[ ] **3.** Withhold the stool softener until it is needed.
[ ] **4.** Give the antiosteoporitic drug with milk.

The nurse initiates a teaching plan for the client with Parkinson's disease.

42. Which teaching instruction should be the nurse's priority in this situation?
[ ] **1.** Steps to enhance the client's immune system
[ ] **2.** Importance of maintaining a balanced diet
[ ] **3.** Need to remove all safety hazards
[ ] **4.** Importance of social interactions

43. Which goal is most realistic for a client diagnosed with Parkinson's disease?
[ ] **1.** To reverse the symptoms and cure the disease
[ ] **2.** To stop the progression of the disease process
[ ] **3.** To maintain optimal muscle and motor function
[ ] **4.** To prepare for a progressive terminal disease

44. Because the client with Parkinson's disease is prone to constipation, the nurse should encourage her to eat more of which food?
[ ] **1.** Raw fruits
[ ] **2.** Wheat pasta
[ ] **3.** Cured meats
[ ] **4.** Canned peas

An older female client with dementia is admitted to the Alzheimer's unit of an extended-care facility.

45. The nurse knows that which characteristic is found in Alzheimer's disease that distinguishes it from other dementias?
[ ] **1.** Destruction of brain cells from hypoxia
[ ] **2.** Destruction of brain cells from a stroke
[ ] **3.** Neurofibrillary tangles and plaques in the brain
[ ] **4.** A superficial infection in the meninges of the brain

46. When the client is observed wandering about the facility, which nursing intervention is most appropriate for the client's safety?
[ ] **1.** Keep the client confined to her room.
[ ] **2.** Attach an identity tag with a phone number to her clothes.
[ ] **3.** Lock all the outside doors in the facility.
[ ] **4.** Make sure she is dressed appropriately.

47. What approach is best when managing the care of a client with dementia who insists on carrying a purse with her at all times?
[ ] **1.** Ask the client where her purse can be stored.
[ ] **2.** Ensure that she has her purse with her.
[ ] **3.** Inform the client that her purse may be lost.
[ ] **4.** Find out why the client feels the need for a purse.

48. The client repeatedly asks for her mother. Which response by the nurse would be best to prevent client frustration and agitation?
[ ] **1.** Explain that her mother has been dead several years.
[ ] **2.** Tell her that her mother will visit a little later.
[ ] **3.** State, "You miss your mother. What was she like?"
[ ] **4.** Ask the client when she last saw her mother.

A 48-year-old female client experiences an exacerbation of multiple sclerosis from which she has been asymptomatic for the past 6 months.

49. How can the nurse best help the client deal with her fears at this time?
[ ] **1.** Encourage her to verbalize her feelings.
[ ] **2.** Provide an accurate explanation of the disease.
[ ] **3.** Tell her about her physical assessment findings.
[ ] **4.** Explain that the disease may become periodically acute.

50. When assisting the client with her activities of daily living (ADLs), which approach is best?
[ ] **1.** Complete all ADLs as quickly as possible.
[ ] **2.** Eliminate whatever the client cannot perform.
[ ] **3.** Let the client rest between the activities.
[ ] **4.** Perform all the client's ADLs for her.

51. What should the nurse warn a client with multiple sclerosis to avoid?
[ ] **1.** Hot weather
[ ] **2.** Wet climates
[ ] **3.** Dry environments
[ ] **4.** Cold temperatures

The physician prescribes interferon beta-1a (Avonex) by the subcutaneous route for a client with multiple sclerosis.

52. When the nurse alternates injection sites on the client's upper arms, how far apart should the injections be spaced?
[ ] **1.** ¼″ (0.6 cm)
[ ] **2.** ½″ (1.3 cm)
[ ] **3.** 1″ (2.5 cm)
[ ] **4.** 2″ (5 cm)

53. The nurse who instructs the client about subcutaneous injections before discharge correctly explains that the client should rotate injections between which two areas?
[ ] **1.** Thighs and hips
[ ] **2.** Forearms and hips
[ ] **3.** Thighs and abdomen
[ ] **4.** Abdomen and buttocks

54. Which nursing action would be most appropriate if the client develops anorexia and nausea while taking interferon beta-1a (Avonex)?
[ ] **1.** Withhold the medication.
[ ] **2.** Offer frequent mouth care.
[ ] **3.** Administer the drug after meals.
[ ] **4.** Provide small, frequent meals.

During a physical assessment, the nurse notes that in addition to the client's weakness, she has numbness in parts of her body.

55. Which measure for preventing impaired skin integrity is appropriate to add to the care plan at this time?
[ ] **1.** Use an air-fluidized (Clinitron) bed.
[ ] **2.** Change the client's positions every 2 hours.
[ ] **3.** Rub any reddened areas every 2 hours.
[ ] **4.** Add alcohol to the client's bath water.

The nurse is caring for an older man who develops myasthenia gravis.

56. Which sign or symptom in the client's medical history would most likely indicate when the client's disease became evident?

[ ] **1.** Sudden hearing loss
[ ] **2.** Sensitivity to light
[ ] **3.** Drooping eyelids
[ ] **4.** Protruding tongue

57. Which assessment finding is especially important to monitor when caring for a client with myasthenia gravis?
[ ] **1.** Breathing
[ ] **2.** Range of motion
[ ] **3.** Appetite
[ ] **4.** Hygiene

58. When planning care for this client, which equipment is most important to keep at the bedside?
[ ] **1.** A pole for administering I.V. fluid
[ ] **2.** A cardiac defibrillator in case of cardiac arrest
[ ] **3.** A suction machine in case of compromised swallowing
[ ] **4.** An electronic pump for administering tube feedings

The physician orders pyridostigmine bromide (Mestinon) for the client. The dosage will be adjusted according to the client's response.

59. Which assessment finding suggests that the dose of pyridostigmine bromide (Mestinon) may be excessive for this client?
[ ] **1.** The client cannot open his mouth.
[ ] **2.** The client cannot make a fist.
[ ] **3.** The client has urinary incontinence.
[ ] **4.** The client talks incoherently.

60. Which nursing action is best for controlling the symptoms of the client diagnosed with myasthenia gravis?
[ ] **1.** Ensure that the client has regular bowel and bladder elimination.
[ ] **2.** Administer each dose of medication at the precise scheduled time.
[ ] **3.** Encourage the client to exercise twice daily for 30 minutes.
[ ] **4.** Provide nutritional supplements between each meal and at bedtime.

The client's care plan indicates that he is to use Credé's method to promote urination.

61. Which action by the client demonstrates that he is performing Credé's method correctly?
[ ] **1.** Running tap water in the sink by the toilet
[ ] **2.** Holding his hand in a bowl of cool water
[ ] **3.** Pouring warm water over his lower abdomen
[ ] **4.** Applying hand pressure over his bladder

A 60-year-old client in the late stage of amyotrophic lateral sclerosis (Lou Gehrig disease) is admitted to the hospital.

62. Based on the course of this disease, which nursing diagnosis is most likely included in the client's care plan?
[ ] **1.** *Sexual dysfunction*
[ ] **2.** *Disturbed body image*
[ ] **3.** *Impaired adjustment*
[ ] **4.** *Self-care deficit*

63. When teaching the children of a client diagnosed with Huntington's chorea, which statement by the nurse is most appropriate?
[ ] **1.** "Genetic testing is advisable before having children."
[ ] **2.** "It's wise to store sperm in a bank for the future."
[ ] **3.** "Have children before you reach the age of 30."
[ ] **4.** "You might consider adopting all your children."

Nursing Care of Clients with Cerebrovascular Disorders

The nurse makes a home health visit to evaluate a 79-year-old client.

64. Which symptom suggests that the client may be having transient ischemic attacks (TIAs)?
[ ] **1.** Brief periods of unilateral weakness
[ ] **2.** Brief periods of mental depression
[ ] **3.** Brief periods of photosensitivity
[ ] **4.** Brief periods of stabbing head pain

65. After the nurse gathers more data concerning the TIAs, which action is most appropriate?
[ ] **1.** Explain the phenomenon in understandable language.
[ ] **2.** Refer the client for immediate medical evaluation.
[ ] **3.** Recommend taking a baby aspirin once daily.
[ ] **4.** Teach the client to avoid dietary sources of fat.

An older man is admitted after emergency medical personnel were called to his home and found him unconscious.

66. When checking this client's pupils, which technique is correct?
[ ] **1.** Ask the client to look directly at the light source.
[ ] **2.** Cover one of the client's eyes, then the other eye.
[ ] **3.** Dim the lights in the examination area.
[ ] **4.** Observe for extraocular eye movement.

The physician orders a computed tomography (CT) scan of the client's brain with contrast dye.

67. When asked about allergies, the client's wife reports that he is allergic to certain foods. Which one must be reported to the physician before the CT scan?
[ ] **1.** Tomatoes
[ ] **2.** Shellfish
[ ] **3.** Chocolate
[ ] **4.** Strawberries

It is determined that the client has had a stroke. The nursing team begins developing a care plan.

68. Which nursing goal is most important to the client's rehabilitation?
[ ] **1.** To regulate bowel and bladder elimination
[ ] **2.** To prevent contractures and joint deformities
[ ] **3.** To deal with problems of altered body image
[ ] **4.** To facilitate positive outcomes from grieving

69. When the nurse monitors the client's neurologic status, which finding is most suggestive that the client's intracranial pressure is increasing?
[ ] **1.** Systolic pressure increases and diastolic pressure decreases.
[ ] **2.** Systolic pressure decreases and diastolic pressure increases.
[ ] **3.** Apical heart rate is greater than the radial rate.
[ ] **4.** Radial pulse rate is greater than the apical rate.

The charge nurse enters the nursing diagnosis Ineffective airway clearance related to decreased level of consciousness and inability to swallow *on the client's care plan.*

70. Which nursing intervention is most appropriate for managing the identified problem?
[ ] **1.** Keeping the client supine
[ ] **2.** Removing all head pillows
[ ] **3.** Performing oral suctioning
[ ] **4.** Providing oral hygiene

The nurse teaches the client's wife how to perform passive range-of-motion (ROM) exercises.

71. When teaching the client's wife, which instruction is most accurate?
[ ] **1.** Move the paralyzed limbs in as many directions as possible.
[ ] **2.** Move all extremities in as many directions as possible.
[ ] **3.** Move the upper extremities in as many directions as possible.
[ ] **4.** Move the lower extremities in as many directions as possible.

The nurse attaches a footboard to the client's bed.

72. Which statement best describes how the nurse positions the client's feet when a footboard is used?
[ ] **1.** The soles are perpendicular to the board.
[ ] **2.** The soles are parallel to the board.
[ ] **3.** The ankles are flexed less than 90 degrees.
[ ] **4.** The ankles are extended more than 90 degrees.

The nurse determines that the client has expressive aphasia.

73. Which nursing intervention is best for communicating with the client at this time?
[ ] **1.** Stimulating the client's hearing by turning on the television
[ ] **2.** Having the client point to key phrases printed on a clipboard
[ ] **3.** Avoiding talking to the client because conversation is impossible
[ ] **4.** Encouraging the client to speak rather than using gestures

74. The client's wife will be caring for him at home upon discharge. The physician has written a new prescription for warfarin (Coumadin). Which teaching topics should the nurse cover before discharge? Select all that apply.
[ ] **1.** Dietary restrictions
[ ] **2.** Driving restrictions
[ ] **3.** Ways to prevent edema of the lower extremities
[ ] **4.** Missed doses
[ ] **5.** Bruising or blood in urine
[ ] **6.** Difficulty sleeping

The nurse is caring for a client who was recently diagnosed with hemiplegia. Assessment reveals that he has hemianopsia.

75. Which intervention should be added to client's care plan in relation to this latest finding?
[ ] **1.** Have the client wear dark glasses when in bright light.
[ ] **2.** Cover the client's affected eye with a dark patch.
[ ] **3.** Approach the client from his unaffected side.
[ ] **4.** Instruct the client to look from near to far to see clearly.

76. When the client is stable enough to transfer from his bed to a wheelchair, which nursing action is correct?
[ ] **1.** Instruct the client about how to balance with a walker.
[ ] **2.** Position the wheelchair perpendicular to the bed.
[ ] **3.** Stand behind the locked wheelchair.
[ ] **4.** Brace the paralyzed foot and knee.

A client with a leaking cerebral aneurysm is being treated conservatively with complete bed rest, anticonvulsants, and sedatives.

77. Of the following nursing observations, which is most important to address in light of the client's condition?
[ ] **1.** The client has a chronic cough.
[ ] **2.** The client is becoming bored.
[ ] **3.** The client has a diminished appetite.
[ ] **4.** The client wants to talk with his wife.

78. The nurse is preparing to examine a client with a cerebral aneurysm. Place all of the following assessment areas in order of priority, listing the top priority first. Use all the options.

1. Bowel movements	
2. Motor strength	
3. Vital signs	
4. Skin integrity	
5. Urine output	
6. Level of conciousness (LOC)	

The client with a cerebral aneurysm tells the nurse that the nonopioid analgesic he received 2 hours ago has not adequately relieved his headache.

79. If the drug is administered every 3 to 4 hours, which nursing action is most appropriate in response to the client's statement?
[ ] **1.** Administer another dose of the nonopioid analgesic immediately.
[ ] **2.** Explain that frequent analgesia administration will mask symptoms.
[ ] **3.** Consult the physician about ordering an opioid analgesic.
[ ] **4.** Use a nondrug intervention such as listening to a guided imagery tape.

Nursing Care of Clients with Tumors of the Neurologic System

A client with a suspected brain tumor is scheduled for positron emission tomography (PET).

80. When preparing the client for his upcoming PET scan, the nurse should instruct him to avoid which substance the day before the test?
[ ] **1.** Caffeine
[ ] **2.** Food dyes
[ ] **3.** Diuretics
[ ] **4.** Antibiotics

81. Which discharge instruction is most appropriate following the PET scan?
[ ]   **1.** Take a mild laxative tonight.
[ ]   **2.** Increase your fluid intake.
[ ]   **3.** Get at least 8 hours of sleep.
[ ]   **4.** Report any abdominal discomfort.

PET confirms a brain tumor, and the client is scheduled for a craniotomy.

82. Which preoperative assessment is most important to document as a basis for postoperative comparison?
[ ]   **1.** Motor strength in all extremities
[ ]   **2.** Anterior and posterior skin integrity
[ ]   **3.** Knowledge of potential surgical risks
[ ]   **4.** Appetite and food preferences

83. When placing a retention catheter in a male client undergoing a craniotomy, to what depth will the nurse insert the catheter?
[ ]   **1.** 2″ to 4″ (5 to 10 cm)
[ ]   **2.** 4″ to 6″ (10 to 15 cm)
[ ]   **3.** 6″ to 8″ (15 to 20 cm)
[ ]   **4.** 8″ to 10″ (20 to 25.5 cm)

The nurse begins skin preparation for the client before his craniotomy.

84. Part of the skin preparation involves shaving the hair from the client's head. When is the best time to shave the client?
[ ]   **1.** The night before surgery
[ ]   **2.** In the morning, after his shower
[ ]   **3.** Before he receives preoperative sedation
[ ]   **4.** Before surgery, in the operating room area

85. How should the nurse dispose of the client's shaved hair?
[ ]   **1.** Dispose of it in a biologic waste container.
[ ]   **2.** Place it in a plastic-lined wastebasket.
[ ]   **3.** Put it in a paper bag and give it to the family.
[ ]   **4.** Flush the hair away in a large waste hopper.

The client is returned to the nursing unit after 6 hours of surgery.

86. During the immediate postoperative assessment, the nurse notes that the client's dressing is moist. Which action is most appropriate to take first?
[ ]   **1.** Change the dressing.
[ ]   **2.** Reinforce the dressing.
[ ]   **3.** Remove the dressing.
[ ]   **4.** Document the findings.

After the craniotomy, the client has periods of confusion.

87. Which nursing intervention is best during these confusion episodes?
[ ]   **1.** Reading a newspaper or magazine to the client
[ ]   **2.** Informing the client that confusion is temporary
[ ]   **3.** Withholding verbal communication temporarily
[ ]   **4.** Reorienting the client to place and situation

The physician orders a clear liquid diet for the client and restricts his oral intake to no more than 1,000 mL.

88. Before requesting the clear liquids prescribed by the physician, which assessment information is essential to know?
[ ]   **1.** Condition of oral mucous membranes
[ ]   **2.** Ability to self-feed
[ ]   **3.** Status of dental hygiene
[ ]   **4.** Ability to swallow effectively

89. When the client asks why he cannot drink fluids freely, which explanation is best?
[ ]   **1.** Oral fluid may contribute to vomiting.
[ ]   **2.** The kidneys need to conserve fluid output.
[ ]   **3.** Fluid restriction reduces the volume in the cranium.
[ ]   **4.** The prescribed volume is sufficient for relieving thirst.

Nursing Care of Clients with Nerve Disorders

A client is diagnosed with trigeminal neuralgia (tic douloureux).

90. Based on factors that cause the client to experience paroxysmal pain, which intervention is most appropriate to include in this client's care plan?
[ ]   **1.** Direct a fan toward the client's face.
[ ]   **2.** Avoid care that involves touching the client's face.
[ ]   **3.** Keep ice chips available at the client's bedside.
[ ]   **4.** Apply warm facial compresses for pain.

The physician treats the client with carbamazepine (Tegretol).

91. Because this drug can cause liver dysfunction, the client's discharge plan should include instructions to report which symptom?
[ ]   **1.** Unusual bleeding
[ ]   **2.** Black stools
[ ]   **3.** Pale urine
[ ]   **4.** Mottled skin

Drug therapy is unsuccessful for a client with trigeminal neuralgia. The physician severs one of the branches of the trigeminal nerve and orders eye irrigations postoperatively.

92. If the eye irrigation is performed correctly, the nurse instills the eye irrigant in which direction?
[ ] **1.** Lower conjunctiva toward the corneal surface
[ ] **2.** Outer canthus of the eye to the inner canthus
[ ] **3.** Nasal corner of the eye toward the temple
[ ] **4.** Margin of the eyelashes to the folds of the lids

A female client develops Bell's palsy due to inflammation around the seventh cranial nerve.

93. When the nurse performs a physical assessment, which finding is most indicative of the client's disorder?
[ ] **1.** Quivering eye movement
[ ] **2.** Muscle spasms about the lips
[ ] **3.** Sudden loss of olfactory function
[ ] **4.** Unilateral facial paralysis

94. Which intervention is most appropriate for a client with Bell's palsy?
[ ] **1.** Reduce the amount of light within the room.
[ ] **2.** Advise the client to drink liquids from a cup.
[ ] **3.** Inspect the buccal pouch for food after eating.
[ ] **4.** Discourage the client from looking in a mirror.

A home health nurse evaluates a client's response to treatment for postherpetic neuralgia following an outbreak of shingles (herpes zoster).

95. When the client asks the nurse about the source of her condition, the most accurate explanation is that the symptoms result from a reactivation of which infectious agent?
[ ] **1.** Rubella
[ ] **2.** Rubeola
[ ] **3.** Chickenpox
[ ] **4.** Influenza

A client who experiences recurrent pain along the sciatic nerve is scheduled for a myelogram.

96. When the nurse describes the myelogram procedure to the client, which statement is most accurate?
[ ] **1.** "Part of the test involves a lumbar puncture."
[ ] **2.** "You will be asked to change positions frequently."
[ ] **3.** "Dye is instilled into a vein in your arm."
[ ] **4.** "Light anesthesia is administered during the test."

The myelogram shows that the client has a herniated intervertebral lumbar disk.

97. The nurse begins developing a teaching plan for the client. Which instruction is most applicable after symptoms are relieved?
[ ] **1.** Carry heavy objects away from your center of gravity.
[ ] **2.** Lift with your knees bent and your back straight.
[ ] **3.** Create a base of support by keeping your feet together.
[ ] **4.** Select a soft, spongy mattress for your bed.

The client eventually undergoes spinal surgery for his herniated disk.

98. When changing the client's position postoperatively, which nursing action is best?
[ ] **1.** Raise the client with a mechanical lift.
[ ] **2.** Logroll the client from side to side.
[ ] **3.** Have the client flex his legs and lift.
[ ] **4.** Pull the client's arms and then his legs.

99. The nurse is completing a history on a client who has been having right sciatic pain. Identify the area where sciatic pain originates.

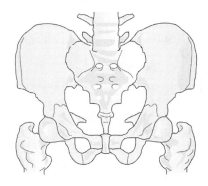

A client who underwent spinal surgery is fitted with a thoracolumbar sacro-orthotic (TCSO) brace.

100. Which statement offers the best evidence that the client understands how to prevent skin breakdown while wearing a TCSO brace?
[ ] **1.** "I need to dust my skin with talc every morning."
[ ] **2.** "I should apply a lubricant to the brace hinges."
[ ] **3.** "I need to wear a cotton shirt under my brace."
[ ] **4.** "I should rub my skin with alcohol every night."

Correct Answers and Rationales

Nursing Care of Clients with Infectious and Inflammatory Conditions

1. 2. Meningitis is an inflammation of the meninges. Neck stiffness, also called nuchal rigidity, is a common symptom among those who contract meningitis. Another symptom is photosensitivity, not double vision. Meningeal irritation may be accompanied by a severe headache but not joint aches. Thirst may be a consequence of a high temperature and dehydration, but it is not a common complaint.

> *Client Needs Category—Physiological integrity*
> *Client Needs Subcategory—Physiological adaptation*

2. 3. A lumbar puncture is completed by placing an aspiration needle into the subarachnoid space of the spinal cord, usually in the lumbar area at the level of the fourth intervertebral space. The client is typically positioned on his side, with the neck and knees acutely flexed to increase the space between the vertebrae. It is anatomically difficult for the physician to perform this test with the client in a knee-chest, orthopneic, or left lateral position.

> *Client Needs Category—Physiological integrity*
> *Client Needs Subcategory—Reduction of risk potential*

3. 4. To prevent complications and allow time for more cerebrospinal fluid to form, clients are kept flat in bed for several hours following lumbar puncture. Increasing fluids helps reform cerebrospinal fluid at a faster rate. To apply pressure on the puncture site, a supine position is preferred. Ambulating the client is unsafe; it can lead to a severe headache or neurologic complications.

> *Client Needs Category—Physiological integrity*
> *Client Needs Subcategory—Physiological adaptation*

4. 1. There are only three categories of transmission-based precautions: airborne, droplet, and contact precautions. Because most forms of meningitis are spread from the droplets of infected persons, droplet precautions are most appropriate. Airborne and contact precautions are not used for clients with meningitis. Standard precautions are followed when caring for all clients, regardless of their infectious status.

> *Client Needs Category—Safe, effective care environment*
> *Client Needs Subcategory—Safety and infection control*

5. 2. To protect the client's skin, there should be a layer of light cloth between the client and the cooling blanket. The pad is placed beneath the client. Distilled water is used to fill the fluid chamber. Ice is not used; the distilled water is chilled electronically.

> *Client Needs Category—Safe, effective care environment*
> *Client Needs Subcategory—Safety and infection control*

6. 1. Keeping the room dark and quiet helps relieve photophobia and the potential for seizures. The room should also be cool and well-ventilated because this helps restore and maintain normal body temperature. A warm environment is least appropriate for clients with meningitis.

> *Client Needs Category—Physiological integrity*
> *Client Needs Subcategory—Reduction of risk potential*

7. 3. Encephalitis is caused by bacteria, fungi, or viruses and causes changes in the white and gray matter of the spinal cord and brain. Severe inflammation of the brain occurs. The best sign of improvement is when a previously unresponsive client now responds when hearing his name called. When checking the pupils, a normal finding is that they constrict when stimulated with light. A swallowing reflex is just that—a reflex. It is not a measure of cognitive improvement.

> *Client Needs Category—Physiological integrity*
> *Client Needs Subcategory—Physiological adaptation*

8. 1. Guillain-Barré syndrome is characterized by an acute autoimmune inflammatory destruction of the myelin sheath covering the peripheral nerves, which causes rapid, progressive symmetrical loss of motor function; however, the sensory nerves remain intact. The exact cause of Guillain-Barré syndrome is unknown, but there seems to be a relationship to prior exposure to infectious agents via an actual infection or their attenuated form in an immunization. This condition is not associated with spider bites, unpasteurized milk, or insecticides.

> *Client Needs Category—Physiological integrity*
> *Client Needs Subcategory—Physiological adaptation*

9. 4. When planning client care, it is important to know that weakness often begins in the extremities and progresses to the upper areas, including the lungs. The pulse oximetry reading, which can be monitored continuously, is the most accurate technique for assessing whether a client is breathing effectively. The pulse rate increases with hypoxemia, but tachycardia can be due to other causes such as anxiety. Cyanosis is not an early sign of hypoxemia. RBC count may increase in response to hypoxemia, but this occurs more in chronic conditions than in acute situations.

Client Needs Category—Physiological integrity
Client Needs Subcategory—Basic care and comfort

10. 2. Tube feedings utilize the normal route for digestion, absorption, and elimination of nutrients. NG tube feedings are less invasive than gastrostomy tube feedings. Crystalloid I.V. fluid does not supply all the nutrients that a person needs to maintain a healthy state. TPN requires a more invasive technique for administration than NG tube feedings.
Client Needs Category—Physiological integrity
Client Needs Subcategory—Physiological adaptation

11. 2. Although OPV is the preferred method for immunizing infants against poliomyelitis, there have been rare cases in which children immunized in this way have actually developed vaccine-related paralysis. The theory is that the live virus in the oral vaccine is capable of causing the disease. Killed virus is unable to cause the disease. If immunization schedules are followed, OPV is given at 2, 4, and 6 months of age. A booster is given before entry to school. Although OPV is usually given at the same time as diphtheria, pertussis, and tetanus immunizations, there is nothing in the literature to suggest that the disease can develop if OPV is given with rubella vaccine.
Client Needs Category—Health promotion and maintenance
Client Needs Subcategory—None

12. 3. Human immunodeficiency virus encephalopathy, also known as *AIDS dementia complex,* occurs in at least two-thirds of clients with AIDS. It is characterized by a progressive decline in cognitive, behavioral, and motor function. The best technique to clear up the client's confusion is to reorient him to person, place, and circumstances. Reorientation may have to be repeated frequently. Encouraging the family to turn on the television, play the client's favorite music, or look at a photo album with the client are techniques for providing sensory stimulation and do not help with confusion.
Client Needs Category—Physiological integrity
Client Needs Subcategory—Basic care and comfort

Nursing Care of Clients with Seizure Disorders

13. 3. Autonomic manifestations of a seizure include an increase in epigastric secretions, pallor, sweating, flushing, piloerection, pupillary dilation, and tachycardia. Numbness and tingling and changes in taste and speech are somatosensory changes. Psychic changes include an aura that may be associated with a smell, noise, or sensation.
Client Needs Category—Physiological integrity
Client Needs Subcategory—Physiological adaptation

14. 3. An EEG is a record of the brain's electrical activity. To ensure that the electrodes of the EEG remain attached to the skull, hair should be clean and dry. Fasting is not required, although beverages containing caffeine are restricted 8 hours before an EEG. The blood pressure is assessed before the test; however, it is unnecessary to have the client lie down and then sit during the assessment. Drugs that affect brain activity, such as sedatives, are withheld for 24 to 48 hours because they can affect the test outcome. To increase the chances of recording seizure activity, it is sometimes recommended that the client be deprived of sleep.
Client Needs Category—Physiological integrity
Client Needs Subcategory—Physiological adaptation

15. 4. To protect a client with a known or suspected seizure disorder, the bedside rails are usually padded with bath blankets to prevent injury. Keeping the room brightly lit is unnecessary, and can be disturbing to the client; in fact, bright lights and noise can precipitate a seizure in some people. Although glass or metal utensils on a tray may injure a client, they are not usually restricted. The nurse may be able to observe the client more closely if nearer to the nursing station, but such room arrangements are not always available.
Client Needs Category—Safe, effective care environment
Client Needs Subcategory—Safety and infection control

16. 4. When a client begins to convulse, the highest priority is establishing a patent airway. Turning the client on her side, which allows saliva and vomitus (if present) to drain from the mouth, is the easiest method. Turning also prevents the tongue from blocking the airway. Oxygen is administered after the airway is open and clear. Vital signs are taken after the seizure is completed. A client is never restrained while having a seizure because restraint could cause musculoskeletal injuries.
Client Needs Category—Physiological integrity
Client Needs Subcategory—Reduction of risk potential

17. 2. Although the time that the seizure started is important information to document, it is not as valuable to the diagnostic process as identifying the seizure's duration. The client's mood before the seizure and comments afterward may be diagnostic, but they are not higher priorities than documenting the duration of the seizure.
Client Needs Category—Physiological integrity
Client Needs Subcategory—Physiological adaptation

18. 4, 5, 6. When responding to the client who is experiencing a tonic-clonic seizure, safety and maintaining the airway are the priority concerns. Rolling the client's whole body to the side facilitates any drainage that may occur from the mouth and keeps the airway open. Objects or situations that could harm the client should be removed from the environment. The emergency response system should be activated for additional support, such as oxygen therapy and transport to the hospital.

Inserting objects into the client's mouth may damage the oral mucosa and teeth. Also, the jaw is typically clenched during a seizure. Calling out the client's name is not essential because she may lose consciousness for up to several minutes during a seizure. Holding the client during the seizure activity can harm the client and does nothing to stop it.

Client Needs Category—Physiological integrity
Client Needs Subcategory—Physiological adaptation

19. 2. In the event of a lawsuit, it is important to prove that safety standards were being followed. The best evidence is noting that the signal cord was within the client's reach. This information may relieve the nurse from liability. It is important to document the vital signs at the time that the client was found. The time that the client was last observed is more pertinent legally than what the client was doing when observed. Having a client assigned to a licensed nurse does not relieve the nurse from liability. Safety precautions must be followed.

Client Needs Category—Safe, effective care environment
Client Needs Subcategory—Safety and infection control

20. 3. A tonic-clonic (grand mal) seizure involves both a tonic phase and a clonic phase. Within the tonic phase, loss of consciousness, dilated pupils, and muscular stiffening are common clinical manifestations. This period lasts approximately 20 to 30 seconds. The clonic phase of the grand mal seizure results in repetitive movements of muscle contraction. The grand mal seizure ends with confusion, drowsiness, and resumption of regular respirations. Jerking in one extremity is a clinical manifestation of a partial seizure. A petit mal seizure, which frequently goes unnoticed, involves staring with brief loss of consciousness. Seizures do not include paralysis of the facial muscles or drooling.

Client Needs Category—Physiological integrity
Client Needs Subcategory—Physiological adaptation

21. 2. A priority nursing measure during the postictal phase of a seizure is to assess the client's breathing pattern for an effective rate, rhythm, and depth. Oxygen may be necessary. Assessing the levels of consciousness and arousability as well as reorientation to person, place, and time is important to complete after a patent airway and regular respiratory pattern have been established. The client does not need to be placed on a hard surface unless cardiopulmonary respiration is needed.

Client Needs Category—Physiological integrity
Client Needs Subcategory—Physiological

adaptation

22. 1. All the drugs listed are used as anticonvulsants to treat a variety of seizure disorders. However, the drug of choice for treating status epilepticus is diazepam (Valium) by the I.V. route.

Client Needs Category—Physiological integrity
Client Needs Subcategory—Pharmacological therapies

23. 3. Phenytoin sodium (Dilantin) causes gingival hyperplasia. Thorough oral hygiene, gum massage, daily flossing, and regular dental care are essential. Therefore, brushing the teeth becomes especially important for preventing oral infections. Shampooing the hair, trimming the fingernails, and bathing the skin are important components of good hygiene for all clients.

Client Needs Category—Health promotion and maintenance
Client Needs Subcategory—None

Nursing Care of Clients with Neurologic Trauma

24. 4. All assessment findings identified are possible with a head injury, but the most serious is observing serous drainage from the ears. Serous drainage from the ears or nose suggests the meninges have been lacerated and the drainage is cerebrospinal fluid.

Client Needs Category—Physiological integrity
Client Needs Subcategory—Physiological adaptation

25. 1. As long as the accident victim is breathing and alert, it is best to keep his head and neck from moving. Movement may further damage the neck and spinal cord. Therefore, ambulating or moving the victim before he is immobilized in a neck brace is potentially unsafe. Covering the victim with a light blanket is appropriate if the environmental temperature is cold or the client is manifesting signs of shock. Water is generally withheld until the need for surgery is ruled out.

Client Needs Category—Physiological integrity
Client Needs Subcategory—Physiological adaptation

26. 2. According to most Good Samaritan laws, after stopping to provide aid, nurses have an obligation to remain with the victim until someone else with comparable knowledge and skills arrives. The other options describe actions that are legal but unethical.

Client Needs Category—Safe, effective care environment
Client Needs Subcategory—Safety and infection control

27. 2. Keeping the head elevated 30 to 45 degrees aids in promoting venous return, which helps to reduce in-

tracranial pressure. None of the other positions allows for elevation of the victim's head and, therefore, will not help to reduce or stabilize the intracranial pressure.
   Client Needs Category—*Physiological integrity*
   Client Needs Subcategory—*Physiological adaptation*

28. 4. Changes in pupil response indicate increasing intracranial pressure and provide vital information regarding the client's neurologic status. Preventing and stabilizing intracranial pressure is a priority because elevated intracranial pressure could lead to brain damage. The other assessments are appropriate when caring for any client, but they do not provide information about the client's neurologic status.
   Client Needs Category—*Physiological integrity*
   Client Needs Subcategory—*Physiological adaptation*

29. 3. A change in the client's level of consciousness is the most sensitive indication that intracranial pressure is increasing and possible secondary brain damage is imminent. The information in the other options is important to document, but it is not significant enough to notify the physician.
   Client Needs Category—*Physiological integrity*
   Client Needs Subcategory—*Physiological adaptation*

30. 3. Flexing the neck interferes with venous outflow from the brain. Venous congestion raises intracranial pressure. Fluids are generally restricted for a client with a head injury to reduce the potential for raising intracranial pressure. Being frequently disturbed interferes with the client's sleep pattern, but that is not as significant a consequence as identifying the relationship between neck flexion and increased intracranial pressure. A full bladder causes autonomic dysreflexia in a client with a spinal cord injury.
   Client Needs Category—*Physiological integrity*
   Client Needs Subcategory—*Physiological adaptation*

31. 1. Mannitol (Osmitrol) is a potent osmotic diuretic to reduce cerebrospinal pressure. Monitoring urine output is one of the data that indicate the client's response to drug therapy. Adverse effects associated with mannitol therapy include dehydration, electrolyte loss, vomiting, and diarrhea. The other options are not related to mannitol (Osmitrol).
   Client Needs Category—*Physiological integrity*
   Client Needs Subcategory—*Pharmacological therapies*

32. 3. The client is correct in stating that he will retain function above the chest; however, with a complete transection of the spinal cord at the T5 level, he will have permanent paraplegia. At the present time, there has been some success in restoring neuromuscular functions in laboratory animals. Human experimentation has not been attempted.

Client Needs Category—*Physiological integrity*
Client Needs Subcategory—*Physiological adaptation*

33.

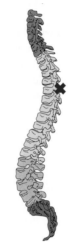

Understanding the area of injury and the neurologic deficits that accompany it are important aspects of nursing care. At the top of the vertebral column are the cervical vertebrae (C1-C8), followed by the thoracic vertebrae (T1-T12), then the lumbar vertebrae (L1-L5), and the sacral vertebrae (S1-S5). The correct placement of the X is at the level of T5 where the injury occurred.
   Client Needs Category—*Physiological integrity*
   Client Needs Subcategory—*Physiological adaptation*

34. 2. All the goals are appropriate, but the highest priority for maintaining the client's physical abilities is to strengthen and retain as much upper body function as possible. Upper body strength is key to ensuring the client's mobility and self-care. Managing pain, addressing the client's denial of his condition, and allowing the client to verbalize his feelings are important, but not the priority.
   Client Needs Category—*Health promotion and maintenance*
   Client Needs Subcategory—*None*

35. 4. Autonomic dysreflexia is an acute emergency that occurs as a result of exaggerated autonomic responses to stimuli. It occurs after spinal shock has been resolved and is often triggered by a full bladder or fecal impaction. Therefore, of the four options, checking the client's catheter for patency is the most appropriate action to take. Autonomic dysreflexia can have life-threatening consequences if unrelieved. An alert client is not likely to tolerate an oral airway. Relieving the client's anxiety is appropriate, but it is not the most appropriate action to take first. Compressing the client's abdomen will not relieve the symptoms of autonomic dysreflexia.
   Client Needs Category—*Physiological integrity*
   Client Needs Subcategory—*Physiological adaptation*

36. **2.** Adding bulk to the stool promotes regular stool elimination. Fiber makes a moister stool, which reduces or prevents fecal impaction. The presence of fecal impaction may also cause autonomic dysreflexia. Some paraplegics perform manual disimpaction on a regular basis to promote bowel elimination. Daily enemas are excessive; however, if an enema is necessary, it is more effective if administered after a meal, when the gastrocolic reflex is more active. Changing disposable undergarments and padding the bedpan promote skin integrity, but these measures will not help manage bowel elimination.

Client Needs Category—Physiological integrity
Client Needs Subcategory—Physiological adaptation

37. **2.** A wheelchair ramp will promote mobility by enabling the client to get in and out of the house easily. A hospital bed will assist with positioning the client. A handicapped parking sticker ensures that the client will not have to travel long distances to get in and out of public facilities, but it does not ultimately promote mobility. Supportive shoes help to prevent contractures, but the client will most likely never use his legs for ambulating again.

Client Needs Category—Health promotion and maintenance
Client Needs Subcategory—None

Nursing Care of Clients with Degenerative Disorders

38. **1.** Assessing the client's ability to carry out various ADLs facilitates planning interventions for which the client will require assistance. It also allows for properly planning with the various disciplines that will be involved in the client's care. All the other data are important to the care of the client, but physiological needs are a higher priority.

Client Needs Category—Safe, effective care environment
Client Needs Subcategory—Coordinated care

39. **2.** The first sign of Parkinson's disease is usually fine motor tremors. The client is often the first person to notice this sign. Muscle rigidity is the second sign. Due to the tremors and muscle rigidity, muscle deterioration and muscle weakness may occur if the muscles are not regularly used.

Client Needs Category—Physiological integrity
Client Needs Subcategory—Physiological adaptation

40. **4.** Offering a few sips of water before placing the capsule in the client's mouth should help moisten the oral cavity and help the client swallow the medication. Capsules are never softened by placing them in water before administration or by having the client hold the capsule in her mouth. An opened capsule at the least is unpleasant to taste. At the worst, an opened capsule may be absorbed at an undesirable rate.

Client Needs Category—Safe, effective care environment
Client Needs Subcategory—Safety and infection control

41. **2.** Pyridoxine (vitamin B_6), which is present in most multivitamins, reduces the effectiveness of levodopa (Dopar). Therefore, it is best to hold the multivitamin while checking the drug order with the physician. Stool softeners are generally given on a routine basis to facilitate the ease of passing feces. The antiosteoporitic drug can be given with or without milk.

Client Needs Category—Physiological integrity
Client Needs Subcategory—Pharmacological therapies

42. **3.** The primary focus of teaching the client with Parkinson's disease is safety because much of the disease progression renders the client at risk for falling. The client typically has a propulsive unsteady gait, characterized by a tendency to take increasingly quicker steps while walking. The client may have difficulty beginning to walk, then difficulty returning to a seated position.

Client Needs Category—Safe, effective care environment
Client Needs Subcategory—None

43. **3.** The most realistic goal is to help the client function at her best. This includes muscle and motor function. Intensity and duration of symptoms may vary due to the client's status from day to day or between medication doses. There is no known cure for Parkinson's disease and no way to stop its progression. However, many clients live with the disease for years.

Client Needs Category—Health promotion and maintenance
Client Needs Subcategory—None

44. **1.** Raw fruits and vegetables are good sources of fiber, which increases the bulk and water content of the stool. Almost all pasta is made from some type of refined wheat flour. Whole grains are a better source of fiber. Cured meat, such as frankfurters and ham, contains fiber and a great deal of sodium. The serving size of meat is likely to be smaller in volume and less healthy than a piece of raw fruit. Cooking softens the fiber in vegetables and fruit; consequently, the cooking process reduces the indigestible bulk.

Client Needs Category—Health promotion and maintenance
Client Needs Subcategory—None

45. 3. Neurofibrillary tangles and plaques are found in postmortem examinations of clients with Alzheimer's disease. This clinical manifestation makes Alzheimer's disease different from other types of dementias. Hypoxia of the brain cells may result from a cerebrovascular accident or stroke or any type of ischemic insult. Evidence of infection of the meninges is common in meningitis.

Client Needs Category—Physiological integrity
Client Needs Subcategory—Physiological adaptation

46. 2. Make sure the client can be identified and returned to the care-providing agency. The Alzheimer's Association distributes identification tags and keeps a registry of client names as well. Confining the client to her room is inappropriate. Locking the outside doors is a safety hazard. It is better to install doors that sound an alarm when opened. Keeping the client dressed appropriately preserves the client's dignity but does not ensure safety.

Client Needs Category—Safe, effective care environment
Client Needs Subcategory—Safety and infection control

47. 2. The purse may be a symbol of security for the client. Therefore, it is best to accommodate the client's idiosyncrasy. Trying to alter the client's behavior may increase her confusion and lead to aggressive behavior. The client may not have the cognitive ability to offer a reason, choose a storage place, or understand the concept of loss.

Client Needs Category—Psychosocial integrity
Client Needs Subcategory—None

48. 3. Clients with dementia can sometimes be distracted from their original thoughts. In many cases, their short-term memory has deteriorated; however, the long-term memory may be intact. Reminding the client that her mother is dead may distress her. Lying to the client is unethical. The client whose memory is impaired may become frustrated when asked to identify when she last saw her mother.

Client Needs Category—Psychosocial integrity
Client Needs Subcategory—None

49. 1. Being able to verbalize feelings of fear and frustration about her debilitating disease can be extremely therapeutic for the client. Sharing possibly irrational fears with a caring individual may help put them in a more realistic light. Giving accurate information, identifying assessment findings, and validating that her health experience is common are appropriate nursing measures once the client verbalizes her fears.

Client Needs Category—Psychosocial integrity
Client Needs Subcategory—None

50. 3. A client with multiple sclerosis is typically weak and tires easily. Scheduling rest periods between activities will help manage these symptoms; it may also facilitate more self-care measures and elevate the client's self-esteem. The client is entitled to have her basic needs met; if she cannot meet her own needs, then staff must carry out the responsibility. Hurrying through tasks would probably tire the client. Doing tasks that the client is capable of performing is demeaning to her.

Client Needs Category—Physiological integrity
Client Needs Subcategory—Basic care and comfort

51. 1. Hot weather, even hot baths, increases the weakness common among clients with multiple sclerosis. Clients are not usually as adversely affected by rainy, dry, or cold environments.

Client Needs Category—Health promotion and maintenance
Client Needs Subcategory—None

52. 3. Subcutaneous injections are placed no closer than 1″ in all directions from another recent injection.

Client Needs Category—Safe, effective care environment
Client Needs Subcategory—Safety and infection control

53. 3. The thighs and abdomen are commonly used for administering subcutaneous interferon injections because they are more accessible for self-administration than the arms.

Client Needs Category—Health promotion and maintenance
Client Needs Subcategory—None

54. 4. Interferon beta-1a (Avonex) is essential for reducing the frequency of exacerbations in relapsing forms of multiple sclerosis. The drug slows the progression of physical disability. Therefore, withholding the drug because of anorexia and nausea is not an option. Mouth care improves the client's appetite, but it will not relieve the client's nausea. Administering the drug after meals will neither improve the client's appetite nor will it relieve nausea. Therefore, the best approach is to meet the client's nutritional needs by providing small, frequent meals.

Client Needs Category—Physiological integrity
Client Needs Subcategory—Basic care and comfort

55. 2. Clients with multiple sclerosis may experience numbness or decreased sensations; consequently, they may be unable to tell when an area of pressure is developing. Changing the client's position every 2 hours is sufficient in most circumstances to maintain skin that is still intact. An air-fluidized bed is appropriate for clients who are totally immobile or who have already developed stage 3 or 4 pressure ulcers. Rubbing a reddened skin area is inappropriate because this further damages the skin.

> ***Client Needs Category**—Physiological integrity*
> ***Client Needs Subcategory**—Basic care and comfort*

56. 3. Myasthenia gravis is a neuromuscular disorder characterized by severe weakness of one or more skeletal muscles. Ptosis, which is drooping of the eyelids, is one of the more common signs of this disease and probably would be noticed by the client. Other common signs of generalized weakness include difficulty swallowing and inarticulate speech. The client's hearing and papillary reflex would be unaffected by the disease. The client may have some problems moving his tongue during speech, but the tongue does not generally protrude.

> ***Client Needs Category**—Physiological integrity*
> ***Client Needs Subcategory**—Physiological adaptation*

57. 1. Clients with myasthenia gravis are prone to upper body muscular weakness that can compromise the ability to breathe. Because ventilation is critical to life, this assessment is the most appropriate and critical to make. The others are components of any client's assessment.

> ***Client Needs Category**—Physiological integrity*
> ***Client Needs Subcategory**—Basic care and comfort*

58. 3. An oral suction machine is best kept at the bedside of a client with myasthenia gravis. Suctioning may be needed quickly if the client cannot clear his airway. A tube-feeding pump may be needed eventually, but its acquisition could be delayed temporarily. An I.V. pole is easily acquired when, and if, it is needed. A cardiac defibrillator should remain centrally located near the nursing station when not in use.

> ***Client Needs Category**—Physiological integrity*
> ***Client Needs Subcategory**—Reduction of risk potential*

59. 1. Pyridostigmine bromide (Mestinon) prolongs the action of acetylcholine, which sustains muscle contraction. Signs of pyridostigmine bromide overdose include clenched jaws, abdominal cramps, and muscle rigidity. An inability to make a fist is a sign that the dose is insufficient. Urinary incontinence and talking incoherently are not drug-related in this case.

> ***Client Needs Category**—Physiological integrity*
> ***Client Needs Subcategory**—Pharmacological therapies*

60. 2. Administering medications for myasthenia gravis at precise times prevents the worsening of symptoms as the medication wears off. Getting adequate nourishment is a healthy behavior, but dietary measures do not affect the symptoms of myasthenia gravis. Exercise may actually precipitate muscular weakness.

Ensuring elimination is an appropriate nursing measure for managing the consequences of myasthenia gravis, but not for controlling the muscular weakness that causes elimination problems.

> ***Client Needs Category**—Physiological integrity*
> ***Client Needs Subcategory**—Physiological adaptation*

61. 4. Leaning forward from the waist and pressing over the bladder area is the proper way to perform Credé's method. The remaining options describe other methods that are sometimes used to promote urination.

> ***Client Needs Category**—Health promotion and maintenance*
> ***Client Needs Subcategory**—None*

62. 4. As amyotrophic lateral sclerosis progresses, clients generally become totally dependent on family or health care workers for all of their basic needs; therefore, the nursing diagnosis *Self-care deficit* is likely to be included in the client's care plan. Death is usually a consequence of respiratory failure or pneumonia. *Sexual dysfunction, Disturbed body image,* and *Impaired adjustment* may be in the care plan, depending on the client's circumstances.

> ***Client Needs Category**—Physiological integrity*
> ***Client Needs Subcategory**—Physiological adaptation*

63. 1. Huntington's chorea is a fatal hereditary disease that manifests around age 30. Genetic testing can identify who will eventually develop the disease and pass it on to their children. Those who have inherited the gene can take measures to prevent conception of infants who may also be affected. All remaining statements would be inappropriate for the nurse to make.

> ***Client Needs Category**—Health promotion and maintenance*
> ***Client Needs Subcategory**—None*

Nursing Care of Clients with Cerebrovascular Disorders

64. 1. A client who is experiencing a TIA may have weakness, dizziness, speech disturbances, visual loss, or double vision. Depression is common among older adults, but it is not unique to TIAs. Although the client may report visual changes, photosensitivity is not one of them. Stabbing head pain is more characteristic of a cerebral hemorrhage.

> ***Client Needs Category**—Physiological integrity*
> ***Client Needs Subcategory**—Physiological adaptation*

65. 2. A TIA signals that a stroke may occur in the very near future; it is therefore contraindicated to ignore the symptoms. Providing an explanation is appropriate, but referring the client for immediate medical evaluation is the nurse's priority. Taking a baby aspirin daily may prevent vascular thrombosis; however, it does not supersede seeking evaluation and treatment of the underlying cause of symptoms. Although a low-fat diet promotes a healthy lifestyle, the client has probably been developing atherosclerosis for a long time; dietary restrictions alone are unlikely to correct the problem.

Client Needs Category—*Physiological integrity*
Client Needs Subcategory—*Reduction of risk potential*

66. 3. To obtain valid assessment data, the nurse should dim the lights in the examination area. If conscious, the client is typically instructed to stare into the distance, not directly at the light. Both eyes are open, and the response of each eye is observed separately before the opposite eye is directly stimulated. The nurse is primarily observing for constriction of the stimulated pupil, not extraocular eye movement.

Client Needs Category—*Physiological integrity*
Client Needs Subcategory—*Physiological adaptation*

67. 2. An allergy to shellfish indicates sensitivity to iodine, which is a component in many contrast dyes. To avoid a reaction, an allergy to shellfish must be reported. None of the other allergic substances affects the CT procedure.

Client Needs Category—*Physiological integrity*
Client Needs Subcategory—*Reduction of risk potential*

68. 2. The long-term outcomes following a stroke are often determined by aggressive nursing efforts to maintain musculoskeletal function. Rehabilitation begins on admission with functional positioning, active and passive exercise, and early physical and occupational therapies. Managing bowel and bladder elimination does not have the same impact as preventing the development of musculo-skeletal deformities. Helping the client cope with altered body image and grieving are appropriate nursing responsibilities; however, even if those concerns are positively resolved, the client's rehabilitation would be delayed if contractures and joint immobility develop.

Client Needs Category—*Physiological integrity*
Client Needs Subcategory—*Reduction of risk potential*

69. 1. A widened pulse pressure is an ominous sign that accompanies increased intracranial pressure. Pulse pressure is the difference between systolic and diastolic blood pressures. A pulse pressure between 30 and 50 mm Hg is considered normal. A widened pulse pressure is one that exceeds 50 mm Hg. If a trend is developing, however, it should be reported early rather than waiting until the pulse pressure equals or exceeds 50 mm Hg.

Client Needs Category—*Physiological integrity*
Client Needs Subcategory—*Physiological adaptation*

70. 3. Suctioning is required whenever a client cannot clear his own airway. An unconscious client should be positioned on his side rather than supine. Removing pillows is inconsequential to maintaining a clear airway. Oral hygiene is an appropriate nursing measure for meeting the client's basic needs, but it does not clear the airway.

Client Needs Category—*Physiological integrity*
Client Needs Subcategory—*Physiological adaptation*

71. 2. Passive ROM exercises are performed on a routine basis to prevent paralyzed extremities from forming contractures. Passive ROM exercises are performed on all of the joints that the client does not move actively. For an unconscious client, this principle applies to all extremities.

Client Needs Category—*Health promotion and maintenance*
Client Needs Subcategory—*None*

72. 2. To ensure the maximum potential use of the feet, they are maintained in a functional position, which correlates with a person's position when standing. When standing, the soles of the feet are flat against the supporting surface. Therefore, the soles of the client's feet should be parallel to the footboard when he is in bed. The ankles are neither flexed less than 90 degrees nor extended more than 90 degrees.

Client Needs Category—*Physiological integrity*
Client Needs Subcategory—*Reduction of risk potential*

73. 2. Expressive aphasia means that the client can understand what is said but cannot respond using spoken language. An appropriate alternative is to use some nonverbal method by which the client can communicate, such as a written or printed list of key words that he can point to. A television may be useful as a diversion, but it is not therapeutic in restoring speech. Encouraging the client to speak is likely to cause frustration because his loss of language is not from a lack of effort or practice. Despite the client's inability to respond verbally, it is still appropriate for the nurse to speak to the client.

Client Needs Category—*Psychosocial integrity*
Client Needs Subcategory—*None*

74. 1, 4, 5. Warfarin (Coumadin) is an orally administered blood thinner that reduces the clotting time by causing a deficiency of prothrombin. Discharge instructions should cover the following: dietary restrictions (foods high in vitamin K, including avocado, green leafy vegetables, and broccoli, can reverse or reduce drug effects); missed doses (the client should not double the dose if missed, but should call the physician); and bruising or blood in the urine (if the client experiences signs of bleeding, the physician should be notified immediately). There are no driving restrictions associated with warfarin (Coumadin) use. Usual adverse effects of the medication include signs of bleeding, not edema in the lower extremities or difficulty sleeping.

> *Client Needs Category—Physiological integrity*
> *Client Needs Subcategory—Physiological adaptation*

75. 3. Hemianopsia is blindness in one half of the vision field. Therefore, to accommodate the client's residual peripheral vision, it is best to approach the client from his unaffected side. The interventions listed in the other options have no therapeutic value when caring for a client with hemianopsia.

> *Client Needs Category—Safe, effective care environment*
> *Client Needs Subcategory—Safety and infection control*

76. 4. A client with hemiplegia is best assisted from bed to a wheelchair by bracing the disabled foot and knee. The client with hemiplegia is unable to use a walker unless there is some residual strength in the paralyzed arm. The wheelchair is placed parallel to the bed. The nurse stands in front of the client to facilitate bracing and balancing him.

> *Client Needs Category—Physiological integrity*
> *Client Needs Subcategory—Reduction of risk potential*

77. 1. Coughing increases intracranial pressure and thereby increases the potential for cerebral bleeding. The other identified problems require the nurse's attention, but reducing or eliminating coughing should be the highest priority.

> *Client Needs Category—Physiological integrity*
> *Client Needs Subcategory—Reduction of risk potential*

78.

6. Level of conciousness (LOC)
2. Motor strength
3. Vital signs
5. Urine output
1. Bowel movements
4. Skin integrity

The first assessment that the nurse should make is to evaluate the client's LOC. This is the best indicator of brain function; any deterioration in the client's condition would alter his LOC. Motor strength, the second assessment performed, is an indication of the brain's ability to control voluntary actions. Any changes in the ability to follow commands might signify deterioration. Vital signs are measured next (they should be measured frequently in a client with a cerebral aneurysm). Signs of a leaking aneurysm include increased pulse rate, respiratory changes, and elevated blood pressure. Urine output, bowel movements, and skin integrity are assessed last. Decreased urine output may signal decreased kidney perfusion. Bowel movements are assessed regularly to ensure that the client is not straining to defecate. Skin integrity must be assessed for evidence of breakdown caused by the client's limited activity.

> *Client Needs Category—Physiological integrity*
> *Client Needs Subcategory—Physiological adaptation*

79. 4. Using nondrug interventions such as guided imagery in combination with an analgesic increases the drug's therapeutic effect. Most oral analgesics are administered at 3- or 4-hour intervals; giving another dose sooner would be contraindicated. The goal of pain management is to relieve the symptoms of pain, thereby making the client more comfortable. If the physician was concerned with masking symptoms, he would not have prescribed the pain medication. Opioid analgesics are generally avoided in most neurologic conditions because they can alter the client's pupil response, level of consciousness, bowel pattern, and breathing. Mild nonopioid analgesics can be safely used to treat pain experienced by neurologic clients.

> *Client Needs Category—Physiological integrity*
> *Client Needs Subcategory—Physiological adaptation*

Nursing Care of Clients with Tumors of the Neurologic System

80. 1. The client should be instructed to eliminate caffeine, alcohol, tobacco, tranquilizers, and sedatives for 24 hours before a PET scan. Diuretics, food dyes, and antibiotics don't affect PET results.

> *Client Needs Category—Physiological integrity*
> *Client Needs Subcategory—Reduction of risk potential*

81. 2. Consuming extra fluids helps excrete the radioisotope used during the examination. There is no specific reason to recommend taking a laxative, getting sleep, or reporting abdominal discomfort.

> *Client Needs Category—Physiological integrity*
> *Client Needs Subcategory—Physiological adaptation*

82. 1. The nurse must frequently monitor the neurologic status of a client who had a craniotomy. One of the most important assessments involves checking the client's extremities for movement and motor strength. Any decrease in strength or ability to move usually indicates that the intracranial pressure is increasing. Although the other assessments are appropriate to note, they are not as significant to the client's critical condition.
Client Needs Category—*Physiological integrity*
Client Needs Subcategory—*Physiological adaptation*

83. 3. When catheterizing an adult man, the device is usually inserted a distance of 6″ to 8″ (15 to 20 cm), or until urine begins to flow. A catheter that is inserted less than 6″ or inflated before urine flows might not be properly located in the bladder. Urethral damage may occur if the tip of the catheter and the bulb are not fully within the bladder.
Client Needs Category—*Physiological integrity*
Client Needs Subcategory—*Physiological adaptation*

84. 4. To preserve the client's dignity and to reduce the potential for infection, the hair of someone undergoing a craniotomy is usually shaved after the client has been transferred from the nursing unit to the surgical department. Shaving the night before facilitates colonization of microorganisms within the skin abrasions. If skin preparation is done on the nursing unit, it is best done before administering sedation. The head is shaved before a shower so loose hair can be rinsed away.
Client Needs Category—*Physiological integrity*
Client Needs Subcategory—*Reduction of risk potential*

85. 3. The client's hair is usually bagged in a paper bag and offered to the client's family. They may wish to retain it for sentimental reasons or have it used for constructing a wig. If the family is not interested in keeping the hair, the information is documented. The hair is then disposed of according to facility policies.
Client Needs Category—*Physiological integrity*
Client Needs Subcategory—*Physiological adaptation*

86. 2. To reduce the potential for a wound infection, it is best to reinforce a moist dressing. Usually, the surgeon performs the first dressing change unless otherwise specified in the medical orders. The condition of the dressing and the action taken are important information to document. Removing or changing the dressing would be inappropriate.
Client Needs Category—*Physiological integrity*
Client Needs Subcategory—*Reduction of risk potential*

87. 4. Reorientation is appropriate during periods of confusion. It may be necessary to repeat information several times. Explaining the nature of the confusion to the client or withholding communication would be inappropriate. Reading to the client may help to raise his consciousness, but would not necessarily correct his confusion.
Client Needs Category—*Psychosocial integrity*
Client Needs Subcategory—*None*

88. 4. Before the client receives oral fluids, the nurse must assess the client's ability to swallow. Clients undergoing neurologic surgery may have residual muscular weakness, which creates the potential for aspiration. The other assessments are appropriate, but they are not as important to consuming liquids as the ability to swallow.
Client Needs Category—*Physiological integrity*
Client Needs Subcategory—*Reduction of risk potential*

89. 3. Limiting fluids controls the potential for developing cerebral edema and reduces the client's risk of vomiting, but controlling intracranial pressure is more important. The kidneys automatically adjust the volume of urine excreted according to the client's fluid status. Thirst is a subjective phenomenon. Restricting oral fluids to 1,000 mL does not ensure that the client's thirst will be relieved.
Client Needs Category—*Physiological integrity*
Client Needs Subcategory—*Physiological adaptation*

Nursing Care of Clients with Nerve Disorders

90. 2. The client's care plan must include measures to prevent any stimulation to trigger points that could provoke pain along the ophthalmic, mandibular, and maxillary branches of the trigeminal nerve. Therefore, all contact with the face—including heat, cold, or drafts—should be avoided.
Client Needs Category—*Physiological integrity*
Client Needs Subcategory—*Physiological adaptation*

91. 1. Because the liver produces prothrombin, a substance important to clot formation, signs of unusual bleeding in a client taking carbamazepine (Tegretol) indicate adverse effects to the liver. This drug also causes hematologic changes that may also be evidenced as abnormal bleeding. Clay-colored stools and dark brown urine, not black stools and pale urine, are associated with liver disturbances. Mottled skin is not a sign of liver impairment.
Client Needs Category—*Health promotion and maintenance*
Client Needs Subcategory—*None*

92. 3. Directing the flow across the conjunctiva from the nasal to temporal corners of the eye helps keep the solution from dripping down the client's nose. It also keeps debris from entering the nasolacrimal duct. None of the other anatomic descriptions is accurate.
Client Needs Category—*Physiological integrity*
Client Needs Subcategory—*Physiological adaptation*

93. 4. The seventh cranial nerve is the facial nerve. Inflammation around the facial nerve results in sudden paralysis of skeletal muscles about the face. The paralysis is usually unilateral. The other assessment findings are not commonly associated with Bell's palsy.
Client Needs Category—*Physiological integrity*
Client Needs Subcategory—*Physiological adaptation*

94. 3. Food may become trapped in the buccal pouch of a client with Bell's palsy. Therefore, the nurse should inspect this area after each meal, assess for mechanical trauma, and remove any debris found. Controlling light has no therapeutic value. Drinking from a cup does not promote better facial muscle function. Although looking in a mirror may be distressing, dealing with the reality of the situation is a component of the grieving process. The nurse may wish to stress that some clients recover muscular function, although the period of recovery may be quite slow.
Client Needs Category—*Physiological integrity*
Client Needs Subcategory—*Physiological adaptation*

95. 3. The same virus that causes chickenpox (herpes) is implicated in the condition called shingles. Latent virus cells are apparently harbored within peripheral nerves. The virus becomes activated by a variety of means, such as a concurrent infection, injury, or injection.
Client Needs Category—*Physiological integrity*
Client Needs Subcategory—*Physiological adaptation*

96. 1. To allow room for instilling dye or air within the vertebral column, approximately 15 mL of spinal fluid is withdrawn via a lumbar puncture. The client is instructed to lie prone on the examination table. The table, however, is tilted to promote movement of the dye. Local anesthesia is used at the site of the lumbar puncture, but no other forms of anesthesia are commonly given.
Client Needs Category—*Physiological integrity*
Client Needs Subcategory—*Physiological adaptation*

97. 2. Bending the knees while keeping the back straight is an excellent technique for using good body mechanics. The back is often strained by lifting objects with the waist bent. Heavy objects are carried close to the center of gravity.
Client Needs Category—*Health promotion and maintenance*
Client Needs Subcategory—*None*

98. 2. Until healing takes place, clients are logrolled following spinal surgery. Logrolling involves moving the client's shoulders and hips as a unit to avoid twisting the spine. None of the other turning options describes a logrolling technique.
Client Needs Category—*Physiological integrity*
Client Needs Subcategory—*Reduction of risk potential*

99.

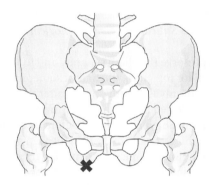

The correct placement of the X is the right ischium, or near the right hipbone. Starting at lumbar segment 3 in the lower back area, the sciatic nerve is the largest in the body. Pressure on the sciatic nerve from a herniated disc is typically the cause of sciatica. The client may experience pain, burning, tingling, or numbness in the leg or buttocks, often accompanied by a shooting pain that makes it hard for the client to stand up.
Client Needs Category—*Physiological integrity*
Client Needs Subcategory—*Physiological adaptation*

100. 3. The most effective technique for maintaining the integrity of the skin is to wear a knit cotton shirt under the brace. Talc helps to absorb moisture from the skin; it does not prevent skin breakdown. Alcohol dries the skin and reduces the presence of microorganisms. The brace does not have hinges that require lubrication.
Client Needs Category—*Health promotion and maintenance*
Client Needs Subcategory—*None*

The Nursing Care of Clients with Disorders of Sensory Organs and the Integument

TEST 3

⇨ Nursing Care of Clients with Eye Disorders
⇨ Nursing Care of Clients with Disorders of Accessory Eye Structures
⇨ Nursing Care of Clients with Ear Disorders
⇨ Nursing Care of Clients with Nasal Disorders
⇨ Nursing Care of Clients with Disorders of the Skin and Related Structures
⇨ Correct Answers and Rationales

Directions: With a pencil, blacken the space in front of the option you have chosen for your correct answer.

Nursing Care of Clients with Eye Disorders

A high-school chemistry student is sent to the school nurse after being splashed in the eyes with a chemical.

1. Which information is most important for the nurse to obtain initially?
[ ] **1.** Whether safety glasses were worn
[ ] **2.** The name of the splashed chemical
[ ] **3.** The treatment already given
[ ] **4.** Whether the client's vision is impaired

The nurse prepares to irrigate the student's irritated eye.

2. Assuming the following solutions are available, which one is best for the nurse to use at this time?
[ ] **1.** Tap water
[ ] **2.** Sodium bicarbonate
[ ] **3.** Normal saline
[ ] **4.** Magnesium sulfate

3. When irrigating the client's eyes, which technique is the best way to direct the flow of irrigating solution?
[ ] **1.** Directly onto the corneal surface
[ ] **2.** Away from the inner canthus
[ ] **3.** Within the anterior chamber
[ ] **4.** Toward the nasolacrimal duct

4. To whom should the nurse refer the student once emergency treatment is completed?
[ ] **1.** An optician
[ ] **2.** An ophthalmologist
[ ] **3.** An optometrist
[ ] **4.** An orthoptist

5. When a foreign body becomes embedded in a person's eye, which action should be taken first before referring the client for emergency treatment?
[ ] **1.** Remove the object with forceps.
[ ] **2.** Ask the person to blink rapidly.
[ ] **3.** Instill antibiotic ointment.
[ ] **4.** Loosely patch both eyes.

6. The nurse is preparing to irrigate a client's eye. What steps are appropriate in completing the irrigation? Select all that apply.
[ ] **1.** Place the solution directly into the center of the eye.
[ ] **2.** Tilt the head toward the opposite eye.
[ ] **3.** Wash the hands and put on gloves.
[ ] **4.** Offer the client a tissue.
[ ] **5.** Place the drops of solution into the conjunctival sac.
[ ] **6.** Continue eye irrigations until all redness is resolved.

A nurse uses a Snellen chart to assess the visual acuity of clients before the physician examines them.

7. When describing the examination procedure to clients, which statement by the nurse is most accurate?
[ ] **1.** "You'll read words that are the size of newsprint."
[ ] **2.** "You'll read letters from a distance of 20 feet."
[ ] **3.** "You'll look at a color picture and identify an image."
[ ] **4.** "You'll look at a screen and tell me when an object appears."

8. How does the nurse in an eye clinic correctly document a client's nearsightedness?
[ ] **1.** Presbyopia
[ ] **2.** Amblyopia
[ ] **3.** Hyperopia
[ ] **4.** Myopia

A nursing assistant confides to the nurse that her father needs eyeglasses but cannot afford them.

9. Which organization can the nurse suggest as a resource to the nursing assistant and her father?
[ ] **1.** The Loyal Order of Moose
[ ] **2.** The American Legion
[ ] **3.** Lions Clubs International
[ ] **4.** The Knights of Columbus

The nurse reads in the medical record that a client has astigmatism.

10. Based on the documented condition, how would the nurse expect the client to report his vision when looking at an object while not wearing corrective glasses or contact lenses?
[ ] **1.** "I see near objects more clearly."
[ ] **2.** "I see a blurry area in front of me."
[ ] **3.** "I see far objects more clearly."
[ ] **4.** "I see two of the same object."

11. When instructing a nursing assistant on the proper technique for cleaning a client's prescription glasses, the nurse recommends washing the lenses with soap and warm water or a commercial glass cleaner and drying them how?
[ ] **1.** With a paper tissue
[ ] **2.** With a soft cloth
[ ] **3.** With a paper towel
[ ] **4.** By air evaporation

12. Which intervention is most appropriate to include in the care plan of an anxious client who is blind or has both eyes patched?
[ ] **1.** Touch the client before speaking.
[ ] **2.** Explain what you plan to do beforehand.
[ ] **3.** Shut the door to his room to decrease noise.
[ ] **4.** Leave the room lights on at all times.

The nurse observes a nursing assistant ambulating a blind client.

13. Which instruction to the nursing assistant is best for maintaining the client's safety and security?
[ ] **1.** Let the client take your arm while walking.
[ ] **2.** Take the client's arm while walking with him.
[ ] **3.** Position the client in front and to your side.
[ ] **4.** Have the client walk independently by your side.

14. Which plan best promotes a blind client's feeling of self-reliance when eating?
[ ] **1.** Help the client locate his food by comparing its placement to clock positions.
[ ] **2.** Ask a hospital volunteer to feed the client so he does not have to ask for help.
[ ] **3.** Order foods that can be sipped from containers rather than those that require eating utensils.
[ ] **4.** Ask the dietary department to serve the client's food on paper plates and in cups.

The nurse is assigned to care for an older man who has bilateral senile cataracts.

15. Which symptom would the nurse expect to note in the client's history that is directly related to his medical condition?
[ ] **1.** Gradual loss of vision
[ ] **2.** Fullness within the eye
[ ] **3.** Ocular pain or discomfort
[ ] **4.** Flashes of light

16. When the nurse inspects the client's eyes, which clinical finding is most indicative of cataracts?
[ ] **1.** Ruptured blood vessels on the eye
[ ] **2.** An irregularly shaped iris
[ ] **3.** A white spot behind the pupil
[ ] **4.** A painless corneal lesion

17. Which statement made by the client best indicates that he understands when surgery is needed?
[ ] **1.** "I'll need surgery when my loss of vision really interferes with my activities."
[ ] **2.** "I'll need surgery when I can't control the pain anymore with eye drops."
[ ] **3.** "I'll need surgery when I start to feel self-conscious about my eye color."
[ ] **4.** "I'll need surgery when my cataracts are at their largest size and no further changes are observed."

The client with bilateral cataracts is scheduled to have a cataract removed from his right eye. Preoperative orders include the following: (1) Scrub face with povidone-iodine (Betadine) for 10 minutes on the morning of surgery; (2) Withhold anticoagulant therapy; (3) Instill dilating drops at least 1 hour before surgery.

18. After reviewing the medical orders, it is essential for the nurse to assess which of the following preoperatively?
[ ] **1.** The client's face for skin lesions
[ ] **2.** The last dose of medication taken by the client
[ ] **3.** The client's right eye for drainage
[ ] **4.** The client's left eye for signs of strain

One hour before surgery, the nurse instills eye drops per the physician's orders.

19. The nurse should instill the eye drops into which part of the client's eye?
[ ] **1.** Onto the cornea
[ ] **2.** At the inner canthus
[ ] **3.** At the outer canthus
[ ] **4.** In the lower conjunctival sac

The nursing team meets to individualize a standardized postoperative nursing care plan for a client who is scheduled for a cataract extraction.

20. Which standing nursing order should be eliminated from this client's care plan?
[ ] **1.** Keep the client's bed in a low position at all times.
[ ] **2.** Reapply antiembolism stockings twice daily.
[ ] **3.** Urge the client to cough every 2 hours while awake.
[ ] **4.** Assist the client when he ambulates in the hall or room.

21. After cataract surgery, the client tells the nurse that he is experiencing severe pain in his operative eye. Which nursing action is most appropriate?
[ ] **1.** Report the finding to the charge nurse.
[ ] **2.** Give the client a prescribed analgesic.
[ ] **3.** Assess the client's pupil response with a penlight.
[ ] **4.** Reposition the client on his operative side.

Before the client is discharged from the hospital, the physician instructs him to wear a metal shield over his operative eye while sleeping.

22. When the client asks the nurse about the purpose of the eye shield, which explanation is best?
[ ] **1.** The shield keeps foreign substances out of the eye.
[ ] **2.** The shield protects the eye from accidental trauma.
[ ] **3.** The shield reduces rapid eye movement when dreaming.
[ ] **4.** The shield promotes dilation of the pupil at night.

23. Which information is most appropriate to include in the discharge instructions for the client who has undergone a cataract extraction?
[ ] **1.** Avoid bending over from the waist.
[ ] **2.** Keep both eyes patched at all times.
[ ] **3.** Sleep with the head slightly elevated.
[ ] **4.** Expect bleeding to decrease in 1 week.

A nurse is assigned to care for an older woman with chronic open-angle glaucoma.

24. Which common characteristic of open-angle glaucoma is this client most likely to report?
[ ] **1.** Itching and burning eyes
[ ] **2.** Headaches while reading
[ ] **3.** Seeing halos around lights
[ ] **4.** Loss of central vision

The nurse prepares to assist the physician during the client's examination.

25. If the physician wants to check the client's intraocular pressure (IOP), which instrument should the nurse have available?
[ ] **1.** Ophthalmoscope
[ ] **2.** Tonometer
[ ] **3.** Retinoscope
[ ] **4.** Speculum

26. Which symptom related to the chronic progression of disease is a client with untreated glaucoma most likely to report to the nurse?
[ ] **1.** Tunnel vision
[ ] **2.** Double vision
[ ] **3.** Bulging eyes
[ ] **4.** Bloodshot eyes

27. The nurse has been instructed to administer eye ointment to a client. Identify the correct area to begin applying the ointment.

A client with chronic open-angle glaucoma is given a prescription for timolol maleate (Timoptic) 1 gtt in each eye daily. The nurse provides client instructions.

28. Which comment strongly suggests that the client needs more teaching?
[ ] **1.** "I must wash my hands before instilling the drops."
[ ] **2.** "This drug decreases the formation of fluid in my eye."
[ ] **3.** "I'll need to take this until my eye pressure is normal."
[ ] **4.** "The cap on the container should be replaced immediately."

29. The nurse must withhold medication administration and notify the physician if which drug is ordered for a client with glaucoma?
[ ]   **1.** Atropine sulfate (Sal-Tropine)
[ ]   **2.** Morphine sulfate (Roxanol)
[ ]   **3.** Magnesium sulfate (Epsom salts)
[ ]   **4.** Ferrous sulfate (Feosol)

30. Which assessment finding is commonly noted when the IOP of a client with angle-closure glaucoma becomes dangerously high?
[ ]   **1.** Spots in the visual field
[ ]   **2.** Severe eye pain
[ ]   **3.** Pinpoint pupils
[ ]   **4.** Bulging eyes

31. The nurse compares the characteristics of open-angle glaucoma with those of angle-closure glaucoma. In which ways are they similar? Select all that apply.
[ ]   **1.** The symptoms appear suddenly.
[ ]   **2.** The visual field examination demonstrates a loss of vision.
[ ]   **3.** Clients are initially treated with medications.
[ ]   **4.** Blurred vision is a common manifestation.
[ ]   **5.** Attacks are self-limiting but are more harmful with each episode.
[ ]   **6.** Surgery is often required.

Once the intraocular pressure has been temporarily reduced, the physician performs an iridectomy on a client with angle-closure glaucoma.

32. When the nurse assesses the client's operative eye following surgery, which finding is most expected?
[ ]   **1.** The pupil appears cloudy and gray.
[ ]   **2.** The pupil is a fixed size and shape.
[ ]   **3.** The entire iris lacks color.
[ ]   **4.** A section of the iris appears black.

The nurse documents the health history of a client with a retinal detachment.

33. Of the following information provided by the client, which factor is most likely to cause a retinal detachment?
[ ]   **1.** The client is younger than age 40.
[ ]   **2.** The client fell within the last day.
[ ]   **3.** The client has multiple allergies.
[ ]   **4.** The client is recovering from pneumonia.

The nurse applies patches to both of the client's eyes, as instructed by the physician.

34. Which of the nurse's actions is most appropriate when applying eye patches?

[ ]   **1.** Occluding all sources of room light
[ ]   **2.** Ensuring that both patches exert tight pressure on the eyes
[ ]   **3.** Maintaining the client's eyelids in a closed position
[ ]   **4.** Making sure the client can see while the patches are in place

The nurse delivers a phone message to a hospitalized client with retinal detachment. The client is on strict bed rest with the head of the bed slightly elevated.

35. Before leaving the room, which of the following nurse's actions best preserves the client's dignity?
[ ]   **1.** The nurse straightens the client's linens.
[ ]   **2.** The nurse informs the client when leaving the room.
[ ]   **3.** The nurse offers to give the client a back rub.
[ ]   **4.** The nurse shares some current events with the client.

After a few days of continual bed rest, the client tells the nurse, "I'm not having any pain, and I'm not dying. Why can't I just get up once to go to the bathroom?"

36. Which response by the nurse is best in this situation?
[ ]   **1.** "Gravity helps to reattach the separated retina."
[ ]   **2.** "You don't want to be permanently blind, do you?"
[ ]   **3.** "I can get you a sedative if it's hard to lay still."
[ ]   **4.** "The doctor knows what's best for you, and you should listen."

The client with a detached retina undergoes a scleral buckling procedure.

37. Postoperatively, which client problem should be the nurse's highest priority?
[ ]   **1.** Pain
[ ]   **2.** Vomiting
[ ]   **3.** Anxiety
[ ]   **4.** Boredom

A client with myopia has a laser keratotomy (LASIK) procedure.

38. Which statement is the best evidence that the client understands the anticipated outcome of this procedure?
[ ]   **1.** "I'll have better night vision."
[ ]   **2.** "I'll correctly identify colors."
[ ]   **3.** "I'll see well without glasses."
[ ]   **4.** "I'll use both eyes when reading."

A nurse is asked to assess a person who says he has "pinkeye."

39. Upon inspecting the eye, the nurse will note which symptom of conjunctivitis in addition to erythema?
[ ] **1.** Dried drainage along the eyelid
[ ] **2.** Lack of pupil response to light
[ ] **3.** Bulging of the eye from the orbit
[ ] **4.** Loss of moisture on the cornea

40. Which health teaching instruction is most important for a client with conjunctivitis?
[ ] **1.** Eat a well-balanced, nutritious diet.
[ ] **2.** Always wear sunglasses in bright light.
[ ] **3.** Do not share towels and washcloths with other family members.
[ ] **4.** Avoid aspirin-containing products.

The physician asks the nurse to assist with applying a stain to the eye of a client who may have a foreign body in or injury to the cornea.

41. The nurse correctly hands the physician a vial containing which solution?
[ ] **1.** Povidone-iodine (Betadine)
[ ] **2.** Gentian violet
[ ] **3.** Methylene blue
[ ] **4.** Fluorescein

42. What images will a female client with macular degeneration most likely describe having an ability to see?
[ ] **1.** Those that are close to her face
[ ] **2.** Those that are at a far distance
[ ] **3.** Those that are in her outer peripheral fields
[ ] **4.** Those that are in her central field of vision

A nurse makes home visits to several older adult clients with chronic health problems.

43. To identify problems that may compromise the client's vision, the nurse recommends regular eye examinations by an ophthalmologist to which client?
[ ] **1.** A client who takes aspirin daily
[ ] **2.** A client who has diabetes mellitus
[ ] **3.** A client who has lactose intolerance
[ ] **4.** A client who uses a potassium supplement

A client with a malignant eye tumor has consented to have an enucleation of the eye.

44. Which statement provides the best evidence that the client understands the postoperative outcome of this surgery?
[ ] **1.** "My vision will be restored with a plastic prosthesis."
[ ] **2.** "The prosthetic eye will be inserted during surgery."
[ ] **3.** "I will have to remove my prosthesis for cleaning."
[ ] **4.** "I will have a permanently empty eye socket."

45. Which sign most suggests that a client who had a corneal transplant is experiencing rejection of the donor tissue?
[ ] **1.** Excessive tearing
[ ] **2.** Change in vision
[ ] **3.** Itching of the eye
[ ] **4.** Frequent blinking

Nursing Care of Clients with Disorders of Accessory Eye Structures

An older client's lower eyelid margins droop outward, exposing the conjunctival membrane and lower portion of the eye.

46. Based on the anatomic changes in the tone of the eyelid, the nurse would expect the client to experience which problem?
[ ] **1.** Double vision
[ ] **2.** Photophobia
[ ] **3.** Lid spasms
[ ] **4.** Dry eyes

The nurse observes that a client has inflamed eyelid margins and patchy dandruff-like flakes that cling to the eyelids and eyelashes.

47. Which recommendation by the nurse is most appropriate if the client's condition is caused by hypersecretion of the sebaceous glands?
[ ] **1.** Increasing attention to hygiene
[ ] **2.** Limiting oral fluid intake
[ ] **3.** Reducing frequent eyestrain
[ ] **4.** Eating more deep yellow vegetables

48. When a client with a stye (hordeolum) asks a nurse to suggest measures to relieve his discomfort, which is the best advice the nurse can offer?
[ ] **1.** Squeeze the lesion to express the exudate.
[ ] **2.** Apply warm, moist compresses to the area.
[ ] **3.** Pierce the lesion with the tip of a pin.
[ ] **4.** Cover the lesion with a dry gauze dressing.

The physician diagnoses swelling within the inner surface of a client's eyelid as a chalazion, a gland obstructed with sebum.

49. The nurse correctly tells the client to expect which problem if the tissue continues to proliferate?
[ ] **1.** Blindness may occur.
[ ] **2.** Lashes may fall out.
[ ] **3.** Surgery may be necessary.
[ ] **4.** Pain may be severe.

Nursing Care of Clients with Ear Disorders

While performing a nursing admission interview, the nurse notes that a client continues to ask her to repeat questions.

50. If the client worked at the following occupations, which one is most likely to have contributed to the hearing loss?
[ ] **1.** Telephone operator
[ ] **2.** Computer programmer
[ ] **3.** Musician
[ ] **4.** Accountant

A client is embarrassed when the nurse inspects his ear canal. He says, "Please bring me something so I can clean the earwax from my ears."

51. Which response is best for the purpose of health teaching?
[ ] **1.** "It's best to use the corner of a soapy washcloth."
[ ] **2.** "Do you prefer a short or long cotton-tipped applicator?"
[ ] **3.** "Have you ever tried removing earwax with a hairpin?"
[ ] **4.** "I can refer you to a physician who will clean them."

52. Which instrument is most appropriate for the nurse to use to test a client's hearing acuity?
[ ] **1.** Otoscope
[ ] **2.** Tuning fork
[ ] **3.** Reflex hammer
[ ] **4.** Stethoscope

A client tells the nurse that he has been experiencing continuous ringing in his ears.

53. Which question is most appropriate for the nurse to ask at this time?
[ ] **1.** "What childhood diseases have you had?"
[ ] **2.** "What's your present occupation?"
[ ] **3.** "Do you eat a well-balanced diet?"
[ ] **4.** "How much aspirin do you take?"

A client who wears a hearing aid is frustrated by the loud and shrill noise (feedback) that he hears occasionally.

54. Which nursing action is most helpful for reducing or eliminating feedback?
[ ] **1.** Repositioning the hearing aid within the ear
[ ] **2.** Cleaning the hearing aid with a soft cloth
[ ] **3.** Replacing the battery in the hearing aid
[ ] **4.** Turning down the volume in the hearing aid

55. If a client who has recently experienced diminished hearing takes drugs from each of the following drug categories, which one is most likely to have affected his hearing?
[ ] **1.** Nonsteroidal anti-inflammatory drugs
[ ] **2.** Beta-adrenergic blockers
[ ] **3.** Aminoglycoside antibiotics
[ ] **4.** Histamine-2 (H_2) antagonists

56. When instilling prescribed medication into the ear of an adult, which is the correct technique for the nurse to use to straighten the ear canal?
[ ] **1.** Pull the ear upward and backward.
[ ] **2.** Pull the ear downward and forward.
[ ] **3.** Pull the ear upward and forward.
[ ] **4.** Pull the ear downward and backward.

57. After instilling medication into the client's ear, which instruction is most appropriate?
[ ] **1.** Remain in position for at least 5 minutes.
[ ] **2.** Pack a cotton pledget tightly in your ear.
[ ] **3.** Do not blow your nose for at least 1 hour.
[ ] **4.** Avoid drinking very warm or cold beverages.

A person who is considering having her earlobes pierced consults a nurse on self-care techniques if the procedure is performed.

58. Which information is most helpful for reducing the potential for infection?
[ ] **1.** Use earrings made of 14-karat gold.
[ ] **2.** Leave the earrings in for 2 weeks.
[ ] **3.** Turn the earrings frequently.
[ ] **4.** Swab the earlobes daily with alcohol.

When inspecting a client's ear, the nurse finds that the ear canal is red, swollen, and tender. The tympanic membrane is intact.

59. Which other assessment finding is most indicative of an infection in the external ear?
[ ] **1.** Foul-smelling drainage
[ ] **2.** Head trauma from a fall
[ ] **3.** Diminished hearing
[ ] **4.** Enlarged lymph nodes

A client asks the nurse why adults do not experience middle ear infections as frequently as children do.

60. The client demonstrates understanding of the nurse's teaching when he identifies which as the reason that organisms travel more easily from the nasopharynx to the middle ear in a child?
[ ] **1.** Because the ear canal is shorter and straighter
[ ] **2.** Because the ear canal is longer and straighter

[ ] **3.** Because the ear canal is shorter and more curved

[ ] **4.** Because the ear canal is longer and more curved

A client arrives at the physician's office complaining of pain in the left ear. A middle ear infection is diagnosed.

61. The nurse uses an illustration to explain to the client the structure of the ear and the area of infection. Identify where the middle ear is situated.

62. Which is the best evidence that the antibiotic the nurse is administering for the treatment of acute otitis media is having a therapeutic effect?

[ ] **1.** The ear feels less warm to the touch.

[ ] **2.** Ringing sounds within the ear stop.

[ ] **3.** Ear drainage is thin and watery.

[ ] **4.** Ear discomfort is relieved.

63. If a client with a middle ear infection reports the following symptoms, which one is most indicative that the infection has spread to the inner ear?

[ ] **1.** Temporal headaches

[ ] **2.** A sore throat

[ ] **3.** Nasal congestion

[ ] **4.** Postural dizziness

A physician intends to perform a myringotomy on a client with a middle ear infection.

64. When the nurse prepares the client for the myringotomy, which statement best explains the procedure's purpose?

[ ] **1.** A myringotomy prevents permanent hearing loss.

[ ] **2.** A myringotomy provides a pathway for drainage.

[ ] **3.** A myringotomy aids in administering medications.

[ ] **4.** A myringotomy maintains motion of the ear bones.

65. When planning the client's discharge instructions, it is most appropriate for the nurse to provide which instruction concerning the cotton pledget in his ear canal?

[ ] **1.** Leave the cotton pledget in place until it is saturated.

[ ] **2.** Keep the cotton pledget placed loosely within the ear canal.

[ ] **3.** Soak the cotton pledget in peroxide before insertion.

[ ] **4.** Remove the cotton pledget when the cotton becomes dry.

A middle-aged woman is seen in the physician's office for diminished hearing caused by otosclerosis.

66. Which common health history finding would the nurse expect of a client with otosclerosis?

[ ] **1.** Hearing loss started in childhood.

[ ] **2.** Previous upper respiratory infections were commonly accompanied by high fevers.

[ ] **3.** Tonsils and adenoids were removed.

[ ] **4.** One or more relatives have been similarly diagnosed.

The client asks the nurse to explain what the physician meant by saying that she had a conductive hearing loss.

67. Which statement by the nurse most accurately explains the pathophysiology of the client's conductive hearing loss?

[ ] **1.** Sound waves do not travel to the inner ear.

[ ] **2.** There is a malfunction of inner ear structures.

[ ] **3.** The eighth cranial nerve is permanently damaged.

[ ] **4.** Electric conversion of sound is not produced.

The team leader responsible for the client's initial care plan makes a nursing diagnosis of Risk for impaired verbal communication related to hearing loss.

68. When the team leader asks the admitting nurse to assist with developing a goal for the identified diagnosis, which goal best fits the situation?

[ ] **1.** The client will state she can understand staff communication.

[ ] **2.** The staff will improve verbal communication techniques.

[ ] **3.** The client will demonstrate the ability to express herself.

[ ] **4.** The client will be able to communicate basic needs.

The nurse helps the team leader plan appropriate interventions to ensure effective communication with the client.

69. Which intervention is most appropriate to include in the care plan?
[ ] **1.** Speak directly into the client's ear.
[ ] **2.** Face the client when speaking to her.
[ ] **3.** Drop your voice at the end of each sentence.
[ ] **4.** Raise the pitch of your voice an octave higher.

The client is scheduled for a stapedectomy, but she does not seem to understand the verbal information the physician provided about the surgery.

70. Which nursing intervention is the next best alternative for helping the client comprehend the details of the procedure at this time?
[ ] **1.** Providing her with a printed pamphlet on the topic
[ ] **2.** Asking another stapedectomy client to talk with her
[ ] **3.** Refering the client to someone who can translate the communication in sign language
[ ] **4.** Writing all the information in longhand

The client expresses her concerns about the impending stapedectomy and says to the nurse, "There are so many awful complications that can happen with this surgery."

71. Which response by the nurse is most therapeutic to the client in this situation?
[ ] **1.** "You've got the best surgeon on the staff."
[ ] **2.** "Tell me more about how you're feeling."
[ ] **3.** "Don't worry. Those things hardly ever happen."
[ ] **4.** "Let's think about something more pleasant."

72. After the stapedectomy, which is the most appropriate technique for assessing whether the client's facial nerve function is intact?
[ ] **1.** Ask the client to identify familiar odors.
[ ] **2.** Ask the client to smile or raise her eyebrows.
[ ] **3.** Ask the client to stick out her tongue.
[ ] **4.** Ask the client to read printed information.

73. How should the client be positioned for the first 24 hours after a stapedectomy?
[ ] **1.** Supine with the head elevated and the client lying on the nonoperative ear.
[ ] **2.** With the head raised and facing forward and the knees in the flexed position.
[ ] **3.** Supine with the head of the bed elevated and the head resting on the occiput.
[ ] **4.** Prone with the head positioned toward the operated side.

The day after the stapedectomy, the client is discouraged because her hearing is more impaired than it was preoperatively.

74. Which statement by the nurse most accurately explains the client's hearing loss?
[ ] **1.** The client will have a temporary hearing loss until edema and packing in the operative area are gone.
[ ] **2.** The client will have a temporary hearing loss until the nerve regenerates.
[ ] **3.** The client will have a temporary hearing loss until she is fitted with a molded plastic hearing aid.
[ ] **4.** The client will have a temporary hearing loss until the prosthesis becomes stabilized with new bone.

75. Which instruction by the nurse will best prevent dislodgment of the client's internal prosthesis following her stapedectomy?
[ ] **1.** When chewing food, keep your mouth closed.
[ ] **2.** When blowing your nose, use a paper tissue.
[ ] **3.** When sneezing, keep your mouth wide open.
[ ] **4.** When coughing, turn your head to the side.

76. The nurse correctly advises other staff assigned to care for the client postoperatively that the client is at risk for injury due to which side effect?
[ ] **1.** Fatigue
[ ] **2.** Diplopia
[ ] **3.** Vertigo
[ ] **4.** Pain

77. The nurse knows that the client who underwent a stapedectomy understands her discharge instructions when she states that she must avoid which activity for the next 6 months?
[ ] **1.** Listening to music
[ ] **2.** Flying in an airplane
[ ] **3.** Driving an automobile
[ ] **4.** Singing in the choir

The nurse is assessing a male client who was admitted to the hospital for possible Ménière's disease.

78. Which subjective symptom is the client most likely to report to the nurse?
[ ] **1.** Burning
[ ] **2.** Pressure
[ ] **3.** Vertigo
[ ] **4.** Pain

The client is told that he will undergo a caloric test.

79. Which information provided by the nurse will best prepare the client for what to expect with caloric testing?
[ ] **1.** Cold water and warm water will be instilled into each of your ears.
[ ] **2.** You will wear earphones through which sounds are transmitted.
[ ] **3.** The room will be darkened, and scalp electrodes will be attached to your head.
[ ] **4.** Your blood will be drawn from a vein and examined microscopically.

80. Which response will the nurse most likely observe during the caloric test if the client has Ménière's disease?
[ ] **1.** Onset of severe symptoms
[ ] **2.** No response or change in symptoms
[ ] **3.** Nystagmus and slight dizziness
[ ] **4.** Aphasia and loss of consciousness

The client is positively diagnosed with Ménière's disease. During rounds, the nurse observes that the client seems anxious whenever a member of the nursing staff enters his room.

81. The nurse suspects that the client's anxiety is due to fear that nursing care will intensify his symptoms. Which nursing intervention is most appropriate to add to the care plan at this time?
[ ] **1.** Let the client suggest ways to carry out his care.
[ ] **2.** Discontinue nursing care measures at this time.
[ ] **3.** Restrict care to nutrition and elimination needs only.
[ ] **4.** Carry out nursing activities quickly and efficiently.

The client asks the nurse to clarify the physician's explanation about the cause of Ménière's disease.

82. The nurse is most accurate in stating that the cause of Ménière's disease is unknown but that the symptoms are related to which disorder?
[ ] **1.** An electrolyte deficit
[ ] **2.** An excess of fluid
[ ] **3.** A vitamin deficiency
[ ] **4.** A genetic defect

83. When caring for a client with Ménière's disease, which nursing action is most helpful in preventing nausea and vomiting?
[ ] **1.** Increasing the client's intake of oral fluids
[ ] **2.** Changing the client's position frequently
[ ] **3.** Keeping the room lights dim
[ ] **4.** Avoiding jarring the bed

The client with Ménière's disease responds to conservative treatment and will be discharged today.

84. The nurse should stress to the client the importance of adhering to which dietary restriction?
[ ] **1.** Fats
[ ] **2.** Sodium
[ ] **3.** Potassium
[ ] **4.** Cholesterol

85. Which statement by the client indicates that he requires additional teaching about Ménière's disease?
[ ] **1.** "I'll feel well between attacks."
[ ] **2.** "Future attacks may last minutes or days."
[ ] **3.** "My hearing will gradually improve."
[ ] **4.** "Ménière's disease is incurable."

Nursing Care of Clients with Nasal Disorders

86. When the nurse assesses a newly admitted client, which finding is most suggestive that the client may have had a fractured nose in the past?
[ ] **1.** Multiple polyps noted on nasal mucous membranes
[ ] **2.** A red-skinned nose, unusually large and bulbous
[ ] **3.** A deviated septum to the side, narrowing one naris
[ ] **4.** Serous drainage within the nares and pharynx

An older man comes to the emergency department with a severe nosebleed.

87. Based on the following assessment findings, which finding most likely caused or contributed to the client's nosebleed?
[ ] **1.** Pulse rate of 110 beats/minute
[ ] **2.** Blood pressure of 200/104 mm Hg lying down
[ ] **3.** Temperature of 97.6° F (36.4° C) orally
[ ] **4.** Respirations of 24 breaths/minute

88. Which nursing action is best for controlling the client's nosebleed?
[ ] **1.** Have the client lie down slowly and swallow frequently.
[ ] **2.** Have the client lie down and breathe through his mouth.
[ ] **3.** Have the client lean forward and apply direct pressure to the nose.
[ ] **4.** Have the client lean forward and clench his teeth.

The client is frightened by the amount of blood that has collected on his shirt as a result of the nosebleed.

89. How can the nurse best relieve the client's fear and anxiety at this time?
[ ] **1.** Have the client recline so he will not see his clothes.
[ ] **2.** Give the client a popular magazine to read.
[ ] **3.** Replace the client's clothing with a hospital gown.
[ ] **4.** Cover the client's eyes with a bath towel.

The physician uses silver nitrate to chemically cauterize the client's nasal area to stop the nosebleed.

90. Before the client leaves the emergency department, which nursing instruction related to preventing nosebleeds is essential?
[ ] **1.** Advise the client to limit his dietary intake to fluids.
[ ] **2.** Tell the client to sleep in a recliner or with his head up.
[ ] **3.** Show the client how to take his carotid pulse at hourly intervals.
[ ] **4.** Warn him to avoid blowing his nose for several hours.

A male client consults the physician concerning nasal polyps.

91. During the initial assessment, the nurse can best assist the physician to determine the etiology of the client's problem by asking whether he has a history of which condition?
[ ] **1.** Recent nasal injury
[ ] **2.** Respiratory allergies
[ ] **3.** Previous nasal surgery
[ ] **4.** A past tonsillectomy

The client undergoes a nasal polypectomy and has nasal packing in place when he returns from surgery.

92. Besides blood on the anterior end of the packing, which other sign or symptom would suggest that the client is bleeding from the operative site?
[ ] **1.** Frequent swallowing
[ ] **2.** Impaired appetite
[ ] **3.** Hoarseness
[ ] **4.** Diminished hearing

A middle-aged woman is having a rhinoplasty procedure to improve the appearance of her nose.

93. When the nurse collects the following postoperative data, which finding is most indicative that the client requires frequent oral care?
[ ] **1.** The client says her throat is sore.
[ ] **2.** The client's dressing is bloody.
[ ] **3.** The client is slightly nauseated.
[ ] **4.** The client is mouth-breathing.

After the rhinoplasty, the client asks the nurse how she looks.

94. Which response by the nurse is best at this time?
[ ] **1.** "I'm sure you will look absolutely gorgeous."
[ ] **2.** "I didn't think you were unattractive before."
[ ] **3.** "Your face is swollen with bruises around the eyes."
[ ] **4.** "Your personality is more important than your looks."

Nursing Care of Clients with Disorders of the Skin and Related Structures

A 20-year-old man is brought to the emergency department with second- and third-degree burns covering more than 25% of his body.

95. Which immediate nursing interventions are appropriate for this client? Select all that apply.
[ ] **1.** Place ice packs on the burned areas.
[ ] **2.** Pour normal saline solution over the burned areas before dressing care.
[ ] **3.** Begin an I.V. infusion of lactated Ringer's solution.
[ ] **4.** Administer a tetanus injection.
[ ] **5.** Administer pain medication.
[ ] **6.** Administer oxygen therapy.

A nurse stops to give first aid to a female burn victim who is seen running from her home. The victim's clothing is on fire.

96. Which action is the nurse's priority?
[ ] **1.** Rub petroleum jelly into the burned areas.
[ ] **2.** Wrap the affected areas with a clean cloth.
[ ] **3.** Apply ice to the affected burned areas.
[ ] **4.** Roll the victim to smother the flames.

The nurse notes that the victim's chest and neck are burned.

97. Which nursing action is most appropriate at this time?
[ ] **1.** Obtaining the client's pulse and blood pressure
[ ] **2.** Monitoring the client for respiratory distress
[ ] **3.** Identifying the client's next of kin
[ ] **4.** Determining the extent of the burn

In the emergency department, it is determined that the burn victim has deep partial- and full-thickness burns over 35% of her upper body.

98. The nurse who documents the burn injury is accurate in identifying the full-thickness burns as those that are what in appearance?
[ ] **1.** White and leathery
[ ] **2.** Pink and blistered
[ ] **3.** Red and painful
[ ] **4.** Mottled and wet

99. Once her blood pressure is stabilized, the best way to assess the client's response to the initial burn treatment is by checking for which sign?
[ ] **1.** Normal body temperature
[ ] **2.** Minimal level of pain
[ ] **3.** Adequate urine output
[ ] **4.** Ability to perform range-of-motion exercises

The client's treatment plan includes using the open method of burn wound management.

100. It is most appropriate for the nurse to monitor a client being treated by the open method for which potential problem?
[ ] **1.** Infection
[ ] **2.** Hyperthermia
[ ] **3.** Depression
[ ] **4.** Malnutrition

The physician orders the application of mafenide (Sulfamylon) to the burn wound.

101. The nurse who applies Sulfamylon (Mafenide) understands that which is the chief disadvantage of using this drug?
[ ] **1.** Skin discoloration
[ ] **2.** Pain on application
[ ] **3.** Fluid volume deficit
[ ] **4.** Contact dermatitis

The burn wound is periodically debrided using hydrotherapy.

102. Shortly before each debridement, which nursing intervention is essential?
[ ] **1.** Keeping the client in a fasting state
[ ] **2.** Witnessing a signed consent form
[ ] **3.** Administering a prescribed analgesic
[ ] **4.** Weighing the client on a bed scale

The health care team is informed that skin autografting is planned for the burn client.

103. Which action is most appropriate to include in the postoperative care plan when a client has skin grafts?
[ ] **1.** Minimize the client's movement to prevent graft disruption.
[ ] **2.** Change the dressing over the graft every 8 hours.
[ ] **3.** Reinforce the graft dressing if drainage occurs.
[ ] **4.** Apply wet soaks to the graft every 4 hours.

Before the burn client is discharged, she is fitted for an elasticized pressure garment that covers the burned areas of skin.

104. Which statement best indicates that the client understands the purpose of wearing the pressure garment?
[ ] **1.** It prevents subsequent wound infection.
[ ] **2.** It prevents exposure to the sun.
[ ] **3.** It reduces the severity of scar formation.
[ ] **4.** It reduces the potential for social rejection.

During the nurse's initial physical assessment of an older male client who was just transferred from a nursing home, the nurse notes that the client has a stage III pressure ulcer on his left hip and sacrum.

105. Based on the nurse's understanding of the etiology of pressure ulcers, the nurse should plan for which intervention to promote the client's skin integrity?
[ ] **1.** Apply a skin-toughening agent to susceptible areas.
[ ] **2.** Massage skin areas that remain persistently red.
[ ] **3.** Keep the head of the bed elevated 30 degrees.
[ ] **4.** Reposition the client every 2 hours.

An elderly female client has been approved for admission to a long-term care facility for recuperation following open-heart surgery. The client will be discharged to the care of her daughter with whom she resides. The charge nurse receives a brief physical history that includes cardiovascular disease, recent coronary artery bypass graft surgery, rheumatoid arthritis, and a sacral pressure ulcer.

106. Prior to the client's arrival, which services should the nurse anticipate adding to the care plan? Select all that apply.
[ ] **1.** Dietary
[ ] **2.** Physical therapy
[ ] **3.** Enterostomal therapy
[ ] **4.** Psychiatric therapy
[ ] **5.** Physician consult
[ ] **6.** Occupational therapy

An elderly bedridden man is frequently found at the bottom of the bed with his feet hanging over the footboard. The nurses typically pull him up in bed and reposition him for comfort.

107. Because the immobile client slides down in bed, the nurse is correct to assess for which type of injury?

[ ] **1.** An injury resulting from continuous pressure

[ ] **2.** An injury resulting from a shearing force

[ ] **3.** A superficial skin injury from friction

[ ] **4.** A secondary injury from agitation in bed

108. To promote wound healing, which nursing intervention is best to add to the care plan of a client with a venous stasis ulcer?

[ ] **1.** Elevate the lower extremities at all times.

[ ] **2.** Keep the legs covered with warm blankets.

[ ] **3.** Assess peripheral pulse sites every shift.

[ ] **4.** Advise and assist the client to sit in a chair three times per day.

A home health nurse visits the home of a family being treated for pediculosis (head lice).

109. Which of the mother's statements indicates that she needs more teaching?

[ ] **1.** "One use of medicated shampoo eliminated the lice."

[ ] **2.** "I've washed all the bed linens in soap and hot water."

[ ] **3.** "None of my children share each other's combs."

[ ] **4.** "I hope no other classmates have acquired lice."

A biopsy reveals that a scalp lesion on a white male client is a basal cell carcinoma.

110. Which of the client's biographical data most likely contributed to developing skin cancer?

[ ] **1.** The client is a chronic cigarette smoker.

[ ] **2.** The client has male pattern baldness.

[ ] **3.** The client eats few vegetables.

[ ] **4.** The client bathes with a deodorant soap.

The nurse is instructing a client about potential skin disorders.

111. What is the most common profile of a client with malignant melanoma?

[ ] **1.** An African American client with dark skin and dark hair

[ ] **2.** A Scandinavian client with freckles and blue eyes

[ ] **3.** A Mexican client with tan skin and dark brown hair

[ ] **4.** A Caucasian client with brown hair and brown eyes

112. Which area of health teaching is essential when a female client is prescribed isotretinoin (Accutane) for treating acne vulgaris?

[ ] **1.** Breast self-examination techniques

[ ] **2.** Techniques for avoiding pregnancy

[ ] **3.** Methods for predicting ovulation

[ ] **4.** Information on preventing sexual transmission

113. What is the best nursing advice for individuals who have frequent outbreaks of tinea pedis (athlete's foot)?

[ ] **1.** Never go barefoot when outdoors.

[ ] **2.** Cut the nails straight across.

[ ] **3.** Wear different shoes each day.

[ ] **4.** Avoid wearing white cotton socks.

A client with shingles (herpes zoster) takes acyclovir (Zovirax).

114. When the client asks about the cause of shingles, the nurse answers correctly with which cause of the disease?

[ ] **1.** The reactivation of a dormant virus

[ ] **2.** A vector-borne insect such as a tick

[ ] **3.** A toxin from a bacterial infection

[ ] **4.** An antibody response to a drug allergen

115. Which health-teaching information is most appropriate for a client with a herpes simplex virus type 1 infection?

[ ] **1.** Apply petroleum jelly to the lesions to prevent spreading the virus to adjacent areas.

[ ] **2.** Use good personal hygiene to prevent spreading the virus to other body parts.

[ ] **3.** Avoid using soap and water on open lesions.

[ ] **4.** Remove the scabs daily by soaking with hot compresses.

A nurse assesses a female client with psoriasis at a dermatology clinic.

116. When examining the client's skin, which finding would the nurse expect to observe?

[ ] **1.** Weeping skin lesions on the trunk of the body.

[ ] **2.** Red skin patches covered with silvery scales.

[ ] **3.** Fluid-filled blisters surrounded by crusts.

[ ] **4.** A red rash containing raised pustules.

The client states that she is ashamed of the patches of psoriasis on her lower arms and asks, "What's causing this condition?"

117. The nurse correctly teaches the client that psoriasis is an inflammatory dermatosis that results from which skin condition?

[ ] **1.** A superficial skin infection
[ ] **2.** The effects of dermal abrasion
[ ] **3.** A proliferation of epidermal cells
[ ] **4.** An infection of the hair follicles

A nursing assistant with an allergy to latex asks the nurse for advice on carrying out standard precautions for preventing the transmission of blood-borne viruses.

118. What is the best advice the nurse can offer the nursing assistant?
[ ] **1.** "Rinse your latex gloves with running tap water before putting them on."
[ ] **2.** "Apply a petroleum ointment to both hands before putting on latex gloves."
[ ] **3.** "Don't wear gloves, but wash your hands vigorously with alcohol after client contact."
[ ] **4.** "Wear two pairs of vinyl gloves when there's a potential for contact with blood."

A man who had prolonged exposure to cold consults a nurse about first-aid measures for treating frostbite.

119. Which measure is best for the nurse to recommend?
[ ] **1.** Soak affected body parts in a warm solution that is approximately 100° F (37.8° C).
[ ] **2.** Begin the rewarming process by first applying cold skin compresses.
[ ] **3.** Apply a heating pad on the highest setting to the affected body parts.
[ ] **4.** Flood the affected skin surface with hot water at a temperature of approximately 140° F (60° C).

120. Which nursing measure is most appropriate to relieve discomfort in a client who develops pruritus?
[ ] **1.** Use hypoallergenic or glycerin soap for bathing.
[ ] **2.** Add extra wool blankets to the bedding for warmth.
[ ] **3.** Take showers rather than tub baths.
[ ] **4.** Rub the skin dry after bathing.

A nurse is working in a wound clinic and treats different types of wounds daily.

121. When developing nursing care plans, the nurse is careful to classify which type of wound as a chronic wound?
[ ] **1.** A gunshot wound with tissue damage
[ ] **2.** A slow-healing diabetic foot ulcer
[ ] **3.** A stage I pressure ulcer on the coccyx
[ ] **4.** A 7-day-old infected surgical wound

Correct Answers and Rationales

Nursing Care of Clients with Eye Disorders

1. 3. Immediate action is important when treating chemical injuries to the eyes. Therefore, it is important for the nurse to determine what treatment was given at the time of injury. This information provides a baseline for further treatment. Diluting and removing the chemical reduces the potential for corneal damage. Identifying the chemical is important; taking time to determine what, if anything, will neutralize the chemical does not compromise immediate treatment. Liability is affected if safety glasses are not worn, but the priority is treating the chemical splash if that has not already been done. It's too soon to evaluate the extent of sensory damage.
Client Needs Category—Physiological integrity
Client Needs Subcategory—Physiological adaptation

2. 1. Water is typically used in an emergency to flush the eyes and dilute the chemical. Tap water from a faucet or shower is generally available. The other chemical solutions may be appropriate depending on the specific chemical that caused the trauma, but they may need to be diluted to a specific strength to prevent additional damage to the eye. Delaying first-aid measures wastes valuable time.
Client Needs Category—Physiological integrity
Client Needs Subcategory—Physiological adaptation

3. 2. The irrigating solution is directed so that it flows from the inner canthus toward the outer canthus. This is an especially important principle to follow so that substances in one eye do not come in contact with the tissue of the other eye. It is best to instill the force of the water on the conjunctiva rather than onto the sensitive cornea, which may cause discomfort or reflex blinking. The anterior chamber is not an external eye structure. The nasolacrimal duct lies in the area of the inner canthus.
Client Needs Category—Physiological integrity
Client Needs Subcategory—Physiological adaptation

4. 2. An ophthalmologist is a physician who is licensed to diagnose and treat eye diseases and traumatic injuries. An optician fills prescriptions for corrective lenses. An optometrist tests vision and prescribes glasses or contact lenses to correct visual acuity. An orthoptist is a person who helps strengthen the extraocular muscles of the eye.
Client Needs Category—Health promotion and maintenance
Client Needs Subcategory—None

5. 4. The eyes are patched loosely with the lids closed to reduce further injury by blinking and eye movement. Instilling antibiotic ointment interferes with the medical examination, although it may be prescribed after the object is removed. Attempts to remove an embedded object are left to those with specialized medical training.

Client Needs Category—*Physiological integrity*
Client Needs Subcategory—*Physiological adaptation*

6. 3, 4, 5. The nurse should wash her hands and wear gloves to prevent the transmission of microorganisms. She should offer the client a tissue, or pad the shoulder area to absorb solution as it drains from the eye. The solution should be directed from the inner canthus to the outer canthus of the eye to prevent contaminating the unaffected eye. The solution should not be directed into the center of the eye because this can harm the cornea. The client's head should be tilted toward the affected eye to facilitate drainage and prevent contamination of the unaffected eye. The eye will remain reddened after irrigation due to the irritant nature of the chemical. In a chemical exposure, the eye should be irrigated for at least 10 minutes.

Client Needs Category—*Physiological integrity*
Client Needs Subcategory—*Physiological adaptation*

7. 2. A Snellen chart is used to test far vision. Therefore, clients stand 20′ (6 m) from the chart and are asked to read letters that progressively become smaller. Jaeger's chart is used to test near vision. Ishihara's plates are used to test color vision. A tangent screen, which is used to assess the peripheral visual field, requires the client to indicate when he sees a stimulus in his peripheral vision.

Client Needs Category—*Health promotion and maintenance*
Client Needs Subcategory—*None*

8. 4. The term for nearsightedness is myopia. Clients with myopia hold objects closer to their eyes to see them well. Presbyopia is a type of farsightedness associated with aging. It is caused by loss of elasticity in the lenses. Amblyopia is commonly referred to as lazy eye. Untreated, amblyopia results in the loss of vision in one eye from lack of use. Hyperopia is farsightedness.

Client Needs Category—*Health promotion and maintenance*
Client Needs Subcategory—*None*

9. 3. The Lions Clubs International organization has vision and hearing improvement as its major goal. Local or state chapters can provide information and assistance to those who need but cannot afford glasses, a guide dog, hearing aid, or surgery. The other organiza-

tions are both fraternal and philanthropic, but they have not named vision or hearing assistance as their projects.

Client Needs Category—*Health promotion and maintenance*
Client Needs Subcategory—*None*

10. 2. Due to an irregularly shaped cornea or lens, a person with astigmatism has unequal refraction of images on the retina. Therefore, there will be an area where objects appear more blurred or distorted (wider or taller) than they actually are. People with hyperopia see far objects more clearly. People with myopia can see near objects more clearly. No visual acuity disorder causes objects to appear unusually small.

Client Needs Category—*Physiological integrity*
Client Needs Subcategory—*Physiological adaptation*

11. 2. Glasses are washed first and wiped with a soft cloth to avoid scratching the surface with dirt and dust. Paper products should not be used for drying because they are made from wood pulp, which could scratch the lenses. Plastic lenses scratch easily. Air-drying is tedious and likely to leave the glasses streaked.

Client Needs Category—*Safe, effective care environment*
Client Needs Subcategory—*Coordinated care*

12. 2. Anxiety occurs because a person feels threatened by an unexpected or unfamiliar situation. Hearing an explanation of care beforehand prepares a person for what is about to take place. The nurse should always speak to a blind client before touching him. Shutting the door increases a client's feeling of isolation and fear that help will be unavailable. Having adequate light helps partially sighted clients, not those who cannot see.

Client Needs Category—*Psychosocial integrity*
Client Needs Subcategory—*None*

13. 1. A blind person feels safer and more secure by following the lead of someone who is sighted. This is best accomplished by having the blind person stand slightly behind and to the side while taking the sighted person's arm. Safety is a higher priority than total independence in an unfamiliar environment.

Client Needs Category—*Safe, effective care environment*
Client Needs Subcategory—*Safety and infection control*

14. 1. Using the imagery of a clock helps a blind client to locate food and feed himself. Feeding a client who has the ability to feed himself does not promote self-reliance. Ordering liquid forms of nourishment without collaborating first with the client implies that he is not capable of eating like an adult and may lower his self-esteem. Beverages in paper cups are more likely to spill during the client's attempts to eat independently and may reinforce a feeling of inadequacy.

> ***Client Needs Category**—Psychosocial integrity*
> ***Client Needs Subcategory**—None*

15. **1.** As senile cataracts form, they cause progressively diminished vision. The visual change is due to degeneration of the eye lenses as a result of aging. Fullness and ocular pain or discomfort are more likely due to trauma or an inflammatory process. Seeing flashes of light is a symptom described by someone with a detached retina.

> ***Client Needs Category**—Physiological integrity*
> ***Client Needs Subcategory**—Reduction of risk potential*

16. **3.** When the eyes of someone with cataracts are examined, the usually black pupil appears white, gray, or yellow. This is due to an opacity of the lens, which lies behind the pupil, the opening in the center of the iris. Ruptured blood vessels on the eye are associated with conditions in which the blood pressure has been suddenly elevated, such as when performing Valsalva's maneuver while vomiting or defecating. An irregularly shaped iris can be the result of surgery performed for the treatment of glaucoma. Abnormal tissue may appear as a growth on the cornea.

> ***Client Needs Category**—Physiological integrity*
> ***Client Needs Subcategory**—Physiological adaptation*

17. **1.** The time for cataract removal is left to the client. It largely depends on the person's tolerance of the condition and the degree in which vision impairment interferes with his quality of life. Cataracts are painless. The opinions of others should have no bearing on the timing of surgery. Postponing surgery until a cataract ripens is no longer considered a standard of care.

> ***Client Needs Category**—Health promotion and maintenance*
> ***Client Needs Subcategory**—None*

18. **2.** Upon reviewing the preoperative orders, it is especially important to note the discontinuation of anticoagulant therapy. This is essential to reduce the risk of retrobulbar hemorrhage. Reviewing the last dose and time of medication allows the nurse to assess if the client has withheld the medication for the appropriate amount of time. Assessing for facial lesions and right eye drainage is appropriate to document preoperatively, but they are not as critical as documenting the last dose of medication. Eyestrain is a subjective finding that may also be documented preoperatively.

> ***Client Needs Category**—Health promotion and maintenance*
> ***Client Needs Subcategory**—None*

19. **4.** Eyedrops and ointments are placed in the exposed lower conjunctival sac. By pulling downward below the eye on the lower eyelid, the sac is exposed, thus opening the conjunctival sac. If they are placed on the cornea, they may cause discomfort and reflex blinking. Medication is systemically absorbed when instilled at the inner canthus. Placing eye drops and ointments at the outer canthus makes it difficult to distribute them in the eye.

> ***Client Needs Category**—Safe, effective care environment*
> ***Client Needs Subcategory**—Safety and infection control*

20. **3.** Coughing and other activities, such as straining or squeezing the eyelids together, are avoided to prevent an increase in intraocular pressure. Raising intraocular pressure strains the delicate sutures and may dislodge an implanted intraocular lens. All other interventions are appropriate for this client.

> ***Client Needs Category**—Physiological integrity*
> ***Client Needs Subcategory**—Physiological adaptation*

21. **1.** Severe pain is an indication that intraocular hemorrhage is occurring. It is essential to report this finding to the charge nurse or surgeon immediately. Giving an analgesic will mask the symptom, thereby diminishing its significance as a serious complication. Assessing the pupils will not reveal the cause of the symptom. The pupils will most likely be dilated and not respond to light. Postoperatively, cataract clients are not positioned on their operative side.

> ***Client Needs Category**—Physiological integrity*
> ***Client Needs Subcategory**—Physiological adaptation*

22. **2.** A metal eye shield, called a *Fox shield,* is applied at night or before naps to prevent accidental injury to the operative eye. Although the shield is a mechanical barrier between the environment and the eye, its primary purpose is to prevent traumatic injury. Patching the eyes will not prevent the rapid eye movements that occur during sleep. If pupil dilation is necessary, drugs will be used to paralyze the ciliary muscle.

> ***Client Needs Category**—Health promotion and maintenance*
> ***Client Needs Subcategory**—None*

23. **1.** Bending over is contraindicated for approximately 2 weeks after eye surgery because it puts strain on the operative sutures. It is unnecessary to keep both eyes patched at all times. The client may sleep with or without a pillow, but should be instructed to sleep only on his unaffected side for about 1 week to prevent pressure on the operative eye and reduce tissue edema. External bleeding is not expected at any time postoperatively. Intraocular bleeding, indicated by sudden eye pain, is considered a complication that necessitates immediate examination.

> ***Client Needs Category***—*Health promotion and maintenance*
> ***Client Needs Subcategory***—*None*

24. **3.** People with chronic or acute glaucoma generally describe the appearance of rainbow halos or rings, particularly around lights. Other medical symptoms include optic nerve damage, visual field defects, and ocular pain. Itching and burning are most likely allergic responses. Headaches may occur when a client in need of corrective lenses strains to read. The loss of central vision is a symptom of macular degeneration.

> ***Client Needs Category***—*Physiological integrity*
> ***Client Needs Subcategory***—*Physiological adaptation*

25. **2.** The symptoms of glaucoma occur as a result of increased intraocular pressure. This condition is diagnosed using an instrument called a *tonometer*. An ophthalmoscope is used for viewing the fundus or back portion of the eye. A retinoscope is used to measure visual acuity and determine refractory errors. A speculum is an instrument that widens a cavity.

> ***Client Needs Category***—*Safe, effective care environment*
> ***Client Needs Subcategory***—*Coordinated care*

26. **1.** Chronic glaucoma causes a gradual loss of peripheral vision. If untreated, the visual field is reduced to only the image that is focused directly on the macula. Clients typically describe this as looking through a tube or tunnel. Double vision is due to neurologic diseases or a weakness in eye muscles. Bulging eyes, also called *exophthalmos*, accompanies hyperthyroidism. Inflamed eyes can be attributed to various irritating substances.

> ***Client Needs Category***—*Physiological integrity*
> ***Client Needs Subcategory***—*Physiological adaptation*

27.

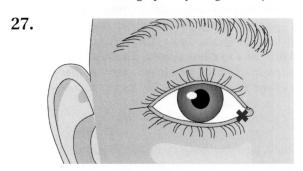

The correct procedure is to apply a thin ribbon of ointment into the conjunctival pocket beginning at the inner corner or inner canthus and moving to the outer canthus.

> ***Client Needs Category***—*Health promotion and maintenance*
> ***Client Needs Subcategory***—*None*

28. **3.** Glaucoma is a chronic disease characterized by increased intraocular pressure resulting in atrophy of the optic nerve and possibly leading to blindness. Glaucoma requires lifelong treatment unless the client is treated surgically. Hand washing and replacing the cap of the prescription container are aseptic measures that prevent the transmission of organisms within the eye. Timolol maleate (Timoptic) is a beta-adrenergic blocker that decreases aqueous humor formation without constricting the pupil.

> ***Client Needs Category***—*Health promotion and maintenance*
> ***Client Needs Subcategory***—*None*

29. **1.** Atropine sulfate (Sal-Tropine) and other anticholinergic drugs dilate the pupil. This blocks the drainage of aqueous humor. If administered, it may cause an acute attack by precipitating high intraocular pressure, which if left untreated can cause permanent blindness. Morphine sulfate (Roxanol) is an opioid analgesic. Magnesium sulfate is known as Epsom salts. Ferrous sulfate (Feosol) is an iron preparation. None of these last three substances is contraindicated for clients with glaucoma.

> ***Client Needs Category***—*Physiological integrity*
> ***Client Needs Subcategory***—*Pharmacological therapies*

30. **2.** A client who experiences an acute increase in IOP will have severe eye pain, nausea, vomiting, and loss of vision. Dangerously high ocular pressure is an emergency. A client with retinal detachment or hypertension typically describes seeing spots in the visual field. During an acute attack of angle-closure glaucoma, the pupils are widely dilated; treatment involves administering drugs that both constrict the pupils and eliminate intraocular fluid. The eyes appear normal in size even during an acute attack of angle-closure glaucoma.

> ***Client Needs Category***—*Physiological integrity*
> ***Client Needs Subcategory***—*Physiological adaptation*

31. **2, 3, 6.** In both open-angle glaucoma and angle-closure glaucoma, the visual field examination indicates a loss of vision. Also, clients with either type of glaucoma are initially treated with medication. Surgical management is required if medication therapy is unsuccessful.

In some cases, clients with open-angle glaucoma (a chronic form of the disease) are asymptomatic and may not realize they have glaucoma until undergoing a routine eye examination. However, many clients experience eye discomfort, temporary blurred vision, the appearance of halos or lights, and reduced peripheral vision. Clients with angle-closure glaucoma (an acute condition also known as *narrow-angle glaucoma*) experience symptoms suddenly. The eyes become rock hard and painful, and nausea and vomiting may occur. Each subsequent attack harms the eye.

Client Needs Category—Physiological integrity
Client Needs Subcategory—Physiological adaptation

32. **4.** An iridectomy involves removing a piece of the iris to allow aqueous humor to flow from the posterior chamber into the anterior chamber and out Schlemm's canal. Intense heat is used to create this opening for drainage. The iris no longer appears perfectly round postoperatively; the missing section appears black.
Client Needs Category—Physiological integrity
Client Needs Subcategory—None

33. **2.** Retinal detachment, the separation of retinal pigment epithelium from the sensory layer, has multiple etiologies. Common causes include trauma (such as occurs with a fall or a blow to the head), myopia, and degenerative changes. Aging is a factor, but the most common period for retinal detachment is between ages 50 and 60. There is no causal relationship between retinal detachment and infection or allergies.
Client Needs Category—Physiological integrity
Client Needs Subcategory—Reduction of risk potential

34. **3.** The purpose for patching the eyes of a client with a detached retina is to keep the eyes at rest; therefore, patches are applied to both eyes with the eyelids closed. Keeping the eyelids closed also protects them from contact with dust or fibers and prevents the eyes from becoming dry because blinking is difficult once the eyes are patched. Light is not necessarily harmful, but it may cause the client to look about when he should be resting his eyes. Gravity rather than pressure has some therapeutic value when treating a detached retina. Patching the eyes but facilitating vision is a contradiction in therapeutic principles.
Client Needs Category—Physiological integrity
Client Needs Subcategory—Reduction of risk potential

35. **2.** It is important for the nurse to indicate when she is leaving because the client whose eyes are patched has no visual cue as to whether the nurse is still in the room. The client would find it frustrating and embarrassing to carry on a conversation if no one is there to respond to him. Straightening the client's linens, offering a back rub, and sharing current events are offerings of kindness and good nursing care but do not specifically help to maintain the client's dignity.
Client Needs Category—Psychosocial integrity
Client Needs Subcategory—None

36. **1.** Bed rest and bilateral patching is a conservative treatment that relies on the principle of gravity to help reattach the separated retina. This approach is commonly tried before surgical alternatives are considered. Explaining the purpose of bed rest may help the client to comply with the prescribed therapy. Asking whether the client wants to be permanently blind may heighten his anxiety. Although sedatives are sometimes prescribed, this situation does not warrant the added risks caused by sedation. Responding in a superficial, belittling manner, as in the last example, implies that the client's question is frivolous.
Client Needs Category—Psychosocial integrity
Client Needs Subcategory—None

37. **2.** Scleral buckling is a surgical procedure that shortens the sclera and allows contact between the choroid and the retina, thereby repairing a detached retina. An increase in intraocular pressure, which occurs with vomiting, could damage the surgical site; therefore, vomiting requires prompt treatment. The client requires an antiemetic; if one was not ordered, the nurse must notify the charge nurse or physician immediately. Pain is expected after surgery for a detached retina. Although pain causes discomfort, its treatment should not affect the outcome of the surgical procedure. Anxiety and boredom are not physiological problems and therefore do not rank as high on the list of priorities.
Client Needs Category—Physiological integrity
Client Needs Subcategory—Reduction of risk potential

38. **3.** Radial keratotomy is performed to reshape the cornea so visual images converge directly on the retina. If the procedure is successful, the client should no longer require corrective lenses. Radial keratotomy does not improve night vision, correct color blindness, or facilitate binocular vision.
Client Needs Category—Physiological integrity
Client Needs Subcategory—Physiological adaptation

39. **1.** A client with pinkeye, which is a common name for conjunctivitis, will have an obviously inflamed conjunctiva, sticky or crusty drainage that collects on the lid, itching or burning of the eyes, and possible edema of the eyelid. The disorder does not affect pupil response. The eyelid may be swollen, but the eye itself should not protrude. Tearing may be excessive.
Client Needs Category—Physiological integrity
Client Needs Subcategory—Physiological adaptation

40. **3.** Using individual bath linen and performing frequent hand washing are techniques for preventing the transmission of infectious microorganisms present in the inflammatory secretions. Eating a nutritious diet and wearing sunglasses to filter ultraviolet light are healthful behaviors, but they are unrelated to the client's disorder. The use of aspirin is not contraindicated; in fact, a mild analgesic may relieve some of the client's discomfort.
Client Needs Category—Health promotion and maintenance
Client Needs Subcategory—None

41. **4.** Fluorescein is a tissue-staining substance that is applied topically to assess the condition of the cornea, including the presence of foreign bodies or lesions. Povidone-iodine (Betadine) and gentian violet are used for their antimicrobial properties rather than for diagnostic purposes. Methylene blue is used to stain pathology slides.
> *Client Needs Category—Physiological integrity*
> *Client Needs Subcategory—Physiological adaptation*

42. **3.** Having lost macular function, which is the point where light rays converge to provide the clearest and most distinct visual information, clients are left with what appears to them as a bull's-eye visual defect. Peripheral vision remains, but it is insufficient to read or perform other activities that require acute vision.
> *Client Needs Category—Physiological integrity*
> *Client Needs Subcategory—None*

43. **2.** Clients with diabetes mellitus are at risk for developing vascular pathology in the retina. Their retinal blood vessels tend to weaken and bleed. Loss of vision is delayed or prevented when weakened and bleeding retinal blood vessels are treated early with photocoagulation using a laser or having a vitrectomy performed. Clients who take aspirin, have lactose intolerance, or use potassium supplements are not at any higher risk for ophthalmologic complications than the general population.
> *Client Needs Category—Health promotion and maintenance*
> *Client Needs Subcategory—None*

44. **3.** Following an enucleation, clients are taught how to remove, cleanse, and replace the shell-shaped prosthetic eye. The prosthetic eye is only cosmetic, not functional. A conformer, which is a round implant, is inserted during surgery to maintain the shape of the eye. The conformer remains permanently in place; the prosthetic eye is not inserted until healing takes place, which typically is approximately 4 to 6 weeks postoperatively.
> *Client Needs Category—Health promotion and maintenance*
> *Client Needs Subcategory—None*

45. **2.** Signs of corneal transplant rejection include redness, loss of vision, and sensitivity to light. Tearing, blinking, and itching would require medical assessment; however, they are not the usual indications of tissue rejection.
> *Client Needs Category—Physiological integrity*
> *Client Needs Subcategory—Reduction of risk potential*

Nursing Care of Clients with Disorders of Accessory Eye Structures

46. **4.** Incomplete closure of the eyelids leads to dry eyes. The tarsal muscles within the lids are generally atonic due to age; consequently, lid spasms are unlikely. Topical medications are used to treat the symptoms, but surgery provides a more permanent cosmetic and functional solution. Neither double vision nor light sensitivity is a common manifestation of structural disorders of the lids.
> *Client Needs Category—Physiological integrity*
> *Client Needs Subcategory—Physiological adaptation*

47. **1.** Blepharitis, an inflammation of the eyelid margin, is commonly associated with excessive oiliness of the skin, face, and scalp. In most cases, more frequent washing of the face and hair relieves the symptoms. In chronic or severe conditions, clients improve with the additional use of a topical antibiotic ointment. Modifying fluid and food intake and reducing eyestrain throughout the day are unlikely to prove therapeutic in managing the signs and symptoms of blepharitis.
> *Client Needs Category—Physiological integrity*
> *Client Needs Subcategory—Physiological adaptation*

48. **2.** Warm, moist heat improves circulation to the area that is inflamed and swollen. Vasodilation relieves the edema and promotes a reduction in exudate via absorption or phagocytosis. Incision and drainage may become necessary, but a physician should do this, not the client. Covering the lesion disguises the appearance of the stye, but it does not provide any therapeutic benefit.
> *Client Needs Category—Physiological integrity*
> *Client Needs Subcategory—None*

49. **3.** A chalazion and other eyelid disorders tend to be minor. If gentle massage fails to relieve the obstruction, office surgery is performed to excise the cystlike growth of tissue. A chalazion is more likely to produce a sensation of pressure than of pain. The eyelashes are lost from seborrheic blepharitis, not a chalazion. Blindness is not commonly associated with a chalazion.
> *Client Needs Category—Physiological integrity*
> *Client Needs Subcategory—Reduction of risk potential*

Nursing Care of Clients with Ear Disorders

50. **3.** Musicians and others who are exposed to excessively loud sounds without ear protection can acquire sensorineural hearing loss. There is no significant evidence that occupations involving computer programming, using the telephone, or accounting are associated with impaired hearing.

***Client Needs Category**—Physiological integrity*
***Client Needs Subcategory**—Basic care and comfort*

51. 1. The accumulation of normal cerumen is best removed by washing the ears with soapy water and a soft cloth. Hard and sharp objects can injure the ear canal or tympanic membrane. A medical referral is appropriate only if the cerumen is excessively hard or impacted.
   ***Client Needs Category**—Health promotion and maintenance*
   ***Client Needs Subcategory**—None*

52. 2. A tuning fork is used to test for conductive and sensorineural hearing loss. Weber's test is performed by striking the tuning fork and placing it centrally on the forehead. The Rinne test is performed by striking the tuning fork and placing it on the mastoid bone and beside the ear. An otoscope is used to inspect the physical structures in the external ear. A reflex hammer is used to test deep tendon responses. A stethoscope is used to auscultate body sounds.
   ***Client Needs Category**—Health promotion and maintenance*
   ***Client Needs Subcategory**—None*

53. 4. Tinnitus, ringing or buzzing in the ears, is a common symptom experienced by people who take repeated, high dosages of aspirin. Although tinnitus is associated with many ear disorders and a few occupations, the other questions posed by the nurse do not necessarily help to establish a cause-and-effect relationship with the client's symptom.
   ***Client Needs Category**—Physiological integrity*
   ***Client Needs Subcategory**—Reduction of risk potential*

54. 1. Feedback, a loud shrill noise, occurs when a hearing aid is positioned incorrectly within the ear. Cleaning, replacing the battery, and regulating the volume are important considerations for the client with a hearing aid, but they do not affect feedback.
   ***Client Needs Category**—Health promotion and maintenance*
   ***Client Needs Subcategory**—None*

55. 3. The aminoglycoside family of antibiotics, of which gentamicin sulfate (Garamycin) is one example, is ototoxic and nephrotoxic. Beta-adrenergic blockers cause vertigo but do not affect hearing acuity. Neither nonsteroidal anti-inflammatory drugs nor H_2 antagonists are known to be ototoxic.
   ***Client Needs Category**—Physiological integrity*
   ***Client Needs Subcategory**—Pharmacological therapies*

56. 1. The correct technique for straightening the ear canal of an adult is to pull the ear upward and backward. For a child, the ear is pulled downward and backward.
   ***Client Needs Category**—Physiological integrity*
   ***Client Needs Subcategory**—Pharmacological therapies*

57. 1. Maintaining a position, such as the head tilted to the side or a side-lying position, facilitates the movement of the medication to the lowest area of the ear canal. Cotton is loosely inserted within the ear to collect drainage and any excess volume of medication. The eustachian tube does connect the middle ear with the pharynx. However, if the tympanic membrane is intact, blowing the nose will not displace the medication. The temperature of beverages does not affect the instillation of eardrops.
   ***Client Needs Category**—Physiological integrity*
   ***Client Needs Subcategory**—Pharmacological therapies*

58. 4. Swabbing the earlobes mechanically removes microorganisms from the area. The use of alcohol, which is an antimicrobial agent, inhibits the growth of pathogens that remain. Using quality metal, such as 14-karat gold, tends to reduce local inflammation due to hypersensitivity. Leaving the earrings in place temporarily and turning them facilitates the formation of a well-healed channel.
   ***Client Needs Category**—Health promotion and maintenance*
   ***Client Needs Subcategory**—None*

59. 1. The presence of drainage, called *otorrhea*, is most suggestive that an inflammatory process is the underlying problem. Because the drainage is foul smelling, the inflammation is most likely due to a pathogen. Hearing is diminished from swelling and drainage that block the transmission of sound on air currents, but other preinfectious factors can also cause a loss of hearing. Although trauma can rupture the eardrum, the client's eardrum is intact in this situation. Injuring the head is unlikely related to an infection. Enlarged lymph nodes are indicative of a systemic inner ear infection.
   ***Client Needs Category**—Physiological integrity*
   ***Client Needs Subcategory**—Physiological adaptation*

60. 1. Organisms travel more easily through a pathway that is short and straight, which is the case in infants and children. With growth, the ear canal changes to a 45-degree angle. This natural curve provides a barrier against ascending pathogens.
   ***Client Needs Category**—Health promotion and maintenance*
   ***Client Needs Subcategory**—None*

61.

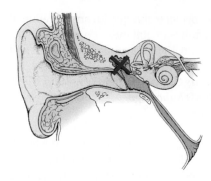

The middle ear, which is the client's site of infection, is a small, air-filled cavity in the temporal bone. The eustachian tube extends from the floor of the middle ear to the pharynx and is lined with mucous membrane. A chain of three small bones—the malleus, the incus, and the stapes—stretches across the middle ear cavity from the tympanic membrane to the oval window.

> *Client Needs Category*—*Physiological integrity*
> *Client Needs Subcategory*—*Physiological adaptation*

62. **4.** Antibiotic efficacy is most evident when the client's ear discomfort is relieved. The inflamed area in the middle ear is beyond the reach of the fingers; therefore, assessing the temperature of the tissue by touch is impossible. Tinnitus, or disturbing sounds, is not generally a problem for a person during the acute phase of a middle-ear infection. Watery or purulent drainage is an indication that the eardrum is perforated.

> *Client Needs Category*—*Physiological integrity*
> *Client Needs Subcategory*—*Pharmacological therapies*

63. **4.** Signs of labyrinthitis (inflammation of the labyrinth of the inner ear) include dizziness, nausea, vomiting, and nystagmus. Headaches indicate the infection has extended to the meningeal area of the brain. Sore throat and nasal congestion are more likely caused by the primary upper respiratory infection, which commonly precedes a middle-ear infection.

> *Client Needs Category*—*Physiological integrity*
> *Client Needs Subcategory*—*Physiological adaptation*

64. **2.** A *myringotomy*, which is the term for incising the tympanic membrane or eardrum, provides a pathway for drainage from the middle ear. As the exudate drains, the client's discomfort is reduced. A surgical incision is preferable to the spontaneous rupture of the eardrum because a surgical incision heals better. Although hearing may be permanently diminished, it is less affected with an incised tympanic membrane. Systemic antibiotics rather than topical drugs are more effective in treating a middle-ear infection. Incising the eardrum is not done to preserve motion of the ossicles in the middle ear.

> *Client Needs Category*—*Physiological integrity*
> *Client Needs Subcategory*—*Physiological adaptation*

65. **2.** Loosely packed cotton is more likely to absorb drainage than tightly packed cotton. The client should be instructed to follow a regular schedule for replacing the cotton pledget when it is moist, not totally saturated. The ear canal is generally cleaned before inserting the dry cotton.

> *Client Needs Category*—*Health promotion and maintenance*
> *Client Needs Subcategory*—*None*

66. **4.** Otosclerosis is the result of bony overgrowth of the stapes, a bone of the middle ear, and a common cause of hearing impairments in adults. Although the cause of otosclerosis is unknown, most of those affected have a family history of this condition. The onset of this disorder usually becomes apparent when clients are in their 20s or 30s. High fever and removal of the tonsils or adenoids have no relationship to the development of otosclerosis.

> *Client Needs Category*—*Physiological integrity*
> *Client Needs Subcategory*—*Physiological adaptation*

67. **1.** A conductive hearing loss occurs when there is a barrier in the transmission of vibrating sound waves from the external and middle ear to the inner ear. Common causes of conductive hearing loss include otosclerosis, otitis media, and a ruptured tympanic membrane. The other options all describe the causes of sensorineural hearing loss.

> *Client Needs Category*—*Physiological integrity*
> *Client Needs Subcategory*—*Physiological adaptation*

68. **1.** Indicating an ability to understand staff is a measurable, client-centered goal. Accomplishing this goal indicates that the approaches used by the staff to communicate with the hearing-impaired client are effective. The goal should not indicate what the nursing team hopes to accomplish. The client with normal speech but decreased hearing does not have difficulty verbally communicating to staff.

> *Client Needs Category*—*Safe, effective care environment*
> *Client Needs Subcategory*—*Coordinated care*

69. **2.** It is best to face a hearing-impaired client so that lip movements and facial expressions are seen because most hearing-impaired persons learn to adapt by lip reading or speech reading. Speaking into the client's ear distorts the words and masks the visual cues. Dropping the voice causes some of the words to be missed. Raising or lowering the voice pitch helps persons with hearing loss in one or the other vocal registers. High tones are generally more difficult to hear.

> *Client Needs Category*—*Physiological integrity*
> *Client Needs Subcategory*—*Basic care and comfort*

70. 1. As long as the client is literate and not visually impaired, reading a descriptive pamphlet is an appropriate alternative. Another stapedectomy client should not be the primary resource for explaining technical information. The client with otosclerosis probably is not so profoundly deaf that she uses sign language. Writing short sentences or words is appropriate, but writing lengthy technical information is too tedious and time-consuming.
Client Needs Category—Physiological integrity
Client Needs Subcategory—Physiological adaptation

71. 2. Encouraging the client to discuss her feelings is therapeutic. Endorsing or defending the surgeon's expertise will not relieve the client's fears about the risks she faces. Giving advice, offering a reassuring cliché, and changing the subject are nontherapeutic communication techniques.
Client Needs Category—Psychosocial integrity
Client Needs Subcategory—None

72. 2. The facial nerve, which is cranial nerve VII, is assessed by having the client smile or raise her eyebrows. Facial asymmetry suggests damage to this nerve. By asking the client to identify familiar odors, the olfactory nerve is assessed. By having the client stick out her tongue, the hypoglossal nerve is tested. By determining if the client can see, the optic nerve is tested.
Client Needs Category—Physiological integrity
Client Needs Subcategory—None

73. 1. Keeping the client flat with the head of the bed elevated and the operative ear up helps to maintain the placement of the prosthetic stapes and reduce the occurrence of vertigo. The client should not lie on the operative ear but should be positioned with the head resting on the nonoperative ear. None of the other positional choices accomplishes this goal.
Client Needs Category—Physiological integrity
Client Needs Subcategory—Reduction of risk potential

74. 1. Both rebound swelling and packing within the ear contribute to a diminished hearing acuity after a stapedectomy. This setback is only temporary and eventually subsides in the absence of any complications. The success of the surgery is evident in a matter of weeks. If the surgery is successful, the client will not need a hearing aid. The prosthetic stapes is secured to the incus by a fine wire loop or hook; it moves without any bone formation around it.
Client Needs Category—Physiological integrity
Client Needs Subcategory—Physiological adaptation

75. 3. To avoid displacing the device that replaces the stapes, the client should keep her mouth widely open when a sneeze is unavoidable. Aesthetically, chewing food with a closed mouth shows good etiquette. To prevent transmitting infectious organisms, it is best to enclose the exudate from the nose in a paper tissue and dispose of it in a lined refuse container. Turning the head also reduces the potential for droplet transmission of pathogens.
Client Needs Category—Health promotion and maintenance
Client Needs Subcategory—None

76. 3. Stapedectomy clients commonly experience vertigo due to a loss of perilymph, or labyrinthitis. To prevent injury, the nurse should ensure that the client's bedside rails are kept raised and that the client is assisted with ambulation. The client undergoing stapedectomy is generally young or middle-aged and unlikely to feel exceptionally tired. Diplopia is not associated with the effects of this surgery. Although some discomfort is anticipated following surgery, this is not generally considered a major postoperative problem that predisposes the client to injury.
Client Needs Category—Safe, effective care environment
Client Needs Subcategory—Coordinated care

77. 2. Flying in an airplane is temporarily contraindicated after a stapedectomy because of the potential damaging effects that may occur with sudden changes in air pressure. For the same reason, scuba diving is also avoided. None of the other activities are specifically contraindicated for a client who has had a stapedectomy.
Client Needs Category—Evaluation
Client Needs Subcategory—Health promotion and maintenance

78. 3. The major symptom of Ménière's disease is severe vertigo. Typically, the client will describe this as a sensation of seeing and feeling motion or rotation, not just a case of dizziness. Ménière's disease encompasses a group of symptoms that includes progressive deafness, ringing in the ears, dizziness and a feeling of pressure or fullness in the ears. The other symptoms are unrelated to Ménière's disease.
Client Needs Category—Physiological integrity
Client Needs Subcategory—Physiological adaptation

79. 1. A caloric test, used to assess vestibular function, involves instilling cold and warm solutions separately into each ear. Warm water elicits rotatory nystagmus. Cold water elicits nystagmus on the opposite side. An audiometric test requires headphones. Electrodes are used for electroencephalography and electronystagmography. A specimen of blood is not used in a caloric test.
Client Needs Category—Physiological integrity
Client Needs Subcategory—None

80. **1.** A client with Ménière's disease develops a sudden onset of severe symptoms, such as vertigo, nausea, vomiting, and tinnitus, during a caloric test. No response to the instillation of warm or cold solution within the ear indicates an auditory nerve tumor. People without Ménière's disease experience slight dizziness and nystagmus during a caloric test. Aphasia and loss of consciousness are unrelated to the mechanics or physiology of a caloric test.
>*Client Needs Category*—*Physiological integrity*
>*Client Needs Subcategory*—*Physiological adaptation*

81. **1.** Allowing the client to participate in the planning and implementation of nursing activities maintains an independent locus of control. The client, more than anyone, knows what movement will cause him the least discomfort. Discontinuing or restricting nursing activities does not reflect a high standard of care. Performing nursing activities quickly heightens the client's anxiety because unexpected movements can induce or aggravate his symptoms.
>*Client Needs Category*—*Psychosocial integrity*
>*Client Needs Subcategory*—*None*

82. **2.** Ménière's disease seems to be related to an increase in endolymphatic fluid within the spaces of the labyrinth in the inner ear. Electrolyte deficits, vitamin deficiencies, and genetics do not play a role in the development of Ménière's disease.
>*Client Needs Category*—*Physiological integrity*
>*Client Needs Subcategory*—*Physiological adaptation*

83. **4.** Sudden movement of the client's head or sudden body movements can precipitate an attack that includes nausea and vomiting. Decreasing the client's fluid intake is beneficial. Frequent changing of positions should be avoided. The intensity of room lights is not a factor in controlling the symptoms of Ménière's disease.
>*Client Needs Category*—*Physiological integrity*
>*Client Needs Subcategory*—*Reduction of risk potential*

84. **2.** Most clients with Ménière's disease can be successfully treated with diet and medication therapy. Many clients can control their symptoms by avoiding sodium and adhering to a low-sodium diet. The amount of sodium is one of the many factors that regulate the balance of fluid within the body. Sodium and fluid retention disrupts the delicate balance between endolymph and perilymph in the inner ear. Limiting the amount of fat intake and cholesterol in the diet is a good health practice but not essential with Ménière's disease. Strict potassium requirements are unnecessary.
>*Client Needs Category*—*Physiological integrity*
>*Client Needs Subcategory*—*Reduction of risk potential*

85. **3.** Hearing loss associated with Ménière's disease becomes progressively worse with each subsequent attack. The period of time that symptoms last is unpredictable. Between attacks, the client generally resumes normal activities and feelings of wellness. Surgery is performed in advanced cases to eliminate the vertigo, nausea, and vomiting. However, permanent deafness is a consequence of most surgical procedures.
>*Client Needs Category*—*Physiological integrity*
>*Client Needs Subcategory*—*Physiological adaptation*

Nursing Care of Clients with Nasal Disorders

86. **3.** Without proper medical attention, fractures and other nose injuries can bend the septum to one side or the other. Nasal polyps are generally due to chronic inflammation. An enlarged, red, bulbous nose may be from a skin condition such as acne rosacea. Serous drainage indicates concurrent irritation from an allergen or pathogen.
>*Client Needs Category*—*Physiological integrity*
>*Client Needs Subcategory*—*Physiological adaptation*

87. **2.** Nosebleeds occur when the arterial blood pressure becomes high. The hypertension causes capillaries in the nasal membrane to rupture and bleed. Therefore, a pulse rate of 110 beats/minute is the result, not the cause, of blood loss. Anxiety causes a transient elevation in both the heart and respiratory rate. An oral temperature of 97.6° F (36.4° C) is slightly lower than normal. However, a low temperature is not likely to cause the nosebleed.
>*Client Needs Category*—*Physiological integrity*
>*Client Needs Subcategory*—*Physiological adaptation*

88. **3.** The best first-aid measure for controlling a nosebleed is to apply direct pressure. Leaning forward allows blood to drain from the nose rather than down the nasopharynx into the throat. An upright position tends to lower the blood pressure. Swallowing, mouth breathing, and teeth clenching do not control bleeding.
>*Client Needs Category*—*Physiological integrity*
>*Client Needs Subcategory*—*Physiological adaptation*

89. **3.** Fear is an emotional response to a real or imagined danger. It occurs when a person feels helpless or powerless to control the situation in which he is involved. Eliminating or reducing the fear-provoking stimulus—in this case the bloody clothing—will probably diminish his fear. Having the client recline is inappropriate because the first-aid treatment for a nosebleed involves having the client lean forward. A towel is unlikely to stay in place unless the client is reclining. An anxious or fearful person probably will not be able to concentrate on reading.

Client Needs Category—*Psychosocial integrity*
Client Needs Subcategory—*None*

90. **4.** Blowing the nose retraumatizes the ruptured nasal capillaries, causing bleeding to recur. There is no need to restrict fluid intake. Taking the carotid pulse is unnecessary. Being told to keep his head up to help lower blood pressure is helpful, but it is not the most essential information the client requires in this situation.

> *Client Needs Category*—*Physiological integrity*
> *Client Needs Subcategory*—*Reduction of risk potential*

91. **2.** Nasal polyps are associated with chronic inflammation of the nasopharynx, which is caused by inhalant allergies or upper respiratory infections. Nasal injuries are more correlated with a deviated septum. A history of nasal surgery or tonsillectomy is incidental to the development of nasal polyps.

> *Client Needs Category*—*Physiological integrity*
> *Client Needs Subcategory*—*Physiological adaptation*

92. **1.** Swallowing at frequent intervals is common when blood accumulates posteriorly in the pharynx. The client feels the need to continue to swallow as the blood accumulates. Impaired appetite, hoarseness, and diminished hearing are abnormal assessment findings, but they are not directly related to nasal bleeding.

> *Client Needs Category*—*Physiological integrity*
> *Client Needs Subcategory*—*Reduction of risk potential*

93. **4.** Breathing through the mouth is drying to the oral mucous membranes. Frequent mouth care, including moistening the area with swabs, is necessary. A sore throat is relieved by offering cool or warm liquids or by using a medicated gargle. A bloody dressing indicates a need to change or reinforce the dressing. Many clients feel nauseated from swallowing blood; however, mouth care will not relieve the client's discomfort.

> *Client Needs Category*—*Physiological integrity*
> *Client Needs Subcategory*—*Physiological adaptation*

94. **3.** Remaining objective and limiting the response to a description of the client's external appearance is the most appropriate approach. Predicting that the client will look gorgeous is considered false reassurance because body image is a personal concept. The client most likely felt unattractive before the surgery; contradicting her opinion might cause her to mistrust the nurse. Telling the client that personality is more important also expresses the nurse's subjective opinion. It borders on giving advice, which is a nontherapeutic communication technique.

> *Client Needs Category*—*Psychosocial integrity*
> *Client Needs Subcategory*—*None*

Nursing Care of Clients with Disorders of the Skin and Related Structures

95. **3, 4, 5, 6.** When a client with a burn arrives in the emergency department, the medical team works quickly to stabilize the body systems and assess the extent of the injury. Team members ensure adequate ventilation by administering oxygen or inserting an endotracheal tube. Fluid resuscitation with lactated Ringer's solution and administration of pain medication is completed via an I.V. infusion. The client also receives a tetanus injection and antibiotics at this time. Ice and normal saline solution would not be placed on the wound because they may lead to hypothermia or further tissue damage.

> *Client Needs Category*—*Physiological integrity*
> *Client Needs Subcategory*—*Physiological adaptation*

96. **4.** The first response in helping a victim who is in flames is to smother the fire either by rolling the victim on the ground or covering the flames with a blanket or some other dense material. Nothing but cool water is applied to the skin until the physician examines the victim. A clean cloth is used to cover the burn wound, but this would be done only after the flames are under control. The use of ice is contraindicated because it causes hypothermia or further thermal injury to the burned tissue.

> *Client Needs Category*—*Physiological integrity*
> *Client Needs Subcategory*—*Reduction of risk potential*

97. **2.** Whenever a burn involves the head, neck, or chest, establishing and maintaining a patent airway is vitally important. Many burn victims, regardless of the area that is burned, inhale smoke, which irritates the air passages and results in increased respiratory secretions and edema of the air passages. Taking the pulse and blood pressure is important, but this assessment can be delayed until determining that the airway is patent. Identifying the next of kin and determining the extent of burns are less important than ensuring the victim can breathe.

> *Client Needs Category*—*Physiological integrity*
> *Client Needs Subcategory*—*Physiological adaptation*

98. **1.** Full-thickness burns include the epidermis, dermis, and subcutaneous layers of skin. Previously identified as third- or fourth-degree burns, these burns are generally white, cherry red, tan, dark brown, or black. The tissue is generally leathery and painless. Partial-thickness burns are pink to rosy red, dull white or tan, blistered, and painful.

> *Client Needs Category*—*Physiological integrity*
> *Client Needs Subcategory*—*Physiological adaptation*

99. 3. The first major complication of a burn is hypovolemic shock. Therefore, urine output is monitored hourly to evaluate the effectiveness of fluid replacement therapy. Burn clients initially receive massive volumes of fluid to replace what is lost from the intracellular space and what is transferred from the intravascular space to the interstitial space. Although body temperature is difficult to regulate during the initial stages after a burn injury, the client's temperature must be monitored to track the course of infection that typically occurs in later phases of burn management. Clients with full-thickness burns do not experience as much pain as those with partial-thickness burns over a similar percentage of body surface area. Range of motion is not an initial concern but becomes a priority when contractures develop during the healing phases of burn care.
> ***Client Needs Category***—*Physiological integrity*
> ***Client Needs Subcategory***—*Physiological adaptation*

100. 1. Infection is a common complication when the burn wound is exposed to microorganisms in the environment and those present and residing in the client's own tissues, secretions, and excretions. Hypothermia, rather than hyperthermia, occurs due to leaving the burn wound undressed. Depression about the potential change in body image and malnutrition occur regardless of the method used to manage the burn wound.
> ***Client Needs Category***—*Physiological integrity*
> ***Client Needs Subcategory***—*Reduction of risk potential*

101. 2. Mafenide (Sulfamylon) is an excellent antimicrobial for preventing and treating postburn wound infections. However, the pain it causes on application is an obvious disadvantage. Another topical antimicrobial, silver sulfadiazine (Silvadene), does not cause pain but can cause a rash. Silver nitrate, which is used for burn wound management, stains tissue and everything else it contacts. It also causes stinging on application and increases the potential for electrolyte imbalance.
> ***Client Needs Category***—*Physiological integrity*
> ***Client Needs Subcategory***—*Pharmacological therapies*

102. 3. Because debridement causes pain, it is essential to administer an analgesic no sooner than 30 minutes before the procedure. In the case of hydrotherapy when a whirlpool is used, the client does not need to refrain from ingesting food or fluids. If the client requires surgical debridement under anesthesia, a consent form must be obtained and the client needs to fast.
> ***Client Needs Category***—*Physiological integrity*
> ***Client Needs Subcategory***—*Physiological adaptation*

103. 1. Minimal movement of the grafted area is best for approximately 48 hours to ensure that the graft is not displaced. Disturbance of the graft may result in such problems as failure of the graft to adhere to underlying tissues, infection, and tissue necrosis. The graft dressing is only changed or reinforced by the physician. Wet soaks are not applied to the graft because this disturbs the contact between the graft and underlying tissues.
> ***Client Needs Category***—*Physiological integrity*
> ***Client Needs Subcategory***—*Physiological adaptation*

104. 3. Pressure garments are worn for as long as 2 years to promote a smooth appearance to the burn scar and help prevent or reduce wound contractures. Pressure garments are not used for preventing wound infection, exposure to sunlight, or social rejection, although the latter two are considered secondary benefits.
> ***Client Needs Category***—*Health promotion and maintenance*
> ***Client Needs Subcategory***—*None*

105. 4. Repositioning the client every 2 hours is the best method of restoring or maintaining skin integrity. Application of a skin-toughening agent would be ineffective if the client's position is not changed at frequent intervals. Keeping the head of the bed elevated is of no value in preventing skin breakdown; a sitting position creates a shearing force that contributes to skin impairment. Massaging skin that does not blanch when pressure is relieved is contraindicated because it causes further skin disruption and damage.
> ***Client Needs Category***—*Physiological integrity*
> ***Client Needs Subcategory***—*Reduction of risk potential*

106. 1, 2, 3, 5, 6. A dietary consult would be helpful to increase protein in the diet for wound healing for both the sacral pressure ulcer and the coronary artery bypass graft incision. Physical therapy and occupational therapy promote movement and activity, thereby eliminating continuous pressure on the sacral area and helping the client to return to her presurgical status more quickly. An enterostomal therapist, a specialist in skin and wound care, can be helpful in planning treatment for her pressure ulcer. Physician consultations are necessary as a follow-up to surgery and to monitor the client's general health and recovery. Nothing in the scenario provided indicates that the client requires psychiatric services.
> ***Client Needs Category***—*Safe, effective care environment*
> ***Client Needs Subcategory***—*Coordinated care*

107. 2. Although all of the options could be a factor in causing injury to the client, sliding down in bed most commonly results in shearing of soft tissues, resulting in skin impairment.

Client Needs Category—*Physiological integrity*
Client Needs Subcategory—*Reduction of risk potential*

108. **1.** Interventions to prevent pooling and congestion of blood are a priority when planning the nursing care of a client with a venous stasis ulcer. Therefore, elevating the legs is best among the choices for promoting venous circulation. Covering the legs with warm blankets promotes warmth and vasodilation, but the fibers may adhere to the ulcer and disrupt wound healing when removed. A bed cradle is used to keep the legs covered and warm while preventing contact between the skin and woven fabrics. Assessing arterial circulation does not promote venous circulation. Sitting contributes to venous congestion if the legs are not elevated.
Client Needs Category—*Physiological integrity*
Client Needs Subcategory—*Physiological adaptation*

109. **1.** At least two applications of a shampoo containing a pediculicide, such as lindane (gamma benzene hexachloride), are necessary to eradicate lice. The first application kills the adult lice, but a subsequent treatment is necessary to kill the lice that hatch from nits that adhere to the hair. As long as nits are seen, shampooing must be repeated.
Client Needs Category—*Health promotion and maintenance*
Client Needs Subcategory—*None*

110. **2.** Male pattern baldness places fair-skinned individuals at risk for chronic exposure to ultraviolet radiation. Smoking cigarettes is a risk factor for other types of cancer. Dark green and yellow vegetables contain beta-carotene, which is considered an antioxidant that contributes to cellular integrity; avoiding them is not as strongly a suggestive link to skin cancer as sun exposure. Although exposure to chemicals is a factor in causing cancer, deodorant soap is considered a safe product.
Client Needs Category—*Physiological integrity*
Client Needs Subcategory—*None*

111. **2.** Malignant melanoma is a malignant, darkly pigmented mole or tumor of the skin. The common risk factors for malignant melanoma include fair-skinned or freckled, blue-eyed, light-haired clients of Celtic or Scandinavian origin. Such clients usually burn easily and do not tan; they may even have a significant history of severe sunburn.
Client Needs Category—*Physiological integrity*
Client Needs Subcategory—*None*

112. **2.** Because birth defects are associated with isotretinoin (Accutane), its use is contraindicated during pregnancy. There is no known relationship between breast cancer or ovulation and increased vulnerability to the drug's adverse effects. Acne vulgaris is not a sexually transmitted disease.
Client Needs Category—*Health promotion and maintenance*
Client Needs Subcategory—*None*

113. **3.** Wearing a different pair of shoes each day provides time for shoe moisture to evaporate. The fungus growth that causes tinea pedis is supported in a dark, moist, and warm environment. Eliminating one or more of these factors may reduce the frequency of tinea pedis. Avoiding bare feet, cutting the nails straight across, and wearing colored socks will not promote or eliminate tinea pedis.
Client Needs Category—*Health promotion and maintenance*
Client Needs Subcategory—*None*

114. **1.** Shingles results from a reactivation of the varicella-zoster virus, which lies dormant in the sensory ganglia after a previous infection with chickenpox. The individual with shingles usually reports a history of chickenpox in childhood. Shingles also occurs in those who have not had chickenpox but who come in contact with someone who has chickenpox or is immunocompromised. Shingles is not caused by the bite of an insect, a bacterial toxin, or an antibody response.
Client Needs Category—*Physiological integrity*
Client Needs Subcategory—*Physiological adaptation*

115. **2.** Clients with herpes simplex virus type 1, also known as *cold sores* or *fever blisters,* are cautioned to use good personal hygiene to prevent the spread of the infection to other areas, such as the eyes and genitals. The application of petroleum jelly delays healing but does not prevent the spread of the infection. Any scabs that form should be allowed to dry and fall off. When cleaning the affected areas, clients should take care to use tissues or gauze to gently clean and remove any fluid that has formed on the lesions. The tissues or gauze should be used only once and then discarded.
Client Needs Category—*Health promotion and maintenance*
Client Needs Subcategory—*None*

116. **2.** Characterized by areas of redness covered with silvery scales, psoriasis is a common chronic disease of the skin in which erythematous papules form plaques with distinct borders. Areas affected usually include the elbows, knees, and scalp, although other areas may also be affected.
Client Needs Category—*Physiological integrity*
Client Needs Subcategory—*Physiological adaptation*

117. **3.** Psoriasis is a chronic, noninfectious, inflammatory skin disease in which epidermal cells are produced at a rate about six to nine times faster than normal. The cells in the basal layer divide too quickly, and the newer formed cells move so rapidly to the skin surface that they become evident as profuse scales or plaques of epidermal tissue. Infections of the skin and hair follicles as well as dermal abrasion are not contributing factors to psoriasis.

Client Needs Category—Physiological integrity
Client Needs Subcategory—Physiological adaptation

118. 4. Vinyl gloves may be substituted for latex gloves; however, because vinyl is more permeable, two pairs should be worn. Neither rinsing the gloves with tap water nor applying petroleum-based ointment eliminates an allergic reaction to latex. It is unsafe for nurses and other health care workers to care for clients without proper protection when there is a potential for contact with body fluids that contain blood.

Client Needs Category—Safe, effective care environment
Client Needs Subcategory—Coordinated care

119. 1. Soaking with a warm solution between 100° and 106° F (37.7° and 41.1° C) is recommended for the treatment of frostbite. Cold applications are contraindicated because this delays effective treatment. A heating pad or hot water is not used because either can cause further tissue damage.

Client Needs Category—Physiological integrity
Client Needs Subcategory—Reduction of risk potential

120. 1. Hypoallergenic or glycerin soap decreases skin irritation and therefore lessens itching. Regular soap removes skin oils, which can contribute to or cause itching. Rough fibers such as wool irritate the skin and contribute to the itching sensation. Tepid water, rather than hot or cold water, is recommended for bathing. Patting the skin dry, rather than rubbing, reduces skin irritation and itching.

Client Needs Category—Physiological integrity
Client Needs Subcategory—Physiological adaptation

121. 2. Chronic wounds are longstanding wounds that are resistant to healing, such as a slow-healing diabetic foot ulcer. In many cases, such chronic wounds begin healing but characteristically fail to continue the healing process. Although the gunshot and surgical wounds mentioned may be slow to heal, the wounds are not necessarily considered chronic; their slow healing is secondary to infection or tissue damage. A stage I pressure ulcer involves only the first layer of skin and does not necessarily progress to a deeper wound.

Client Needs Category—Physiological integrity
Client Needs Subcategory—Physiological adaptation

The Nursing Care of Clients with Endocrine Disorders

⇨ **Nursing Care of Clients with Disorders of the Pituitary Gland**
⇨ **Nursing Care of Clients with Disorders of the Thyroid Gland**
⇨ **Nursing Care of Clients with Disorders of the Parathyroid Glands**
⇨ **Nursing Care of Clients with Disorders of the Adrenal Glands**
⇨ **Nursing Care of Clients with Pancreatic Endocrine Disorders**
⇨ **Correct Answers and Rationales**

Directions: With a pencil, blacken the space in front of the option you have chosen for your correct answer.

Nursing Care of Clients with Disorders of the Pituitary Gland

Following head trauma, a female client develops signs and symptoms of diabetes insipidus.

1. Which characteristic symptom of the client's disorder would the nurse expect to find during an assessment?
[ ] **1.** Hyponatremia
[ ] **2.** Polyuria
[ ] **3.** Glycosuria
[ ] **4.** Hyperglycemia

2. How does the nurse expect the urine that she collects for a routine urinalysis to appear?
[ ] **1.** Tea-colored
[ ] **2.** Pale yellow
[ ] **3.** Colorless
[ ] **4.** Light pink

3. Which nursing intervention is essential for monitoring the client's condition?
[ ] **1.** Measuring intake and output
[ ] **2.** Analyzing blood glucose levels
[ ] **3.** Counting caloric intake
[ ] **4.** Assessing vital signs

The nursing care plan indicates that the client must be weighed each day.

4. When directing the nursing assistant to weigh the client, which instruction is most important for obtaining accurate data?

[ ] **1.** Have the client stand on a bedside scale.
[ ] **2.** Weigh the client at the same time each day.
[ ] **3.** Ask the client to remove her slippers when being weighed.
[ ] **4.** Ask the client to identify her predisease weight.

The client is treated with intranasal lypressin (Diapid), 2 sprays q.i.d. and as needed.

5. The nurse observes the client self-administering the medication. Which action indicates that the client is using the medication correctly?
[ ] **1.** The client shakes the medication vigorously before using.
[ ] **2.** The client tilts her head to the side.
[ ] **3.** The client inverts the drug container.
[ ] **4.** The client inhales with each spray.

6. When instructing the client about lypressin (Diapid), the nurse advises her that the best indication for self-administering an as-needed dose is when she experiences which symptom?
[ ] **1.** Increased thirst
[ ] **2.** Onset of a headache
[ ] **3.** Dark yellow urine
[ ] **4.** A runny nose

The nurse is assessing a male client who is experiencing signs and symptoms related to his diagnosis of acromegaly.

7. During the physical assessment of this client, which finding is the nurse most likely to observe?
[ ] **1.** Exceptional height
[ ] **2.** Enlarged hands
[ ] **3.** Gonadal atrophy
[ ] **4.** Loss of teeth

8. Which nursing diagnosis should the nursing team consider when developing this client's care plan?
[ ] **1.** *Activity intolerance*
[ ] **2.** *Acute confusion*
[ ] **3.** *Ineffective breathing*
[ ] **4.** *Impaired swallowing*

The client is scheduled for a transsphenoidal hypophysectomy following a short course of bromocriptine (Parlodel) to treat his acromegaly.

9. Because bromocriptine (Parlodel) may cause orthostatic hypotension, what does the nurse instruct the client to do?
[ ] **1.** Lie down for ½ hour after taking the medication
[ ] **2.** Avoid taking hot showers
[ ] **3.** Slowly rise from a sitting or lying position
[ ] **4.** Have his blood pressure taken once per week

The night before surgery, the nurse provides the client with information on what to expect during the postoperative period.

10. Which statement by the client indicates that he has misunderstood the expected outcome of his surgery?
[ ] **1.** "My appearance will gradually become normal."
[ ] **2.** "I'll need to take replacement hormones."
[ ] **3.** "I'll need to see my physician regularly."
[ ] **4.** "The surgical incision will be inconspicuous."

11. Immediately after surgery, the nurse assesses the client for bleeding. Where is the best location to assess for bleeding?
[ ] **1.** The skull
[ ] **2.** The nose
[ ] **3.** Behind the ear
[ ] **4.** Above the eyelid

Nursing Care of Clients with Disorders of the Thyroid Gland

A 35-year-old woman seeks medical attention to determine why she has stopped menstruating. The physician orders a radioactive iodine uptake test.

12. After the test, the nurse provides the client with instructions. Which nurse's statement is accurate?
[ ] **1.** "You must remain isolated until the radiation level decreases sufficiently."
[ ] **2.** "You're free to go without further precautionary instructions."
[ ] **3.** "You must follow special precautions for a short period of time."
[ ] **4.** "You'll be given an antidote for reducing the radioactivity level."

The results of the diagnostic tests confirm that the client has myxedema.

13. In addition to amenorrhea, which other sign of myxedema is the nurse likely to observe in this client?
[ ] **1.** Hoarse, raspy voice
[ ] **2.** Oily skin with large pores
[ ] **3.** Thin trunk and extremities
[ ] **4.** Extreme restlessness

14. When the nurse conducts an admission history, which subjective symptom is the client likely to describe?
[ ] **1.** Difficulty urinating
[ ] **2.** Intolerance to cold
[ ] **3.** Profuse perspiration
[ ] **4.** Excessive appetite

The client with myxedema is treated with levothyroxine (Synthroid), one tablet P.O. every day.

15. Which statement provides the best evidence that the client understands her prescribed drug therapy?
[ ] **1.** "I must take this drug after meals."
[ ] **2.** "I should avoid driving when sleepy."
[ ] **3.** "I'll need to take this drug for the rest of my life."
[ ] **4.** "I can skip a dose if I'm nauseated."

A female client seeks medical attention because she notices an area of fullness in her neck. After several diagnostic tests, an endemic goiter is diagnosed.

16. To prevent a goiter from developing in other family members, the nurse recommends increasing dietary intake of which food?
[ ] **1.** Green leafy vegetables
[ ] **2.** Iodized table salt
[ ] **3.** Whole grains
[ ] **4.** Citrus fruits

17. Which symptom related to goiter would the nurse expect to find while reviewing this client's medical history?
[ ] **1.** Gradual weight loss
[ ] **2.** Slight hand tremors
[ ] **3.** Trouble swallowing
[ ] **4.** Sparse hair loss

A female client is undergoing treatment for Graves' disease.

18. Which characteristic facial feature would the nurse expect to note during a physical examination of this client?

[ ] **1.** Bulging eyes
[ ] **2.** Bulbous nose
[ ] **3.** Thick lips
[ ] **4.** Large tongue

The physician prescribes propylthiouracil (Propyl-Thyracil) to treat the client's condition.

19. Before administering this medication, what is essential for the nurse to ask the client?
[ ] **1.** If she has trouble swallowing
[ ] **2.** If she prefers a liquid form
[ ] **3.** If she has digestive disorders
[ ] **4.** If she might be pregnant

20. Because propylthiouracil (Propyl-Thyracil) can cause agranulocytosis, the nurse advises the client to notify the physician if which problem occurs?
[ ] **1.** Persistent sore throat
[ ] **2.** Occasional heart palpitations
[ ] **3.** Intolerance to fatty foods
[ ] **4.** Prolonged bleeding with trauma

A client with Graves' disease was just informed that he will have to undergo a subtotal thyroidectomy. The physician prescribes Lugol's solution 4 gtt P.O. to be taken for 10 days before the scheduled surgery.

21. When instructing the client on how to self-administer Lugol's solution, which nurse's direction is most appropriate?
[ ] **1.** Swallow the drug quickly.
[ ] **2.** Take the drug before meals.
[ ] **3.** Dilute the drug in fruit juice.
[ ] **4.** Chill the drug before taking it.

The client asks the nurse to explain the purpose of his preoperative drug therapy.

22. Which response by the nurse about Lugol's solution is correct?
[ ] **1.** It firms the gland so it is easily removed.
[ ] **2.** It decreases the postoperative recovery time.
[ ] **3.** It decreases the risk of postoperative bleeding.
[ ] **4.** It eliminates the need for hormone replacement.

23. Preoperatively, which information is most important to teach the client before his subtotal thyroidectomy?
[ ] **1.** Techniques for changing positions
[ ] **2.** Reasons for performing leg exercises
[ ] **3.** Purpose of measuring intake and output
[ ] **4.** Postoperative mealtime schedule

24. To prepare for potential postoperative complications related to the thyroidectomy, which item is necessary to keep at the client's bedside?
[ ] **1.** Dressing change kit
[ ] **2.** Tracheostomy tray
[ ] **3.** Ampule of epinephrine
[ ] **4.** Mechanical ventilator

After surgery, the client is returned to the nursing unit in stable condition.

25. In which position should the client be maintained following his subtotal thyroidectomy?
[ ] **1.** Supine
[ ] **2.** Sims'
[ ] **3.** Semi-Fowler's
[ ] **4.** Recumbent

26. Postoperatively, the nurse should consult the physician before encouraging the client to perform which action?
[ ] **1.** Routinely cough
[ ] **2.** Deep breathe
[ ] **3.** Ambulate
[ ] **4.** Dangle his legs

27. Which intervention is most appropriate to add to the client's care plan when monitoring for incisional bleeding after a subtotal thyroidectomy?
[ ] **1.** Pass a flashlight across the incisional dressing.
[ ] **2.** Assess for dampness at the back of the client's neck.
[ ] **3.** Remove the dressing to directly inspect the wound.
[ ] **4.** Weigh all gauze dressings before and after changing.

28. Which assessment technique is most appropriate when checking for laryngeal nerve damage in a client who has had a thyroidectomy?
[ ] **1.** Turning the client's head from side to side
[ ] **2.** Observing the client swallowing
[ ] **3.** Looking for tracheal deviation
[ ] **4.** Asking the client to say "Ah"

29. The nurse should assess for hypocalcemia based on which client statement following a subtotal thyroidectomy?
[ ] **1.** "I don't have much of an appetite."
[ ] **2.** "My lips feel numb and tingly."
[ ] **3.** "Light seems to bother my eyes."
[ ] **4.** "I feel weak when I walk."

The client's care plan indicates that the nurse should assess for Chvostek's sign if hypocalcemia is suspected.

30. Which technique best describes how Chvostek's sign is elicited?
[ ] **1.** The nurse lightly taps over the client's facial nerve.
[ ] **2.** The nurse strokes the sole of the client's foot.
[ ] **3.** The nurse dorsiflexes each of the client's feet.
[ ] **4.** The nurse asks the client to touch his nose.

31. Manifestation of which sign is most indicative that the postoperative thyroidectomy client is developing thyroid crisis?
[ ] **1.** High fever
[ ] **2.** Falling blood pressure
[ ] **3.** Regular noisy respirations
[ ] **4.** Hand spasms

32. At the beginning of thyroid replacement therapy following a thyroidectomy, the nurse must monitor the client closely for side effects. Which findings would the nurse expect to assess? Select all that apply.
[ ] **1.** Hyperglycemia
[ ] **2.** Tachycardia
[ ] **3.** Insomnia
[ ] **4.** Hirsutism
[ ] **5.** Tremors
[ ] **6.** Hypertension

Nursing Care of Clients with Disorders of the Parathyroid Glands

A client who develops a benign parathyroid tumor manifests signs of hyperparathyroidism.

33. When the nurse reviews the client's history, which assessment finding is closely associated with the client's diagnosis?
[ ] **1.** Nightly leg cramps
[ ] **2.** Recurrent kidney stones
[ ] **3.** Loose bowel movements
[ ] **4.** Difficulty falling asleep

The nursing assistant assigned to this client asks why the care plan indicates that the client is at risk for injury.

34. The best explanation by the nurse would be that which side effect is one of the consequences of hyperparathyroidism?
[ ] **1.** The inability to maintain balance
[ ] **2.** The risk of developing seizures
[ ] **3.** Fainting when changing positions
[ ] **4.** Pathologic bone fractures

The client has three of the four lobes of her parathyroid gland surgically removed.

35. After the client returns from surgery and resumes eating, the nurse should encourage her to eat foods from which food group?
[ ] **1.** Bread and cereals
[ ] **2.** Milk and cheese
[ ] **3.** Meat and seafood
[ ] **4.** Fruit and vegetables

A client diagnosed with hypoparathyroidism develops tetany and comes to the emergency department for treatment.

36. Which I.V. medication can the nurse expect the physician to order to treat the client's condition?
[ ] **1.** Calcium gluconate
[ ] **2.** Ferrous sulfate
[ ] **3.** Potassium chloride
[ ] **4.** Sodium bicarbonate

Nursing Care of Clients with Disorders of the Adrenal Glands

The nurse cares for a client with Addison's disease.

37. Which characteristic finding would the nurse expect to assess in a client with Addison's disease?
[ ] **1.** Enlarged abdomen
[ ] **2.** Skin blemishes
[ ] **3.** Moon-shaped face
[ ] **4.** Bronzed skin

38. Which nursing assessment is most helpful in evaluating the status of a client with Addison's disease?
[ ] **1.** Blood pressure
[ ] **2.** Bowel sounds
[ ] **3.** Breath sounds
[ ] **4.** Heart sounds

The client's care plan indicates that the nurse should assist the client in selecting foods that are good sources of sodium as part of the treatment for Addison's disease.

39. If the following foods are available, which one should the nurse recommend?
[ ] **1.** Graham crackers
[ ] **2.** Cheddar cheese
[ ] **3.** Raw carrots
[ ] **4.** Canned peaches

The nurse documents that the client has recurrent episodes of hypoglycemia.

40. If a regular diet is ordered, which between-meal snack should the nurse offer to help regulate the client's blood glucose level?

[ ] **1.** Lemonade and peanuts
[ ] **2.** Cola and potato chips
[ ] **3.** Coffee and a muffin
[ ] **4.** Milk and crackers

41. Because this client is at risk for developing addisonian crisis, a life-threatening condition, what does the nurse correctly instruct him to avoid?
[ ] **1.** Stress-producing situations
[ ] **2.** Consuming alcoholic beverages
[ ] **3.** Eating complex carbohydrates
[ ] **4.** Getting too little sleep

A 38-year-old female client is hospitalized after developing symptoms that resemble Cushing's syndrome.

42. Based on the client's condition, which finding is the nurse most likely to document at the initial physical assessment?
[ ] **1.** The client has very thin legs.
[ ] **2.** The client looks emaciated.
[ ] **3.** The client has bulging eyes.
[ ] **4.** The client's skin is pale.

The physician orders a 24-hour urine collection to aid in the diagnosis of Cushing's syndrome.

43. The nurse is most accurate in telling the client that the urine collection will begin when?
[ ] **1.** With the client's next voiding
[ ] **2.** After the client's next voiding
[ ] **3.** After drinking a pitcher of water
[ ] **4.** With the first voiding in the morning

44. Which statement is correct concerning the collection of urine for a 24-hour specimen?
[ ] **1.** The volume of each voiding is measured and recorded.
[ ] **2.** The urine is placed in a container of preservative.
[ ] **3.** Each voiding is taken immediately to the laboratory.
[ ] **4.** The client voids directly into the specimen container.

After the health care team meets to discuss the client's nursing needs, the nursing diagnosis Disturbed body image *is added to the care plan.*

45. The best rationale for adding this nursing diagnosis to the care plan is that female clients with Cushing's syndrome typically experience which adverse effect?
[ ] **1.** Masculine characteristics
[ ] **2.** Heavy menstrual flow
[ ] **3.** Extreme weight loss
[ ] **4.** Large, pendulous breasts

Diagnostic tests confirm that the client's adrenal glands are producing excessive amounts of adrenocortical hormones.

46. When the nurse reinforces the physician's explanation of the disorder to the client's spouse, it is accurate to stress that the client is also likely to experience which side effect?
[ ] **1.** Anxiety and occasional panic attacks
[ ] **2.** Depression and suicidal tendencies
[ ] **3.** Impulsiveness and poor self-control
[ ] **4.** Forgetfulness and memory changes

The physician orders a low-sodium diet to help treat the client's Cushing's syndrome.

47. Which action by the nurse provides the best data for monitoring the client's therapeutic response to sodium restriction?
[ ] **1.** Monitoring the percentage of sodium eaten
[ ] **2.** Measuring abdominal girth
[ ] **3.** Assessing skin integrity
[ ] **4.** Weighing the client

48. Which nursing intervention is most appropriate for managing the basic needs of a client with Cushing's syndrome?
[ ] **1.** Have the client sleep on a convoluted foam mattress.
[ ] **2.** Ambulate the client at frequent intervals.
[ ] **3.** Reduce environmental stimuli such as noise.
[ ] **4.** Offer high-carbohydrate nourishment.

Eventually, the client undergoes a bilateral adrenalectomy to correct her Cushing's syndrome.

49. Which documentation finding provides the best indication that the client has successfully avoided an adrenal (addisonian) crisis following surgery?
[ ] **1.** Urine output is approximately 2,000 mL/day.
[ ] **2.** Pain is controlled at a tolerable level.
[ ] **3.** Capillary blood glucose level is within normal limits.
[ ] **4.** Vital signs are within preoperative ranges.

50. Based on the knowledge that clients with Cushing's syndrome heal slowly, which nursing measure is most appropriate during the client's postoperative period?
[ ] **1.** Monitoring infusion of I.V. antibiotics
[ ] **2.** Removing tape toward the incision site
[ ] **3.** Increasing the client's dietary protein intake
[ ] **4.** Covering the wound with gauze

51. Which statement provides the best evidence that the client understands her postoperative course?
[ ] **1.** "I should avoid people with infectious diseases."
[ ] **2.** "I need to limit my fluid intake to 1 quart per day."
[ ] **3.** "My appearance will never be the same as it was before."
[ ] **4.** "No other treatment is necessary after I recover from surgery."

A client with pheochromocytoma, a tumor of the adrenal medulla, is scheduled to have the tumor surgically removed.

52. During the admission assessment, which finding is the nurse most likely to observe?
[ ] **1.** Hyperkalemia
[ ] **2.** Hypertension
[ ] **3.** Hyperinsulinism
[ ] **4.** Hyperthermia

53. If the following are served on the dietary tray of the client with pheochromocytoma, which one is most appropriate for the nurse to remove?
[ ] **1.** Hot tea
[ ] **2.** Ice water
[ ] **3.** Skim milk
[ ] **4.** Apple juice

Nursing Care of Clients with Pancreatic Endocrine Disorders

A 23-year-old woman manifests symptoms of hyperinsulinism.

54. During the nursing history, the client is most likely to describe experiencing symptoms that typically occur when?
[ ] **1.** After fasting more than 6 hours
[ ] **2.** About 2 hours after eating a meal
[ ] **3.** Late in the evening, before bedtime
[ ] **4.** Early in the morning, before breakfast

A 5-hour glucose tolerance test is ordered to determine if the client has functional hypoglycemia.

55. Which statement by the nurse concerning the test procedure is most accurate?
[ ] **1.** "You need to eat a large meal just before the test."
[ ] **2.** "Bring a voided urine specimen to the laboratory."
[ ] **3.** "You may drink liquids, such as coffee, before the test."
[ ] **4.** "You will be given a sweetened drink before the test."

56. To reduce or eliminate the symptoms that a client with functional hypoglycemia experiences, it is best for the nurse to recommend eating five or six small meals containing which nutrient?
[ ] **1.** Simple sugars
[ ] **2.** Complete proteins
[ ] **3.** Complex carbohydrates
[ ] **4.** Unsaturated fats

57. The best evidence that the dietary measures to control functional hypoglycemia are therapeutic is that the client experiences fewer incidences of which side effect?
[ ] **1.** Weakness and tremors
[ ] **2.** Thirst and dry mouth
[ ] **3.** Muscle spasms and fatigue
[ ] **4.** Hunger and abdominal cramps

A nurse participates in a community-wide screening to identify adults who may have undiagnosed diabetes mellitus.

58. If the screening includes a measurement of postprandial blood glucose, the nurse is correct in explaining that blood will be drawn at which time?
[ ] **1.** Approximately 2 hours before breakfast
[ ] **2.** Approximately 2 hours after a meal
[ ] **3.** Approximately 2 hours before bedtime
[ ] **4.** Approximately 2 hours after fasting

59. Which statement indicates that a client with an elevated 2-hour postprandial blood glucose level understands the significance of the screening test?
[ ] **1.** "I need to eat less frequently."
[ ] **2.** "I need to stop eating candy."
[ ] **3.** "I need to consult my physician."
[ ] **4.** "I need to begin taking insulin."

60. Which signs and symptoms are most appropriate for the nurse to investigate when screening adults who have come to have their blood glucose tested?
[ ] **1.** Diarrhea, anorexia, and weight gain
[ ] **2.** Constipation, weight loss, and thirst
[ ] **3.** Polycholia, polyemia, and polyplegia
[ ] **4.** Polyuria, polydipsia, and polyphagia

After the screening test, one client was referred to her physician for additional follow-up. Further diagnostic tests confirm that the client has type 2 diabetes mellitus.

61. When the client demonstrates a shocked response to the news of her diagnosis, which nursing action is most appropriate at this time?
[ ] **1.** Emphasizing the importance of treatment
[ ] **2.** Reassuring the client that injections are easy
[ ] **3.** Explaining that many people live with diabetes
[ ] **4.** Listening as she expresses her current feelings

The newly diagnosed client with type 2 diabetes mellitus is referred to the diabetic clinic for teaching.

62. When the client asks the nurse why regular exercise is recommended for diabetic clients, the best answer is that exercise tends to facilitate which positive outcome?
[ ] **1.** Controlled weight gain
[ ] **2.** Decreased appetite
[ ] **3.** Reduced blood glucose level
[ ] **4.** Improved circulation to the feet

A dietitian explains how to use the American Diabetes Association exchange list.

63. Which statement by the client provides the best evidence that she understands the principle of an exchange list for meal planning?
[ ] **1.** "I can eat one serving from each category on the exchange list per day."
[ ] **2.** "Measured amounts of food in each category are equal to one another."
[ ] **3.** "The number of servings from the exchange list is unlimited."
[ ] **4.** "I need to use the exchange list to determine the nutrition in food."

64. The nurse knows the diabetic client understands that "free" foods are those foods or beverages that can be consumed as often as she wants when she excludes which beverage from her meal plan?
[ ] **1.** Iced tea
[ ] **2.** Mineral water
[ ] **3.** Light beer
[ ] **4.** Club soda

65. Using the Dietary Exchange Plan for a client who has diabetes and is on a 1,500-calorie diet, which item is appropriate for the client to have in the mid-afternoon?

	Starch/ bread	Meat	Vegetable	Fruit	Milk	Fat
Breakfast	2			1	1	1
Lunch	2	1	1	1		1
Snack				1		
Dinner	2	2	1	1		2
Bedtime	1			1	1	

[ ] **1.** An 8-oz carton of milk
[ ] **2.** Two graham crackers
[ ] **3.** A medium apple
[ ] **4.** A 2-oz slice of turkey

The physician prescribes glyburide (DiaBeta) orally for the client to treat her diabetes.

66. When the client asks why her diabetic uncle cannot take his insulin orally, what is the best answer?
[ ] **1.** Insulin is inactivated by digestive enzymes.
[ ] **2.** Insulin is absorbed too quickly in the stomach.
[ ] **3.** Insulin is irritating to the gastric mucosa.
[ ] **4.** Insulin is incompatible with many foods.

67. The nurse instructs the client taking glyburide (DiaBeta) to avoid which food because of the risk of a food-drug interaction?
[ ] **1.** Chocolate
[ ] **2.** Pecans
[ ] **3.** Yogurt
[ ] **4.** Alcohol

68. The diabetic client tells the nurse that she never eats breakfast. Which response by the nurse is most appropriate?
[ ] **1.** "If you drink a glass of milk, it will be sufficient for breakfast."
[ ] **2.** "You should eat each meal and between-meal snacks at a consistent time."
[ ] **4.** "If you omit breakfast, eat a high-calorie snack at mid-morning."
[ ] **5.** "Wait to take your medication until you eat your first meal of the day."

After the diabetic client is discharged from the hospital, the physician wants her to continue monitoring her response to the diet and medication plan.

69. If the client lives on a limited income, which monitoring approach is most helpful to recommend?
[ ] **1.** Testing the urine with a chemical reagent strip
[ ] **2.** Using a glucometer to check capillary blood glucose levels
[ ] **3.** Having laboratory personnel draw venous blood samples
[ ] **4.** Arranging for testing by a home health agency nurse

Emergency medical personnel bring a client who is lethargic and confused to the emergency department. A tentative diagnosis of type 1 diabetes mellitus and diabetic ketoacidosis (DKA) is made.

70. Which assessment findings would the nurse expect to document if the client has DKA?
[ ] **1.** The client is hypertensive and tachycardic.
[ ] **2.** The client is dyspneic and hypotensive.
[ ] **3.** The client breathes noisily and smells of acetone.
[ ] **4.** The client stares blankly and smells of alcohol.

The nurse plans to monitor the client's response to insulin therapy closely with an electronic glucometer.

71. Which technique is correct when using an electronic glucometer to monitor the client's blood glucose level?
[ ] **1.** Clean the client's finger with povidone-iodine (Betadine).
[ ] **2.** Wrap a rubber band around the test finger.
[ ] **3.** Pierce the central pad of the client's finger.
[ ] **4.** Apply a large drop of blood to a test strip or area.

72. If the glucometer indicates that the client's blood glucose reading is 58 mg/dL and he is shaky and dizzy, what is the most appropriate nursing action?
[ ] **1.** Administer the next scheduled dose of insulin.
[ ] **2.** Give the client sweetened fruit juice.
[ ] **3.** Report the client's symptoms to the physician.
[ ] **4.** Perform a complete head-to-toe assessment.

The physician orders sliding scale regular insulin for the client.

73. How soon after administering the client's dose of regular insulin should the nurse assess for signs of hypoglycemia?
[ ] **1.** 5 minutes later
[ ] **2.** 30 minutes later
[ ] **3.** 6 hours later
[ ] **4.** 10 hours later

The client with type 1 diabetes must learn to combine two insulins—regular and intermediate-acting—and self-administer the injection before being discharged.

74. Which action best indicates that the client needs more practice in combining two insulins in one syringe?
[ ] **1.** The client rolls the vial of intermediate-acting insulin to mix it with its additive.
[ ] **2.** The client instills air into both the fast-acting and intermediate-acting insulin vials.
[ ] **3.** The client instills the intermediate-acting insulin into the vial of rapid-acting insulin.
[ ] **4.** The client inverts each vial prior to withdrawing the specified amount of insulin.

75. When the client practices self-administration of the insulin, which action is correct?
[ ] **1.** Piercing the skin at a 30-degree angle
[ ] **2.** Using a syringe calibrated in minims
[ ] **3.** Using a 2″ needle on the syringe
[ ] **4.** Rotating the sites of each injection

76. The nurse receives an order to administer Novolin R 10 units with Novolin N 20 units to be given subcutaneously at 0730. Place the following actions in correct sequence to show how the nurse would mix the medications. Use all the options.

1. Instill 20 units of air in the vial of Novolin N.

2. Instill 10 units of air in the vial of Novolin R.

3. Withdraw 20 units of insulin from the vial of Novolin N.

4. Withdraw 10 units of insulin from the vial of Novolin R.

The nurse implements a diabetes teaching plan in anticipation of the client's discharge.

77. Which statement indicates that the client has misunderstood the nurse's teaching?
[ ] **1.** "I may need more insulin during times of stress."
[ ] **2.** "I may need more food when exercising strenuously."
[ ] **3.** "My insulin needs may change as I get older."
[ ] **4.** "My dependence on insulin may stop eventually."

78. The nurse teaches a client with newly diagnosed diabetes mellitus about the signs and symptoms of hypoglycemia. Which of the following should the nurse stress in teaching? Select all that apply.
[ ] **1.** Sleepiness
[ ] **2.** Shakiness
[ ] **3.** Thirst
[ ] **4.** Hunger
[ ] **5.** Diaphoresis
[ ] **6.** Disturbed cognition

79. When the client asks how to store insulin, where does the nurse correctly respond that it may be stored?
[ ] **1.** In the bathroom close to the shower
[ ] **2.** In the refrigerator
[ ] **3.** At room temperature
[ ] **4.** In a home freezer

The nurse includes foot care as a component of diabetes teaching.

80. Which statement by the client about foot care indicates the need for further teaching?
[ ] **1.** "I need to inspect my feet daily."
[ ] **2.** "I should soak my feet each day."
[ ] **3.** "I need to wear shoes whenever I'm not sleeping."
[ ] **4.** "I need to schedule regular appointments with the podiatrist."

After 3 months, the client returns for a follow-up appointment with his physician to evaluate his self-care.

81. Which information is most important for the nurse to elicit from the client in order to effectively evaluate his compliance with the prescribed therapy?
[ ] **1.** The dosage and frequency of his insulin administration
[ ] **2.** The client's glucose monitoring records for the past week
[ ] **3.** The client's weight and vital signs before the office interview
[ ] **4.** The symptoms he experienced in the past month

82. Which laboratory test result is most important for the nurse to monitor to determine how effectively the client's diabetes is being managed?
[ ] **1.** Fasting blood glucose
[ ] **2.** Blood chemistry profile
[ ] **3.** Complete blood count
[ ] **4.** Glycosylated (A1c) hemoglobin

The nurse meets with a type 1 diabetic client to discuss managing his disorder with a continuous insulin infusion pump.

83. The nurse teaches the client how the infusion pump operates and correctly points out that the infusion is typically administered in which location?
[ ] **1.** In a vein within the nondominant hand
[ ] **2.** In the muscular tissue of the thigh
[ ] **3.** In the subcutaneous tissue of the abdomen below the belt line
[ ] **4.** In an implanted I.V. catheter threaded into the neck

The nurse cares for an older male client who is insulin-dependent and in a nursing home.

84. When developing the client's care plan, which intervention is most appropriate to add?
[ ] **1.** Encourage the client to use an electric razor.
[ ] **2.** Tell the client to file rather than cut his toenails.
[ ] **3.** Make sure that the client receives mouth care twice per day.
[ ] **4.** Advise the client to use deodorant soap when bathing.

85. The nurse has prepared 24 units of Humulin N insulin for subcutaneous administration. Identify the preferred location for insulin administration to facilitate rapid absorption.

86. Which sign is most suggestive that a client with type 2 (non-insulin-dependent) diabetes is developing hyperosmolar hyperglycemic nonketotic syndrome (HHNS)?
[ ] **1.** The client's blood glucose level is 200 mg/dL.
[ ] **2.** The client urinates copious amounts.
[ ] **3.** The client's skin is warm and dry.
[ ] **4.** The client's urine contains acetone.

87. The nurse discusses the long-term effects of diabetes mellitus with the client and realizes that he needs further teaching when he incorrectly states that he could develop which complication as a result of his illness?
[ ] **1.** Blindness
[ ] **2.** Stroke
[ ] **3.** Renal failure
[ ] **4.** Liver failure

An insulin-dependent diabetic client is treated in the emergency department for diabetic ketoacidosis (DKA). The nurse documents that Kussmaul's respirations were detected during the initial assessment.

88. Which respiratory pattern best describes the client's breathing?
[ ] **1.** Fast, deep, labored respirations
[ ] **2.** Shallow respirations, alternating with apnea
[ ] **3.** Slow inhalation and exhalation through pursed lips
[ ] **4.** Shortness of breath with pauses

A client with type 1 diabetes comes to the clinic complaining of persistent bouts of nausea, vomiting, and diarrhea for the past 4 days. The client states that he has skipped his insulin injections because he has not been eating and cannot keep anything down.

89. Which instruction should the nurse give the client about insulin administration during sick days?
[ ] **1.** Monitor blood glucose levels every 2 to 4 hours.
[ ] **2.** Eat candy or sugar frequently.
[ ] **3.** Attempt to drink a high-calorie beverage every hour.
[ ] **4.** Test urine daily for protein.

90. During change of shifts, a nurse discovers that a hospitalized client with diabetes received two doses of insulin. After notifying the physician, which nursing action is most appropriate?
[ ] **1.** Completing an incident report
[ ] **2.** Calling the intensive care unit (ICU)
[ ] **3.** Performing frequent neurologic checks
[ ] **4.** Monitoring the client's blood glucose level

Correct Answers and Rationales

Nursing Care of Clients with Disorders of the Pituitary Gland

1. **2.** Diabetes insipidus is a disorder of the posterior lobe of the pituitary gland that results in excessive urination caused by inadequate amounts of antidiuretic hormone, or vasopressin. It can occur secondary to head trauma, brain tumors, or such infections as meningitis. Clients with diabetes insipidus may excrete as much as 20 L per day of very dilute urine; consequently, they need to compensate for fluid loss and may drink up to 20 to 40 L per day, resulting in frequent voiding that poses limits on activity. Weakness, dehydration, and weight loss will result. They also experience polydipsia (intense thirst) and hypernatremia. Hyponatremia, glycosuria, and hyperglycemia are not characteristic of this disorder.
 Client Needs Category—*Physiological integrity*
 Client Needs Subcategory—*Physiological adaptation*

2. **3.** The urine of someone with diabetes insipidus is so dilute that it appears colorless. The specific gravity may be 1.002 or less. Dark tea or cola-colored urine is commonly associated with glomerulonephritis (a renal disorder), not diabetes insipidus (an endocrine disorder). Normal urine appears pale yellow. Light pink urine indicates hematuria (blood in the urine), which can result from irritation, infection, or renal disorders.
 Client Needs Category—*Physiological integrity*
 Client Needs Subcategory—*Physiological adaptation*

3. **1.** To prevent dehydration, it is essential to replace fluids based on the deficit between the client's intake and output. Glucose metabolism is unaffected in diabetes insipidus; therefore, monitoring blood glucose values is unnecessary. Although a client with diabetes insipidus might not eat well because of his constant drinking, maintaining an adequate fluid volume—not counting calories—is the primary nursing concern. Vital signs are important to assess, but monitoring intake and output is critical in this situation.
 Client Needs Category—*Physiological integrity*
 Client Needs Subcategory—*Reduction of risk potential*

4. **2.** For the sake of comparison, clients are weighed at the same time each day, on the same scale and wearing similar clothing each time. Nothing in the situation indicates whether a standing scale was used or whether the client wore slippers during previous weight assessments. The client's predisease weight has no bearing on her current condition except as a point of reference.

Client Needs Category—Physiological integrity
Client Needs Subcategory—Basic care and comfort

5. 4. Lypressin (Diapid) is a synthetic hormone prescribed because of its antidiuretic effects. The client should maintain her head in an upright position when administering lypressin (Diapid) because the tip of the container is inserted upright into a nostril. The client then inhales while compressing the container and releasing the spray. Vigorous shaking does not improve the medication's effectiveness and, therefore, is unnecessary.

Client Needs Category—Physiological integrity
Client Needs Subcategory—Pharmacological therapies

6. 1. The need to administer additional doses of lypressin (Diapid) is based on increased thirst and frequency of urination. If more than the prescribed number of doses is required, the interval between routine administrations is generally decreased while the number of sprays at each dose remains the same. Someone with diabetes insipidus would have urine that is colorless, not dark yellow; a dark yellow color indicates that the urine is concentrated and has a high specific gravity. A runny nose is a side effect of excessive use of the nasal spray. Headaches are not typically associated with this disorder.

Client Needs Category—Physiological integrity
Client Needs Subcategory—Pharmacological therapies

7. 2. Acromegaly results from an overproduction of growth hormone. When the disorder occurs in adulthood, the bones of the hands, jaw, feet, and forehead enlarge but do not lengthen. Acromegaly that develops at or before puberty generally results in gigantism. Males with acromegaly are likely to experience impotence, but their testes are not unusually small. Although the disorder may cause wide gaps between the teeth due to jaw changes, acromegaly is not known to cause tooth loss.

Client Needs Category—Physiological integrity
Client Needs Subcategory—Physiological adaptation

8. 1. Despite his large size, a client with acromegaly is likely to suffer from *Activity intolerance* because of muscle weakness, joint pain, and joint stiffness. Cognitive functions are not usually affected unless there is metastatic disease involving the cortex. Pulmonary functions generally remain adequate. Clients with acromegaly have difficulty chewing because of the malformations in their jaw and teeth, but swallowing is unaffected.

Client Needs Category—Safe and effective care environment
Client Needs Subcategory—Coordinated care

9. 3. The client may experience dizziness when his blood pressure falls due to rapid positional changes. Lying down after taking the medication and avoiding hot showers will not prevent orthostatic hypotension. It is appropriate to have the blood pressure monitored, but this assessment should be performed first in a supine position and then upright, which this option does not specify. If orthostatic hypotension is a concern, frequent monitoring of blood pressure is necessary. Blood pressure should be monitored at least every 4 hours and with activity changes.

Client Needs Category—Physiological integrity
Client Needs Subcategory—Pharmacological therapies

10. 1. Unfortunately, a client with acromegaly will never regain his normal appearance despite successful treatment of the disease. Hormone replacement therapy is necessary following surgery or irradiation of the anterior pituitary gland. The client should wear a medical alert tag and see his physician regularly. The surgical incision is made through the nose and is invisible.

Client Needs Category—Physiological integrity
Client Needs Subcategory—Physiological adaptation

11. 2. The surgical incision is made through the upper gingival mucosa, along one side of the nasal septum and through the sphenoid sinus. Postoperatively, the nose is packed with gauze. In addition to checking the saturation and appearance of the gauze packing, the nurse inspects the pharynx, where blood or cerebrospinal fluid may drain posteriorly. Examining the client's skull, behind the ear, or above the eyelid will not help with the assessment.

Client Needs Category—Physiological integrity
Client Needs Subcategory—Reduction of risk potential

Nursing Care of Clients with Disorders of the Thyroid Gland

12. 3. The amount of radiation used in a radioactive iodine uptake test is minute, but special precautions (such as flushing the toilet twice after use, rinsing the bathroom sink and tub, and using separate bath linens) are generally suggested. These precautions are only needed for a few days. Although there is no antidote for radioactive iodine, there is no justification for isolating the client because of the minute exposure.

Client Needs Category—Safe, effective care environment
Client Needs Subcategory—Reduction of risk potential

13. 1. Common signs of myxedema include a hoarse and raspy voice, slow speech, lethargy, expressionless face, protruding tongue, coarse and sparse hair, weight gain, and dry skin.

> ***Client Needs Category**—Physiological integrity*
> ***Client Needs Subcategory**—Physiological adaptation*

14. 2. Due to their lowered rate of metabolism, individuals with myxedema do not generate the same amount of energy and body heat as those with a normal metabolism. Consequently, clients typically complain of being excessively cold. The disorder is not associated with difficulty in urination, profuse perspiration, or excessive appetite.

> ***Client Needs Category**—Physiological integrity*
> ***Client Needs Subcategory**—Physiological adaptation*

15. 3. Thyroid replacement therapy is maintained during the course of a client's lifetime. A low dose is given initially, then increased or decreased based on the drug levels in the blood. Dosage adjustments are also made periodically during a client's lifetime based on the client's liver and kidney function, other medications that the client may be taking, and the client's clinical presentation of signs and symptoms. The physician prescribed the drug to be taken once per day, not after each meal. Levothyroxine (Synthroid) is more likely to cause insomnia than fatigue or sleepiness. The client should consult her physician before omitting or discontinuing the drug, regardless of the reason.

> ***Client Needs Category**—Physiological integrity*
> ***Client Needs Subcategory**—Pharmacological therapies*

16. 2. One of the causes of endemic (colloid, or simple) goiter is a deficiency of iodine in the diet. One method of ensuring an adequate supply of iodine is to use iodized salt, not plain table salt. Leafy vegetables, whole grains, and citrus fruits are not good sources of iodine.

> ***Client Needs Category**—Health promotion and maintenance*
> ***Client Needs Subcategory**—None*

17. 3. An endemic goiter is unlikely to cause any symptoms unless it becomes so large that it creates pressure on the airway or esophagus. If this occurs, the client would have difficulty breathing or swallowing. Weight is unaffected by the disorder. Hand tremors are a sign of toxic goiter (Graves' disease). Sparse loss of hair is characteristic of myxedema.

> ***Client Needs Category**—Physiological integrity*
> ***Client Needs Subcategory**—Physiological adaptation*

18. 1. Exophthalmos (bulging or enlarged eyes) is a common characteristic among clients with Graves' disease, or toxic diffuse goiter. The other facial features described are not directly related to this thyroid disorder.

> ***Client Needs Category**—Physiological integrity*
> ***Client Needs Subcategory**—Physiological adaptation*

19. 4. Antithyroid drugs such as propylthiouracil (Propyl-Thyracil) can cause cretinism (hypothyroidism) in a developing fetus. Therefore, asking about the client's pregnancy status is essential. Although the client may have trouble swallowing and the drug may cause gastrointestinal side effects, ensuring the safety of the client and her fetus is the nurse's priority. Propylthiouracil (Propyl-Thyracil) is not available in a liquid form, but the client may be instructed to crush the tablet and mix it with food.

> ***Client Needs Category**—Physiological integrity*
> ***Client Needs Subcategory**—Pharmacological therapies*

20. 1. A sore throat, fever, and malaise may indicate that the client has insufficient white blood cells to prevent infection. Heart palpitations, a symptom of Graves' disease, become infrequent as treatment with propylthiouracil (Propyl-Thyracil) continues. The client may experience nausea, vomiting, and epigastric distress; however, these symptoms may occur regardless of which foods the client ingests, including fatty foods. Prolonged bleeding is evidence of thrombocytopenia, but this is not a sign of agranulocytosis.

> ***Client Needs Category**—Physiological integrity*
> ***Client Needs Subcategory**—Pharmacological therapies*

21. 3. Diluting the strong Lugol's iodine solution in fruit juice or water tends to disguise its unpleasant taste. Although swallowing the drug quickly may ensure that all of the drug is taken, this is not the best advice. There is no real reason to recommend chilling the drug or taking it before meals.

> ***Client Needs Category**—Physiological integrity*
> ***Client Needs Subcategory**—Pharmacological therapies*

22. 3. Preoperative therapy with antithyroid drugs reduces the potential for postoperative bleeding and the development of a thyroid crisis, or storm. Even though the treatment reduces the size of the gland, this is not the underlying reason for the drug therapy. The postoperative recovery period is shortened if complications are prevented, but reducing the potential for bleeding is a more accurate answer. Thyroid replacement therapy may still be required after a subtotal thyroidectomy despite preoperative antithyroid drug therapy.

Client Needs Category—*Physiological integrity*
Client Needs Subcategory—*Pharmacological therapies*

23. **1.** Preoperative instructions must include how to support the head and neck when turning or rising to a sitting or standing position. This prevents tension on the sutures in the neck. The other information is important to include, but it is not as essential for the client to know.
Client Needs Category—*Physiological integrity*
Client Needs Subcategory—*Basic care and comfort*

24. **2.** Airway obstruction is a potential postoperative complication for clients who undergo thyroidectomy. Therefore, a common standard of practice is to keep a tracheostomy tray in the client's room. A mechanical ventilator will probably be unnecessary once airway patency is reestablished. A dressing change kit can be easily obtained; it is not an emergency item. Epinephrine may be necessary if the client develops a life-threatening cardiac arrhythmia, but this drug is usually stocked in emergency carts.
Client Needs Category—*Physiological integrity*
Client Needs Subcategory—*Reduction of risk potential*

25. **3.** Semi-Fowler's position, with the head elevated 30 to 45 degrees, is best for reducing postoperative incisional edema and facilitating ventilation. None of the other identified positions is therapeutic for accomplishing this goal.
Client Needs Category—*Physiological integrity*
Client Needs Subcategory—*Reduction of risk potential*

26. **1.** Coughing may precipitate bleeding in and around the surgical area and increase the risk of airway obstruction. Therefore, it is best to consult the physician before encouraging the client to cough postoperatively. The client is encouraged to take deep cleansing breaths, ambulate, and dangle his legs from the side of the bed, as tolerated.
Client Needs Category—*Physiological integrity*
Client Needs Subcategory—*Reduction of risk potential*

27. **2.** Gently placing a gloved hand behind the client's neck and checking for dampness allows the nurse to determine if blood or drainage is oozing from the incisional wound. The pillow, bed linen, and dressing should also be inspected for fresh drainage each time the client is turned. Passing a flashlight across the dressing is unreliable; it may reveal Betadine stains or dried surgical blood. Initially, the physician removes the postoperative dressing to inspect the wound. Weighing the dressing is

unnecessary because the physician asks for the number, not the weight, of soiled dressings.
Client Needs Category—*Physiological integrity*
Client Needs Subcategory—*Reduction of risk potential*

28. **4.** Although hoarseness may be temporary after a subtotal thyroidectomy, laryngeal nerve damage is manifested by persistent voice changes or the inability to make vocal sound. None of the other techniques is appropriate for assessing laryngeal nerve function.
Client Needs Category—*Physiological integrity*
Client Needs Subcategory—*Reduction of risk potential*

29. **2.** Tingling and numbness around the mouth and extremities are characteristic of hypocalcemia. These are commonly the first symptoms noted by a client following a subtotal thyroidectomy. The remaining complaints (loss of appetite, weakness, and sensitivity to light) are not usually associated with hypocalcemia.
Client Needs Category—*Physiological integrity*
Client Needs Subcategory—*Reduction of risk potential*

30. **1.** A client with hypocalcemia will manifest Chvostek's sign, facial muscle spasms elicited when the cheek over the facial nerve is gently tapped. Stroking the sole of the foot is a means of assessing the Babinski response. Homans' sign is assessed by dorsiflexing the foot. Closing the eyes and touching the nose is a method for testing proprioception, the ability to identify the location of a body part without looking at it.
Client Needs Category—*Physiological integrity*
Client Needs Subcategory—*Physiological adaptation*

31. **1.** Exaggerated signs of increased metabolism are a manifestation of thyroid crisis (also called *thyroid storm*). Some signs include hyperpyrexia (fever), hypertension, severe tachycardia, chest pain, and an altered level of consciousness. Carpal spasms are a sign of hypocalcemia. Noisy respirations may indicate laryngospasm due to hypocalcemia or a partial airway obstruction. Hypotension is not a sign of thyroid crisis.
Client Needs Category—*Physiological integrity*
Client Needs Subcategory—*Reduction of risk potential*

32. **2, 3, 5, 6.** Thyroid replacement therapy can increase metabolism, causing symptoms similar to hyperthyroidism. Until the client adjusts to the replacement therapy or the optimum dosage is determined, the client may experience stimulation of the cardiovascular system, which is manifested by tachycardia and hypertension. Metabolic stimulation can also result in

insomnia and tremors. Hyperglycemia and hirsutism are side effects of corticosteroid therapy.
   Client Needs Category—*Physiological integrity*
   Client Needs Subcategory—*Pharmacological therapies*

Nursing Care of Clients with Disorders of the Parathyroid Glands

33. **2.** A parathyroid tumor usually causes hypercalcemia and a loss of calcium from the bones to the blood. This leads to the formation of kidney stones and other renal complications. Hypocalcemia or other etiologies cause leg cramps. Constipation, not loose stools, is more common among clients with hyperparathyroidism. Insomnia is not commonly associated with hyperparathyroidism.
   Client Needs Category—*Physiological integrity*
   Client Needs Subcategory—*Physiological adaptation*

34. **4.** Loss of calcium from the bones weakens the skeletal system, which potentiates the risk of pathologic fractures. Impaired equilibrium, seizures, and syncope are not common among clients with hyperparathyroidism.
   Client Needs Category—*Safe, effective care environment*
   Client Needs Subcategory—*Safety and infection control*

35. **2.** Postoperatively, it is therapeutic to include sources of calcium in the client's diet because the function of the parathyroid gland is suddenly and severely compromised. Foods that are good sources of calcium include milk and cheese. Calcium gluconate may be administered I.V. if the client experiences severe hypocalcemia.
   Client Needs Category—*Physiological integrity*
   Client Needs Subcategory—*Basic care and comfort*

36. **1.** Hypoparathyroidism is caused by inadequate secretion of parathyroid hormone, which leads to increased phosphorus levels and a deficiency in blood calcium levels. This deficiency results in hypocalcemia and leads to tetany, the chief symptom of hypoparathyroidism. Tetany is a general muscular condition that results in tremors and spastic, uncoordinated movements. When tetany occurs, calcium gluconate or calcium chloride is the drug of choice for I.V. administration. Ferrous sulfate is a source of iron; it is administered orally to treat anemia. Potassium chloride is given to prevent or relieve hypokalemia. Sodium bicarbonate is administered to maintain normal acid-base balance.

   Client Needs Category—*Physiological integrity*
   Client Needs Subcategory—*Pharmacological therapies*

Nursing Care of Clients with Disorders of the Adrenal Glands

37. **4.** Addison's disease is caused by a deficiency of cortical hormones that develops from adrenal insufficiency. Clients appear unusually tan, bronze, or darkly pigmented. Other signs and symptoms include fatigue, emaciation, hypotension, decreased glucose and sodium levels, and increased potassium level. A moon-shaped face, skin blemishes, and obesity are more characteristic of a hyperfunctioning adrenal cortex or endogenous steroid therapy.
   Client Needs Category—*Physiological integrity*
   Client Needs Subcategory—*Physiological adaptation*

38. **1.** If inadequately treated, Addison's disease leads to dehydration and hypotension. If unresolved, it can lead to addisonian crisis, which is characterized by cyanosis, fever, and the classic signs of shock. Monitoring the blood pressure and its subsequent trends provides some of the best data for evaluating the client's health status. Bowel, breath, and heart sounds are not generally abnormal in Addison's disease.
   Client Needs Category—*Physiological integrity*
   Client Needs Subcategory—*Physiological adaptation*

39. **2.** A client with Addison's disease has low sodium levels; therefore, replacing dietary sodium is important. Milk products, such as cheese, and other sources of animal protein are high in natural sodium content. Although baked goods also contain hidden sodium, two graham crackers have half the amount of sodium as 1 ounce of cheddar cheese. Fruits and vegetables are considered low in sodium when compared with other food sources.
   Client Needs Category—*Physiological integrity*
   Client Needs Subcategory—*Basic care and comfort*

40. **4.** Clients with Addison's disease are prone to developing low blood glucose levels (hypoglycemia). Snacks such as milk and crackers contain complex carbohydrates that take longer to metabolize than simple sugars. Therefore, they are more likely to help maintain a stable blood glucose level. To reduce episodes of hypoglycemia, it is appropriate to schedule at least six small meals per day or between-meal snacks. Although the other choices contain some complex carbohydrates, they also contain sources of quickly metabolized sugars.

Client Needs Category—*Physiological integrity*
Client Needs Subcategory—*Basic care and comfort*

41. **1.** Stress and any of the following factors—salt deprivation, infection, trauma, exposure to cold, or overexertion—can overwhelm the client's ability to maintain homeostasis. This imbalance can lead to the development of addisonian crisis, a life-threatening condition. Alcohol consumption, eating complex carbohydrates, and sleep deprivation are not relevant factors in Addison's disease.
Client Needs Category—*Physiological integrity*
Client Needs Subcategory—*Reduction of risk
potential*

42. **1.** Cushing's syndrome is the result of excessive corticosteroid production. When this occurs, the client develops several multisystem clinical manifestations, including thin extremities (from muscle wasting and weakness) and a heavy trunk. Other common signs and symptoms include moon face, buffalo hump, ruddy complexion, thin and fragile skin, bruising, striae, peripheral edema, hypertension, hirsutism (in women), mood changes, depression, and psychosis.
Client Needs Category—*Physiological integrity*
Client Needs Subcategory—*Physiological
adaptation*

43. **2.** To be precise, a 24-hour urine collection begins after a client empties his bladder and ends with a final voiding at the same time the following day.
Client Needs Category—*Safe, effective care environment*
Client Needs Subcategory—*Coordinated care*

44. **2.** To avoid chemical changes in the contents of the urine, a 24-hour specimen is deposited in a container with preservative. Generally, the urine is refrigerated or placed on ice during the collection period. The collection container is usually kept in the client's room or bathroom. It is unnecessary to measure each voided volume; if this is done, it is for reasons other than specimen collection. Clients generally void into a urinal or container suspended in the toilet; the urine is then added to the collection container.
Client Needs Category—*Physiological integrity*
Client Needs Subcategory—*Reduction of risk
potential*

45. **1.** Female clients with Cushing's syndrome acquire masculine characteristics, such as a deep voice and excessive growth of body hair, including facial hair. If premenopausal, they may also develop amenorrhea. Large breasts, heavy menstruation, and severe weight loss are not characteristic of Cushing's syndrome.

Client Needs Category—*Physiological integrity*
Client Needs Subcategory—*Physiological
adaptation*

46. **2.** Depression is common among clients with Cushing's syndrome because of the severity of physical changes; this places clients at increased risk for suicide. The other emotional symptoms are not necessarily associated with Cushing's syndrome, although they may occur randomly in some clients for other psychophysiologic reasons.
Client Needs Category—*Psychosocial adaptation*
Client Needs Subcategory—*None*

47. **4.** A sodium-restricted diet is prescribed to reduce the potential for excess fluid volume and increased serum sodium levels. One of the best ways to monitor the effects of sodium restriction is by weighing the client daily. The client's skin turgor and abdominal girth are unlikely to change as much as her weight from one day to the next. Monitoring the amount of sodium that the client consumes from the dietary tray is appropriate to document, but it does not provide as objective an assessment as the daily weight.
Client Needs Category—*Safe, effective care environment*
Client Needs Subcategory—*Coordinated care*

48. **1.** Clients with Cushing's syndrome have thin, fragile, easily traumatized skin that is susceptible to the effects of prolonged pressure. Therefore, it is appropriate to exercise gentleness when turning and repositioning the client and to use pressure-relieving devices such as a convoluted foam mattress. The client needs rest more than activity to accommodate her weakness and fatigue. Controlling environmental stimuli is not more important for this client than for other clients. The client's carbohydrate intake should be limited because of the tendency for hyperglycemia.
Client Needs Category—*Physiological integrity*
Client Needs Subcategory—*Physiological
adaptation*

49. **4.** Extreme hypotension, fever, vomiting, diarrhea, abdominal pain, profound weakness, headache, and restlessness are all signs of addisonian crisis, which occurs from a sudden drop in adrenocortical hormones. Therefore, the client's ability to maintain vital signs within preoperative ranges is the best indication that addisonian crisis has been avoided. An adequate urine output, normal blood glucose level, and comfort are all positive outcomes of nursing care, but they are not the best evidence that addisonian crisis has been prevented.
Client Needs Category—*Physiological integrity*
Client Needs Subcategory—*Physiological
adaptation*

50. 2. Because of the client's thin, fragile skin and tendency to heal slowly, it is necessary to pull tape toward the suture line rather than away from it when changing dressings. This will prevent the sutures from separating. Although it is true that protein promotes healing, and that the nurse needs to monitor I.V. antibiotics and cover the client's wound with gauze, these nursing measures are not as critical to the healing process as preserving an intact incisional site.
Client Needs Category—Physiological integrity
Client Needs Subcategory—Basic care and comfort

51. 1. Preoperatively and postoperatively, a client with Cushing's syndrome is at increased risk for acquiring infections because of the anti-inflammatory effects of corticosteroid hormones, which may mask the common signs of inflammation and infection. Therefore, avoiding people with infectious diseases is prudent. The client is also at risk for fluid volume deficits and should maintain an adequate fluid intake. The client's cushingoid appearance should slowly recede as hormone levels are reestablished at lower-than-preoperative levels. After a bilateral adrenalectomy, hormone replacement therapy is a lifelong necessity. In fact, a medical alert tag should be worn at all times.
Client Needs Category—Health promotion and maintenance
Client Needs Subcategory—None

52. 2. The adrenal medulla secretes epinephrine and norepinephrine. A tumor involving the adrenal medulla produces signs of sympathetic nervous system stimulation, such as severe hypertension, tachycardia, anxiety, insomnia, tremors, headache, and diaphoresis (sweating). Hyperglycemia—not hyperinsulinism—is more apt to occur. Although the client may have heat intolerance and diaphoresis, the body temperature would not be extremely increased. Hyperkalemia is not associated with pheochromocytoma.
Client Needs Category—Physiological integrity
Client Needs Subcategory—Physiological adaptation

53. 1. Caffeine in any form—tea, coffee, cola—compounds the systemic stimulation already manifested as a result of pheochromocytoma. Ice water, skim milk, and apple juice are not as potentially dangerous as caffeine for this client.
Client Needs Category—Physiological integrity
Client Needs Subcategory—Reduction of risk potential

Nursing Care of Clients with Pancreatic Endocrine Disorders

54. 2. Hyperinsulinism, also known as *functional hypoglycemia*, is caused by an overproduction of insulin, which occurs about 2 hours after eating a meal, especially one containing refined sugar or simple carbohydrates. This results in a drop in blood glucose levels.
Client Needs Category—Physiological integrity
Client Needs Subcategory—Physiological adaptation

55. 4. A container of 75 to 100 g of glucose is consumed orally or administered I.V. before the glucose tolerance test begins. Otherwise, the client fasts before and during the test. Only water is allowed during the test. Urine specimens are collected before the glucose is administered and when subsequent blood samples are taken. The client is instructed to consume an adequate diet containing carbohydrates for at least 3 days before the diagnostic test, then fast for 12 hours before the test.
Client Needs Category—Physiological integrity
Client Needs Subcategory—Basic care and comfort

56. 3. To maintain stable blood glucose levels, it is best for clients with functional hypoglycemia to consume small, frequent meals that contain high-fiber complex carbohydrates. Some examples include fruits, vegetables, legumes, and whole grains. Simple sugars, such as glucose, fructose, and galactose, tend to stimulate the release of insulin and lower the blood glucose level drastically. Complete proteins and unsaturated fats in moderate amounts are components of a healthy diet, but they are not as therapeutic for stabilizing the blood glucose.
Client Needs Category—Health promotion and maintenance
Client Needs Subcategory—None

57. 1. If dietary measures are appropriate, clients experience fewer symptoms of hypoglycemia, such as weakness, tremors, headache, nausea, hunger, malaise, excess perspiration, confusion, and personality changes. The other choices do not relate to functional hypoglycemia.
Client Needs Category—Health promotion and maintenance
Client Needs Subcategory—None

58. 2. The term postprandial means after eating a meal. The meal acts as a glucose challenge. The blood glucose level normally increases in response to the intake of carbohydrates. Two hours later, the blood glucose level of nondiabetics should return to normal. If the blood glucose level remains elevated 2 hours after eating, this suggests a metabolic disorder such as diabetes mellitus.

Client Needs Category—*Health promotion and maintenance*
Client Needs Subcategory—*None*

59. 3. Positive screening test results are an indication that the client requires further evaluation by a physician. Because several factors and disease pathologies can cause hyperglycemia, it is always best to refer hyperglycemic individuals to a physician. Comments about taking insulin or avoiding candy should alert the nurse that the client requires further education about his condition.

Client Needs Category—*Health promotion and maintenance*
Client Needs Subcategory—*None*

60. 4. Polyuria (excessive secretion and voiding of urine), polydipsia (excessive thirst), and polyphagia (increased appetite) are the classic signs and symptoms of diabetes mellitus. Polycholia (increased secretion of bile), polyemia (increased amount of circulating blood), polyplegia (paralysis of several muscles), diarrhea, constipation, and anorexia are not considered signs and symptoms of this endocrine disorder. Weight gain or loss is seen in some people with diabetes.

Client Needs Category—*Health promotion and maintenance*
Client Needs Subcategory—*None*

61. 4. The client needs time to accept the diagnosis and to talk about fears and concerns. Listening is the most therapeutic intervention at this point. Stressing the importance of treatment is likely to increase her fears. The client with type 2 diabetes may be required to self-administer injections. Telling the client that others manage their diabetes ignores the fact that this disorder is unique to the newly diagnosed diabetic.

Client Needs Category—*Psychosocial integrity*
Client Needs Subcategory—*None*

62. 3. Exercise has many beneficial effects, such as controlling weight, reducing appetite, improving circulation, and lowering heart rate, regardless of a person's health status. For a client with diabetes, however, one of the primary benefits is a reduced blood glucose level. If the blood glucose level decreases with exercise, drug treatment with oral hypoglycemic agents or insulin may be delayed, reduced, or eliminated.

Client Needs Category—*Health promotion and maintenance*
Client Needs Subcategory—*None*

63. 2. The main advantage of using an exchange list is that it eliminates the need to count calories. Instead, clients are prescribed the number of exchanges they may use in particular categories. They can choose among items of equal nutritional value, provided they consume the serving size the list specifies.

Client Needs Category—*Health promotion and maintenance*
Client Needs Subcategory—*None*

64. 3. "Lite" or "light" is a food-labeling term that means the product contains one-third fewer calories than a similar unaltered item. Thus, light beer contains calories or grams of nutrients that must be calculated in the diabetic's diet and exchange list.

Client Needs Category—*Health promotion and maintenance*
Client Needs Subcategory—*None*

65. 3. A medium apple is the most appropriate choice for this client. The 1,500-calorie Dietary Exchange Plan indicates that a client can have one fruit exchange as a mid-afternoon snack.

Client Needs Category—*Physiological integrity*
Client Needs Subcategory—*Basic care and comfort*

66. 1. Insulin is administered parenterally because it is a protein substance readily destroyed in the GI tract. None of the other choices accurately describes the rationale for excluding insulin administration by the oral route.

Client Needs Category—*Physiological integrity*
Client Needs Subcategory—*Pharmacological therapies*

67. 4. Clients who take glyburide (DiaBeta) and consume alcohol may have a disulfiram-like reaction. Disulfiram (Antabuse), a drug commonly given to treat alcoholism, interacts with alcohol to produce flushing, throbbing head pain, respiratory difficulty, nausea, vomiting, sweating, thirst, chest pain, palpitations, tachycardia, hypotension, syncope, blurred vision, and confusion. The remaining choices are not known to cause food-drug interactions.

Client Needs Category—*Physiological integrity*
Client Needs Subcategory—*Reduction of risk potential*

68. 2. To maintain stable control of blood glucose levels, it is essential to take medication, eat, and exercise at regular, consistent times each day. Implying that the therapeutic regimen is flexible predisposes clients to develop unstable blood glucose levels and metabolic complications.

Client Needs Category—*Health promotion and maintenance*
Client Needs Subcategory—*None*

69. **1.** Urine testing using reagent tablets or strips is the most economical of diabetic monitoring techniques. A home glucometer is more accurate and preferred for poorly controlled diabetic clients. Self-monitoring with a glucometer is costly but less expensive than the added charges for the services of laboratory personnel or a home health nurse.

Client Needs Category—Health promotion and maintenance
Client Needs Subcategory—None

70. **3.** An acetone (sometimes described as sweet or fruity) breath odor, weakness, thirst, anorexia, vomiting, drowsiness, abdominal pain, rapid and weak pulse, hypotension, flushed skin, and Kussmaul's (rapid, deep, and noisy) respirations are manifested by persons with DKA. In severe cases, the client may be comatose or semi-comatose.

Client Needs Category—Physiological integrity
Client Needs Subcategory—Physiological adaptation

71. **4.** It is best to let the blood flow passively by gravity onto the test strip or reflecting area of the electronic glucometer. The skin is usually cleaned with soap and water. A rubber band is not applied. In fact, some recommend that the nurse avoid squeezing the tissue to promote bleeding. Piercing the central pad of a finger is avoided; the margin around the digit produces less pain.

Client Needs Category—Safe, effective care environment
Client Needs Subcategory—Safety and infection control

72. **2.** A blood glucose reading below 70 mg/dL is a sign of hypoglycemia. Assuming the glucometer reading is accurate and the client is symptomatic, the best action is to implement some means of increasing the client's blood glucose level. This may be done with a variety of substances, such as sweetened fruit juice, honey, hard candy, cake icing, or packets of granulated sugar. Insulin will drop the blood glucose level further; therefore, it is inappropriate in this case. A complete head-to-toe assessment may be done, but will prolong treatment. The physician is usually notified, but only after the nurse implements some method to increase the blood glucose level. The physician may prescribe parenterally administered glucose or glucagon if the client is unresponsive.

Client Needs Category—Physiological integrity
Client Needs Subcategory—Physiological adaptation

73. **2.** The onset of action of most rapid-acting insulins (regular insulin in particular) is within 30 to 90 minutes after administration. Hypoglycemia is even more likely to occur when insulin reaches its peak effect. For regular insulin, this peak is approximately 2 to 5 hours later. The duration of regular insulin is approximately 8 hours.

Client Needs Category—Physiological integrity
Client Needs Subcategory—Pharmacological therapies

74. **3.** The client needs to take care to avoid mixing the intermediate-acting insulin, which contains an additive, with the additive-free insulin. The additive-free insulin is always withdrawn first. The actions described in the other options are safe and appropriate for mixing two different types of insulins.

Client Needs Category—Safe, effective care environment
Client Needs Subcategory—Safety and infection control

75. **4.** To prevent lipodystrophy and lipoatrophy and promote appropriate absorption of insulin, it is correct to rotate insulin injection sites. Insulin is prepared in an insulin syringe calibrated in units. The needle length is ½″ to ⅝″. Insulin is injected at a 45- or 90-degree angle, depending on the client's size.

Client Needs Category—Health promotion and maintenance
Client Needs Subcategory—None

76.

1.	Instill 20 units of air in the vial of Novolin N.
2.	Instill 10 units of air in the vial of Novolin R.
4.	Withdraw 10 units of insulin from the vial of Novolin R.
3.	Withdraw 20 units of insulin from the vial of Novolin N.

When insulins are mixed, air is instilled in the vial with the longer-acting insulin first. The syringe is removed, and then air is added to the short-acting insulin. The prescribed amount of the short-acting insulin is immediately withdrawn into the syringe after instilling the air. The syringe is then returned to the vial of longer-acting insulin, and the prescribed amount is withdrawn into the syringe. The principle is: "clear to cloudy," which means the clear (Novolin R, in this example) in-

sulin is placed in the syringe first before adding the cloudy (Novolin N, in this example) to the syringe.
Client Needs Category—Physiological integrity
Client Needs Subcategory—Pharmacological therapies

77. 4. Insulin-dependent clients are likely to remain so for the rest of their lives. Therefore, further instruction is needed if the client believes that he may eventually stop taking the medication. Even some clients with type 2 diabetes eventually become insulin-dependent. The client is correct in understanding that insulin needs increase during times of stress, such as infections and emotional crises. Although exercise is beneficial, clients may need additional calories to prevent symptoms of hypoglycemia.
Client Needs Category—Health promotion and maintenance
Client Needs Subcategory—None

78. 2, 4, 5, 6. A client with diabetes must learn to recognize the signs of hypoglycemia. Shakiness and disturbed cognition—two classic signs—occur when the central nervous system, which relies entirely on glucose for energy, has insufficient glucose circulating in the blood. The body releases epinephrine in response to low blood glucose, causing such symptoms as palpitations and diaphoresis. Hunger, a homeostatic response, promotes the consumption of calories. Signs of hyperglycemia (not hypoglycemia) include thirst and sleepiness.
Client Needs Category—Physiological integrity
Client Needs Subcategory—Reduction of risk potential

79. 3. Insulin deteriorates if exposed to excessive heat or light. It is best kept at room temperature or stored in a cool area. Unopened vials may be kept refrigerated. Insulin should never be frozen.
Client Needs Category—Health promotion and maintenance
Client Needs Subcategory—None

80. 2. Soaking the feet tends to soften the skin and predisposes it to trauma. The feet are washed daily with soap and water, and then dried thoroughly before the client dons clean socks and supportive shoes. Clients with diabetes should inspect their feet daily for signs of injury or poor circulation. Going barefoot is contraindicated because this predisposes the client to foot injuries. The client should see a podiatrist regularly to have the toenails cut and filed.
Client Needs Category—Health promotion and maintenance
Client Needs Subcategory—None

81. 2. The most objective evidence for evaluating how well the client is managing therapy is a record of glucose monitoring values. Some glucometers store the data so that results can be retrieved and evaluated. Otherwise, clients are asked to keep a written record of their monitoring results. Identifying the dosage and frequency of insulin administration does not indicate that the client is actually self-administering the insulin. Maintaining or gradually losing weight is good evaluative information, but it is not as specific as glucose monitoring values. Some clients are not as self-aware of symptoms, and some have an exaggerated awareness of their body functions. Therefore, subjective symptoms are not as valuable as hard objective data.
Client Needs Category—Health promotion and maintenance
Client Needs Subcategory—None

82. 4. A glycosylated (A1c) hemoglobin test reveals the effectiveness of diabetic therapy for the preceding 8 to 12 weeks. A fasting blood glucose provides information on the blood glucose status for the immediate period of time. Blood chemistry includes a blood glucose measurement as well as several other diagnostic test results. A complete blood count indicates the status of the client's hematopoietic functions.
Client Needs Category—Health promotion and maintenance
Client Needs Subcategory—None

83. 3. Continuous insulin infusions are administered by the subcutaneous route, usually in abdominal tissue. However, any of the subcutaneous sites (such as the buttocks, thighs, arms, and sections of the back) may be used. An insulin infusion pump delivers regular insulin at a carefully regulated rate. Insulin is absorbed too quickly when instilled I.V. or I.M.
Client Needs Category—Health promotion and maintenance
Client Needs Subcategory—None

84. 2. Clients with diabetes should consult their physician about trimming or cutting the toenails. An abrasive file may be used to keep the nails short, but it is best to refer clients to a podiatrist for nail maintenance or other foot problems. The other hygiene measures are good to implement, but they are not as pertinent to the care of a client with diabetes.
Client Needs Category—Health promotion and maintenance
Client Needs Subcategory—None

85.

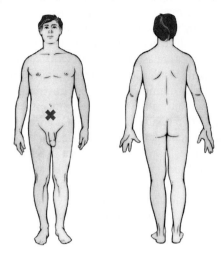

The abdomen is the preferred site for insulin administration to facilitate the most rapid rate of absorption. Absorption is somewhat slower in the arms, slower still in the legs, and slowest in the hip or buttocks area. The abdomen is also generally easier to access for self-administration, and the absorption rate is constant.

Client Needs Category—Physiological integrity
Client Needs Subcategory—Pharmacological
*   therapy*

86. 2. HHNS is characterized by extremely high blood glucose levels—between 600 and 1,000 mg/dL—without signs of ketoacidosis. The severe hyperglycemia causes fluid to shift from the intracellular space to the extracellular space, and copious amounts of urine are excreted. Warm, dry skin from dehydration is a normal finding. Acetone is not present in the urine of clients experiencing HHNS; it is typically found in the urine of those with ketoacidosis.

Client Needs Category—Physiological integrity
Client Needs Subcategory—Safety and infection
*   control*

87. 4. Clients with diabetes are prone to many systemic vascular and neurologic complications. These include a higher incidence of premature cataract formation, retinal hemorrhage and blindness, stroke, myocardial infarction, renal failure, peripheral neurovascular disease and amputations, and sexual dysfunction. Liver disease is atypical among clients with diabetes mellitus.

Client Needs Category—Health promotion and
*   maintenance*
Client Needs Subcategory—None

88. 1. Kussmaul's respirations, a common sign of DKA, are a compensatory mechanism to eliminate carbon dioxide from the body and prevent a further drop in pH. Respirations are typically fast, rapid, deep, and

labored with a longer expiration. The other options are not characteristic of Kussmaul's respirations.

Client Needs Category—Physiological integrity
Client Needs Subcategory—Physiological adaptation

89. 1. Insulin is a hormone that regulates glucose in the blood. During times of sickness, dehydration (from persistent vomiting and diarrhea) and the stress of illness can cause the glucose level to increase. This is especially critical for an insulin-dependent diabetic, who may not have enough insulin in his system to counteract the rising glucose level. Therefore, it is important for the nurse to teach the client about the effects of dehydration and the need for blood glucose monitoring and insulin administration when ill. Blood glucose levels should be monitored every 2 to 4 hours during sick times. Eating candy or drinking high-calorie beverages will cause the blood glucose level to rise, especially if there is no insulin on board to counteract the glucose. Testing the urine daily for protein is not typically done during times of illness.

Client Needs Category—Health promotion and
*   maintenance*
Client Needs Subcategory—None

90. 4. Insulin lowers blood glucose levels. Because the client received two doses of insulin, he is at risk for developing hypoglycemia and possible diabetic coma. Therefore, the nurse should monitor the client's blood glucose level frequently. In addition, if the client is conscious, the nurse may offer orange juice with added sugar, a carbonated beverage, milk, candy, or a glucose gel. If the client is unconscious, the nurse should prepare to start an I.V. dextrose infusion. Because a medication error was made, an incident report must be completed; however, this should not take priority over the client's well-being. Calling ICU is unnecessary unless the client's glucose level drops dangerously low and treatment is ineffective. Performing neurologic checks and taking vital signs are prudent measures, but they are not as important as frequent blood glucose monitoring in this situation.

Client Needs Category—Physiological integrity
Client Needs Subcategory—Pharmacological
*   therapies*

The Nursing Care of Clients with Cardiac Disorders

⇨ **Nursing Care of Clients with Hypertensive Heart Disease**
⇨ **Nursing Care of Clients with Coronary Artery Disease**
⇨ **Nursing Care of Clients with Myocardial Infarction**
⇨ **Nursing Care of Clients with Congestive Heart Failure**
⇨ **Nursing Care of Clients with Conduction Disorders**
⇨ **Nursing Care of Clients with Valvular Disorders**
⇨ **Nursing Care of Clients with Infectious and Inflammatory Disorders of the Heart**
⇨ **Correct Answers and Rationales**

Directions: With a pencil, blacken the space in front of the option you have chosen for your correct answer.

Nursing Care of Clients with Hypertensive Heart Disease

A nurse volunteers to do blood pressure screenings at a local community hospital's annual health fair.

1. Which modification is most appropriate when taking the blood pressure of a person who weighs 250 pounds?
[ ] 1. The nurse takes the blood pressure on the client's thigh.
[ ] 2. The nurse has the client lie down during the assessment.
[ ] 3. The nurse pumps the manometer up to 250 mm Hg.
[ ] 4. The nurse uses an extra-large blood pressure cuff.

2. The nurse obtains adult blood pressure readings on four separate clients. Which client should have a follow-up blood pressure check within 2 months?
[ ] 1. The client whose blood pressure is 138/88 mm Hg
[ ] 2. The client whose blood pressure is 132/98 mm Hg
[ ] 3. The client whose blood pressure is 120/80 mm Hg
[ ] 4. The client whose blood pressure is 118/78 mm Hg

At the health fair, the nurse teaches the wife of a man with hypertension how to take and document her husband's blood pressure.

3. The nurse tells the wife that which is the correct time to note the diastolic blood pressure reading?
[ ] 1. When the loud knocking sounds become muffled
[ ] 2. When the last loud knocking sound is heard
[ ] 3. When the swishing sound becomes loud
[ ] 4. When the swishing sound becomes faint

While getting his blood pressure checked, an African American man asks the nurse why it is important for him to control his hypertension.

4. Which response by the nurse is most accurate?
[ ] 1. Sustained hypertension decreases the life span of many blood cells.
[ ] 2. Sustained hypertension leads to the formation of venous blood clots.
[ ] 3. Sustained hypertension compromises blood flow to many vital organs.
[ ] 4. Sustained hypertension predisposes to narrowing of the cardiac valves.

5. When obtaining a health history from this client, which finding strongly suggests that he is hypertensive?
[ ] 1. Unexplained nosebleeds
[ ] 2. Difficulty sleeping all night
[ ] 3. Blood in the urine
[ ] 4. Occasional heart palpitations

The nurse suggests to the client that he seek medical attention immediately. The client makes an appointment to see his physician.

6. When the nurse reviews the client's medical record, which finding best indicates that his heart has been affected by sustained high blood pressure?
[ ] **1.** The client has a strong S_1 heart sound.
[ ] **2.** The client's heart rate is 100 beats/minute when active.
[ ] **3.** The client's heart is moderately enlarged.
[ ] **4.** The client has an irregular heart rhythm.

The physician of a client with hypertension recommends that the client follow a low-sodium diet.

7. The best evidence that the client understands his dietary restrictions is if he says he must avoid which food?
[ ] **1.** Soy sauce
[ ] **2.** Lemon juice
[ ] **3.** Maple syrup
[ ] **4.** Onion powder

8. If the client with hypertension is willing to implement lifestyle changes to reduce his blood pressure, which change would be most beneficial?
[ ] **1.** Eating more fiber
[ ] **2.** Balancing rest with exercise
[ ] **3.** Taking time for more leisure activities
[ ] **4.** Giving up smoking cigarettes

The client with hypertension will begin taking furosemide (Lasix) 40 mg orally every day. However, prior to giving the first oral dose, the physician orders 60 mg I.M. STAT.

9. If the furosemide (Lasix) comes prepared in an ampule labeled 50 mg/2 mL, the nurse would expect to administer how many milliliters?
[ ] **1.** 0.24
[ ] **2.** 0.4
[ ] **3.** 1
[ ] **4.** 2.4

10. When preparing to withdraw furosemide (Lasix) from the ampule, which technique should the nurse use?
[ ] **1.** Allow the ampule to stand undisturbed for a few minutes after shaking it
[ ] **2.** Tap the ampule stem with the fingernail a few times
[ ] **3.** Hold the ampule upside down, then quickly turn it right-side up
[ ] **4.** Roll the ampule gently between the palms of the hands

11. Which observation best indicates that the furosemide (Lasix) has had a therapeutic effect on the client?
[ ] **1.** His pulse becomes slower.
[ ] **2.** His blood pressure stabilizes.
[ ] **3.** His urine output increases.
[ ] **4.** His anxiety is diminished.

12. When preparing discharge instructions for this client, the nurse should instruct him to take his oral furosemide (Lasix) at what time of day?
[ ] **1.** Before bedtime
[ ] **2.** When arising in the morning
[ ] **3.** With his main meal
[ ] **4.** In the late afternoon

13. When teaching the client about the side effects of furosemide (Lasix), the nurse instructs him that he will need to eat foods high in which mineral?
[ ] **1.** Potassium
[ ] **2.** Sodium
[ ] **3.** Calcium
[ ] **4.** Iron

14. The nurse instructs the client to monitor his urine output while taking furosemide (Lasix) at home because it may lead to which condition?
[ ] **1.** Dehydration
[ ] **2.** Fluid overload
[ ] **3.** Hypernatremia
[ ] **4.** Hyperkalemia

Nursing Care of Clients with Coronary Artery Disease

The nurse working on a medical-surgical unit identifies several clients who have been diagnosed with coronary artery disease (CAD).

15. Which of the following client risk factors is most significant for developing CAD?
[ ] **1.** Drinking a nightly cocktail
[ ] **2.** History of mitral valve repair
[ ] **3.** Rheumatic fever during childhood
[ ] **4.** Obesity

The physician tells a client at risk for CAD that his high cholesterol level needs to be lowered and advises him to follow a low-cholesterol diet.

16. When the client asks the nurse how cholesterol acts as a cardiac risk factor, what is the best explanation?

[ ] **1.** Excess fat in the blood expands the circulating blood volume.

[ ] **2.** Excess fat in the blood thickens the lining of the arteries.

[ ] **3.** Excess fat in the blood causes slower blood clotting.

[ ] **4.** Excess fat in the blood stimulates the heart to beat faster.

The client tells the nurse that his usual breakfast includes sausage, eggs, hash browns, and white bread and butter.

17. When providing dietary instructions for this client, which healthful alternative should the nurse recommend?

[ ] **1.** Wheat toast for white bread

[ ] **2.** Margarine for butter

[ ] **3.** Cereal for eggs

[ ] **4.** Ham for sausage

Lifestyle changes prove insufficient for reducing the client's cholesterol level, and the physician prescribes the antihyperlipidemic drug atorvastatin calcium (Lipitor).

18. After providing medication instructions, the best evidence that the client knows this drug's potential side effects is when he says it may cause which adverse effect?

[ ] **1.** Muscle pain

[ ] **2.** Palpitations

[ ] **3.** Visual changes

[ ] **4.** Weight loss

The client is scheduled for a stress electrocardiogram (ECG).

19. When the client asks why the physician ordered the ECG, how does the nurse correctly explain its purpose?

[ ] **1.** It will show how the heart performs during exercise.

[ ] **2.** It will determine the client's potential target heart rate.

[ ] **3.** It will verify how much the client needs to improve his fitness.

[ ] **4.** It will help predict whether the client will have a heart attack soon.

A client with CAD experiences periodic chest pain and is diagnosed with angina pectoris.

20. If the client is typical of others who have angina pectoris, the nurse would expect the client to report that his chest pain is best relieved by which nonpharmacologic measure?

[ ] **1.** Taking a deep breath

[ ] **2.** Resting in a chair

[ ] **3.** Applying heat to the chest

[ ] **4.** Rubbing the chest

The client informs the nurse that the physician just gave him a prescription to take sublingual nitroglycerin tablets whenever he experiences chest pain.

21. The nurse informs the client that the correct way to administer nitroglycerin is to place one tablet where?

[ ] **1.** Between his gum and cheek

[ ] **2.** At the back of his throat

[ ] **3.** Under his tongue

[ ] **4.** Between his teeth

22. Which side effect is most closely associated with the use of nitroglycerin tablets?

[ ] **1.** Headache

[ ] **2.** Backache

[ ] **3.** Diarrhea

[ ] **4.** Jaundice

The nurse explains to the client that nitroglycerin tablets lose their potency if exposed to light and air.

23. The nurse knows that the client understands how to determine when the nitroglycerin tablets need replacing when he makes which statement?

[ ] **1.** "The tablets will smell like vinegar."

[ ] **2.** "The tablets will be discolored."

[ ] **3.** "They won't tingle when I put them in my mouth."

[ ] **4.** "They'll disintegrate when I touch them."

24. The nurse correctly instructs the client that, if his chest pain is not relieved after taking one nitroglycerin tablet, he should take which action?

[ ] **1.** Take another tablet in 5 minutes

[ ] **2.** Drive to the emergency department

[ ] **3.** Call his physician immediately

[ ] **4.** Swallow two additional tablets

Because the client has repeated episodes of angina that have not been relieved with sublingual nitroglycerin, the physician prescribes a nitroglycerin transdermal patch (Nitrodisc).

25. Which nursing action is most appropriate when applying a new transdermal patch?

[ ] **1.** Rotate the application site.

[ ] **2.** Clean the skin with alcohol before applying the patch.

[ ] **3.** Tape the patch to the client's chest.

[ ] **4.** Take the client's blood pressure after placing the patch.

26. Which assessment finding should signal the nurse to withhold applying the client's nitroglycerin patch and notify the physician?

[ ] **1.** Temperature of 99.8° F (37.6° C)
[ ] **2.** Respiratory rate of 24 breaths/minute at rest
[ ] **3.** Apical heart rate of 90 beats/minute
[ ] **4.** Blood pressure of 94/62 mm Hg

A client diagnosed with angina has been advised to reduce his consumption of saturated fat and calories to control the progression of CAD.

27. The best evidence that the client is complying with his diet therapy is that he reports using which type of fat for cooking?

[ ] **1.** Margarine
[ ] **2.** Shortening
[ ] **3.** Coconut oil
[ ] **4.** Corn oil

The client tells the nurse that he is particularly fond of hot apple pies like those sold at a fast-food restaurant and that he eats several per week. He asks the nurse how many calories are in one pie.

28. If the literature supplied by the fast-food chain indicates that one hot apple pie contains 2 g of protein, 14 g of fat, and 31 g of carbohydrates, the nurse would be correct to tell him that one hot apple pie is equal to how many calories?

[ ] **1.** 47
[ ] **2.** 199
[ ] **3.** 258
[ ] **4.** 343

Because this client has been experiencing an increased number of anginal episodes, the physician prescribes an oral long-acting nitrate, isosorbide dinitrate (Isordil), to reduce the occurrences.

29. Which symptom reported by the client indicates that his isosorbide dinitrate (Isordil) dosage probably needs to be adjusted?

[ ] **1.** Nausea
[ ] **2.** Anorexia
[ ] **3.** Drowsiness
[ ] **4.** Dizziness

The client is scheduled to undergo a heart catheterization and coronary arteriogram.

30. Which nursing action can best help reduce the client's anxiety in this situation?

[ ] **1.** Teach the client how CAD is usually treated.
[ ] **2.** Listen to the client express his feelings about his condition.
[ ] **3.** Explain that the procedure has been very helpful for other clients.
[ ] **4.** Avoid discussing the heart catheterization until the client has relaxed.

The nurse implements the teaching plan for cardiac catheterization and coronary arteriogram.

31. Which statement by the client indicates that he understands what will happen during the testing procedure?

[ ] **1.** "I'll be able to hear my heart beating in my chest."
[ ] **2.** "I'll feel a heavy sensation all over my body."
[ ] **3.** "I'll be anesthetized and will not feel any discomfort."
[ ] **4.** "I'll feel a warm sensation as the dye is instilled."

32. Prior to the heart catheterization and coronary arteriogram, it is essential for the nurse to ask the client if he is allergic to iodine or which other substance?

[ ] **1.** Penicillin
[ ] **2.** Morphine
[ ] **3.** Shellfish
[ ] **4.** Eggs

During the procedure, the physician uses the femoral artery to thread the heart catheter.

33. After the coronary arteriogram, the nurse must keep the client flat in bed with his affected leg in which position?

[ ] **1.** Extended
[ ] **2.** Flexed
[ ] **3.** Abducted
[ ] **4.** Adducted

34. After the femoral artery has been cannulated and the client is returned to his room, what should the nurse plan to do?

[ ] **1.** Palpate the client's distal peripheral pulses.
[ ] **2.** Auscultate the client's heart and breath sounds.
[ ] **3.** Percuss all four quadrants of the client's abdomen.
[ ] **4.** Inspect the skin integrity in the client's groin.

35. The nurse provides discharge instructions for a client who has recovered following a cardiac catheterization. Which instructions should be included? Select all that apply.

[ ] **1.** Take a shower rather than a tub bath until the puncture site heals.

[ ] **2.** Perform leg exercises by flexing and extending your affected leg every 2 hours while awake.

[ ] **3.** Drink a generous amount of fluids for the next 24 hours.

[ ] **4.** Report worsening of pain in the leg that was catheterized.

[ ] **5.** Double-flush all eliminated urine or stool for 24 hours.

[ ] **6.** Change the dressing over the puncture site daily until it heals.

Based on the results of the coronary arteriogram, the physician recommends that the client undergo percutaneous transluminal coronary angioplasty (PTCA).

36. The nurse knows that the client understands the physician's explanation of the PTCA procedure when he makes which statement?

[ ] **1.** "A balloon-tipped catheter will be inserted into my coronary artery."

[ ] **2.** "A Teflon graft will be used to replace an area of weakened heart muscle."

[ ] **3.** "A section of my leg vein will be grafted around a narrowed coronary artery."

[ ] **4.** "A battery-operated pacemaker will be implanted to maintain my heart rate."

While waiting to undergo PTCA, the client takes propranolol (Inderal).

37. When the client asks the nurse how propranolol (Inderal) helps to prevent angina, what is the best explanation?

[ ] **1.** Propanolol promotes excretion of body fluid.

[ ] **2.** Propanolol reduces the rate of heart contraction.

[ ] **3.** Propanolol alters pain receptors in the heart.

[ ] **4.** Propanolol dilates the major coronary arteries.

38. While the client takes propranolol (Inderal), how would the nurse expect the client's pulse rate to be?

[ ] **1.** Faster than usual

[ ] **2.** Stronger than before

[ ] **3.** Temporarily irregular

[ ] **4.** Slower than in the past

The client is also advised by his physician to take 81 mg of aspirin daily while waiting for his scheduled PTCA.

39. What is the best explanation for the drug therapy in this situation?

[ ] **1.** Aspirin tends to relieve chest pain.

[ ] **2.** Aspirin tends to prevent blood clots.

[ ] **3.** Aspirin tends to lower the blood pressure.

[ ] **4.** Aspirin tends to dilate the coronary arteries.

40. When the client returns to his room after the PTCA procedure, which assessment finding should be reported immediately to the physician?

[ ] **1.** Urine output of 100 mL/hour

[ ] **2.** Blood pressure of 108/68 mm Hg

[ ] **3.** Dry mouth

[ ] **4.** Chest pain

The client who previously had a PTCA is now having coronary artery bypass graft (CABG) surgery. Shortly after the procedure, the client is returned to his room and assessed by the nurse.

41. The nurse checking the client's leg incision is aware that which is the most common blood vessel used in CABG surgery?

[ ] **1.** The saphenous vein

[ ] **2.** The femoral artery

[ ] **3.** The popliteal vein

[ ] **4.** The iliac artery

The nurse asks the nursing assistant to take the client's vital signs.

42. Which action by the nursing assistant indicates that more instruction is needed to accurately assess the client's pulse rate?

[ ] **1.** The nursing assistant places her thumb over the radial artery.

[ ] **2.** The nursing assistant counts the pulse rate for 1 full minute.

[ ] **3.** The nursing assistant rests the client's arm on his abdomen.

[ ] **4.** The nursing assistant presses the radial artery against the bone.

The client complains that he is having acute pain in his incisional area.

43. Based on the client's complaint, the nurse would expect the pain to have which possible effect on his vital signs?

[ ] **1.** Temperature may be elevated.

[ ] **2.** Pulse rate may become rapid.

[ ] **3.** Respiratory rate may slow.

[ ] **4.** Blood pressure may fall.

The physician orders a patient-controlled analgesia (PCA) infusion pump for the client after CABG surgery.

44. When the nurse informs the client about the use of the PCA pump, which instruction is most important to include?
[ ] **1.** "Press the control button whenever you feel you need pain medication."
[ ] **2.** "Call the nurse each time you need to use the PCA pump."
[ ] **3.** "Use the PCA pump only when the pain is severe."
[ ] **4.** "Don't use the PCA pump too frequently, as it can cause addiction."

45. Which information about the client's use of a PCA pump is most important to communicate to the staff on the next shift?
[ ] **1.** Name of the client's physician
[ ] **2.** Purpose of using the pump
[ ] **3.** Number of doses administered
[ ] **4.** The client's need for further teaching

46. After the CABG surgery, which assessment finding provides the best evidence that collateral circulation at the donor graft site is adequate?
[ ] **1.** The client is free from chest pain.
[ ] **2.** The client's toes are warm and nonedematous.
[ ] **3.** The client moves his leg easily.
[ ] **4.** The client's heart rate remains regular.

Nursing Care of Clients with Myocardial Infarction

A 65-year-old client with severe chest pain is evaluated in the emergency department. A tentative diagnosis of myocardial infarction (MI) is made.

47. Which assessment finding is most closely correlated with an evolving MI?
[ ] **1.** Profuse sweating
[ ] **2.** Facial flushing
[ ] **3.** Severe headache
[ ] **4.** Coughing up pink-tinged mucus

48. When obtaining this client's health history, which question about pain is least helpful?
[ ] **1.** "How long have you been in pain?"
[ ] **2.** "Where is your pain located?"
[ ] **3.** "What were you doing when your pain started?"
[ ] **4.** "When was the last time you had anything to eat or drink?"

49. If the client's severe chest pain is typical of other people who experience an MI, he is most likely to tell the nurse that his discomfort radiates where?

[ ] **1.** To the flank
[ ] **2.** To the groin
[ ] **3.** To the abdomen
[ ] **4.** To the shoulder

50. Which description of chest pain is most characteristic of a client experiencing an MI?
[ ] **1.** "The pain comes and goes."
[ ] **2.** "The pain came on slowly."
[ ] **3.** "The pain is tingling in nature."
[ ] **4.** "The pain has remained continuous."

51. If the client's pain is due to an MI, which prescribed medication would be most helpful?
[ ] **1.** A nonsteroidal anti-inflammatory drug such as ibuprofen (Advil)
[ ] **2.** A nonsalicylate such as acetaminophen (Tylenol)
[ ] **3.** A salicylate such as acetylsalicylic acid (aspirin)
[ ] **4.** An opioid such as meperidine (Demerol)

The client's wife tells the nurse that her husband delayed seeking medical attention for his chest pain because he thought his discomfort was due to strained muscles from doing yard work.

52. The nurse understands that the client's hesitation in going to the hospital is an example of which coping technique?
[ ] **1.** Regression
[ ] **2.** Projection
[ ] **3.** Denial
[ ] **4.** Undoing

53. Which risk factor is least likely to have predisposed the client to having an MI?
[ ] **1.** Smoking cigarettes
[ ] **2.** Eating fatty foods
[ ] **3.** Working under emotional stress
[ ] **4.** Drinking an occasional cocktail

54. Which laboratory results would the nurse expect to be elevated if the client had an MI?
[ ] **1.** Isoenzymes and troponin
[ ] **2.** Sodium and potassium
[ ] **3.** Red blood cells and platelets
[ ] **4.** Plasminogen and lactic acid

Based on the laboratory test results and the occurrence of symptoms for only a few hours, the physician instructs the nurse to administer streptokinase (Streptase).

55. The nurse correctly explains to the client's wife that streptokinase (Streptase) is being given to achieve which effect?

[ ] **1.** To dissolve blood clots
[ ] **2.** To slow the client's heart rate
[ ] **3.** To improve heart contraction
[ ] **4.** To lower the client's blood pressure

56. When a client receives streptokinase (Streptase), the nurse must monitor for which adverse effect?
[ ] **1.** Hypertension
[ ] **2.** Hyperthermia
[ ] **3.** Bleeding
[ ] **4.** Tachypnea

57. Which drug should the nurse have on hand in case the client develops an allergic reaction to the streptokinase (Streptase)?
[ ] **1.** Vitamin K (Synkayvite)
[ ] **2.** Heparin (Liquaemin sodium)
[ ] **3.** Diphenhydramine (Benadryl)
[ ] **4.** Warfarin (Coumadin)

58. Which symptom would the nurse expect to observe if the client is having an allergic reaction to streptokinase (Streptase)?
[ ] **1.** Urticaria
[ ] **2.** Dysuria
[ ] **3.** Hemoptysis
[ ] **4.** Dyspepsia

A 65-year-old woman collapses in the hospital elevator while coming to visit a family member. She is unresponsive.

59. Which action is the nurse's priority upon finding this unresponsive victim?
[ ] **1.** Open the victim's airway.
[ ] **2.** Give two breaths.
[ ] **3.** Shake the victim gently.
[ ] **4.** Call a code blue.

60. Which technique is most appropriate for the nurse to use to open the airway of a victim who is not breathing?
[ ] **1.** Elevate the neck.
[ ] **2.** Lift the chin.
[ ] **3.** Press on the jaw.
[ ] **4.** Clear the mouth.

61. Which is the best method for determining if the victim requires rescue breathing?
[ ] **1.** Observe the victim's skin color.
[ ] **2.** Feel for pulsations at the neck.
[ ] **3.** Listen for spontaneous breathing.
[ ] **4.** Blow air into the victim's mouth.

62. How should the nurse deliver an effective volume of air into the lungs of a victim who is not breathing?

[ ] **1.** Press on the victim's trachea.
[ ] **2.** Remove the victim's dentures.
[ ] **3.** Pinch the victim's nose shut.
[ ] **4.** Squeeze the victim's cheeks.

The nurse further assesses the client and finds that she is unresponsive and pulseless. The nurse begins chest compressions.

63. Where is the correct placement for the nurse's hands before administering cardiac compressions?
[ ] **1.** On the lower half of the sternum
[ ] **2.** Below the tip of the xiphoid process
[ ] **3.** Over the costal cartilage
[ ] **4.** Directly above the manubrium

64. During cardiopulmonary resuscitation (CPR), the nurse compresses the chest of an adult victim at which rate?
[ ] **1.** No less than 15 compressions per minute
[ ] **2.** No less than 40 compressions per minute
[ ] **3.** No less than 80 compressions per minute
[ ] **4.** No less than 100 compressions per minute

After the nurse calls for help, a second health care provider arrives to assist with CPR.

65. When two rescuers perform CPR, what is the rate of compressions to ventilations?
[ ] **1.** 15 compressions to 2 breaths
[ ] **2.** 5 compressions to 1 breath
[ ] **3.** 1 compression for each breath
[ ] **4.** 1 compression to 5 breaths

66. Which finding best indicates that cardiac compressions can be discontinued?
[ ] **1.** The victim's color improves.
[ ] **2.** The pupils become dilated.
[ ] **3.** A pulse can be palpated.
[ ] **4.** The victim begins to vomit.

67. After the client has been successfully resuscitated, the nurse correctly places her in which body position while she is awaiting transfer to the emergency department?
[ ] **1.** Supine with her head elevated
[ ] **2.** On her side
[ ] **3.** Prone with her head lowered
[ ] **4.** Flat with her knees raised

Once the client has been transferred and admitted to the intensive care unit (ICU), the nurse attaches ECG leads to the chest and connects her to a cardiac monitor.

68. When the client is startled by an alarm caused by a loose lead, the nurse knows that which is the best approach for relieving her anxiety?
[ ] 1. Describe her current heart rhythm.
[ ] 2. Explain the reason the alarm sounded.
[ ] 3. Give her a prescribed tranquilizer.
[ ] 4. Allow her to look at a tracing of her heart pattern.

The physician diagnoses a myocardial infarction (MI) and writes the following medication order: Diltiazem (Cardizem) 30 mg P.O. a.c.

69. The nurse correctly carries out the drug order by administering the medication at which time?
[ ] 1. At bedtime
[ ] 2. Before meals
[ ] 3. After meals
[ ] 4. As necessary

The client says to the ICU nurse, "This scares me. I'm concerned about what could have happened to me."

70. Which response by the nurse is most appropriate at this time?
[ ] 1. "What are your concerns?"
[ ] 2. "Why are you so scared?"
[ ] 3. "Your doctor says you're doing just fine."
[ ] 4. "You need to concentrate on getting well."

Once the client recovers from the MI, she is transferred to the medical-surgical unit for continued recovery and rehabilitation.

71. The nursing team develops a care plan and expected outcomes for the client's recovery. Which expected outcomes are most important? Select all that apply.
[ ] 1. The client will not gain weight.
[ ] 2. The client's activity tolerance will increase.
[ ] 3. The client will comply with her low-sodium, low-fat diet.
[ ] 4. The client will avoid caffeine and carbonated beverages.
[ ] 5. The client will verbalize fears and anxieties freely.
[ ] 6. The client will maintain pressure over the femoral access site.

Before discharge, the physician requests that the client receive dietary instructions about a calorie-restricted, low-fat, low-sodium diet as well as instructions about necessary activity restrictions.

72. The best evidence that the client understands the nurse's dietary instructions is that she says she should avoid eating which food?

[ ] 1. Pepperoni pizza
[ ] 2. Vinegar and oil salad dressing
[ ] 3. Liver and onions
[ ] 4. Lemon-peppered chicken

73. After hearing the nurse's instructions about activity restrictions and the potentially dangerous consequences of certain activities, the client correctly states that she knows she should avoid engaging in which activity?
[ ] 1. Carrying groceries from the car
[ ] 2. Straining during a bowel movement
[ ] 3. Bathing in warm water
[ ] 4. Having intercourse

At the client's follow-up clinic visit 1 week after discharge, the physician orders an echocardiogram to evaluate the damage done to the client's heart.

74. The nurse assumes that the client understands how an echocardiogram is performed when she tells the nurse that this examination involves imaging the heart using which type of waves?
[ ] 1. Heat
[ ] 2. Sound
[ ] 3. Radiation
[ ] 4. Electric

Nursing Care of Clients with Congestive Heart Failure

75. Using the following cardiac structures, trace the normal pathway in which blood circulates on the left side of the heart. Use all the options.

1. Aorta	
2. Left ventricle	
3. Pulmonary veins	
4. Left atrium	
5. Mitral valve	

A 78-year-old woman is admitted to the hospital with left-sided heart failure.

76. When obtaining a health history from the client, the nurse would expect to learn that which was the client's earliest symptom?
[ ] 1. Anorexia
[ ] 2. Dyspnea
[ ] 3. Nausea
[ ] 4. Headaches

77. While auscultating the client's lungs, what is the nurse most likely to hear?
[ ] **1.** Clear breath sounds
[ ] **2.** Diminished breath sounds
[ ] **3.** Crackles
[ ] **4.** Wheezes

78. Which body position is most beneficial for the client at this time?
[ ] **1.** Back-lying
[ ] **2.** Face-lying
[ ] **3.** Side-lying
[ ] **4.** Semi-sitting

79. The nurse anticipates that the client will most likely demonstrate which emotional response in relation to her heart failure?
[ ] **1.** Depression
[ ] **2.** Anxiety
[ ] **3.** Anger
[ ] **4.** Stoicism

After assessing the client's degree of heart failure, the physician orders supplemental oxygen therapy.

80. Which assessment finding best indicates that the oxygen therapy is effective?
[ ] **1.** The client's face is flushed.
[ ] **2.** Capillary refill is 6 seconds.
[ ] **3.** The client states she can breathe easier.
[ ] **4.** The apical pulse is less bounding.

The client's left-sided heart failure worsens, and she develops severe pulmonary edema. The nurse prepares to transfer the client to the intensive care unit (ICU).

81. The client tells the nurse that she is extremely frightened. What is the most appropriate action for the nurse to take at this time?
[ ] **1.** Stay with the client.
[ ] **2.** Notify the physician.
[ ] **3.** Tell her she will be OK.
[ ] **4.** Record the collected data.

82. To provide adequate care for the client with worsening left-sided heart failure, the ICU nurse should monitor which of the following on a daily basis?
[ ] **1.** Pupil response
[ ] **2.** Peripheral edema
[ ] **3.** Appetite
[ ] **4.** Weight

The nurse monitors the client's laboratory values because of the large doses of diuretics the client received to treat her pulmonary edema.

83. Which value should the nurse report immediately to the physician?
[ ] **1.** Sodium: 137 mEq/L
[ ] **2.** Potassium: 2.5 mEq/L
[ ] **3.** Chloride: 97 mEq/L
[ ] **4.** Bicarbonate: 25 mEq/L

84. Which assessment finding best indicates that the client is developing right-sided heart failure?
[ ] **1.** Her urine contains glucose.
[ ] **2.** Her ankles are swollen.
[ ] **3.** She has an irregular pulse.
[ ] **4.** She has a chronic cough.

85. Which additional assessment finding would support the possibility of right-sided heart failure?
[ ] **1.** Jugular vein distention
[ ] **2.** Bradycardia
[ ] **3.** Dry, hacking cough
[ ] **4.** Flushed, red face

The physician orders digoxin (Lanoxin). After the digitalizing loading doses have achieved their therapeutic effect, the physician prescribes a daily maintenance dosage of 0.125 mg of digoxin P.O.

86. If each tablet of digoxin (Lanoxin) contains 0.25 mg, how much should the nurse administer to the client each day?
[ ] **1.** ½ tablet
[ ] **2.** One tablet
[ ] **3.** Two tablets
[ ] **4.** Three tablets

87. Before administering the digoxin (Lanoxin) to the client, what is essential for the nurse to assess?
[ ] **1.** The client's heart rate
[ ] **2.** The client's blood pressure
[ ] **3.** The client's heart sounds
[ ] **4.** The client's breath sounds

88. If the client develops digoxin toxicity, what would the nurse expect her to exhibit?
[ ] **1.** Anorexia and nausea
[ ] **2.** Dizziness and insomnia
[ ] **3.** Pinpoint pupils and double vision
[ ] **4.** Ringing in the ears and itchy skin

The nursing team establishes the nursing diagnosis Decreased cardiac output related to tachycardia, decreased stroke volume, and increased vascular volume, and enters this into the client's care plan. The team also includes the following goal: The client will have an improvement in cardiac output.

89. How can the nurse best measure whether the client has achieved the goal?
[ ] 1. The client will have vital signs within normal parameters.
[ ] 2. The client will lose no more than 5 lb per day.
[ ] 3. The client will have decreased peripheral edema.
[ ] 4. The client will have a 24-hour urine output of 1,000 mL.

Nursing Care of Clients with Conduction Disorders

The physician orders a 24-hour Holter monitor for a client who has been experiencing brief fainting spells. The nurse provides instructions for the client regarding the purpose and use of the Holter monitor.

90. Which client instruction made by the nurse is most beneficial for helping the physician interpret the information collected by the Holter monitor?
[ ] 1. "Record the time and type of physical activities you perform."
[ ] 2. "Take your radial pulse rate every hour during the next day."
[ ] 3. "Try to relax and limit your exercise as much as possible."
[ ] 4. "Keep your lower extremities elevated while sitting."

91. To prevent electrical interference with the Holter monitor, it is most appropriate to recommend that the client avoid which action?
[ ] 1. Standing close to a microwave oven
[ ] 2. Driving under overhead power lines
[ ] 3. Shaving with an electric razor
[ ] 4. Using a cellular telephone

After evaluating the 24-hour Holter monitor tracings, the physician admits the client to the hospital for an abnormal heart rhythm. On admission, the nurse notes that the client has an irregularly fast heart rate and notifies the physician. The physician schedules the client for cardioversion.

92. The nurse knows that the client understands the cardioversion procedure when he states that it involves which action?
[ ] 1. Administering an electric current to the heart
[ ] 2. Threading a thin, plastic catheter into the heart
[ ] 3. Evaluating blood flow to areas of heart muscle
[ ] 4. Scanning the heart after injecting a radioisotope

93. Before cardioversion is attempted, the nurse appropriately withholds which prescribed medication?

[ ] 1. Diazepam (Valium)
[ ] 2. Digoxin (Lanoxin)
[ ] 3. Heparin (Lipo-sodium)
[ ] 4. Warfarin (Coumadin)

94. Which finding would strongly indicate that the cardioversion procedure has been successful?
[ ] 1. The client regains consciousness immediately.
[ ] 2. Normal sinus cardiac rhythm is restored.
[ ] 3. The apical heart rate equals the radial rate.
[ ] 4. The pulse pressure is approximately 40 mm Hg.

Because the client continues to have an irregular heart rate, the physician schedules the insertion of an artificial pacemaker.

95. If the client understands the nurse's explanation of the heart's conduction system, which structure will he identify as the site of the natural pacemaker?
[ ] 1. Purkinje fibers
[ ] 2. Bundle of His
[ ] 3. Atrioventricular (AV) node
[ ] 4. Sinoatrial (SA) node

96. To assess the area where the permanent pacemaker battery has been implanted, the nurse knows to examine which area of the skin?
[ ] 1. Beneath the left nipple
[ ] 2. Near the brachial artery
[ ] 3. In the midsternum
[ ] 4. Below the clavicle

97. As part of the discharge instructions, the nurse correctly instructs the client that which symptom is a sign of artificial pacemaker malfunction?
[ ] 1. Tingling in the chest area
[ ] 2. Dizziness during activity
[ ] 3. Pain radiating to the arm
[ ] 4. Tenderness beneath the skin

Nursing Care of Clients with Valvular Disorders

During a routine pre-employment physical examination, a physician discovers that a 28-year-old woman has a heart murmur.

98. If the heart murmur is related to valve damage caused by a childhood infection, the nurse would expect the client to report having had which disease?
[ ] 1. Varicella (chickenpox)
[ ] 2. Rubella (German measles)
[ ] 3. Rheumatic fever
[ ] 4. Whooping cough

After a diagnostic workup, the physician informs the client that she has mitral valve stenosis.

99. The nurse accurately describes the mitral valve as being located between which heart structures?
[ ] **1.** The right ventricle and pulmonary artery
[ ] **2.** The left atrium and left ventricle
[ ] **3.** The right atrium and right ventricle
[ ] **4.** The left ventricle and aorta

100. Where is the best anatomic area for the nurse to auscultate mitral valve sounds?
[ ] **1.** At the fifth intercostal space in the left midclavicular line
[ ] **2.** At the fourth intercostal space to the left of the sternum
[ ] **3.** At the second intercostal space to the right of the sternum
[ ] **4.** At the second intercostal space to the left of the sternum

The physician prescribes 250 mg of nafcillin (Unipen) P.O. daily to treat the client's mitral valve stenosis.

101. Which statement by the nurse best explains why the client needs to take the prescribed medication?
[ ] **1.** "It may destroy the virus causing your disease."
[ ] **2.** "It may reduce the scar tissue on the valve."
[ ] **3.** "It may stop blood clots from forming."
[ ] **4.** "It may prevent future bacterial infections."

Over a period of 10 years, the client has been taking diuretics and digoxin for the long-term treatment of her mitral valve stenosis. Her condition has progressively worsened, and she is now scheduled to have surgery for a mitral valve replacement.

102. Which statement best indicates that the client understands the surgical procedure involving mitral valve replacement?
[ ] **1.** "My blood will be circulated through a heart-lung machine."
[ ] **2.** "The surgeon will enlarge my valve by inserting a stent."
[ ] **3.** "My chest will be opened during surgery, but my heart will not."
[ ] **4.** "A piece of my leg vein will be used to replace the diseased valve."

Postoperatively, the client is placed on fluid restriction.

103. Which nursing intervention is most appropriate to add to the care plan to alleviate the client's thirst?

[ ] **1.** Offer hard, sour candy.
[ ] **2.** Give ice chips frequently.
[ ] **3.** Provide clear liquid foods.
[ ] **4.** Chill all oral fluids.

Postoperatively, the client experiences shortness of breath with moderate activity. The physician writes an order stating that the client may sit up in a chair if she can tolerate the increased activity.

104. Which nursing action would best reduce the client's energy expenditure?
[ ] **1.** Administering oxygen when the client is dyspneic.
[ ] **2.** Planning to perform routine care activities over the course of several hours.
[ ] **3.** Providing analgesic medications when necessary.
[ ] **4.** Restricting visitors to brief periods of time.

105. Which assessment finding offers the best evidence that the client can tolerate the activity involved in getting out of bed?
[ ] **1.** Her appetite has improved.
[ ] **2.** She has more restful sleep.
[ ] **3.** Her heart rate is stable.
[ ] **4.** She can get out of bed without assistance.

The client is disappointed that she is not progressing from her mitral valve replacement as quickly as she thinks she should. One day, she pushes away her lunch tray and it falls to the floor.

106. Which nursing response is most appropriate at this time?
[ ] **1.** Cleaning up the floor and say nothing
[ ] **2.** Finding out what food she would prefer
[ ] **3.** Allowing the client to talk about her feelings
[ ] **4.** Leaving her alone until she feels better

The nurse is caring for a client who was recently diagnosed with aortic stenosis.

107. The client asks the nurse to explain what part of his heart is affected. Locate the aortic valve on the illustration below.

108. Which sign will adults with chronic cardiac diseases most frequently manifest?
[ ] **1.** Barrel-shaped chest
[ ] **2.** Flushed facial skin
[ ] **3.** Clubbed fingertips
[ ] **4.** Chest pain

Nursing Care of Clients with Infectious and Inflammatory Disorders of the Heart

A pulmonary artery catheter was used to monitor pressure within the heart of a client after cardiac surgery. The client is now suspected of having bacterial endocarditis.

109. Which assessment finding documented by the nurse provides the best evidence that the client has a bacterial infection?
[ ] **1.** Chest pain
[ ] **2.** Dry cough
[ ] **3.** Fever
[ ] **4.** Dyspnea

A 63-year-old man with liver cancer is admitted to the medical-surgical unit with a diagnosis of pericarditis.

110. When auscultating the client's heart and breath sounds during a routine shift assessment, which action by the nurse is most appropriate?
[ ] **1.** Asking the client to hold his breath
[ ] **2.** Turning the television off momentarily
[ ] **3.** Positioning the client flat in bed
[ ] **4.** Locating the xiphoid process

111. Which sound is the nurse most likely to hear when auscultating the chest of a client with pericarditis?
[ ] **1.** Weak, thready heart sounds
[ ] **2.** Heart rate greater than 120 beats/minute
[ ] **3.** A pericardial friction rub
[ ] **4.** A clicking heart murmur

112. Which assessment finding best supports the assumption that the client's cardiac stroke volume is reduced?
[ ] **1.** The client faints with activity.
[ ] **2.** The client develops hypertension.
[ ] **3.** The client manifests bradycardia.
[ ] **4.** The client has a bounding pulse.

A 50-year-old man is scheduled for a heart transplantation tomorrow. The night nurse is asked to review the surgical procedure with the client. Because of the client's anxiety, he has difficulty comprehending the nurse's information.

113. Which nursing action is it most appropriate to perform next?
[ ] **1.** The nurse notifies the physician, requesting a hypnotic or sedative.
[ ] **2.** The nurse provides a video of the surgery for the client to watch.
[ ] **3.** The nurse asks the client to call his wife, then describes the surgery when husband and wife are together.
[ ] **4.** The nurse talks to the client about his fears concerning surgery and rehabilitation.

114. During the postoperative period, why does the nurse frequently assesses the client's fluid status?
[ ] **1.** Because urine retention is common after a heart transplantation
[ ] **2.** Because urine output is an indication of perfusion to the kidneys
[ ] **3.** Because hydration determines when the client needs to be transfused
[ ] **4.** Because hydration indicates when fluids should be increased

Correct Answers and Rationales

Nursing Care of Clients with Hypertensive Heart Disease

1. 4. The nurse can assume that an obese client will need a larger than usual adult cuff. A common guide is to select a cuff with a bladder that encircles at least two-thirds of the limb at its midpoint and is as wide as 40% of the midlimb circumference. If the cuff is too narrow, the blood pressure will be higher than its true measurement; if too wide, the measurement will be lower than the true pressure.

A normal-sized cuff will not fit around the obese client's thigh. Having the client lie down would have no bearing on the cuff size, but it could affect a client's blood pressure reading; in this case, the cuff is too small anyway. Pumping the manometer to 250 mm Hg is also incorrect. The blood pressure manometer should be pumped up to approximately 30 mm Hg above the baseline blood pressure. The American Heart Association recommends the following: Inflate the cuff while palpating the brachial artery, note when the pulse disappears, deflate the cuff, wait, and reinflate the cuff to 30 mm Hg above the point at which the palpation disappeared.

Client Needs Category—Health promotion and maintenance
Client Needs Subcategory—None

2. 2. Normal blood pressure is less than 120/80 mm Hg. Therefore, the clients mentioned in options 1 and 3 fall within ranges that do not require follow-up. A systolic reading greater than or equal to 140 mm Hg or a diastolic reading greater than or equal to 90 mm Hg is the definition of hypertension. The Joint National Committee on Detection, Evaluation, and Treatment of High Blood Pressure (2003) recommends that an initial diastolic pressure between 90 and 99 mm Hg be rechecked in 2 months even if the systolic pressure is less than 140 mm Hg. Although the client in option 4 has a slightly lower systolic and diastolic blood pressure reading, this may be normal for that client.

Client Needs Category—Health promotion and maintenance
Client Needs Subcategory—None

3. 2. Phase V of Korotkoff sounds (the point at which the last sound is heard before a period of continuous silence) is considered the best reflection of adult diastolic pressure. In some cases, two diastolic pressures are recorded: The pressure at which the loud knocking sound becomes muffled and the last sound heard.

Client Needs Category—Health promotion and maintenance
Client Needs Subcategory—None

4. 3. Untreated hypertension tends to cause fibrous tissue formation in systemic arterioles. The fibrous tissue leads to decreased tissue perfusion, which is especially dangerous when it affects target organs, such as the heart, kidneys, and brain. Hypertension is not linked to a shortened life cycle of blood cells, venous clots, or stenosis of cardiac valves. The nurse should assess risk factors for hypertension at the time that the blood pressure is taken. Risk factors for hypertension include obesity, hypercholesterolemia, smoking, family predisposition, and ethnicity or race. In this case, African American men are at risk for hypertension.

Client Needs Category—Health promotion and maintenance
Client Needs Subcategory—None

5. 1. Hypertension is a serious disorder that is associated with stroke and heart disease. It may be classified as primary (without a known cause) or secondary (a known pathology). Some of the earliest signs and symptoms of hypertension include spontaneous nosebleeds, awakening with a headache, and blurred vision. Other symptoms include a persistent throbbing or pounding headache, dizziness, fatigue, and nervousness. Congestive heart failure, one of the complications of hypertension, can cause dyspnea when lying down, which may affect sleeping; insomnia, however, can have many causes. Hematuria and heart palpitations are not generally associated with hypertension.

Client Needs Category—Physiological integrity
Client Needs Subcategory—Physiological adaptation

6. 3. Myocardial hypertrophy (heart enlargement) is the direct consequence of the heart having to pump against increased peripheral vascular resistance due to hypertension. A strong S_1 heart sound is a healthy finding. A heart rate of 100 beats/minute is within normal limits, especially with activity. Hypertension is not usually associated with an irregular heart rhythm, which can have multiple causes.

Client Needs Category—Physiological integrity
Client Needs Subcategory—Physiological adaptation

7. 1. Soy sauce is high in sodium and, therefore, is restricted on a low-sodium diet. Lemon juice and onion powder (not onion salt) may be used liberally. Maple syrup is not restricted for its sodium content but may be limited if the client needs to monitor blood glucose levels or lose weight.

Client Needs Category—Health promotion and maintenance
Client Needs Subcategory—None

8. 4. Smoking cessation is the single most therapeutic health change for anyone who has, or is at risk for, cardiopulmonary disease. Although increasing the intake of complex carbohydrates (such as fiber-containing oatmeal and other whole grains) has healthy benefits in lowering blood cholesterol, smoking cessation provides dramatic results in less time. Striking a healthy balance between rest and exercise and taking advantage of more leisure activities are also beneficial, but any one of these cannot compare with the beneficial effects on arterioles achieved by smoking cessation.

Client Needs Category—*Health promotion and maintenance*
Client Needs Subcategory—*None*

9. 2.4. To calculate the correct answer, use the dosage desired/dosage on hand formula:

$$\frac{\text{Dosage desired}}{\text{Dosage on hand}} \times \text{Quantity} = \frac{60}{50} \times 2 \ \text{ or } \ \frac{60}{50} = \frac{50}{2}$$

$$50 = 120X = 2.4 \text{ mL}$$

Client Needs Category—*Safe, effective care environment*
Client Needs Subcategory—*Safety and infection control*

10. 2. The best technique for bringing medication to the base of an ampule is to tap the stem several times with a fingernail. Allowing the ampule to stand, flipping the ampule back and forth, or rolling the ampule does not bring medication trapped in the ampule stem into the base of the container.

Client Needs Category—*Safe, effective care environment*
Client Needs Subcategory—*Safety and infection control*

11. 3. Furosemide (Lasix) is a loop diuretic. Therefore, an increase in urine output indicates that the drug is achieving its desired effect. Eliminating excessive water from the blood volume reduces the work of the heart, resulting in less fluid accumulation in the lungs. Furosemide (Lasix) may lower blood pressure due to the change in fluid volume, but this does not offer the best evidence of the medication's effectiveness. Pulse rate does not change appreciably when furosemide is given. Although improved breathing can help reduce the client's anxiety, this is not the best indication of the drug's effectiveness.

Client Needs Category—*Physiological integrity*
Client Needs Subcategory—*Pharmacological therapies*

12. 2. When given once daily, furosemide (Lasix) is generally administered in the early morning to avoid disturbing the client's sleep with the need to urinate. If

the medication is ordered for twice a day, the first dose is usually given early in the morning at about 0600, and the other dosage in the early afternoon at about 1300.

Client Needs Category—*Health promotion and maintenance*
Client Needs Subcategory—*None*

13. 1. Furosemide (Lasix) typically depletes potassium levels; therefore, the client should eat foods that replace this electrolyte. One banana contains approximately 10 mEq of potassium. Other fruits that are rich sources of potassium include oranges and orange juice, cantaloupe, and nectarines. Although furosemide (Lasix) can also alter sodium levels, the unwanted effect causes potassium depletion. Unless dehydration occurs, the drug will not affect calcium and iron levels.

Client Needs Category—*Health promotion and maintenance*
Client Needs Subcategory—*None*

14. 1. Diuretics are administered to prevent or treat fluid volume overload. They work by increasing the urine output; therefore, dehydration is a potential complication. The client should monitor his urine output as a way of evaluating the medication's effectiveness. A loop diuretic, such as furosemide (Lasix), increases sodium excretion, which can lead to hyponatremia, not hypernatremia. It is also a potassium-depleting drug, which can lead to low levels of potassium (hypokalemia). Many clients who take a loop diuretic replace the lost potassium by eating foods that contain appreciable amounts of this electrolyte or by taking potassium supplements.

Client Needs Category—*Physiological integrity*
Client Needs Subcategory—*Pharmacological therapies*

Nursing Care of Clients with Coronary Artery Disease

15. 4. Obesity, which is often linked with hyperlipidemia, is a risk factor for developing CAD. Drinking a nightly cocktail and undergoing surgery to repair the mitral valve are unrelated to development of CAD. Rheumatic fever is more likely to cause valvular disease than CAD.

Client Needs Category—*Health promotion and maintenance*
Client Needs Subcategory—*None*

16. 2. A buildup of cholesterol causes atherosclerosis. As fat becomes deposited within the lining of arteries, the deposits enlarge to form plaque, which thickens the arterial walls and causes the blood vessels to narrow. Eventually the plaque is infiltrated with calcium, which causes the vessel to become hard and rigid. When a

normal volume of blood is forced through these narrowed, inelastic vessels, the pressure within the vessels increases. The heart is prone to failure because it must work hard to pump against the vascular resistance. Cholesterol neither expands the circulating blood volume, nor causes the heart to beat faster. Blood clots may form quicker due to the narrowing blood vessel. This narrowing can also cause stagnation of the blood.
Client Needs Category—Physiological integrity
Client Needs Subcategory—Physiological adaptation

17. **3.** In keeping with a low-cholesterol diet, the healthiest change is to eat cereal rather than eggs for breakfast. Egg yolk is a rich source of cholesterol. There is not much, if any, appreciable change in cholesterol levels by substituting the foods listed in the other options. Whole grain wheat toast, however, provides additional fiber, which is healthier than white bread.
Client Needs Category—Health promotion and maintenance
Client Needs Subcategory—None

18. **1.** Atorvastatin (Lipitor) lowers low-density lipoprotein and total triglyceride levels and increases the amount of high-density lipoproteins. In doses large enough to lower blood fat components, this drug may cause back pain and muscle pain (myalgia). The nurse must assess for muscle pain, tenderness, or weakness as well as monitor the client's cholesterol levels. Palpitations, visual changes, and weight loss are not known side effects of this drug.
Client Needs Category—Physiological integrity
Client Needs Subcategory—Pharmacological therapies

19. **1.** A stress ECG demonstrates the extent to which the heart tolerates and responds to the additional demands placed on it during exercise. The heart's ability to continue adapting is related to the adequacy of blood supplied to the myocardium through the coronary arteries. If the client develops chest pain, dangerous cardiac rhythm changes, or significantly elevated blood pressure, the diagnostic testing is stopped. Although the test may indicate that further exercise is needed, this is not the primary purpose of testing. An ECG does not predict the occurrence of a heart attack or determine the target heart rate.
Client Needs Category—Physiological integrity
Client Needs Subcategory—Physiological adaptation

20. **2.** Rest generally relieves angina. The chest pain is caused by an inadequate supply of oxygenated blood to the myocardium due to narrowed coronary arteries. Once the myocardium's demand for additional oxygen is reduced through inactivity or rest, the chest pain is relieved. Taking a deep breath and applying heat to the chest or rubbing the chest will not alleviate the pain of angina pectoris. One main difference between stable angina pectoris and a myocardial infarction is that rest relieves the chest pain associated with stable angina.
Client Needs Category—Physiological integrity
Client Needs Subcategory—Physiological adaptation

21. **3.** Sublingual, or under the tongue, is the route by which nitroglycerin tablets are administered. The drug is then quickly absorbed through a rich supply of blood vessels beneath the tongue. Clients who take sublingual nitroglycerin for angina are instructed not to chew or swallow the tablets. Tablets for buccal administration are placed between the gum and cheek. A tablet intended for swallowing is placed on the tongue at the back of the throat. A chewable tablet is placed between the teeth.
Client Needs Category—Physiological integrity
Client Needs Subcategory—Pharmacological therapies

22. **1.** Side effects of nitroglycerin include headache, flushing, and dizziness. These effects are the direct result of vasodilation. Decreasing the drug dosage or taking a mild pain reliever offers relief. The other choices are not associated with nitroglycerin.
Client Needs Category—Physiological integrity
Client Needs Subcategory—Pharmacological therapies

23. **3.** The client should experience a fizzing or tingling in the mouth if nitroglycerin tablets are still fresh. Tablets need to be replaced approximately every 3 months. They do not discolor or disintegrate when they have lost their potency. Old aspirin tablets tend to smell like vinegar.
Client Needs Category—Health promotion and maintenance
Client Needs Subcategory—None

24. **1.** The dose of nitroglycerin may be repeated in 5 minutes, for a total of three doses. However, the client is told to call the physician if the pain is unrelieved after three successive doses because other treatment may be necessary. A client having chest pain should never drive to the hospital alone. Sublingual tablets are never swallowed.
Client Needs Category—Physiological integrity
Client Needs Subcategory—Pharmacological therapies

25. **1.** When topical nitroglycerin ointment or transdermal patches are used, application sites are rotated and the medication may be placed on the chest, back, upper abdomen, or arms. The drug reservoir should not be touched, squeezed, or manipulated in any way. The patch is self-adhering when the adhesive backing is removed. Ointment application papers are covered with plastic wrap and taped in place to prevent soiling and promote drug absorption. It is not necessary to apply ice to the skin or to clean the skin with alcohol before applying. Clipping the chest hair may be necessary, especially if the client is particularly hairy. After removing the old patch or paper, the old ointment should be removed with a dry cloth. It is not standard practice to take the client's blood pressure after application unless the client becomes symptomatic.

Client Needs Category—*Physiological integrity*
Client Needs Subcategory—*Pharmacological therapies*

26. **4.** Nitroglycerin dilates arterial vessels, especially the coronary vessels. This action lowers the blood pressure. Therefore, if the client's blood pressure is already low (as with a pressure of 94/62 mm Hg), the nurse should check with the physician before applying the patch. It is not unusual for a client with an MI to have a slightly elevated temperature. This is probably due to the inflammatory response from the injury to the myocardium. A respiratory rate of 24 breaths/minute and an apical heart rate of 90 beats/minute are within normal limits.

Client Needs Category—*Physiological integrity*
Client Needs Subcategory—*Pharmacological therapies*

27. **4.** Corn oil is an example of a polyunsaturated oil. Using unsaturated fats helps lower blood cholesterol. In limited amounts, it is healthier to consume polyunsaturated fats made from vegetable products than saturated fats, such as grease or lard, or hydrogenated fats, such as solid vegetable shortenings and hard margarines. Coconut and palm oil are more highly saturated than lard.

Client Needs Category—*Health promotion and maintenance*
Client Needs Subcategory—*None*

28. **3.** Protein and carbohydrates both have 4 calories per gram; fat contains 9 calories per gram. Thus, the total calorie count for a pie containing 2 g of protein, 14 g of fat, and 31 g of carbohydrate is 258 calories.

Client Needs Category—*Health promotion and maintenance*
Client Needs Subcategory—*None*

29. **4.** Dizziness is a common side effect of nitrate drugs. Nitrates have a direct relaxing effect on the smooth muscle of blood vessels, thereby producing vasodilation. When blood vessels dilate, the client will experience a drop in blood pressure, resulting in vertigo. Isosorbide dinitrate (Isordil) is administered in a range of 5 to 40 mg. Once the data are reported, the physician may wish to lower the client's dosage or instruct him to take the drug at night before bedtime. In some in-

stances, the side effects diminish or disappear after the drug has been taken over a period of time. Nausea, anorexia, and drowsiness are not recognized as major side effects of this drug.

Client Needs Category—*Physiological integrity*
Client Needs Subcategory—*Pharmacological therapies*

30. **2.** When a client is worried and fearful, the nurse should encourage him to express his feelings and then listen attentively. Most clients feel alone, overwhelmed, and helpless during a crisis; being able to verbalize fears and concerns can help ease the client's mental burden. Listening is an active process, even if the nurse does not make many verbal contributions. Teaching the client about the treatment of CAD is inappropriate because learning is impaired during times of mild to severe anxiety. How others have responded to a diagnostic test or procedure disregards the uniqueness of the client's situation. Avoiding the subject communicates that the nurse does not care.

Client Needs Category—*Psychosocial integrity*
Client Needs Subcategory—*None*

31. **4.** The contrast dye used during the coronary arteriogram causes vasodilation and is experienced as a brief flush or warmth that spreads over the skin surface. Some clients feel fluttering or what is described as "butterflies" as the catheter is passed into the heart, disturbing its rhythm. Heaviness or chest pain, if experienced, is generally treated with nitroglycerin. The client receives sedation but is not anesthetized prior to the diagnostic testing.

Client Needs Category—*Physiological integrity*
Client Needs Subcategory—*Pharmacological therapies*

32. **3.** People who are allergic to shellfish may also be sensitive to iodine. The radiopaque dye used during the arteriogram is iodine-based. The physician must be notified if the client indicates a history of allergies to either substance. At this point, the physician will determine whether to cancel the procedure or prepare to administer an antihistamine or other emergency drugs. Morphine and penicillin are not associated with allergic reactions caused by the dye. Allergy to eggs is related to certain types of vaccines given as immunizations.

Client Needs Category—*Physiological integrity*
Client Needs Subcategory—*Reduction of risk potential*

33. **1.** If the femoral artery was the site used for inserting the heart catheter, the nurse must position the client so that his legs are extended (not bent) to prevent him from flexing his hip for 6 to 8 hours after the procedure. Flexing the hip may lead to bleeding and clot formation. Abduction and adduction have no bearing on the affected leg. Sandbags may be placed over the pressure dressing to decrease discomfort and control bleeding.

Client Needs Category—*Physiological integrity*
Client Needs Subcategory—*Reduction of risk potential*

34. **1.** Peripheral pulses distal to the catheter insertion site are assessed frequently following arteriography. This is performed because of the injury to the artery and subsequent bleeding, which can lead to clot formation. A thrombus could totally occlude the flow of oxygenated blood through the vessel, resulting in the absence of a distal pulse—a medical emergency that must be reported immediately. After checking the client's pulses, the nurse would inspect the skin integrity in the groin because bleeding, hemorrhage, or hematoma formation may occur. Assessing the heart, lungs, and abdomen should be done regardless of whether the arteriogram is performed.

Client Needs Category—*Physiological integrity*
Client Needs Subcategory—*Physiological adaptation*

35. **1, 3, 4, 6.** Following cardiac catheterization, a shower is preferred because it reduces the risk of infection at the puncture site. Consuming fluid promotes the excretion of dye that was instilled intravenously during the procedure. An increase in leg pain may indicate formation of an arterial thrombus and arterial occlusion, which requires immediate intervention. The puncture site should be covered with a dressing until it heals. The client should rest for 3 days and avoid strenuous activity; therefore, leg exercises are contraindicated. There is no need to double-flush urine or stool because excreted waste products contain no toxic or biological hazardous substances.

Client Needs Category—*Physiological integrity*
Client Needs Subcategory—*Reduction of risk potential*

36. **1.** PTCA involves dilating narrowed or occluded coronary arteries with a double-lumen balloon catheter. The pressure from the inflated balloon compresses the fatty plaque that has narrowed the artery. Leg veins are used in coronary artery bypass grafting (CABG) surgery to bypass narrowed coronary arteries. A pacemaker is used when it is difficult to maintain a normal heart rate or rhythm with drug therapy. Grafting skeletal muscle, not Teflon, over scarred areas of the myocardium is now in experimental stages.

Client Needs Category—*Physiological integrity*
Client Needs Subcategory—*Physiological adaptation*

37. **2.** Propranolol (Inderal) is a beta-adrenergic blocker. It blocks the sympathetic receptors for epinephrine. Epinephrine speeds the heart rate, which requires a great deal of oxygen. By blocking the effect of epinephrine, the heart rate is slowed and the myocardium does not need as much oxygen. In addition, at a slower rate, the heart fills with a greater volume of blood. Thus, each time the heart contracts, it delivers a substantial amount of blood to the coronary arteries. As long as the coronary arteries deliver an adequate amount of oxygenated blood to the myocardium, chest pain is prevented. Propranolol (Inderal) does not dilate major coronary arteries, nor does it help with the excretion of urine. Pain receptors are not altered by the use of this drug.

Client Needs Category—*Physiological integrity*
Client Needs Subcategory—*Pharmacological therapies*

38. **4.** Beta-adrenergic blockers such as propranolol (Inderal) interfere with the action of epinephrine. They reduce heart rate. Therefore, the pulse rate tends to be slower than in the nonmedicated period. Some clients develop bradycardia while taking the drug. Propranolol (Inderal) does not produce a stronger heartbeat or irregular heart rhythms.

Client Needs Category—*Physiological integrity*
Client Needs Subcategory—*Pharmacological therapies*

39. **2.** Aspirin is recommended in low daily doses to reduce the potential for forming a blood clot, which could occlude the narrowed opening in a diseased coronary artery. It interferes with platelet aggregation or clumping and, therefore, acts as a prophylactic antithrombotic agent. Aspirin is more useful in relieving headaches and musculoskeletal pain than chest pain. Aspirin will not lower the blood pressure or cause vasodilation of the coronary arteries.

Client Needs Category—*Physiological integrity*
Client Needs Subcategory—*Pharmacological therapies*

40. **4.** Signs of complications after PTCA include chest pain, bleeding from the catheter insertion site, and abnormal heart rhythms. Chest pain indicates that the dilated coronary artery has suddenly closed again. If untreated, an MI could occur. An hourly urine output of 30 to 50 mL or more is considered adequate. A blood pressure of 108/68 mm Hg is within the low ranges of normal. A dry mouth is a consequence of fluid restriction and medication administered prior to the procedure. As long as the blood pressure continues to remain within normal ranges, the nurse relieves the discomfort of a dry mouth by giving oral care and administering oral fluids.

Client Needs Category—*Physiological integrity*
Client Needs Subcategory—*Physiological adaptation*

41. **1.** CABG surgery is performed when more than one blood vessel is occluded. The saphenous vein, which is located in the leg, is commonly harvested for grafting. The nurse should assess pulses and the incisional site in the affected leg immediately after surgery. The internal mammary artery, located in the chest, is another vessel sometimes used for CABG surgery. The other vessels mentioned in the remaining options are not typically used for this type of surgery.

Client Needs Category—Physiological integrity
Client Needs Subcategory—Physiological adaptation

42. **1.** Using the thumb to obtain a pulse rate can yield inaccurate data because the health care worker might be feeling her own pulse rather than the client's. It is best to rest or support the client's arm and compress the artery against the bone using the fingertips. Counting the pulse for 1 full minute seems prudent immediately following major cardiovascular surgery.

Client Needs Category—Safe, effective care environment
Client Needs Subcategory—Safety and infection control

43. **2.** A client in acute pain is most likely to have a rapid pulse rate, rapid respiratory rate, and rising blood pressure. Pain is least likely to influence body temperature.

Client Needs Category—Physiological integrity
Client Needs Subcategory—Physiological adaptation

44. **1.** With a PCA pump, the client presses a control button to release a very low dose of an opioid when he feels the need for medication. The dose is low enough to allow for frequent administration. Usually, this results in the client's using less total medication because his discomfort rarely falls below a tolerable level. It is best to use the PCA pump before pain becomes severe. PCA pumps are used only for a few days postoperatively, making addiction unlikely. Because the client can use the machine independently, it frees the nurse to tend to other responsibilities.

Client Needs Category—Physiological integrity
Client Needs Subcategory—Pharmacological therapies

45. **3.** The number of doses the client administered during the current shift is the most important information to communicate to the nurses on the next shift. This serves as a measure of how much pain the client is experiencing. The name of the client's physician is readily available on multiple records. The only reason to use a PCA pump is to relieve pain. The PCA pump allows the client to control his drug dosage, promoting a sense of independence. If the client demonstrates a lack of understanding about the pump's function, this should be communicated to the next shift as well; however, it is not the most important information to convey.

Client Needs Category—Safe, effective care environment
Client Needs Subcategory—Safety and infection control

46. **2.** The saphenous vein is the most common blood vessel used for CABG surgery. Removing a portion of this leg vein can temporarily impair the return of venous blood to the heart. Impaired venous return is manifested by cool skin and edema in the toes, foot, or ankle of the operative leg. Therefore, the fact that the toes are warm and nonedematous is the best evidence that venous blood is adequately returning to the heart through other blood vessels in the leg. The ability to move the leg indicates that neurologic function is intact. A regular heart rate and absence of chest pain are evidence that the newly attached graft is supplying the heart muscle with adequate oxygenated blood.

Client Needs Category—Physiological integrity
Client Needs Subcategory—Physiological adaptation

Nursing Care of Clients with Myocardial Infarction

47. **1.** The chest pain accompanying an MI is usually so severe that the client becomes extremely diaphoretic. Hypotension is apt to make the client's skin appear pale or ashen, not flushed. Headache is more closely associated with stroke. Coughing up pink-tinged mucus is characteristic of clients with congestive heart failure.

Client Needs Category—Physiological integrity
Client Needs Subcategory—Physiological adaptation

48. **4.** The most pertinent data to assess concerning a client's pain are its onset, quality, intensity, location, and duration and what makes the pain better or worse. Therefore, the least important question relates to eating or drinking. Nausea may accompany chest pain, but this does not relate to the chest pain itself.

Client Needs Category—Physiological integrity
Client Needs Subcategory—Physiological adaptation

49. **4.** A client experiencing an MI is most likely to describe the pain as being substernal or radiating to the shoulder, arm, teeth, jaw, or throat. Other signs and symptoms of an MI include tachycardia, increased blood pressure, arrhythmias, cold and mottled skin, tachypnea, dyspnea, anxiety, elevated temperature, increased white blood cell count, and a rise in cardiac enzymes. Women may experience similar symptoms but may also have breast pain, pain in the upper back between the scapulae, and extreme fatigue.

Client Needs Category—Physiological integrity
Client Needs Subcategory—Physiological adaptation

50. 4. Unlike angina pectoris, the pain caused by an acute MI is unrelieved by rest, sublingual nitroglycerin, or other oral nitrate drugs. Many clients describe the pain associated with MI as continuous, and they use such terms as *squeezing, suffocating,* or *crushing.* The pain comes on suddenly and usually is not tingling in nature.
Client Needs Category—Physiological integrity
Client Needs Subcategory—Physiological adaptation

51. 4. An opioid analgesic, such as meperidine (Demerol) or morphine sulfate, is usually required to relieve the severe pain associated with an MI. Nonsteroidal, nonsalicylate, and salicylate analgesics are generally prescribed for minor pain that is not cardiac in origin.
Client Needs Category—Physiological integrity
Client Needs Subcategory—Pharmacological therapies

52. 3. Denial is a coping mechanism used to control anxiety and fear. Denial shuts out the painful awareness of reality. The client refuses to believe that an event, such as a heart attack, is really happening. Regression occurs when a client resorts to a pattern of behavior characteristic of an earlier age. Projection involves blaming a negative situation on someone or something else. Undoing often takes on the form of offering a verbal apology or gift to make up for unacceptable behavior.
Client Needs Category—Psychosocial integrity
Client Needs Subcategory—None

53. 4. Of the factors listed in this question, having an occasional alcoholic beverage is least likely to predispose a client to an MI. One drink of alcohol per day may increase the client's so-called "good" cholesterol (high-density lipoprotein) and will elevate triglyceride levels; however, the relationship of elevated triglyceride levels to heart disease has not been conclusively established. Smoking, working under stress, and eating a diet high in fat and "bad" cholesterol (low-density lipoprotein) are definite risk factors in developing an MI.
Client Needs Category—Health promotion and maintenance
Client Needs Subcategory—None

54. 1. Cardiac enzyme studies are the major tests used to diagnose MI. Cardiac enzymes and isoenzymes are released into the bloodstream when the heart cells die. Isoenzymes include CK-MB, CK-BB, and CK-MM. CK-MB, the isoenzymes most commonly used to diagnose MI, is found in high concentrations in the heart and skeletal muscles and in much smaller amounts in

brain tissue. The creatine kinase (CK) blood level, especially its isoenzyme CK-MB, becomes elevated within 2 hours after an infarction. CK enzymes correlate to the size of the infarct—in other words, the higher the serum CK-MB, the greater the damage to the heart. If an MI is suspected, cardiac enzymes are drawn upon admission and at periodic intervals (every 8 hours) for the next 2 days.

Troponin, a protein necessary for heart conduction, is also quickly elevated during an MI. Therefore, it can be used to rule out or confirm an MI. Troponin levels are usually drawn in the emergency department or even in the ambulance on the way to the hospital.

Sodium and potassium are electrolytes; they are not used to diagnose an MI. Red blood cells and platelets also are not considered diagnostic indicators of an MI. Plasminogen is a protein that prevents clot formation. Lactic acid is a waste product of cellular metabolism and causes sore skeletal muscles. Neither is used to diagnose an MI.
Client Needs Category—Physiological integrity
Client Needs Subcategory—Physiological adaptation

55. 1. Streptokinase (Streptase), a thrombolytic enzyme, is most therapeutic if used within 6 hours after the onset of MI symptoms. It is used to dissolve deep vein and arterial thromboemboli. This and other thrombolytic agents, such as urokinase (Abbokinase), anistreplase (Eminase), alteplase (Activase), and tissue plasminogen activator, activate plasminogen and convert it to plasmin. Plasmin breaks down the fibrin of a blood clot. Thrombolytic agents do not slow the heart rate, improve heart contraction, or lower blood pressure. Thrombolytics are contraindicated for clients who have bleeding disorders, a history of stroke, recent trauma, childbirth, or surgery.
Client Needs Category—Physiological integrity
Client Needs Subcategory—Pharmacological therapies

56. 3. Bleeding is the most common adverse reaction associated with thrombolytic drug therapy. Blood loss may be internal, involving the gastrointestinal or genitourinary tract, or may result in bleeding within the brain. Bleeding may also be external or superficial, manifested as oozing from venipuncture or injection sites, nosebleeds, and skin bruising. Other side effects include hypotension, nausea and vomiting, and cardiac arrhythmias. Hypertension, hyperthermia, and tachypnea are not recognized side effects of this drug.
Client Needs Category—Physiological integrity
Client Needs Subcategory—Pharmacological therapies

57. 3. The antihistamine drug diphenhydramine (Benadryl) is typically used when a client develops an allergic reaction to streptokinase (Streptase). Vitamin K may be given as an antidote when prothrombin levels are beyond the therapeutic range, as in the case of oral anticoagulants such as warfarin (Coumadin). Both heparin (Liquaemin sodium) and warfarin are administered to prevent future blood clots from developing.

> ***Client Needs Category***—*Physiological integrity*
> ***Client Needs Subcategory***—*Pharmacological therapies*

58. **1.** Urticaria is a term for hives. Hives, welts, and rashes are common manifestations of an allergic reaction to streptokinase (Streptase). In addition, the nurse may observe difficulty breathing, wheezing, and hypotension. Dysuria describes painful urination. Hemoptysis refers to coughing up bloody sputum. Dyspepsia is another word for indigestion. Dysuria, hemoptysis, and dyspepsia are not considered allergic reactions to streptokinase (Streptase).

> ***Client Needs Category***—*Physiological integrity*
> ***Client Needs Subcategory***—*Physiological adaptation*

59. **3.** To properly assess the need for resuscitation, the nurse's first action would be to gently shake the victim and shout, "Are you OK?" If the victim remains unresponsive, it is important for the rescuer to call loudly for additional help. If the victim cannot be aroused and is not breathing, the rescuer should open the airway and give two rescue breaths. Calling a code may not be appropriate in all cases; for instance, the victim may have only fainted.

> ***Client Needs Category***—*Safe, effective care environment*
> ***Client Needs Subcategory***—*Safety and infection control*

60. **2.** If the victim is not breathing and neck trauma is not suspected, the nurse would use the chin-lift/head-tilt method to open the airway. This is performed by using one hand to lift the chin upward to maintain position and placing the other hand across the victim's forehead. The jaw thrust method is used only if the chin lift/head-tilt method does not open the airway adequately or if the victim might have a neck injury. Placing a hand under the neck is no longer recommended. After the airway is opened, the mouth is cleared with a finger sweep.

> ***Client Needs Category***—*Safe, effective care environment*
> ***Client Needs Subcategory***—*Safety and infection control*

61. **3.** Once the airway is open, some victims begin breathing spontaneously. The nurse assesses for spontaneous breathing by leaning over the victim's head and listening or feeling for the movement of air from the nose or mouth. The chest or abdomen is also observed

for rising and falling. Skin color is not a dependable indicator of breathing because hypotension is likely to cause the victim to appear pale or ashen. The nurse would check the carotid pulse to determine the need for chest compressions, not rescue breathing. Administering rescue breathing is unnecessary if the victim is spontaneously breathing.

> ***Client Needs Category***—*Safe, effective care environment*
> ***Client Needs Subcategory***—*Safety and infection control*

62. **3.** Pinching the nose shut allows maximum ventilation with no loss of air through the nostrils. If the victim has a mouth injury or it is impossible to prevent air from leaking (in an adult victim), the rescuer may use the mouth-to-nose technique for giving ventilations. When resuscitating an infant or small child, the rescuer makes a seal by covering both the victim's nose and mouth with her mouth. Once the breath is given, the rescuer allows the air to be exhaled passively. Pressing on the trachea may interfere with air passage. Removing dentures and squeezing the victim's cheeks may interfere with maintaining a tight seal during rescue breathing.

> ***Client Needs Category***—*Safe, effective care environment*
> ***Client Needs Subcategory***—*Safety and infection control*

63. **1.** The hands of the rescuer are on top of one another on the lower half of the sternum, two fingerbreadths above the xiphoid process. The costal cartilage connects the ribs to the sternum. Compressing over the costal cartilage could fracture the victim's ribs. The manubrium is the upper portion of the sternum. The hands are placed too high on the chest if positioned above the manubrium. The hands are too low if they are placed below the tip of the xiphoid process. This position could damage the stomach, lacerate the liver, or cause vomiting.

> ***Client Needs Category***—*Safe, effective care environment*
> ***Client Needs Subcategory***—*Safety and infection control*

64. **4.** During CPR, the adult victim's chest is compressed at a rate of 100 times per minute. The sternum is depressed approximately 1½″ to 2″ (3.5 to 5 cm) with each compression. Rates below 100 per minute are unlikely to circulate blood adequately.

> ***Client Needs Category***—*Safe, effective care environment*
> ***Client Needs Subcategory***—*Safety and infection control*

65. 1. The American Heart Association recommends that when two rescuers perform CPR, the ratio is 15 compressions to 2 breaths—the same as is it for one-man CPR. When the client becomes intubated, the ratio of chest compressions to breathing changes to 5:1. CPR is never interrupted for longer than 7 seconds.
> *Client Needs Category—Safe, effective care environment*
> *Client Needs Subcategory—Safety and infection control*

66. 3. If the pulse returns, cardiac compressions are stopped. The carotid pulse is assessed for a full 5 seconds after the first minute of resuscitation and every few minutes thereafter unless consciousness is restored. The victim's color may improve as a consequence of effective resuscitative efforts. Dilated and fixed pupils are an indication that the brain is inadequately oxygenated. Vomiting can occur in a nonbreathing and pulseless victim because of distention with air.
> *Client Needs Category—Safe, effective care environment*
> *Client Needs Subcategory—Safety and infection control*

67. 2. The recovery position following successful CPR is a side-lying position. This position helps protect and maintain the airway and prevents aspiration if the client should vomit. The other choices do not adequately promote the airway.
> *Client Needs Category—Safe, effective care environment*
> *Client Needs Subcategory—Safety and infection control*

68. 2. Hospitalization, for most people, is a unique experience. Therefore, providing clients who are in an unfamiliar environment with information about hospital equipment, clinical procedures, and agency routines helps relieve anxiety. All explanations are given in simple, understandable terms. Once informed, the client has a basis for interpreting the reality of his experiences. The client is unlikely to understand a description of heart rhythm or interpret the pattern on a rhythm strip. Administering a tranquilizer at this time will not help prevent a similar reaction in the future.
> *Client Needs Category—Psychosocial integrity*
> *Client Needs Subcategory—None*

69. 2. The abbreviation *a.c.* means that a medication is administered before meals. The abbreviation for a bedtime administration is *h.s.* If the physician wants the drug administered after meals, the abbreviation *p.c.* is used. Administering a drug as necessary or as needed is indicated with the abbreviation *p.r.n.*

> *Client Needs Category—Safe, effective care environment*
> *Client Needs Subcategory—Safety and infection control*

70. 1. Asking open-ended questions encourages the client to elaborate, which may eventually relieve emotional tension. The best approach is to listen actively, remain nonjudgmental, and avoid offering personal opinions. Asking a client a "why" question is usually nontherapeutic, because the client may not be consciously aware of what is motivating her feelings or behavior. Telling the client that her physician believes she is doing fine implies that the client's fears are unfounded. A nonempathic response may cause the client to terminate further discussion. Giving advice, as in "You need to concentrate on getting well," is also nontherapeutic because it blocks continued communication about the subject.
> *Client Needs Category—Psychosocial integrity*
> *Client Needs Subcategory—None*

71. 1, 2, 3, 5. Heart failure is a common complication following an MI. Gaining more than 2 lb per day is indicative of the heart's inability to pump fluids, which places additional work on the heart. Therefore, no additional weight gain is the goal. Throughout the recovery and rehabilitation phases, the goals of activity and exercise are accomplished by gradual increased conditioning; therefore, increased tolerance to activity is an important outcome. A low-sodium diet decreases fluid volume, thereby reducing the workload of the heart, and a low-fat diet leads to weight reduction, which also decreases the heart's workload. Complying with such a diet is also an appropriate outcome.
 A client with MI is usually anxious for a variety of reasons. During rehabilitation and just before discharge, the client may experience increased anxiety related to returning home, possible recurrence of MI, and necessary health and lifestyle changes. Consequently, being able to verbalize fears and anxieties freely is an appropriate outcome.
 Maintaining pressure over the femoral site is an expected outcome after cardiac catheterization, not during the recovery and rehabilitation phase. Other than a low-sodium, low-fat diet, there are usually no other dietary restrictions, such as caffeine or carbonated beverages.
> *Client Needs Category—Health promotion and maintenance*
> *Client Needs Subcategory—None*

72. 1. Pepperoni pizza contains lots of calories, salt (processed meat), and fat (cheese). That makes this choice unsuitable for the client's low-calorie, low-fat, low-sodium diet. Vinegar and oil salad dressing is appropriate because it is low in sodium and calories. The oil, however, must be used sparingly. Liver and onions are acceptable for this client's dietary restrictions, and the liver may improve iron stores. However, liver contains some cholesterol and should be eaten sparingly. Lemon-peppered chicken is also acceptable on this client's diet because it is low in fat and lemons and pepper are items that can be used freely with this type of diet.

> ***Client Needs Category****—Health promotion and maintenance*
> ***Client Needs Subcategory****—None*

73. 2. Straining during a bowel movement involves holding one's breath and bearing down against a closed glottis. This action, sometimes called Valsalva's maneuver, increases abdominal and arterial pressure. The increase in arterial pressure acts as resistance to the pumping action of the heart. The blood flow through the coronary arteries is temporarily reduced and can cause ischemia and chest pain. If the heart wall is necrotic, the pressure increase could cause the weakened muscle to rupture and the client to hemorrhage to death. Stool softeners are generally ordered prophylactically to eliminate straining when having a bowel movement.

Clients who experience heart attacks can participate in their own self-care activities, such as bathing, provided they do not develop signs of activity intolerance. Signs that indicate the client should rest include becoming short of breath, developing a rapid or irregular heart rate, and experiencing increased blood pressure. Lifting heavy objects, such as groceries, and having intercourse are permitted after discharge. However, clients must usually wait until they can climb two flights of stairs without chest pain before engaging in these activities.

> ***Client Needs Category****—Health promotion and maintenance*
> ***Client Needs Subcategory****—None*

74. 2. An echocardiogram uses ultrasonic (sound) waves to image the heart's structure. The sound waves are reflected back in various ways, depending on the density of the tissues, to produce a replication of the heart that is later evaluated. An X-ray uses radiation. An ECG picks up electrical activity from the heart muscle. Thermography tests sense heat and variations in temperature to formulate images from body structures.

> ***Client Needs Category****—Physiological integrity*
> ***Client Needs Subcategory****—Physiological adaptation*

Nursing Care of Clients with Congestive Heart Failure

75.

3. Pulmonary veins
4. Left atrium
5. Mitral valve
2. Left ventricle
1. Aorta

Oxygenated blood enters the left side of the heart from the pulmonary veins. The oxygenated blood is then deposited into the left atrium. As the mitral valve opens, blood from the left atrium moves into the left ventricle. Then, blood is ejected through the aortic valve into the aorta when the left ventricle contracts.

> ***Client Needs Category****—Physiological integrity*
> ***Client Needs Subcategory****—Physiological adaptation*

76. 2. Heart failure refers to the heart's ineffective ability to pump blood to the tissues and organs to meet the body's metabolic needs. Congestive heart failure (CHF) is the accumulation of blood and fluids in the tissues and organs related to poor circulation. CHF is divided into two types: left-sided, which produces respiratory distress and pulmonary edema, and right-sided, which causes blood congestion throughout the body. Left-sided heart failure causes right-sided heart failure. Early left-sided heart failure is manifested by dyspnea and fatigue. Other classic signs and symptoms include a moist cough, orthopnea, tachycardia, restlessness, and confusion. Anorexia and nausea may have many causes and are not closely associated with CHF. Headaches are related to hypertension, not CHF.

> ***Client Needs Category****—Physiological integrity*
> ***Client Needs Subcategory****—Physiological adaptation*

77. 3. One of the complications of left-sided heart failure is pulmonary edema. In this condition, fluid occupies space within the small airways. As air is moved through the fluid-filled airways, the nurse is likely to hear crackles—high-pitched sounds heard in distant lung areas during inspiration. Some people compare this abnormal sound to that made by a popular rice cereal as it comes in contact with milk. Because of fluid accumulation, the breath sounds are not clear. Pneumonia and other pulmonary diseases can cause diminished breath sounds. Wheezing is closely associated with asthma.

Client Needs Category—Physiological integrity
Client Needs Subcategory—Physiological adaptation

78. 4. A client with heart failure is usually most comfortable, and has the least amount of difficulty with breathing, when placed in either a semi-sitting (semi- or mid-Fowler's), sitting (high-Fowler's), or standing position. Sitting and standing positions cause organs to fall away from the diaphragm, giving more room for the lungs to expand. A face-lying (prone) position will interfere with good lung expansion. Side-lying or back-lying positions are inappropriate because they impede good lung expansion.

Client Needs Category—Physiological integrity
Client Needs Subcategory—Physiological adaptation

79. 2. Clients who are having difficulty breathing, a common symptom in left-sided heart failure, typically feel anxious, apprehensive, and fearful. Appropriate nursing interventions relate to decreasing the client's anxiety and promoting adequate oxygenation. Clients are much less likely to feel depressed, angry, or stoic during this time.

Client Needs Category—Psychosocial integrity
Client Needs Subcategory—None

80. 4. Supplemental oxygen is commonly ordered to decrease the workload of the heart and increase the amount of oxygen in the blood. The cardiac workload is decreased when the apical pulse becomes less bounding and less rapid. Facial flushing can be a sign of fever or hypertension. Normal capillary refill is less than 3 seconds, so a 6-second capillary refill indicates that circulation is impaired. Subjective data related to the client's statement are important to collect, but objective data are more accurate indicators of the effectiveness of this treatment.

Client Needs Category—Physiological integrity
Client Needs Subcategory—Physiological adaptation

81. 1. The presence of another person, especially a health care provider, does much to relieve a client's anxiety. This is especially true when a client perceives herself to be in a helpless, powerless situation. It is essential for the nurse to make sure that the client is not left alone. Notifying the physician of the client's fear is inappropriate because the physician probably will not be able to do anything more in this situation. Telling the client that everything will be OK is meaningless reassurance and nontherapeutic. Recording of data can be temporarily postponed or verbally reported if needed.

Client Needs Category—Psychosocial integrity
Client Needs Subcategory—None

82. 4. Significant weight gain or loss, such as a difference of 2 lb or more in 24 hours, indicates major changes in body fluid distribution. Weight gain indicates fluid retention and impaired renal excretion. Weight loss indicates a therapeutic response to medical and drug therapy. Pupil response and appetite are appropriate to monitor in the daily assessments, but congestive heart failure is not likely to cause major changes in these findings. Edema of the lower extremities is a sign of right-sided heart failure; also, lower extremities should be monitored more often than once per day.

Client Needs Category—Physiological integrity
Client Needs Subcategory—Basic care and comfort

83. 2. Diuretics such as furosemide (Lasix) are potassium-depleting. Therefore, it is important for the nurse to monitor for signs of hypokalemia. Normal serum potassium levels are between 3.5 and 5.0 mEq/L. So a potassium level of 2.5 mEq should signal the need for immediate attention. Normal serum sodium levels are between 135 and 145 mEq/L, making this choice within the normal range. Normal chloride levels are between 90 and 110 mEq/L, also making this value within normal limits. Bicarbonate is a blood gas value. Normal bicarbonate values are between 21 and 28 mEq/L; therefore, this value is also within the normal range.

Client Needs Category—Physiological integrity
Client Needs Subcategory—Pharmacological therapies

84. 2. Swelling of the feet and ankles accompanies right-sided heart failure. Dependent edema occurs because the heart's pumping action is impaired, decreasing blood flow to the kidneys. The combination of heart and kidney impairments causes fluid retention. Excess fluid builds up in the lower extremities and abdomen. Glucose in the urine is associated with diabetes mellitus, not heart failure. An irregular pulse is not unusual in an elderly adult, but its significance should be evaluated. Coughing up frothy, pink-tinged sputum is a sign of left-sided, not right-sided, heart failure. Chronic coughing is usually seen in smokers and clients with chronic obstructive pulmonary disease and chronic bronchitis.

Client Needs Category—Physiological integrity
Client Needs Subcategory—Physiological adaptation

85. 1. If jugular veins distend with the head elevated 45 degrees or more, this indicates that an increased volume of blood is not circulating well through the right side of the heart. Tachycardia—not bradycardia—is associated with heart failure. A dry, hacking cough is an indicator of left-sided, not right-sided, heart failure. A flushed, red face is not commonly associated with congestive heart failure.

Client Needs Category—Physiological integrity
Client Needs Subcategory—Physiological adaptation

86. 1. Half of a 0.25-mg tablet is the correct amount of drug to administer if the prescription is for 0.125 mg. The formula for determining the correct number of tablets is as follows:

$$\frac{\text{Dosage desired}}{\text{Dosage on hand}} \times \text{Quantity} = \text{Amount to administer}$$

$$\frac{0.125}{0.25} \times 1 \text{ tablet} = 0.125/0.25 = 0.5 \text{ mg, or } \frac{1}{2} \text{ tablet}$$

> *Client Needs Category—Safe, effective care environment*
> *Client Needs Subcategory—Safety and infection control*

87. 1. Because digoxin (Lanoxin) preparations affect cardiac automaticity and the conduction system, it is essential that the nurse monitor the client's apical or radial pulse for 1 full minute before each administration of the drug. Assessments of blood pressure, heart sounds, and breath sounds are part of a comprehensive cardiopulmonary assessment, but they are not directly affected by the administration of digoxin (Lanoxin).

> *Client Needs Category—Physiological adaptation*
> *Client Needs Subcategory—Basic care and comfort*

88. 1. GI symptoms associated with digoxin toxicity include anorexia, nausea, vomiting, and diarrhea. The client may also become drowsy and confused or have visual changes, such as blurred vision, disturbance in seeing yellow and green colors, and a halo effect around dark objects. Toxic doses of digoxin (Lanoxin) can also increase cardiac automaticity, causing a rapid heart rate, or depress the conduction of cardiac impulses, causing a slow heart rate. Serum drug levels are used to monitor the client's metabolism of digoxin (Lanoxin). Pinpoint pupils are associated with opiate toxicity. Double vision is associated with myasthenia gravis. Ringing in the ears is a symptom of salicylate toxicity. Itching is a common side effect of many drugs, but it is not related to digoxin toxicity.

> *Client Needs Category—Physiological integrity*
> *Client Needs Subcategory—Physiological adaptation*

89. 1. For the client who exhibits signs and symptoms of heart failure, the main goals include decreasing the heart's workload, improving circulation, and managing fluid retention. The identified goal of "improving circulation" can be measured by assessing the stability of vital signs. Rapid weight loss of 5 lb per day is too much and is inappropriate for this goal. Having a decrease in peripheral edema is too subjective and not easily measured. A 24-hour urine output of 1,000 mL is inadequate; an adequate urine output should be about 2,000 mL per day.

> *Client Needs Category—Physiological integrity*
> *Client Needs Subcategory—Physiological adaptation*

Nursing Care of Clients with Conduction Disorders

90. 1. A Holter monitor is used for 24 hours to gather data about a client's heart rhythm patterns during normal daily activity. For an accurate interpretation, it is important to correlate the recorded data with the performance of physical activity. Instructing the client to keep a log is a good way to do this. The client need not assess his radial pulse; the heart rate is determined from the rhythm strip. The client should not alter his usual activities of daily living to obtain pertinent data. There is no reason that the client's lower extremities should be elevated while the Holter monitor is in place.

> *Client Needs Category—Physiological integrity*
> *Client Needs Subcategory—Physiological adaptation*

91. 3. Using electrical devices, such as electric razors and toothbrushes, may alter the data recorded with a Holter monitor. The other activities are not known to cause electrical interference with a Holter monitor.

> *Client Needs Category—Safe, effective care environment*
> *Client Needs Subcategory—Safety and infection control*

92. 1. Cardioversion is similar to defibrillation, except that cardioversion is a planned procedure whereas defibrillation is used in emergency situations. It involves administering a mild electric shock to the heart to correct rapid arrhythmias. Cardiac catheterization and angiography involve threading a catheter into the heart. Several types of cardiac imaging, such as multigated acquisition and thallium-201 scans, can be used to assess blood flow to the heart muscle.

> *Client Needs Category—Physiological integrity*
> *Client Needs Subcategory—Physiological adaptation*

93. 2. Digoxin (Lanoxin) and diuretics are withheld for 24 to 72 hours before elective cardioversion. Withholding these medications will ensure the heart's normal conduction will not be affected during the procedure. Diazepam (Valium) is generally prescribed as a preprocedural sedative. There are no contraindications for withholding heparin (Lipo-sodium) or warfarin (Coumadin) and anticoagulants.

> *Client Needs Category—Physiological integrity*
> *Client Needs Subcategory—Pharmacological therapies*

94. 2. The purpose of cardioversion is to stop the rapid cardiac rhythm and reestablish the SA node as the pacemaker. If this occurs, the heart beats regularly between 60 and 100 beats/minute. Such drugs as diazepam (Valium) and midazolam hydrochloride (Versed) are used to produce moderate sedation. The client remains awake, but usually has no memory of the experience. Equal apical and radial pulse rates are desirable, but this is not an indication of successful cardioversion. The normal difference between the systolic and diastolic blood pressures, also known as the *pulse pressure,* is approximately 40 mm Hg. Adequate cardiac output is generally reflected in a normal blood pressure measurement. However, the primary expected outcome of cardioversion is the restoration of normal cardiac rhythm.

Client Needs Category—*Physiological integrity*
Client Needs Subcategory—*Physiological adaptation*

95. 4. The SA node is the site of the heart's natural pacemaker. The SA node is called the pacemaker of the heart because it creates the electric impulses that cause the heart to contract. This specialized tissue is located in the wall of the right atrium between the openings of the superior and inferior vena cavae. A properly functioning SA node initiates regular impulses at a rate of 60 to 100 beats/minute. Once an impulse is sent from the SA node, it then travels down several internodal pathways to the AV node, the Bundle of His, the right and left bundle branches, and the Purkinje fibers.

Client Needs Category—*Physiological integrity*
Client Needs Subcategory—*Physiological adaptation*

96. 4. A permanent pacemaker battery is usually implanted beneath the skin below the right clavicle. Sometimes the area below the left clavicle is used. The wire for a temporary pacemaker is inserted through a peripheral vein, not the brachial artery, and then threaded into the right atrium and the right ventricle. Pacemaker wires are placed during cardiac surgery in case a client needs pacing postoperatively. The wires are seen externally from the skin on the chest. The area beneath the nipple is too low for the pacemaker, and most pacemakers are not located in the sternal area.

Client Needs Category—*Physiological integrity*
Client Needs Subcategory—*Physiological adaptation*

97. 2. If the artificial pacemaker does not support a heart rate high enough to maintain adequate cardiac output, the client feels dizzy and possibly faints. Tingling in the chest is unrelated to the artificial pacemaker. Pain that radiates to the arm is a symptom of angina pectoris or myocardial infarction. Tenderness may be caused by an infection.

Client Needs Category—*Physiological integrity*
Client Needs Subcategory—*Physiological adaptation*

Nursing Care of Clients with Valvular Disorders

98. 3. Rheumatic fever commonly causes permanent damage to the heart and valves. About half the clients who had rheumatic fever have narrowed mitral valves.

Varicella, rubella, and whooping cough (pertussis) are acute infections, but they are not known to cause damage to heart valves. Intrauterine rubella infection can cause congenital heart defects.

Client Needs Category—*Physiological integrity*
Client Needs Subcategory—*Physiological adaptation*

99. 2. The mitral valve (or bicuspid valve) is an atrioventricular valve. It is located between the left atrium and left ventricle. The pulmonic valve is between the right ventricle and the pulmonary artery. The tricuspid valve is between the right atrium and right ventricle. The aortic valve is located between the left ventricle and the aorta.

Client Needs Category—*Physiological integrity*
Client Needs Subcategory—*Physiological adaptation*

100. 1. The sound from the mitral valve is best heard by auscultating the apical area, which is at the fifth intercostal space in the left midclavicular line. When assessing heart sounds, the auscultatory areas are not directly over the anatomic locations of the heart valves. The aortic valve is best heard at the second intercostal space to the right of the sternum. The pulmonic valve is best heard at the second intercostal space to the left of the sternum. The tricuspid valve is best heard at the fourth intercostal space to the left of the sternum.

Client Needs Category—*Safe, effective care environment*
Client Needs Subcategory—*Coordinated care*

101. 4. A daily maintenance dose of penicillin, such as nafcillin sodium, is prescribed to prevent future streptococcal infections for some people with a history of rheumatic heart disease. Subsequent streptococcal infections continue to damage the heart. If daily doses of antibiotic are not taken, they are generally prescribed before oral surgery, tooth extractions, or other invasive procedures are performed. Nafcillin will not destroy viruses, reduce scar tissue, or stop blood clots from forming.

Client Needs Category—*Health promotion and maintenance*
Client Needs Subcategory—*None*

102. 1. To maintain adequate perfusion of all the cells in the body during any open heart surgery, including mitral valve replacement, blood is oxygenated and circulated by cardiopulmonary bypass using a heart-lung machine. Porcine (pork) valves and mechanical valves, not harvested leg veins, are used for replacing diseased valvular tissue. Stents are not used to treat defective valves.

Client Needs Category—*Physiological integrity*
Client Needs Subcategory—*Physiological adaptation*

103. **1.** Sucking on hard, sour candy facilitates the production of saliva that keeps the mouth moist and promotes the perception that thirst is quenched. Chilling fluids, especially bitter-tasting liquids, before drinking may make them taste better, but this does not alleviate thirst. Ice chips are not given liberally to clients with fluid restrictions; the ice is calculated within the restricted volume of fluid. Providing clear liquid foods such as gelatin may quench the client's thirst, depending on the fluid restriction.
> ***Client Needs Category****—Physiological integrity*
> ***Client Needs Subcategory****—Basic care and comfort*

104. **2.** Ensuring adequate rest between routine nursing care measures (such as bathing, oral hygiene, and ambulation) helps the client adapt to her activity intolerance. Administering oxygen is appropriate to prevent hypoxemia, but it does not reduce energy expenditure. Analgesics help relieve pain, but they do not relieve shortness of breath. Visits from family and friends are likely to tire the client. However, because most clients benefit from the emotional support of significant others, restricting the client's visitors would not be the first intervention implemented to reduce energy expenditure.
> ***Client Needs Category****—Physiological integrity*
> ***Client Needs Subcategory****—Basic care and comfort*

105. **3.** Evidence of activity intolerance includes rapid or irregular heart rate, hypotension, chest pain, dyspnea, and severe fatigue. If any of these are noted, the nurse is correct in limiting further activity. An improved appetite, restful sleep, and the ability to get out of bed without assistance are all positive signs, but they are not appropriate physiological criteria of a person's ability to tolerate activity.
> ***Client Needs Category****—Physiological integrity*
> ***Client Needs Subcategory****—Reduction of risk potential*

106. **3.** When a client is emotionally upset, it is most therapeutic to allow an opportunity to express feelings. Saying nothing or leaving the room is of little help because these actions are not supportive. In this case, the client is not unhappy with her food. Rather, she is displacing her anger and frustration onto an inanimate object. Finding out her food preferences avoids dealing with the emotional issues.
> ***Client Needs Category****—Psychosocial integrity*
> ***Client Needs Subcategory****—None*

107.

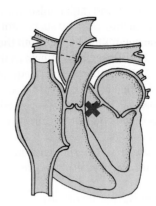

The aortic valve is the valve through which the left ventricle ejects blood. The mitral valve is between the left atrium and left ventricle. The tricuspid valve is between the right atria and the right ventricle. The pulmonic (pulmonary) valve is the valve through which the right ventricle sends blood to the pulmonary arteries and lungs.
> ***Client Needs Category****—Physiological integrity*
> ***Client Needs Subcategory****—Physiological adaptation*

108. **3.** Clubbing of the fingertips is a physical change that occurs after years of poor oxygenation. It is found in people with long-term cardiopulmonary diseases. As the name suggests, the fingertips appear like clubs; they are wider than normal at the distal end. The angle at the base of the nail is greater than the normal 160 degrees. A barrel-shaped chest is most common in clients with chronic obstructive pulmonary disease. Flushed facial skin is seen in clients who are feverish or have hypertension or excess blood volume. Chest pain is a sign of impaired tissue oxygenation. It is not usually associated with chronic cardiac disease.
> ***Client Needs Category****—Physiological integrity*
> ***Client Needs Subcategory****—Physiological adaptation*

Nursing Care of Clients with Infectious and Inflammatory Disorders of the Heart

109. **3.** A fever, one of the primary ways that the body fights an infection, tends to destroy or inhibit the growth and reproduction of microorganisms. Chemicals present in white blood cells, which fight infection, trigger a heat-producing response in the hypothalamus. Chest pain is usually caused by inadequate blood supply to the myocardium. Pneumonia is more likely to cause a moist cough. Dyspnea is a common finding in many cardiopulmonary diseases.
> ***Client Needs Category****—Physiological integrity*
> ***Client Needs Subcategory****—Physiological adaptation*

110. **2.** To enhance the ability to hear auscultated sounds, it is best to reduce or eliminate noise sources in the room, in this case the television. To auscultate both the front and back of the chest, it is necessary for the client to be in a sitting position. Holding the breath may aggravate the client's already compromised ventilation. Locating the xiphoid process will not promote the auscultation of heart or breath sounds.

   Client Needs Category—*Safe, effective care environment*
   Client Needs Subcategory—*Safety and infection control*

111. **3.** A pericardial friction rub is a grating or leathery sound typically heard in clients with pericarditis. It is caused by two layers of tissue moving roughly over each other. Other signs and symptoms of pericarditis include precordial pain, ECG changes, and a drop in systolic blood pressure. Muffled heart sounds (not weak, thready ones) are evident of fluid surrounding the heart. A clicking sound is associated with diseased cardiac valves. A murmur is an abnormal sound made by the turbulent flow of blood through narrow or incompetent valves. Pericarditis is not associated with tachycardia.

   Client Needs Category—*Physiological integrity*
   Client Needs Subcategory—*Physiological adaptation*

112. **1.** Fainting indicates that the volume of blood ejected from the left ventricle is inadequate to keep the brain oxygenated. Reduced stroke volume is also manifested by hypotension, tachycardia, and a weak pulse, which makes the other options inaccurate.

   Client Needs Category—*Physiological integrity*
   Client Needs Subcategory—*Physiological adaptation*

113. **4.** Fear of death is often a cause for increased anxiety in transplant clients. Allowing the client to verbalize fears about death or concerns regarding financial concerns, employment, length of rehabilitation, sexual performance, or immunosuppressive therapy helps decrease anxiety so that learning can take place. If the client's anxiety escalates to the point where he is out of control, requesting an order for a sedative or hypnotic would be appropriate. Providing a video is inappropriate because there is no way to evaluate whether the client has learned anything. Also, the video may provide too much material to comprehend or be too graphic, causing further anxiety. Certainly the spouse should be included in the discussions about the procedure and length of rehabilitation. However, having the spouse at the bedside may not lessen the client's anxiety. Therefore, this choice is not the best option.

   Client Needs Category—*Psychosocial integrity*
   Client Needs Subcategory—*None*

114. **2.** Because the client has had a heart transplant, assessing urine output is a good indicator of the heart's ability to pump and perfuse the kidneys. Monitoring intake and output also helps the nurse determine whether the client has a fluid volume overload or deficit. Usually, heart transplant recipients are fluid-restricted until their condition stabilizes; therefore, fluids are monitored. Hemoglobin values and hematocrit are used to help determine when the client needs transfusions. Urine retention is not common unless several doses of opiate drugs are given for pain.

   Client Needs Category—*Physiological integrity*
   Client Needs Subcategory—*Physiological adaptation*

TEST 6

The Nursing Care of Clients with Peripheral Vascular, Hematologic, and Lymphatic Disorders

➪ *Nursing Care of Clients with Venous Disorders*
➪ *Nursing Care of Clients with Arterial Disorders*
➪ *Nursing Care of Clients with Red Blood Cell Disorders*
➪ *Nursing Care of Clients with White Blood Cell Disorders*
➪ *Nursing Care of Clients with Bone Marrow Disorders*
➪ *Nursing Care of Clients with Coagulation Disorders*
➪ *Nursing Care of Clients with Inflammatory and Obstructive Lymphatic Disorders*
➪ *Correct Answers and Rationales*

Directions: With a pencil, blacken the space in front of the option you have chosen for your correct answer.

Nursing Care of Clients with Venous Disorders

While helping a female client into stirrups for a pelvic examination, the nurse notes that the client has several large protruding leg veins.

1. Which risk factor revealed in the client's health history is most closely related to the development of varicose veins?
[ ] **1.** Her mother also has varicose veins.
[ ] **2.** She has smoked cigarettes for 20 years.
[ ] **3.** She was a track athlete in high school.
[ ] **4.** Her pregnancy history reveals a premature baby.

2. Which statement made by the client best indicates an understanding of her varicose leg veins?
[ ] **1.** "My legs feel heavy and tired by evening."
[ ] **2.** "My feet perspire heavily during the day."
[ ] **3.** "I wake up at night with leg cramps."
[ ] **4.** "I have pain in my shins when I jog."

3. Which nursing instruction is most beneficial in helping relieve the client's symptoms caused by varicose veins?

[ ] **1.** Elevate your legs frequently during the day.
[ ] **2.** Wear a pair of thick cotton socks.
[ ] **3.** Gently massage your calves when experiencing leg cramps.
[ ] **4.** Modify your lifestyle to include sedentary activities.

4. The nurse provides information to the client about varicose veins. Which activity should the client avoid?
[ ] **1.** Walking in high-heeled shoes
[ ] **2.** Wearing nylon pantyhose
[ ] **3.** Sitting with crossed knees
[ ] **4.** Shaving her lower legs

The client is scheduled for a vein-stripping procedure as treatment for her varicose veins. After the surgeon explains the procedure, the client asks the nurse how her blood will circulate in her legs after surgery.

5. Which response by the nurse about blood circulation is most appropriate?
[ ] **1.** Some of the arteries begin to function as veins.
[ ] **2.** New veins grow to replace the ones that were removed.
[ ] **3.** Other veins take over the work of those removed.
[ ] **4.** The healthy vein ends are attached to other veins.

6. When planning this client's postoperative care, which action is the highest priority?

[ ] **1.** Providing the client with protein-rich foods
[ ] **2.** Ambulating the client frequently
[ ] **3.** Monitoring for wound infection
[ ] **4.** Assessing for frequent leg cramping

Postoperatively, the client asks the nurse for pain medication. The physician orders propoxyphene (Darvon), 65 mg, P.O. every 4 hours as needed for pain.

7. When offered the pain medication, the client says to the nurse, "If that's Darvon, I don't want it. It makes me sick to my stomach." What is the most appropriate nursing action at this time?

[ ] **1.** Tell the client that the drug is propoxyphene.
[ ] **2.** Explain that she must take the medication prescribed by the physician.
[ ] **3.** Advise her to take the drug with lots of water.
[ ] **4.** Report the information to the charge nurse.

A 67-year-old client has developed venous stasis ulcers on her lower leg.

8. When assessing the client's lower leg, which finding characteristic of venous stasis ulcers is the nurse most likely to find?

[ ] **1.** Purulent drainage
[ ] **2.** Blanches around the open area
[ ] **3.** Dark brown, dry, and crusty skin
[ ] **4.** Fluid-filled blisters

The physician writes an order for the application of wet-to-dry dressings over the client's leg ulcers.

9. When the client asks why the dressings are being applied, which explanation by the nurse is most accurate?

[ ] **1.** The dressings prevent wound infections.
[ ] **2.** The dressings remove dead cells and tissue.
[ ] **3.** The dressings absorb blood and drainage.
[ ] **4.** The dressings protect the skin from injury.

10. What is the best evidence that a stasis ulcer is healing?

[ ] **1.** The wound size becomes smaller, and more drainage is evident.
[ ] **2.** The wound size becomes smaller, and the client has less discomfort.
[ ] **3.** The wound size becomes smaller, and the cavity appears pink.
[ ] **4.** The wound size becomes smaller, and the wound margins are white.

Eventually the wet-to-dry dressings are discontinued, and the nurse covers the client's leg ulcer with a type of air-occlusive dressing.

11. The nurse correctly informs the client that which is the main advantage of this type of dressing?

[ ] **1.** It will reduce the formation of scar tissue.
[ ] **2.** It will relieve pain from skin irritation.
[ ] **3.** It will be less expensive than gauze dressings.
[ ] **4.** It will speed healing by keeping the wound moist.

12. Which of the following clients are at high risk for acquiring gangrene of the foot? Select all that apply.

[ ] **1.** An insulin-dependent diabetic
[ ] **2.** An elderly man with inadequate circulation
[ ] **3.** A woman who experiences trauma to the toes
[ ] **4.** A homeless person
[ ] **5.** A client who is taking warfarin (Coumadin)
[ ] **6.** A client with a history of myocardial infarction

A nurse gathers admission history from a 57-year-old woman who is scheduled to have an abdominal hysterectomy.

13. Which risk factors associated with thrombophlebitis should the nurse discuss with the physician? Select all that apply.

[ ] **1.** The client weighs 350 lb.
[ ] **2.** The client smokes 2 packs of cigarettes per day.
[ ] **3.** The client has been on bed rest due to congestive heart failure.
[ ] **4.** The client complains of leg fatigue.
[ ] **5.** The client complains of cramping in the lower leg at night.
[ ] **6.** The client complains of pain in the joints.

The woman is recovering from surgery after having an abdominal hysterectomy 2 days earlier.

14. Which nursing observation is most likely to predispose this client to developing venous thrombosis in a lower extremity?

[ ] **1.** The client resists ambulation.
[ ] **2.** The client breathes shallowly.
[ ] **3.** The client requests analgesics frequently.
[ ] **4.** The client drinks coffee excessively.

The client's care plan indicates that she should wear antiembolism stockings.

15. What is the best evidence that the prescribed antiembolism stockings are a correct size and fit for this client?

[ ] **1.** The stockings extend to midcalf.
[ ] **2.** The toes feel warm when touched.
[ ] **3.** The stockings are easily donned.
[ ] **4.** The heels are not reddened.

16. When the nurse assesses the client for Homans' sign, which technique is most accurate?
- [ ] **1.** Have the client push each foot against the mattress.
- [ ] **2.** Have the client extend her legs and flex each foot toward her head.
- [ ] **3.** Ask the client to sit up in bed and point all her toes forward.
- [ ] **4.** Ask the client to contract her thigh muscles.

17. If the client develops a thrombus in one of her leg veins, which client response would the nurse expect when eliciting Homans' sign?
- [ ] **1.** Sharp, immediate calf pain
- [ ] **2.** Sudden numbness in the foot
- [ ] **3.** Inability to bend the knee when asked
- [ ] **4.** Tingling throughout the affected leg

18. Besides a positive Homans' sign, which additional assessment finding best supports the assumption that the client has a thrombus in a leg vein?
- [ ] **1.** The foot on the affected leg is blue.
- [ ] **2.** The affected leg is warmer than the other.
- [ ] **3.** The capillary refill takes 2 seconds.
- [ ] **4.** The lower affected leg is swollen.

Based on data collection, the client has been diagnosed with thrombophlebitis.

19. Which modification is most appropriate to add to the client's care plan at this time?
- [ ] **1.** Ambulate the client twice each shift.
- [ ] **2.** Refrain from massaging the client's legs.
- [ ] **3.** Avoid elevating the client's legs.
- [ ] **4.** Encourage the client to perform active leg exercises.

The physician prescribes warm moist compresses to the affected leg.

20. Which nursing action is most appropriate when applying the warm-moist compress?
- [ ] **1.** Heating the water to 120° F (48.8° C)
- [ ] **2.** Using sterile technique
- [ ] **3.** Inspecting the skin every 4 hours
- [ ] **4.** Covering the wet gauze with a towel

The physician orders heparin (Calciparine) 7,500 units subcutaneously.

21. When the client wants to know why she is receiving the medication, which response by the nurse is most appropriate?
- [ ] **1.** "Heparin helps shrink blood clots."
- [ ] **2.** "Heparin helps dissolve blood clots."
- [ ] **3.** "Heparin prevents more clots from forming."
- [ ] **4.** "Heparin prevents the clot from dislodging."

22. Which laboratory value should the nurse report to the physician before giving the heparin (Calciparine) injection?
- [ ] **1.** Partial thromboplastin time (PTT)
- [ ] **2.** Complete blood count (CBC)
- [ ] **3.** Hemoglobin (Hb)
- [ ] **4.** Prothrombin time (PT)

23. When the nurse withdraws the heparin (Calciparine) from the multidose vial, which technique is correct?
- [ ] **1.** Remove the rubber stopper in the top of the vial.
- [ ] **2.** Instill an equal volume of air as liquid to be withdrawn.
- [ ] **3.** Mix the drug by rolling it between the palms.
- [ ] **4.** Shake the drug vigorously to promote even distribution.

24. If the client is of average weight for her height, which action by the nurse is most appropriate when administering the heparin (Calciparine) subcutaneously?
- [ ] **1.** Selecting the dorsogluteal site
- [ ] **2.** Using a 22-gauge 1½″ needle
- [ ] **3.** Inserting the needle at a 45-degree angle
- [ ] **4.** Massaging the site immediately afterward

25. Which assessment finding, noted several days after the client's daily heparin (Calciparine) injections, should be reported immediately to the physician?
- [ ] **1.** The client says that her abdomen is getting tender.
- [ ] **2.** The client states she is tired of getting stuck with needles.
- [ ] **3.** The client's gums bleed after she brushes her teeth.
- [ ] **4.** The client's stools are light brown.

26. Which drug should the nurse plan to have available in case it becomes necessary to counteract the effects of heparin therapy?
- [ ] **1.** Calcium lactate
- [ ] **2.** Sodium benzoate
- [ ] **3.** Protamine sulfate
- [ ] **4.** Aluminum phosphate

The nurse applies prolonged pressure to an injection site of a woman who is receiving anticoagulant therapy.

27. In this situation, is the nurse's action appropriate or inappropriate?
- [ ] **1.** Inappropriate because it promotes hematoma formation
- [ ] **2.** Inappropriate because it delays drug absorption
- [ ] **3.** Appropriate because it distributes the drug evenly
- [ ] **4.** Appropriate because it diminishes blood loss

The nurse prepares the client's discharge instructions. The client will continue to take warfarin (Coumadin) on a daily basis.

28. Which statement offers the best evidence that this client understands her risk for bleeding?
[ ] **1.** "I'll need to report having dark amber urine."
[ ] **2.** "I must report having tar-colored stools."
[ ] **3.** "I'll call the physician if I have green-tinged emesis."
[ ] **4.** "I'll call the physician if I notice that my skin is turning yellow."

29. The nurse explains to the client that, because she is taking warfarin (Coumadin), she should avoid eating foods containing large amounts of vitamin K. Which foods should the client limit? Select all that apply.
[ ] **1.** Fresh spinach
[ ] **2.** Lettuce
[ ] **3.** Turnip greens
[ ] **4.** Brussels sprouts
[ ] **5.** Peas
[ ] **6.** Corn

30. The client asks the nurse if she can resume taking her dietary supplements and herbal medications after discharge. The nurse responds that much is unknown about dietary supplements and explores the types and dosages of these supplements. Considering the client's condition and medication regimen, which dietary supplements are likely to alter the client's International Normalized Ratio (INR) and prothrombin time (PT)? Select all that apply.
[ ] **1.** Gingko
[ ] **2.** St. John's wort
[ ] **3.** Willow bark
[ ] **4.** Ginger
[ ] **5.** Green tea
[ ] **6.** Creatine

A postoperative client has been receiving I.V. fluids through the same site for several days.

31. Which finding would the nurse expect to document if the client begins developing phlebitis at the I.V. site?
[ ] **1.** The vein is red and feels warm.
[ ] **2.** The vein looks dark and feels cool.
[ ] **3.** The vein is pale and feels hard.
[ ] **4.** The vein looks purplish and feels spongy.

32. What is the first action the nurse should take if she suspects phlebitis at an I.V. site?
[ ] **1.** Elevate the affected extremity on pillows.
[ ] **2.** Apply pressure to the I.V. insertion site.
[ ] **3.** Administer the I.V. solution at a faster rate.
[ ] **4.** Remove the needle or catheter from the current site.

Nursing Care of Clients with Arterial Disorders

A 75-year-old woman in a nursing home has arteriosclerosis.

33. The nurse is aware that which of the following is one of the most common physical assessment findings among clients with arterial insufficiency secondary to peripheral arteriosclerosis?
[ ] **1.** Thick, tough toenails
[ ] **2.** Flushed skin
[ ] **3.** Hyperactive knee jerk reflexes
[ ] **4.** Bounding peripheral pulses

34. Which finding would the nurse expect to note when the client actively exercises?
[ ] **1.** Cyanosis of the feet
[ ] **2.** Burning of the toes
[ ] **3.** Pain in both legs
[ ] **4.** Edema formation in the ankles

35. Which intervention would be most appropriate if the client tells the nurse that her feet are cold?
[ ] **1.** Applying a commercially prepared heat packet
[ ] **2.** Using an electric heating pad
[ ] **3.** Wrapping the client's feet in a warm blanket
[ ] **4.** Elevating the client's feet on a stool

The nurse prepares to use a Doppler ultrasound device to assess blood flow through the client's dorsalis pedis artery.

36. Which technique is correct when using the Doppler device?
[ ] **1.** The nurse places the probe beside the ankle.
[ ] **2.** The nurse applies acoustic gel to the skin.
[ ] **3.** The nurse records the time of capillary refill.
[ ] **4.** The nurse measures the temperature of the skin.

A 36-year-old woman with a 7-year history of Raynaud's disease comes to donate blood during a community blood drive.

37. Considering the client's diagnosis, in which part of the body would the nurse expect the client's symptoms to be chiefly located?
[ ] **1.** Legs
[ ] **2.** Hands
[ ] **3.** Chest
[ ] **4.** Neck

38. Which factor is the client most likely to correlate with the onset of her discomfort?
[ ] **1.** Exposure to heat
[ ] **2.** Exposure to cold
[ ] **3.** Exposure to sun
[ ] **4.** Exposure to wind

39. When preparing this client's teaching plan, the nurse should include information on the importance of avoiding which activity?
[ ] **1.** Wearing gloves
[ ] **2.** Emotional stress
[ ] **3.** Drinking alcoholic beverages
[ ] **4.** Bathing with perfumed soap

A 32-year-old man has been diagnosed with thrombo-angiitis obliterans, also known as Buerger's disease.

40. When the client describes his earliest symptoms, the nurse would expect him to report which symptom?
[ ] **1.** A heavy feeling in his lower extremities
[ ] **2.** Frequent problems with ingrown toenails
[ ] **3.** Leg pain accompanying walking or exercise
[ ] **4.** Swollen feet at the end of the day

41. While palpating the peripheral pulses in the lower extremities, how would the nurse expect this client's pulses to be?
[ ] **1.** Strong
[ ] **2.** Normal
[ ] **3.** Full
[ ] **4.** Weak

42. If the client understands the potential complications related to his disease, he will tell the nurse that it is most important for him to schedule regular appointments with which specialist?
[ ] **1.** Podiatrist
[ ] **2.** Dietitian
[ ] **3.** Dermatologist
[ ] **4.** Ophthalmologist

The physician discusses the possibility of performing a sympathectomy to treat the client's Buerger's disease.

43. The best evidence that the client understands the physician's explanation of the purpose for this surgical procedure is when he says that a sympathectomy will do what?
[ ] **1.** Promote vasodilation.
[ ] **2.** Aid muscle relaxation.
[ ] **3.** Relieve mental stress.
[ ] **4.** Slow his heart rate.

The nurse teaches the client how to perform Buerger-Allen exercises.

44. The nurse observes that the client performs the exercises correctly when he lies flat with his legs elevated for several minutes and then performs which action?
[ ] **1.** He sits on the edge of the bed.
[ ] **2.** He stands and touches his toes.
[ ] **3.** He jogs in place at the bedside.
[ ] **4.** He pretends to climb stairs.

45. When preparing the client's discharge instructions, it is essential for the nurse to warn him to avoid which activity?
[ ] **1.** Heavy lifting
[ ] **2.** Tobacco use
[ ] **3.** Airplane travel
[ ] **4.** Sexual activity

Abdominal X-rays reveal that a 78-year-old man has an abdominal aortic aneurysm.

46. Which finding in the client's history is the most significant factor that predisposes him to formation of an abdominal aortic aneurysm?
[ ] **1.** The client has type 1 diabetes mellitus.
[ ] **2.** The client has chronic hypertension.
[ ] **3.** The client has a sedentary lifestyle.
[ ] **4.** The client takes digoxin (Lanoxin).

47. During the client's physical examination, which assessment finding would the nurse expect to be most evident of his disease?
[ ] **1.** Edema of the feet
[ ] **2.** Hypoactive bowel sounds
[ ] **3.** Multiple abdominal petechiae
[ ] **4.** Pulsating abdominal mass

48. If the client has an accurate understanding of the physician's explanation of his condition, what should he tell the nurse?
[ ] **1.** An aneurysm is a weakened valve in the abdominal aorta.
[ ] **2.** An aneurysm is a stationary blood clot in the abdominal vein.
[ ] **3.** An aneurysm is a fatty deposit in the aorta wall.
[ ] **4.** An aneurysm is an outpouching in the wall of the abdominal aorta.

The client refuses surgical treatment and wishes to stay in the long-term care facility where he lives.

49. Which symptom is the client most likely to exhibit if the aneurysm becomes larger or begins to dissect?
[ ] **1.** Hematuria
[ ] **2.** Indigestion
[ ] **3.** Rectal bleeding
[ ] **4.** Lower back pain

Several years ago, the client prepared an advance directive indicating that he did not want heroic measures performed to sustain his life. The physician wrote a "do-not-resuscitate" (allow natural death) order on his medical record.

50. If the client loses consciousness and remains unresponsive, which nursing action is most appropriate?
[ ] **1.** Have him transferred to the hospital.
[ ] **2.** Call the local ambulance service.
[ ] **3.** Notify his attending physician.
[ ] **4.** Call his next of kin.

Nursing Care of Clients with Red Blood Cell Disorders

The complete blood count (CBC) of a 71-year-old client indicates that his erythrocytes are below normal.

51. Which of the following conditions most likely explains the client's reduced red blood cell count?
[ ] **1.** Mitral valve insufficiency
[ ] **2.** Arteriosclerotic heart disease
[ ] **3.** Peptic ulcer disease
[ ] **4.** Prostatic hypertrophy

52. Once the underlying cause of the client's low red blood cell count is treated, which nursing intervention is most appropriate for reducing his lethargy?
[ ] **1.** Encouraging the client to get at least 8 hours of sleep
[ ] **2.** Having the client exercise twice a day
[ ] **3.** Instructing the client to eat more simple carbohydrates
[ ] **4.** Encouraging the client to rest frequently

An 18-year-old female college student has been feeling extremely tired and makes an appointment at the university's health office.

53. Which laboratory test would the nurse expect to be lower than normal if the cause of the client's fatigue is related to iron deficiency anemia?
[ ] **1.** Prothrombin time (PT)
[ ] **2.** Bleeding time
[ ] **3.** Fibrinogen level
[ ] **4.** Hemoglobin (Hb) level

54. Which information provided by the client is most relevant to her anemia?
[ ] **1.** She has chronic back pain.
[ ] **2.** She experiences menstrual cramps.
[ ] **3.** She feels chilled most of the time.
[ ] **4.** She had rheumatic fever as a child.

When taking the client's dietary history, the nurse learns that the client has been cutting back on foods to lose weight.

55. The elimination of which food group has most likely contributed to the client's iron deficiency anemia?
[ ] **1.** Milk
[ ] **2.** Meat
[ ] **3.** Fruit
[ ] **4.** Vegetables

The physician orders ferrous sulfate (Feosol) 1 tablet orally t.i.d. for the client.

56. Based on the prescription, when should the client take her medication?
[ ] **1.** Between meals
[ ] **2.** With each meal
[ ] **3.** Just before eating
[ ] **4.** Just before bedtime

57. To maximize the absorption of the iron supplement, the nurse correctly advises the client to take the tablet with which beverage?
[ ] **1.** Milk
[ ] **2.** Tea
[ ] **3.** Soft drink
[ ] **4.** Orange juice

58. If the client understands the nurse's explanation about the side effects of iron, she should say that this drug will cause her stools to turn which color?
[ ] **1.** Medium brown
[ ] **2.** Dark black
[ ] **3.** Clay-colored
[ ] **4.** Light green

Three days after going to the clinic, the client phones the health office and explains that she is having difficulty swallowing the large iron capsule. The physician orders a liquid iron preparation.

59. When instructing the client about administration of the liquid iron preparation, the nurse should tell her to perform which action?
[ ] **1.** Use a straw
[ ] **2.** Pour it in a paper cup
[ ] **3.** Take it over ice
[ ] **4.** Mix it with milk

A 42-year-old woman develops anemia due to heavy menstrual blood loss.

60. Which information revealed during the initial interview is most likely related to the client's anemia?
[ ] **1.** She fainted last week at work.
[ ] **2.** She has occasional headaches.
[ ] **3.** Her hemoglobin level is 13 g/dL.
[ ] **4.** Her abdomen is somewhat tender.

61. During the client's physical assessment, which skin assessment finding would the nurse expect to document?
[ ] **1.** The skin appears mottled.
[ ] **2.** The skin is flushed.
[ ] **3.** The skin is pale.
[ ] **4.** The skin has a blue tinge.

The physician instructs the office nurse to administer iron dextran (INFeD) I.M. to the client. The nurse will administer the injection by Z-track (zigzag) technique.

62. The nurse anticipates using which muscle when giving the injection by Z-track technique?
[ ] **1.** Deltoid
[ ] **2.** Trapezius
[ ] **3.** Gluteus medius
[ ] **4.** Latissimus dorsi

63. What is the best reason the nurse can give the client for administering the injection by Z-track technique?
[ ] **1.** Iron dextran stains superficial tissue and needs to be absorbed rapidly.
[ ] **2.** Iron dextran stains superficial tissue and needs to be sealed deeply.
[ ] **3.** Iron dextran stains superficial tissue and needs to be instilled quickly.
[ ] **4.** Iron dextran stains superficial tissue and needs to be massaged vigorously.

64. Just before inserting the needle into the muscle for a Z-track injection, the nurse appropriately pulls the tissue at the injection site in which direction?
[ ] **1.** Laterally
[ ] **2.** Diagonally
[ ] **3.** Downward
[ ] **4.** Upward

A 50-year-old woman is suspected of having pernicious anemia. She is hospitalized for diagnostic purposes.

65. Which question is most appropriate to ask this client while collecting the admission history?

[ ] **1.** "Was all or a portion of your stomach removed?"
[ ] **2.** "Have you ever had any type of hepatitis?"
[ ] **3.** "Were you ever exposed to toxic wastes?"
[ ] **4.** "Do you have severe allergic reactions?"

66. Which entry documented in the nurse's notes during the initial client interview is inappropriate to include?
[ ] **1.** Client states, "I get nauseated when I eat."
[ ] **2.** Has Medicare insurance.
[ ] **3.** Skin over back and buttocks is flushed.
[ ] **4.** Has asked to see a minister.

67. If the client develops neurologic symptoms related to pernicious anemia, the nurse would expect her to report having which symptom?
[ ] **1.** Numbness and tingling in the extremities
[ ] **2.** Morning headaches and sudden dizziness
[ ] **3.** Restlessness and sleep pattern disturbances
[ ] **4.** Periods of temporary amnesia and fainting

The physician orders a Schilling test for the client.

68. The nurse correctly informs the client that a Schilling test involves the collection of what body specimen?
[ ] **1.** Urine
[ ] **2.** Blood
[ ] **3.** Stool
[ ] **4.** Sputum

The Schilling test confirms that the client has pernicious anemia.

69. When the client asks the nurse how her disorder will be treated, which response by the nurse is most appropriate?
[ ] **1.** "The physician will probably prescribe blood transfusions."
[ ] **2.** "The physician will most likely prescribe iron medication."
[ ] **3.** "The physician will probably prescribe vitamin B_{12} injections."
[ ] **4.** "The physician will probably prescribe vitamin K injections."

A 30-year-old man who is experiencing a sickle cell crisis is admitted to the hospital.

70. If this newly admitted client fits the profile of people in the United States with sickle cell anemia, the nurse would expect him to be of which ethnic background?
[ ] **1.** Mexican American
[ ] **2.** Asian American
[ ] **3.** Native American
[ ] **4.** African American

71. During the admission assessment, which finding can the nurse attribute to the client's blood disease?
[ ] **1.** His tongue is white.
[ ] **2.** His urine is cloudy.
[ ] **3.** He is jaundiced.
[ ] **4.** He is nauseated.

72. Which problem would be the nurse's priority during the client's sickle cell crisis?
[ ] **1.** Improving nutrition
[ ] **2.** Controlling pain
[ ] **3.** Assisting ventilation
[ ] **4.** Relieving anxiety

73. If the nurse observes that the client's knee is edematous, which nursing measure is most appropriate to add to the care plan at this time?
[ ] **1.** Help the client to perform passive range-of-motion exercises during each shift.
[ ] **2.** Assist the client in changing positions to achieve comfort.
[ ] **3.** Ambulate the client at frequent intervals.
[ ] **4.** Encourage the client to perform quadriceps-setting exercises.

74. Which nursing intervention is best for maintaining tissue perfusion during a sickle cell crisis?
[ ] **1.** Providing the client with a large quantity of fluids
[ ] **2.** Assisting the client with applying thigh-high elastic stockings
[ ] **3.** Elevating the client's lower extremities
[ ] **4.** Having the client dangle his legs over the side of the bed

The nurse reviews the hereditary implications and precipitating factors of sickle cell anemia with the client.

75. The nurse teaches the client that his sickle cell crisis was most likely triggered by which precipitating factor?
[ ] **1.** Low blood glucose level
[ ] **2.** Fatigue
[ ] **3.** Overexertion
[ ] **4.** Overhydration

76. When the client asks the nurse to elaborate on the significance of having the sickle cell trait, which is the best response?
[ ] **1.** People with sickle cell trait manifest the disease later in life.
[ ] **2.** People with sickle cell trait have a milder form of disease symptoms.
[ ] **3.** People with sickle cell trait do not develop symptoms of the disease.
[ ] **4.** People with sickle cell trait have a much shorter life expectancy.

Nursing Care of Clients with White Blood Cell Disorders

A nurse caring for a 70-year-old man with chronic myelogenous leukemia suspects that the client has an infection.

77. Which assessment finding best indicates a possible infection?
[ ] **1.** Blood in the stool
[ ] **2.** Prolonged vomiting
[ ] **3.** Cloudy urine
[ ] **4.** Extreme fatigue

The nurse notes that the client's mouth bleeds after he brushes his teeth.

78. Which alternative form of oral care is most appropriate at this time?
[ ] **1.** Use foam mouth swabs.
[ ] **2.** Use only dental floss.
[ ] **3.** Use an antiseptic mouthwash.
[ ] **4.** Eliminate the use of toothpaste.

79. When assisting the client with selecting foods from his menu, which food choice should the nurse suggest?
[ ] **1.** Spaghetti with meatballs
[ ] **2.** Grilled cheese sandwich
[ ] **3.** Salad with French dressing
[ ] **4.** Creamed potato soup

The client receives antineoplastic drugs to treat his leukemia.

80. The nurse plans to prepare the client for which common side effect of antineoplastic drugs?
[ ] **1.** Hair loss
[ ] **2.** Rash
[ ] **3.** Constipation
[ ] **4.** Headaches

Laboratory test results indicate that the client has a low platelet count.

81. Based on the client's laboratory results, which nursing intervention is most appropriate at this time?
[ ] **1.** Limiting the client's visitors to family
[ ] **2.** Placing the client in protective isolation
[ ] **3.** Using small-gauge needles for injections
[ ] **4.** Providing rest periods between activities

Several weeks later, the physician informs the client that his leukemia is in remission.

82. Which client statement indicates an understanding of the term *remission?*
[ ] **1.** "I will never need cancer treatment again."
[ ] **2.** "I will need drugs again in a few months."
[ ] **3.** "My disease has responded to treatment."
[ ] **4.** "My disease is cured at the present time."

Two years after the client's initial treatment, he is hospitalized again. Although the client's condition is stable, the physician has discussed with the client and his family that the client will probably not survive more than 6 months.

83. The nurse appropriately refers the client and his family to which organization?
[ ] **1.** The public health department
[ ] **2.** The Centers for Disease Control and Prevention
[ ] **3.** The local hospice organization
[ ] **4.** The local United Way

A female high school student contracts infectious mononucleosis.

84. When the student asks the school nurse to explain how she acquired the condition, the nurse correctly responds that the virus causing this disease is transmitted by which route?
[ ] **1.** Contact with microorganisms in blood
[ ] **2.** Direct contact with an infected person
[ ] **3.** Consuming contaminated food or water
[ ] **4.** Being bitten by a mosquito

85. Which symptom is most likely to have been one of the first experienced by the client?
[ ] **1.** Abdominal discomfort
[ ] **2.** Aching joints
[ ] **3.** Sore throat
[ ] **4.** Intestinal upset

86. Which information is essential for the nurse to address when discussing self-care with this client?
[ ] **1.** Compliance with antibiotic therapy
[ ] **2.** The need to restrict physical activity
[ ] **3.** The importance of taking supplemental vitamins
[ ] **4.** Follow-up blood transfusions

A 32-year-old man with a diagnosis of Hodgkin's disease is admitted to the hospital.

87. If this client is typical of most clients who develop Hodgkin's disease, the nurse would expect to note which characteristic finding during the initial client assessment?
[ ] **1.** Weight gain
[ ] **2.** A large lymph node in the client's neck
[ ] **3.** Frequent headaches
[ ] **4.** Chronic diarrhea

88. If the physical assessment is performed during the early stages of this client's disease, how will the nurse document the appearance of lymph nodes?
[ ] **1.** Enlarged and painless
[ ] **2.** Small and firm
[ ] **3.** Enlarged and painful
[ ] **4.** Fixed and hard

The client is scheduled to undergo external radiation of his cervical and axillary lymph nodes.

89. Which instruction should be included in the teaching plan when preparing the client for radiation therapy?
[ ] **1.** "Avoid getting the skin wet around your neck and under your arms."
[ ] **2.** "Avoid using any deodorants containing aluminum hydroxide."
[ ] **3.** "Shave the hair from your neck and underarms daily."
[ ] **4.** "Apply zinc oxide ointment to the area after each treatment."

90. Which response by the nurse is most appropriate when the client becomes concerned that his skin is reddened?
[ ] **1.** Explain that this is an expected outcome with radiation.
[ ] **2.** Tell him that the heat from radiation causes vasodilation.
[ ] **3.** Inform him that the redness indicates superficial bleeding.
[ ] **4.** Reassure him that the redness is hardly noticeable.

The client will continue his radiation treatment as an outpatient after his discharge from the hospital.

91. Which instruction concerning the outdoors is most important to include in the client's discharge plan?
[ ] **1.** Be sure to wear several layers of warm clothing when outside.
[ ] **2.** Avoid becoming chilled or too warm.
[ ] **3.** Wear a mask when outdoors to filter dust and pollen.
[ ] **4.** Protect your irradiated skin from sunlight.

A client with advanced non-Hodgkin's lymphoma is being treated with antineoplastic drugs to control his disease.

92. Which finding should the nurse report immediately because it indicates that the client requires reverse (protective) isolation?

[ ] **1.** Anorexia and weight loss
[ ] **2.** Frequent diarrhea
[ ] **3.** Low white blood cell count
[ ] **4.** Disorientation and confusion

The client's disease fails to respond to medical treatment. The nurse is present in the room when the physician tells the client that his condition is terminal.

93. Which nursing action is most helpful in assisting the client to deal with his impending death?

[ ] **1.** Providing literature on death and dying
[ ] **2.** Allowing him privacy to think by himself
[ ] **3.** Encouraging him to talk about how he is feeling
[ ] **4.** Suggesting that he get a second opinion

A 24-year-old man makes an appointment with a clinic physician because of unexplained weight loss. When obtaining the client's history, the nurse suspects that the client's signs and symptoms are suggestive of human immunodeficiency virus (HIV) infection.

94. Which of the following signs and symptoms would lead the nurse to suspect HIV infection? Select all that apply.

[ ] **1.** Cough
[ ] **2.** Fever
[ ] **3.** Diarrhea
[ ] **4.** Fatigue
[ ] **5.** Ringed lesion on the face
[ ] **6.** Swollen lymph nodes in the axillae and groin

During a follow-up clinic visit, the client's partner joins him.

95. Which of the following instructions about safe sex practices are appropriate for the nurse to discuss with the client and his partner? Select all that apply.

[ ] **1.** Brush teeth after oral intercourse.
[ ] **2.** Reduce the number of sexual partners to one.
[ ] **3.** Do not reuse condoms.
[ ] **4.** Avoid anal intercourse.
[ ] **5.** Engage in nonpenetrative sexual activities.

96. Which situation would place this client at highest risk for acquired immunodeficiency syndrome (AIDS)?

[ ] **1.** Recent cardiovascular surgery (6 months ago)
[ ] **2.** Recent vacation in Africa
[ ] **3.** Excessive alcohol consumption
[ ] **4.** I.V. drug use

The physician orders several laboratory tests because of suspected AIDS.

97. Which laboratory test is most significant for diagnosing antibodies to HIV?

[ ] **1.** Schick test
[ ] **2.** Dick test
[ ] **3.** Enzyme-linked immunosorbent assay (ELISA)
[ ] **4.** Venereal Disease Research Laboratory (VDRL) test

98. How can the nurse best protect herself from getting AIDS from a client of unknown infectious status?

[ ] **1.** Wear a face mask when changing dressings.
[ ] **2.** Refrain from capping needles after injections.
[ ] **3.** Wear a cover-gown when giving a bed bath.
[ ] **4.** Put on gloves before taking the client's vital signs.

A client with AIDS is admitted to the hospital with an opportunistic respiratory infection. His statements to the nurse imply a sense of hopelessness.

99. When planning care for this client, which approach is most therapeutic?

[ ] **1.** Encourage the client to set small, daily goals.
[ ] **2.** Refer the client to the hospital chaplain.
[ ] **3.** Provide for periodic distractions such as watching television.
[ ] **4.** Recommend that the client contact his next of kin.

Nursing Care of Clients with Bone Marrow Disorders

A client with polycythemia vera has an enlarged spleen.

100. Which position would promote the most comfort for this client?

[ ] **1.** Sitting upright
[ ] **2.** Supine
[ ] **3.** Lateral
[ ] **4.** With legs elevated

101. Which nursing action is most appropriate to prevent the formation of blood clots when a client has polycythemia vera?

[ ] **1.** Administering diuretics as ordered
[ ] **2.** Increasing the client's fluid intake
[ ] **3.** Restricting dietary sodium
[ ] **4.** Encouraging the client to lose weight

The physician informs the client that he requires a phlebotomy and explains the procedure to him.

102. When speaking with the nurse later that day, which statement by the client provides the best evidence that he understood the physician's explanation about the upcoming procedure?
[ ] **1.** "Blood will be removed from my vein."
[ ] **2.** "I'll have tourniquets applied to my arms."
[ ] **3.** "Some veins will be surgically occluded."
[ ] **4.** "I'll receive a blood transfusion."

103. Which symptom should the nurse recognize as a consequence of the client's polycythemia vera?
[ ] **1.** Angina
[ ] **2.** Dyspepsia
[ ] **3.** Dysuria
[ ] **4.** Anorexia

The physician plans to perform a bone marrow aspiration on a 67-year-old woman who has had unexplained low counts of all blood cell components. The physician suspects aplastic anemia.

104. After the nurse explains the anatomic location for bone marrow aspiration to the client, the client correctly identifies the site where the specimen will be taken by pointing to which part of her body?
[ ] **1.** To her posterior hip
[ ] **2.** To her lower spine
[ ] **3.** To her upper arm
[ ] **4.** To her groin area

105. What is one of the nurse's major responsibilities during a bone marrow aspiration?
[ ] **1.** To minimize client discomfort
[ ] **2.** To hold instruments
[ ] **3.** To regulate suction
[ ] **4.** To administer oxygen

106. After completion of the bone marrow aspiration, what is essential for the nurse to monitor?
[ ] **1.** Fluctuations in the client's blood pressure
[ ] **2.** Bleeding from the puncture site
[ ] **3.** Changes in the client's pulse
[ ] **4.** The client's level of consciousness

The results of the bone marrow aspiration confirm that the client has aplastic anemia.

107. When the client is bathing, which nursing observation provides the best indication that she is having difficulty tolerating the current level of activity?
[ ] **1.** She becomes short of breath.
[ ] **2.** She feels extremely nauseated.
[ ] **3.** Her pulse rate drops below 60 beats/minute.
[ ] **4.** Her skin becomes moist and cool.

108. Which assessment finding is most likely due to the client's low platelet count?
[ ] **1.** Multiple bruises
[ ] **2.** Pale skin color
[ ] **3.** Elevated body temperature
[ ] **4.** Cool extremities

109. Considering the client has a reduced leukocyte count, which nursing measure is most important for all caregivers?
[ ] **1.** Performing conscientious hand washing
[ ] **2.** Wearing a gown when providing care
[ ] **3.** Applying direct pressure on all puncture wounds
[ ] **4.** Monitoring the client's heart rate and rhythm each shift

The physician tells the client that she will receive two units of packed blood cells. The client verbalizes concern about becoming HIV-positive from receiving transfusion of publicly donated blood.

110. Which response by the nurse is the most appropriate way to handle the client's comment?
[ ] **1.** "Blood donors are tested for HIV before their blood is accepted."
[ ] **2.** "Donated blood no longer contains the virus causing AIDS."
[ ] **3.** "Donated blood is tested for HIV antibodies after collection."
[ ] **4.** "There's no way to identify the AIDS virus in blood yet."

111. When the client asks how packed cells are different from the usual blood transfusion, which response by the nurse is most accurate?
[ ] **1.** Packed cells contain the same blood cells in less fluid volume.
[ ] **2.** Packed cells contain more blood cells in the same fluid volume.
[ ] **3.** Packed cells are less likely to cause an allergic reaction.
[ ] **4.** Packed cells will stimulate the client's bone marrow to function.

The client has type A Rh-positive blood.

112. Which unit of blood should the nurse refuse to administer knowing that it is incompatible for this client?
[ ] **1.** Type A, Rh-negative
[ ] **2.** Type O, Rh-positive
[ ] **3.** Type O, Rh-negative
[ ] **4.** Type AB, Rh-positive

113. During the first 15 minutes of the infusion, which assessment finding strongly suggests that the client is experiencing a transfusion reaction?

[ ] **1.** The client feels an urgent need to urinate.
[ ] **2.** The client's blood pressure becomes low.
[ ] **3.** The client has localized swelling at the infusion site.
[ ] **4.** The client's skin is pale at the site of the infusing blood.

The client tells the nurse that she has been receiving corticosteroid treatment for more than 1 year in an effort to treat her disease.

114. While the nurse examines the client, which assessment finding is most likely related to the administration of corticosteroids?

[ ] **1.** The client's voice is quite husky.
[ ] **2.** The client's face is moon-shaped.
[ ] **3.** The client's muscles are large.
[ ] **4.** The client's skin looks tanned.

115. Which statement made by the client best supports the nurse's suspicion of a complication resulting from the use of corticosteroids?

[ ] **1.** "I've been experiencing heartburn lately."
[ ] **2.** "I've been taking long naps during the day."
[ ] **3.** "I've lost my appetite."
[ ] **4.** "I've noticed that my urine is light yellow."

Because corticosteroid therapy has not effectively treated her aplastic anemia, the client has consented to have a bone marrow transplant. She undergoes total body irradiation.

116. What is the highest nursing priority for this client immediately before, and for several weeks after, the bone marrow transplantation?

[ ] **1.** Relieving depression
[ ] **2.** Promoting nutrition
[ ] **3.** Preventing infection
[ ] **4.** Monitoring hydration

Nursing Care of Clients with Coagulation Disorders

A physician examines a client with purpura and makes a tentative diagnosis of idiopathic thrombocytopenia.

117. Based on the diagnosis, which finding would the nurse expect to note during a physical assessment of this client?

[ ] **1.** Small skin hemorrhages
[ ] **2.** Dark areas of cyanosis
[ ] **3.** Flushed red skin
[ ] **4.** Protruding veins

118. When the nursing team meets to develop a care plan for the client, which of the following would be considered a nursing priority?

[ ] **1.** Encouraging fluids
[ ] **2.** Promoting activity
[ ] **3.** Restricting visitors
[ ] **4.** Preventing injury

A client with hemophilia experienced a minor closed head injury. Before discharge, the nurse reviews the signs and symptoms that indicate bleeding.

119. The nurse assumes that the client understands his discharge instructions based on his ability to name which symptom as an early indicator of intracranial bleeding?

[ ] **1.** Seizures
[ ] **2.** Drowsiness
[ ] **3.** Ringing in the ears
[ ] **4.** Diminished appetite

Nursing Care of Clients with Inflammatory and Obstructive Lymphatic Disorders

A 78-year-old woman has just been admitted to the nursing home with lymphedema of her right arm.

120. Which history finding most likely contributed to the development of the client's lymphedema?

[ ] **1.** The client has a healed fracture of the humerus.
[ ] **2.** The client had a radical mastectomy years ago.
[ ] **3.** The client is being treated for pernicious anemia.
[ ] **4.** The client was immunized for smallpox as a child.

121. Which intervention is essential to include in the client's care plan?

[ ] **1.** Avoid giving injections in her right arm.
[ ] **2.** Avoid turning the client on her right side.
[ ] **3.** Avoid active exercise of her right arm.
[ ] **4.** Avoid trimming the fingernails on the right hand.

Correct Answers and Rationales

Nursing Care of Clients with Venous Disorders

1. **1.** Heredity is a predisposing factor in the development of varicose veins. Other contributing factors include occupations that require prolonged standing or sitting, obesity, and pressure on veins from an enlarging uterus during the later months of pregnancy. Although smoking is definitely unhealthy, nicotine has a major vasoconstricting effect on arterioles, not veins. An active lifestyle or athletic exercise is beneficial for the cardiovascular system and probably had little to do with the client's developing varicose veins.

Client Needs Category—Physiological integrity
Client Needs Subcategory—Physiological adaptation

2. **1.** Most clients with varicose veins state that their legs ache and feel heavy and tired. Because the impaired circulation is most prominent when the person sits or stands for long periods of time, symptoms are usually relieved during the night. Perspiration is not associated with varicose veins. Leg pain during activity is more likely to be caused by inadequate arterial blood flow or a sport-related injury.

Client Needs Category—Physiological integrity
Client Needs Subcategory—Physiological adaptation

3. **1.** Elevating the legs periodically during the day relieves symptoms associated with varicose veins. Other techniques that improve venous circulation, such as isometric or isotonic exercise, are also helpful. Wearing cotton socks does not provide symptomatic relief from varicose veins; however, wearing elastic support hose is beneficial. Because circulation is already impaired, massaging the legs is not recommended because of the possibility of dislodging a clot. Sitting for long periods of time, as in a sedentary lifestyle, does not promote venous circulation.

Client Needs Category—Health promotion and maintenance
Client Needs Subcategory—None

4. **3.** Clients with varicose veins must avoid anything that promotes venous stasis, such as sitting with crossed knees, standing for long periods of time, and wearing tight undergarments or knee-high stockings. Walking promotes circulation, regardless of whether low- or high-heeled shoes are worn. Pantyhose are better than hose that end at the calf. Shaving the legs is not contraindicated.

Client Needs Category—Health promotion and maintenance
Client Needs Subcategory—None

5. **3.** After a vein-stripping procedure, blood returns to the right side of the heart through other veins deeper in the leg. Arteries cannot transport both oxygenated and unoxygenated blood. New veins do not form as replacements. The ends of the removed veins are sutured closed; they are not reconnected to other blood vessels.

Client Needs Category—Physiological integrity
Client Needs Subcategory—Physiological adaptation

6. **2.** Early and frequent ambulation is essential after vein stripping and vein ligation surgery because it helps promote venous circulation, which is temporarily compromised by the removal of some leg veins. During the immediate postoperative period, walking is ordered hourly while the client is awake. Even during the night, the client is aroused and assisted to walk several times. Although adding protein to the client's diet will help with building and repairing tissue after surgery, this is not the priority intervention at this time. The nurse should always monitor for signs of infection, but this is not the priority following this type of surgery. Leg cramping is not usually associated with vein stripping.

Client Needs Category—Physiological integrity
Client Needs Subcategory—Physiological adaptation

7. **4.** If the client states that she had an unfavorable reaction when taking a particular medication in the past, the nurse should withhold the medication and report the information to the charge nurse or the physician. It would be unethical to try to deceive a client by giving the generic name for a drug she already knows by the trade name. Telling the client that she must take a medication is inappropriate; the physician will likely substitute another drug. Taking the drug with a lot of water is unlikely to reduce or prevent GI upset.

Client Needs Category—Physiological integrity
Client Needs Subcategory—Pharmacological therapies

8. **3.** Stasis ulcers appear darkly pigmented, dry, and scaly. Venous congestion causes edema, and this localized swelling interferes with adequate arterial blood flow, causing poor oxygenation and poor nourishment of skin tissue. This, combined with the retention of metabolic wastes, leads to inflammation of the skin, sometimes referred to as *cellulitis*. The inflamed tissue chronically breaks open, forming craters that are difficult to heal. The remaining descriptions are not characteristic of such ulcers.

Client Needs Category—Physiological integrity
Client Needs Subcategory—Physiological adaptation

9. **2.** Wet-to-dry dressings provide a means for debriding the ulcerated areas of necrotic tissue. Although covering impaired skin reduces the entrance of microorganisms, absorbs drainage, and protects the skin, those benefits are not the primary reasons for the dressing's use.

Client Needs Category—Health promotion and maintenance
Client Needs Subcategory—None

10. 3. The appearance of pink tissue indicates that granulation tissue is forming. Granulation tissue consists of capillaries and fibrous collagen that seal and nourish the tissue. An increase in drainage suggests that cellular death is continuing or the wound is infected. Relief of discomfort is a positive sign; however, venous ulcers are not severely painful even in the acute stage. White or black wound margins suggest an extension of cell death.

Client Needs Category—Physiological integrity
Client Needs Subcategory—Physiological adaptation

11. 4. A moist wound undergoes accelerated healing. An air-occlusive dressing prevents evaporation of wound moisture, thereby allowing the wound to heal by second intention at a more rapid rate. This may then decrease the amount of scar tissue, but this is a secondary benefit of using an air-occlusive dressing and is not the best choice. Some also feel that healing is faster using an air-occlusive dressing because preventing oxygen from reaching the wound externally stimulates capillary growth to the wound. This type of dressing can remain in place for up to 7 days unless it loosens or the client develops signs of an infection. Air-occlusive dressings such as DuoDERM are initially more expensive than traditional gauze dressings; however, the need for less frequent changing tends to reduce the initial cost for some individuals. There is no evidence that this type of dressing will decrease pain related to skin irritation.

Client Needs Category—Health promotion and maintenance
Client Needs Subcategory—None

12. 1, 2, 3. Gangrene (necrosis) of the toes and foot is a result of arterial insufficiency. Gangrene is preceded by arterial ulcers—small, circular, deep ulcerations on the tips of the toes or between the toes—that develop from a combination of ischemia and pressure and lead to tissue necrosis. Clients who have problems with circulation are at highest risk. These include clients with diabetes, clients with inadequate circulation, and those who have experienced trauma to the toes. Although homeless clients may have other risk factors, such as poor nutrition and hygiene issues, they are not at highest risk for acquiring gangrene. Taking warfarin (Coumadin) and having a history of myocardial infarction are not risk factors associated with arterial insufficiency and gangrene.

Client Needs Category—Physiological integrity
Client Needs Subcategory—Physiological adaptation

13. 1, 2, 3. Thrombophlebitis is a condition in which a blood clot totally or partially occludes the venous blood flow. Several risk factors are associated with blood clot formation. They include obesity, smoking, immobilization and bed rest, history of myocardial infarction and congestive heart failure, multiple sclerosis, oral contraceptive use, and cancer of the breast, pancreas, prostate, or ovary. Leg fatigue is associated with varicose veins. Cramping in the lower leg is associated with a vitamin B deficiency. Pain in the joints is associated with sickle cell anemia.

Client Needs Category—Physiological integrity
Client Needs Subcategory—Physiological adaptation

14. 1. Thrombi typically form as a result of venous stasis. A common cause of venous stasis is inactivity. Postoperative clients are encouraged to perform active leg exercises and to ambulate frequently to promote venous circulation. Shallow breathing predisposes a client to pneumonia. Analgesics may make clients lethargic and less willing to ambulate, but relieving pain is not a direct cause of thrombus formation. Caffeine constricts arteries and arterioles, which can impair blood flow. Thrombi generally form in veins.

Client Needs Category—Physiological integrity
Client Needs Subcategory—Physiological adaptation

15. 2. Besides premeasuring the circumference of the calf from the heel to the popliteal space, the best evidence that antiembolism stockings fit correctly and provide adequate circulation is that the toes should feel warm when touched and the capillary refill should occur in less than 3 seconds. Antiembolism stockings should cover the entire calf. Stockings that are easily donned indicate that they are too large for the client. Antiembolism stockings are not intended to prevent redness of the heels.

Client Needs Category—Physiological integrity
Client Needs Subcategory—Physiological adaptation

16. 2. To check Homans' sign, an assessment used to detect venous thrombosis, the nurse would have the client extend each leg separately and dorsiflex the foot (pointing the toes toward the head). A positive Homans' sign is indicated by pain in the calf when the foot is dorsiflexed. None of the actions or positions described in the remaining options are correct.

Client Needs Category—Physiological integrity
Client Needs Subcategory—Physiological adaptation

17. 1. If the client experiences pain in the calf immediately after dorsiflexing the foot (a positive Homans' sign), the discomfort may be due to a thrombus. Numbness, tingling, and impaired function are not classic signs of thrombophlebitis.

Client Needs Category—Physiological integrity
Client Needs Subcategory—Physiological adaptation

18. 4. If the client has a thrombus, the area distal to the thrombus would tend to swell due to the stasis of venous blood and the redistribution of plasma to the interstitial space from increased hydrostatic pressure in the capillaries. Below the thrombus, the leg would feel cool and appear pale. Capillary refilling time is normally less than 3 seconds.
> *Client Needs Category—Physiological integrity*
> *Client Needs Subcategory—Physiological adaptation*

19. 2. When a thrombus is suspected, the legs must not be massaged. Activity is generally restricted because ambulation, exercise, or massage can cause the blood clot to break away from the vessel wall and circulate, possibly to the lung. Although there is some controversy about elevating the legs, raising the legs may relieve local swelling; however, pillows should never be placed under the knees and the bed should not be gatched at the knees.
> *Client Needs Category—Physiological integrity*
> *Client Needs Subcategory—Physiological adaptation*

20. 4. A dry towel and a waterproof cover act as insulators, preventing rapid heat and moisture loss from the compress. To avoid burning the skin, the temperature of the compress solution is between 98° and 105° F (36.6° and 40.5° C). The skin is inspected at least every 30 minutes to monitor for thermal injury. Sterile technique is not necessary as long as the skin is intact.
> *Client Needs Category—Physiological integrity*
> *Client Needs Subcategory—Physiological adaptation*

21. 3. Heparin (Calciparine) prevents future clots from forming and those that have formed from becoming larger. Heparin (Calciparine) is an anticoagulant that inhibits the conversion of fibrinogen to fibrin. Only thrombolytic agents, such as streptokinase (Streptase), will shrink and dissolve clots already formed. The use of thrombolytic agents is extremely hazardous. The risks usually outweigh the benefits in the case of thrombophlebitis. Drug therapy will not prevent a thrombus from becoming dislodged.
> *Client Needs Category—Physiological integrity*
> *Client Needs Subcategory—Physiological adaptation*

22. 1. PTT is used to monitor the client's response to heparin therapy. The therapeutic range is 1.5 to 2.5 times the control time. A CBC reports the number of blood cells, not blood clotting factors. Hb relates to the blood's oxygen-carrying capacity and is unaffected by heparin (Calciparine). PT is a test used to monitor the response of a client who is receiving an oral anticoagulant such as warfarin (Coumadin). Another test used when clients are on warfarin therapy is the International Normalized Ratio.
> *Client Needs Category—Physiological integrity*
> *Client Needs Subcategory—Pharmacological therapies*

23. 2. When a drug is withdrawn from a vial, the nurse instills a volume of air equal to the amount of fluid that will be withdrawn. Adding air to the contents of a vial facilitates withdrawing the drug. If air is not instilled, the partial vacuum created makes it difficult to remove solution. If too much air is instilled, solution will surge into the syringe and, in some cases, force the plunger from the syringe barrel. If the rubber stopper is removed, the drug will not remain sterile. Modified insulins, not heparin, are rotated gently prior to withdrawal to mix the additive and insulin. Heparin (Calciparine) is not shaken before withdrawing it from the vial.
> *Client Needs Category—Safe, effective care environment*
> *Client Needs Subcategory—Safety and infection control*

24. 3. When the adult client is of average or thin size, it is acceptable practice to insert a needle intended for subcutaneous administration at a 45-degree angle to the skin. For obese adults, it is recommended that the nurse use a 90-degree angle to insert the needle. The dorsogluteal site is used for I.M. injections. The needle size for a subcutaneous injection is between ½″ and ⅝″ and 23- to 26-gauge. The injection site should not be massaged after heparin (Calciparine) administration because this increases the tendency for localized bleeding.
> *Client Needs Category—Safe, effective care environment*
> *Client Needs Subcategory—Safety and infection control*

25. 3. Any sign of bleeding in a client receiving anticoagulant therapy must be reported. In this case, bleeding gums should be reported. Clients commonly complain about abdominal tenderness because of repeated subcutaneous sticks to the area. When this happens, the nurse should assess the abdomen for signs of a hematoma; however, abdominal tenderness does not usually require immediate attention. Likewise, clients often complain about the number of times per day they are stuck. This also does not warrant immediate intervention. Having stools that are light brown is normal. Black, tarry stools would require immediate intervention because they could indicate bleeding.
> *Client Needs Category—Physiological integrity*
> *Client Needs Subcategory—Physiological adaptation*

26. 3. Protamine sulfate, a heparin antagonist, is given to counteract the anticoagulant effects of heparin therapy and restore more normal clotting mechanisms. Calcium lactate is a mineral supplement. Sodium benzoate is used as a preservative. Aluminum phosphate is an ingredient in some antacid products.
> *Client Needs Category—Physiological integrity*
> *Client Needs Subcategory—Pharmacological therapies*

27. **4.** When injections of anticoagulant medication cannot be avoided, it is appropriate for the nurse to apply pressure to the injection site for several minutes to prevent oozing of blood or localized bruising. Pressure is not applied to distribute the drug. Hematomas do not form as a result of applying pressure. Drug absorption is not significantly affected by several minutes of local pressure.
> *Client Needs Category—Physiological integrity*
> *Client Needs Subcategory—Physiological adaptation*

28. **2.** Black, sticky, tar-colored stools are a sign of bleeding from the upper GI tract. Dark amber urine is more indicative of low fluid volume. Emesis is usually green-tinged or clear. A coffee-ground appearance to emesis is more suggestive of GI bleeding. Jaundiced skin indicates a liver or biliary disorder or rapid hemolysis of red blood cells.
> *Client Needs Category—Physiological integrity*
> *Client Needs Subcategory—Physiological adaptation*

29. **1, 2, 3, 4.** Green leafy vegetables, such as spinach, lettuce, turnip greens, and brussel sprouts, are among the best food sources of vitamin K. Vitamin K is associated with clotting factors in the blood. Half of the daily requirements of vitamin K comes from the diet, while the bacteria from the intestine manufacture the remaining amounts. Warfarin (Coumadin) is an anticoagulant that prevents clot formation. If foods high in vitamin K are eaten, this will interfere with the main purposes of the drug.
> *Client Needs Category—Health promotion and maintenance*
> *Client Needs Subcategory—None*

30. **1, 2, 3, 4.** Many dietary supplements (including gingko, St. John's wort, willow bark, and ginger) can alter the client's INR and PT. Green tea and creatine, a supplement that increases muscle mass, are not known to alter these levels. The best policy for clients who are taking warfarin (Coumadin) is to avoid all dietary and herbal supplements unless the physician approves. Clients should also avoid vitamin and mineral supplements that contain vitamin K.
> *Client Needs Category—Health promotion and maintenance*
> *Client Needs Subcategory—None*

31. **1.** Signs of phlebitis include redness, tenderness, warmth, and swelling of the vein. An inflamed vein also feels indurated (hard, not soft and spongy) or cordlike, but it does not appear pale, purple, or dark.
> *Client Needs Category—Physiological integrity*
> *Client Needs Subcategory—Physiological adaptation*

32. **4.** The cause of the inflamed vein may be due to the presence of the foreign infusion device, the irritating solution, or trauma to the vein wall. In any case, the infusion should be discontinued to prevent further injury to the vein and to promote healing. Another site would then be chosen to continue the infusion. Elevating the extremity is appropriate to relieve swelling after the needle or catheter has been removed. Applying pressure would not diminish the current problem; rather, it would slow the rate of infusion. Increasing the infusion rate is contraindicated because it has not been medically approved and places the client at risk for fluid volume excess.
> *Client Needs Category—Physiological integrity*
> *Client Needs Subcategory—Physiological adaptation*

Nursing Care of Clients with Arterial Disorders

33. **1.** Individuals with peripheral vascular disease develop trophic changes such as thick, hard nails. Other signs include thin, shiny skin and little hair growth. Trophic changes are the result of chronically impaired blood flow to the epidermal tissues. Flushed skin may be a sign of hypertension, not peripheral vascular disease. The peripheral pulses are often weak and difficult to detect in a client with peripheral vascular disease. Hyperactive knee jerk reflexes are not characteristic of peripheral vascular disease.
> *Client Needs Category—Physiological integrity*
> *Client Needs Subcategory—Physiological adaptation*

34. **3.** When the leg muscles become ischemic, the client with peripheral arterial insufficiency is most likely to report having pain in both legs. The pain goes away with rest, which is the reason the symptom is referred to as intermittent claudication. Cyanosis is more closely associated with venous congestion. Poor distal arterial circulation tends to heighten a person's sensation of being cold. A feeling that the toes are burning is not a common symptom of peripheral arterial insufficiency. Ankle edema is more likely to result because of poor circulation, not active exercise.
> *Client Needs Category—Physiological integrity*
> *Client Needs Subcategory—Physiological adaptation*

35. **3.** Extra clothing or blankets, rather than direct heat applications, are used whenever possible for individuals with peripheral arterial insufficiency. Because of the disease, such clients are typically insensitive to warm temperatures and are at high risk for being burned. Therefore, commercially prepared heat packets or heating pads are contraindicated. Instead, layers of loosely woven fibers, especially of natural material like cotton or wool, help hold pockets of warm air close to the body surface. This promotes a feeling of warmth. Elevating the feet relieves edema but does not necessarily make the feet feel warmer.

Client Needs Category—*Physiological integrity*
Client Needs Subcategory—*Basic care and comfort*

36. 2. The nurse applies acoustic gel to the skin when using a Doppler ultrasound device. The gel helps beam the ultrasound toward the blood vessel being assessed. Movement of red blood cells through an artery produces an intermittent, pulsating sound. Movement of blood through a vein makes a continuous sound, like a whistling wind. The dorsalis pedis artery is on the top of the foot and is often used to assess the strength of the pulse and blood flow to the foot. The posterior tibialis artery is beside the ankle and is used less frequently. When assessing capillary refill, the nurse releases a compressed nail bed and counts the number of seconds it takes for blood to return. A Doppler ultrasound device is not used to measure skin temperature.

Client Needs Category—*Safe, effective care environment*
Client Needs Subcategory—*Safety and infection control*

37. 2. Raynaud's disease is a condition that results in vasospasms to the small arteries and arterioles. Symptoms are generally confined to an individual's hands (most common) or feet and usually result when the client is exposed to cold or emotional upsets. The nose, ears, and chin are less commonly involved. The client experiences periodic episodes during which the affected areas feel cold, painful, numb, and prickly due to poor circulation. The hands usually turn white, then blue and, finally, red. As blood flow resumes, the deprived areas become flushed and warm. A throbbing sensation is then experienced.

Client Needs Category—*Physiological integrity*
Client Needs Subcategory—*Physiological adaptation*

38. 2. Conditions that lead to vasoconstriction, such as exposure to cold or emotional upsets, aggravate or exacerbate the symptoms experienced by individuals with Raynaud's disease. The effect of wind depends on the air temperature. Sun and heat are related to vasodilation and are not associated with this disease.

Client Needs Category—*Physiological integrity*
Client Needs Subcategory—*Physiological adaptation*

39. 2. Stress stimulates the sympathetic nervous system, causing vasoconstriction. When the arterioles narrow, blood flow is impaired, and the client experiences an episodic attack of pain, numbness, and pallor. Therefore, avoiding stressful situations is important in avoiding the onset of symptoms. Wearing warm gloves

while outdoors in cold weather is beneficial and recommended. Drinking alcoholic beverages and bathing with perfumed soap are not necessarily contraindicated for a person with Raynaud's disease.

Client Needs Category—*Health promotion and maintenance*
Client Needs Subcategory—*None*

40. 3. Thromboangiitis obliterans (Buerger's disease) is an acute inflammation of the arteries and veins in the lower extremities. Consequently, a clot forms in the inflamed blood vessel. Smoking causes the disease to worsen. Individuals with the disease commonly report experiencing leg pain or muscle cramps during periods of active movement. Rest can relieve this symptom (referred to as intermittent claudication); however, eventually the pain occurs even while the client is inactive. Clients with varicose veins, not Buerger's disease, report a feeling of heaviness in their legs. Ingrown toenails are not related to the disease. Although edema does occur among clients with Buerger's disease, it is more likely to occur when the disease is far advanced.

Client Needs Category—*Physiological integrity*
Client Needs Subcategory—*Physiological adaptation*

41. 4. Buerger's disease results in decreased blood flow to the legs and feet, although the hands are also sometimes affected. The distal peripheral pulses are frequently found to be weak, diminished, or absent because of impaired circulation. A normal peripheral pulse feels strong or full and is easily felt with only moderate pressure.

Client Needs Category—*Physiological integrity*
Client Needs Subcategory—*Physiological adaptation*

42. 1. Because of impaired arterial and venous circulation, a person with Buerger's disease can easily develop gangrene. A podiatrist is a professional who cares for feet. The services of a podiatrist are used for nail care, treatment of corns and calluses, or other foot problems. Some individuals with this condition eventually undergo amputation when foot lesions become infected or fail to heal. Weight control is important for clients with impaired circulation, but regularly scheduled visits to the dietitian are unnecessary. A dermatologist deals with skin disorders. The client does not need this specialist. An ophthalmologist treats eye disorders; there is no indication that thromboangiitis obliterans affects the eyes.

Client Needs Category—*Health promotion and maintenance*
Client Needs Category—*None*

43. 1. A sympathectomy is a procedure that promotes vasodilation of peripheral arterioles. It involves cutting sympathetic nerve fibers from the autonomic nervous system. Severing these particular nerve fibers will not produce skeletal muscle relaxation, relieve mental stress, or slow the heart rate.

Client Needs Category—Physiological integrity
Client Needs Subcategory—Physiological adaptation

44. **1.** Buerger-Allen exercises help improve and promote collateral circulation and should be done several times per day by the client with Buerger's disease. The client performs them by first lying down and elevating the legs above the heart for 2 to 3 minutes; then, sitting on the edge of the bed or couch, the client lowers his legs to a dependent position. When the legs flush, the client returns to lying flat in bed. After returning to bed, the client should move his feet and toes by dorsiflexion, plantar flexion, and internal and external rotation. Standing and touching the toes, jogging in place, and simulated stair climbing are not part of these exercises.

Client Needs Category—Health promotion and maintenance
Client Needs Subcategory—None

45. **2.** A person with Buerger's disease avoids tobacco because nicotine causes vasoconstriction. There are no contraindications for heavy lifting, traveling by air, or engaging in sexual activity based on the pathology involved in Buerger's disease.

Client Needs Category—Health promotion and maintenance
Client Needs Subcategory—None

46. **2.** An aneurysm is an abnormal dilation (or bulging) of a blood vessel, usually an artery. The dilation typically results from weakness in a portion of the vessel and elevated blood pressure, which is higher in arteries. Several factors can predispose a client to develop an abdominal aortic aneurysm. These include hypertension (which may be secondary to arteriosclerosis), trauma, congenital weakness, smoking, and age. Although diabetes mellitus affects circulation, it is not considered a risk factor. A sedentary lifestyle predisposes clients to many cardiac risks, but it is not as highly correlated with aneurysm formation as hypertension or arteriosclerosis. Digoxin (Lanoxin) is a cardiac glycoside that increases the strength of myocardial contraction and lowers the heart rate. Its use, side effects, and indications have no bearing on aneurysm formation.

Client Needs Category—Physiological integrity
Client Needs Subcategory—Physiological adaptation

47. **4.** When palpating the abdomen of a client with an abdominal aortic aneurysm, it may be possible to feel a pulsating mass. Edema of the feet is not commonly associated with abdominal aneurysms. The extremities are more likely to exhibit signs of diminished circulation, such as paleness, feeling cool, and having faint peripheral pulses. Occasionally, thrombi may form and occlude blood flow to one or both legs, which then causes intense leg or foot pain. Bowel sounds are usually normal. Abdominal petechiae are usually associated with liver or blood disorders.

Client Needs Category—Physiological integrity
Client Needs Subcategory—Physiological adaptation

48. **4.** An aneurysm is a balloon-like outpouching in the wall of an artery, not a vein. Aneurysms commonly occur in the thoracic or abdominal aorta and in cerebral arteries because of the higher blood pressure. Valves are usually seen in veins and they keep the blood flowing in one direction, upward toward the heart. Weakened valves in veins cause blood vessels in the legs to appear distended and twisted. Weakened valves are not associated with abdominal aortic aneurysms. A stationary blood clot (thrombus) may result from altered circulation, but it typically occurs in a vein, not an artery. A fatty deposit in the artery wall (plaque) may build up and lead to arteriosclerosis, which is a risk factor for abdominal aortic aneurysms.

Client Needs Category—Physiological integrity
Client Needs Subcategory—Physiological adaptation

49. **4.** Pressure from an enlarging or dissecting abdominal aortic aneurysm is most likely to be manifested as lower back pain. The client indicates that no position or nursing measure relieves the pain. The client will suffer internal hemorrhage, shock and, possibly, death if the aneurysm becomes so large that it ruptures. Rectal bleeding, hematuria, and indigestion are related to other conditions, not abdominal aortic aneurysms.

Client Needs Category—Physiological integrity
Client Needs Subcategory—Physiological adaptation

50. **3.** If the client has an advance directive indicating his wish for no heroic efforts to sustain life, the nurse would notify the physician of the change in the client's condition. Pertinent assessments, such as vital signs and skin color, should also be reported at this time. If the client is not breathing and is pulseless, it would be unethical to violate his wishes (and the physician's written orders) by performing CPR. Based on the information the nurse communicates, the physician would decide when to transfer the client to the hospital. The physician generally notifies the client's next of kin, but this task may be delegated to the nurse.

Client Needs Category—Safe, effective care environment
Client Needs Subcategory—Safety and infection control

Nursing Care of Clients with Red Blood Cell Disorders

51. 3. Complications of peptic ulcer disease include chronic bleeding or hemorrhage. Blood loss occurs as the ulcer penetrates one or more blood vessels. If the bleeding is slight but continuous, it may go unnoticed until the client becomes weak and fatigued. Mitral valve insufficiency, arteriosclerosis, and an enlarged prostate are not usually associated with chronic or severe red blood cell decreases.

Client Needs Category—Physiological integrity
Client Needs Subcategory—Physiological adaptation

52. 4. Because the client is anemic, he will not have much energy. Balancing rest with activity is one way of maintaining a consistent energy level and avoiding excessive energy expenditures. Adequate sleep, exercise, and eating foods that provide energy are all healthy behaviors, but they are not likely to make as significant an improvement as balancing energy use with rest.

Client Needs Category—Health promotion and maintenance
Client Needs Subcategory—None

53. 4. Iron is necessary for the formation of Hb. Therefore, a low Hb level reflects an iron deficiency. If the Hb level is below 12 g/dL in a woman or 14 g/dL in a man, the person is considered anemic. Because conditions other than iron deficiency can cause a low Hb level, additional diagnostic tests may be necessary. PT, bleeding time, and fibrinogen level are tests commonly performed when a client has a suspected clotting problem or high risk for bleeding. These tests are not typically performed on clients suspected of having anemia.

Client Needs Category—Physiological integrity
Client Needs Subcategory—Physiological adaptation

54. 3. An anemic person is likely to feel colder than usual most of the time. This symptom is most likely due to impaired cellular oxygenation from reduced hemoglobin levels. Without oxygen, the body's ability to produce heat calories during metabolism is affected. Dysmenorrhea, chronic back pain, and a history of rheumatic fever are unrelated to iron deficiency anemia.

Client Needs Category—Physiological integrity
Client Needs Subcategory—Physiological adaptation

55. 2. Omitting meat from the diet can cause iron deficiency anemia. Good food sources of iron include meat, fish, certain beans, iron-enriched cereals, whole grain products, and green leafy vegetables such as spinach. However, iron is more poorly absorbed from vegetables. Milk does not contain iron but is a good source of calcium and protein. Likewise, most fruits do not contain large amounts of iron. Citrus fruits, however, aid in iron absorption and are good sources of potassium and vitamin C.

Client Needs Category—Health promotion and maintenance
Client Needs Subcategory—None

56. 1. Iron is absorbed poorly from the GI tract. Absorption occurs best when the drug is taken on an empty stomach with water. Taking the drug between meals or at least 1 hour before meals is the best routine for maximum benefit. Taking the drug just before eating or with the meal causes the drug to be present in the stomach with food. When food and other drugs such as antacids are taken simultaneously with iron, iron absorption is decreased. If a client experiences GI upset while taking iron, she may reduce the discomfort by taking the ferrous sulfate (Feosol) with food or milk rather than discontinuing the medication. If the client takes the ferrous sulfate (Feosol) only before bedtime, she would not be following the prescribed daily regimen, which is three times per day.

Client Needs Category—Health promotion and maintenance
Client Needs Subcategory—None

57. 4. The presence of vitamin C, found in orange or other citrus juices, improves the absorption of iron. For this reason, some pharmaceutical companies combine iron and vitamin C in the same capsule or tablet. Iron taken with milk interferes with its absorption. Taking iron with tea or a soft drink is not likely to be any more beneficial than taking it with water.

Client Needs Category—Health promotion and maintenance
Client Needs Subcategory—None

58. 2. Most individuals who take iron observe that their stools become black or dark green. Stool is normally a medium brown color. Clay-colored stools are associated with liver or biliary disease. The stool becomes light green with diarrhea, or it assumes this color from eating certain foods.

Client Needs Category—Physiological integrity
Client Needs Subcategory—Physiological adaptation

59. 1. Liquid iron preparations stain the teeth; therefore, drinking the medication through a straw minimizes drug contact with the teeth. Pouring the medication over ice or drinking it from a paper cup does not protect the teeth from unsightly staining. Mixing the medication with milk affects its absorption and does not protect the teeth. However, diluting the liquid iron with at least 2 to 4 ounces of water reduces the potential for staining teeth.

Client Needs Category—Physiological integrity
Client Needs Subcategory—Pharmacological therapies

60. **1.** People who are anemic from blood loss often experience dizziness and fainting. This is probably due to low blood volume or an inability to maintain adequate oxygenation to the brain. Anemia is also likely to cause an individual to feel tired and require more sleep. Headaches are not usually associated with anemia that is related to blood loss, but they may occur in a client with pernicious anemia. Normal hemoglobin levels for a woman are 12 to 14 g/dL; therefore, the client's level is within normal limits and does not indicate anemia. Abdominal tenderness is unrelated to anemia but may occur with menstrual cramping.

Client Needs Category—Physiological integrity
Client Needs Subcategory—Physiological adaptation

61. **3.** The skin of an anemic client is typically pale. This is generally due to the fact that tissue oxygenation, which causes the skin and mucous membranes to appear pink, is impaired from reduced amounts of hemoglobin or red blood cells. Cyanosis, or a bluish color, is more likely caused by the buildup of carbon dioxide in the blood. A flushed appearance is due to such factors as vasodilation, hypertension, increased blood volume, or thermal injury. Mottled skin is a condition characterized by generalized purplish, spotted areas. It is commonly seen in neonates who are chilled or inactive or in clients who are about to die.

Client Needs Category—Physiological integrity
Client Needs Subcategory—Physiological adaptation

62. **3.** The ventrogluteal site, which includes the gluteus medius and gluteus minimus muscles, is the preferred site for administering an injection by Z-track technique. Z-track injections are given deeply into a large muscle because the medication is irritating. The deltoid muscle is used for I.M. injections; however, it is a smaller muscle in comparison to other I.M. injection sites and cannot accommodate large amounts of medication. Neither the trapezius muscle (located in the back and shoulder) nor the latissimus dorsi (the widest muscle in the back) is used for injections.

Client Needs Category—Safe, effective care environment
Client Needs Subcategory—Safety and infection control

63. **2.** Using a Z-track technique allows the nurse to deposit a medication that irritates or stains tissue (such as iron dextran) deeply into the muscle so that the tissue will self-seal, thereby keeping the medication from leaking into subcutaneous tissues. Absorption occurs at the same rate as any other I.M. injection. When giving a medication by Z-track technique, the nurse uses slow, even pressure to inject the drug. After instilling the drug, she waits approximately 10 seconds before removing the needle. The injection site is not massaged afterward.

Client Needs Category—Safe, effective care environment
Client Needs Subcategory—Safety and infection control

64. **1.** When administering an injection using the Z-track technique, the nurse pulls the tissue laterally (to the side) until it is taut, holds the tissue in position during the actual injection, releasing it only after the needle is withdrawn. Upward, downward, or diagonally are inappropriate directions to pull the tissue when using this technique.

Client Needs Category—Safe, effective care environment
Client Needs Subcategory—Safety and infection control

65. **1.** Pernicious anemia is the inability of the body to absorb vitamin B_{12}. This type of anemia occurs because of the lack of intrinsic factor secreted by the gastric mucosa. Therefore, clients who have had a total gastrectomy (removal of the stomach) eventually develop pernicious anemia unless prophylactically treated with injections of vitamin B_{12}. Intrinsic factors are not related to hepatitis, exposure to toxic wastes, or allergic reactions.

Client Needs Category—Physiological integrity
Client Needs Subcategory—Physiological adaptation

66. **2.** Personnel in the admissions or business office are responsible for obtaining information about the client's medical insurance or health coverage. This information should not be entered into the client's chart. The nurse's narrative notes are used for documenting subjective and objective assessment data, nursing care, treatment interventions, and the client's responses. The remaining options are all appropriate to document.

Client Needs Category—Safe, effective care environment
Client Needs Subcategory—Coordinated care

67. **1.** Pernicious anemia impairs peripheral and spinal cord nerve fibers, causing such symptoms as tingling and numbness in the extremities, loss of position sense, a staggering gait, and partial or total paralysis. Other symptoms include a smooth, sore, beefy red tongue, and weakness. Headaches may occur, but they are not a classic complaint among those with pernicious anemia. Restlessness and sleep disturbances are not usually associated with this disorder. Some clients experience confusion, depression, personality changes, and memory loss, but not to the point of amnesia.

Client Needs Category—Physiological integrity
Client Needs Subcategory—Physiological adaptation

68. **1.** A Schilling test, which evaluates the absorption of vitamin B_{12}, is ordered for any client with suspected pernicious anemia. The test involves collecting all of the client's urine for 24 to 48 hours after oral and injected doses of vitamin B_{12}. Subnormal levels of vitamin B_{12} in the urine suggest pernicious anemia. Blood, stool, and sputum are not used for this test.

> *Client Needs Category—Physiological integrity*
> *Client Needs Subcategory—Physiological adaptation*

69. **3.** Pernicious anemia is incurable, but the manifestations of the disease can be treated by lifelong injections of vitamin B_{12}. Blood transfusions are administered to someone who has hemolytic anemia or severely low red blood cell counts and hemoglobin levels. Iron preparations are given when a client has nutritional anemia, or when blood cell counts or hemoglobin levels are low but the condition is not life-threatening. Vitamin K is administered for clotting disorders in which the client's prothrombin level is low.

> *Client Needs Category—Physiological integrity*
> *Client Needs Subcategory—Physiological adaptation*

70. **4.** The gene for sickle-shaped hemoglobin is found in 1 out of every 10 African Americans. In Africa, the sickling effect developed as a genetic adaptation to protect against malaria; the genetic characteristic has continued from generation to generation. Because malaria in the United States is minimal, the genetic phenomenon is detrimental rather than protective. Sickle cell disease also occurs in smaller numbers among people of Mediterranean and Middle Eastern descent. It is not usually associated with Mexican Americans, Asian Americans, or Native Americans.

> *Client Needs Category—Health promotion and maintenance*
> *Client Needs Subcategory—None*

71. **3.** Jaundice is commonly present in individuals with sickle cell anemia. It occurs because sickled red blood cells (RBCs) are destroyed more rapidly than normal RBCs. When RBCs are rapidly destroyed, bilirubin accumulates and causes the jaundiced color. A white, coated tongue indicates a fungal infection or mouth breathing. Cloudy urine is a sign of a urinary tract infection. Nausea has multiple causes, but it is not usually a symptom of sickle cell anemia.

> *Client Needs Category—Physiological integrity*
> *Client Needs Subcategory—Physiological adaptation*

72. **2.** Severe pain is the major problem for clients experiencing a sickle cell crisis. The pain is caused by tissue ischemia secondary to blockage of blood vessels by sickled red blood cells. Pain is most severe in the abdominal area; however, the chest, back, and joints may also be affected. Although the pain is likely to trigger anxiety, if the pain is controlled, anxiety is relieved as

well. Adequate nutrition and ventilation are concerns for all clients. Usually, they are not a major concern in a sickle cell crisis unless complications, such as a cerebral or pulmonary infarction, develop.

> *Client Needs Category—Physiological integrity*
> *Client Needs Subcategory—Physiological adaptation*

73. **2.** Because the client's activity is limited during a sickle cell crisis, it is important to change the client's position frequently to reduce discomfort and prevent complications of immobility. No specific position is ideal; the goal is to relieve pressure and promote comfort. Ambulation and any form of exercise are contraindicated because they increase the client's need for tissue oxygenation at a time when the oxygen-carrying capacity of red blood cells is limited.

> *Client Needs Category—Physiological integrity*
> *Client Needs Subcategory—Physiological adaptation*

74. **1.** Adequate hydration is a major goal for clients in sickle cell crisis. Increasing and maintaining high volumes of fluid by oral or I.V. routes promote the circulation and improve blood flow caused by sickled cells that have occluded the blood vessel. Although elastic stockings would also promote venous return of blood, the client's arterial blood contains the oxygen needed by cells and tissue. Elevating the legs relieves swelling associated with thrombus formation; however, in sickle cell crisis, the client is likely to have many microemboli. Neither elevating the legs nor dangling them helps move red blood cells that accumulate and form thrombi.

> *Client Needs Category—Physiological integrity*
> *Client Needs Subcategory—Physiological adaptation*

75. **3.** A sickle cell crisis occurs when the client has a high demand for oxygen. Factors that can trigger a crisis include overexertion, dehydration, infection, alcohol ingestion, smoking, and exposure to cold weather or high altitudes. Although the client becomes fatigued during a crisis, this is not a precipitating cause. Low blood glucose levels are not known to trigger sickle cell crisis.

> *Client Needs Category—Physiological integrity*
> *Client Needs Subcategory—Physiological adaptation*

76. **3.** People with sickle cell trait inherit one defective gene and one normal gene for hemoglobin. Because the defective gene is a recessive trait, the disease (sickle cell anemia) is never manifested. Those who inherit a set of recessive genes (one defective gene from each parent) will have sickle cell anemia and manifest symptoms. A couple who both carry the recessive trait can produce a normal child (the child acquires a normal gene from both parents), a child who carries the trait (the child acquires one normal gene and one recessive gene), or a child with sickle cell anemia (the child acquires two recessive genes). Sickle cell anemia is usually diagnosed in childhood, not later in life. There is no evidence suggesting that clients who have sickle cell anemia have shorter life spans; however, some clients have died prematurely when they ignored the signs and symptoms of sickle cell crisis.

> *Client Needs Category—Health promotion and maintenance*
> *Client Needs Subcategory—None*

Nursing Care of Clients with White Blood Cell Disorders

77. 3. Cloudy urine is a common sign associated with a urinary tract infection. Other findings that suggest an infection include fever, cough, increased respirations and heart rate, and ulcerated oral mucous membranes. Blood in the stool is associated with altered clotting mechanisms. Prolonged vomiting is a side effect of chemotherapy. Extreme fatigue accompanies reduced numbers of red blood cells, causing anemia.

> *Client Needs Category—Physiological integrity*
> *Client Needs Subcategory—Physiological adaptation*

78. 1. Because the client's gums are bleeding, foam mouth swabs are less likely to traumatize the gums and oral mucous membranes. These swabs are substituted for the toothbrush temporarily. Because the mouth contains organisms that are a source of opportunistic infection, oral hygiene should not be discontinued. Antiseptic mouthwash may be used temporarily to eliminate bacteria, but this is not a permanent alternative to brushing. The risk for injury continues if the nurse eliminates toothpaste but continues to use the toothbrush. Using dental floss can cause further bleeding to the gums.

> *Client Needs Category—Physiological integrity*
> *Client Needs Subcategory—Physiological adaptation*

79. 4. Soft, bland foods, such as creamed soups, cottage cheese, baked fish, macaroni and cheese, custard, and pudding, are recommended for clients with mouth ulcers. These types of foods help maintain nutrition and relieve oral discomfort. Spicy foods (such as spaghetti and French dressing) and coarse and irritating foods (grilled cheese sandwiches) are avoided.

> *Client Needs Category—Physiological integrity*
> *Client Needs Subcategory—Basic care and comfort*

80. 1. The client who receives antineoplastic drugs is likely to experience hair loss. The hair loss is not permanent; hair growth returns when the drug therapy is discontinued. In the meantime, the nurse should allow the client to discuss how he feels about the potential hair loss. If the client is troubled by the loss of hair, the nurse can offers suggestions for disguising the hair loss.

Some possible alternatives include wearing a turban, baseball cap, scarf, or wig. Diarrhea, not constipation, is more closely associated with antineoplastic drugs. Rashes and headaches are not related to this classification of drugs.

> *Client Needs Category—Physiological integrity*
> *Client Needs Subcategory—Physiological adaptation*

81. 3. A low platelet count places the client at risk for bleeding. Using a small-gauge needle for injections reduces the amount of blood loss. Switching to oral medications when possible is even better. When the number of mature white blood cells (not platelets) is low, it is appropriate to place the client in protective isolation and limit contact with visitors who may be infectious. Rest periods are appropriate to counteract the effects of a low red blood cell count.

> *Client Needs Category—Physiological integrity*
> *Client Needs Subcategory—Physiological adaptation*

82. 3. The term *remission* means that the disease has responded to treatment and is not currently progressing; the original signs and symptoms of disease may even be absent. However, this does not mean the condition is cured. Although a remission is a good sign, the client's prognosis continues to be guarded because it is difficult to predict how long the remission will last. Treatment is reinstituted if the disease manifests again. For this reason, it is very important to stress that the client maintain regular checkups with his physician. In the meantime, he should be encouraged to live as fully and normally as possible.

> *Client Needs Category—Health promotion and maintenance*
> *Client Needs Subcategory—None*

83. 3. Hospice organizations offer assistance to dying individuals with fewer than 6 months to live. Pain management and disease management are key goals for the organization. In addition, hospices provide services that assist the family in caring for the terminally ill client's physical and emotional needs at home. They continue working with the family, even after the client's death, to help them resolve their grief. The public health department provides preventive services in the area of immunizations, care of well babies, diagnosing sexually transmitted and other communicable diseases, and inspecting sanitary conditions of buildings and food establishments. The U.S. Centers for Disease Control and Prevention studies the incidence of communicable diseases and recommends practices for controlling their spread. The local United Way is a philanthropic organization that collects and distributes funds to many social welfare organizations in the community.

> *Client Needs Category—Safe, effective care environment*
> *Client Needs Subcategory—Coordinated care*

84. 2. Mononucleosis, an acute viral disease caused by the herpes virus, is transmitted by direct contact with the droplets or saliva of another infected person. Most common among 15- to 25-years-olds, this disease is referred to as the "kissing disease" because the virus passes from one individual to another orally. The incubation period is roughly 30 to 45 days. Sharing eating utensils, cups, and cigarettes are also ways of transmitting this disease. Disease transmission does not occur by eating contaminated food, being bitten by insects, or coming in contact with blood.

Client Needs Category—Physiological integrity
Client Needs Subcategory—Physiological adaptation

85. 3. One of the first signs of infectious mononucleosis is a severe sore throat. Onset of symptoms usually takes 1 to 2 weeks, and the client has flulike symptoms, such as fever, headache, anorexia, fatigue, and generalized aching. In severe cases, the lymph nodes—including the spleen—become enlarged. The symptoms last for 14 to 28 days. If complications develop, jaundice occurs. Abdominal discomfort, aching joints, and intestinal upset are not characteristic of the disorder.

Client Needs Category—Physiological integrity
Client Needs Subcategory—Physiological adaptation

86. 2. Rest is essential for the recovery from infectious mononucleosis. Therefore, activity should be restricted during the course of the illness. Physical activity is likely to intensify symptoms, prolong recovery, or contribute to complications involving the liver, spleen, heart, and nervous system. Nurses should instruct clients with enlarged spleens or livers not to participate in contact sports, such as football or soccer, until the physician has released them from treatment.

Treatment is usually symptomatic, involving oral fluids, analgesics, and antipyretics. Because this is a viral infection, antibiotics are not warranted unless the client has a secondary bacterial infection. Taking vitamins may improve overall health if the client is anorexic, but this is generally unnecessary. Blood transfusions are not indicated for clients who have mononucleosis.

Client Needs Category—Physiological integrity
Client Needs Subcategory—Physiological adaptation

87. 2. Hodgkin's disease is a malignant lymphatic condition chiefly characterized by one or more painlessly enlarged lymph nodes. Other signs and symptoms include pruritus (itching), anorexia, weight loss, fever, night sweats, fatigue, and enlargement of the lymphatic organs (such as the spleen). Bone pain may occur later as the disease progresses. Headaches and diarrhea, if they occur, are not necessarily related to the primary disorder.

Client Needs Category—Physiological integrity
Client Needs Subcategory—Physiological adaptation

88. 1. During the early stages of Hodgkin's disease, the client's lymph nodes are typically enlarged and painless. Enlarged nodes are usually found first in the neck; if the client is untreated, the disease can spread throughout the lymphatic system. The physical change in cervical lymph nodes is generally one of the first abnormal signs of this disease. Later, the axillary and inguinal lymph nodes may also become involved. Regardless of the location in the body, cancerous growths are hardly ever painful in the early stages of the disease. This explains why early warning signs of cancer tend to be ignored. The other choices do not accurately describe the lymph nodes associated with Hodgkin's disease.

Client Needs Category—Physiological integrity
Client Needs Subcategory—Physiological adaptation

89. 2. Deodorants or other skin preparations that contain metals are avoided because they absorb X-rays and increase skin irritation. The skin can be washed with tepid water, mild soap, and a soft washcloth. The hair in the area is not shaved. In fact, shaving may further impair the integrity of the skin, which is somewhat damaged temporarily by the radiation. Zinc oxide contains a metal and, therefore, is not applied to the skin. If the skin does become dry, blistered, or peeling, the physician may prescribe a topical application of vitamin A and D ointment, lanolin, pure aloe vera gel, or cortisone ointment.

Client Needs Category—Safe, effective care environment
Client Needs Subcategory—Safety and infection control

90. 1. Skin reddening or bronzing is expected in the area that is irradiated. It is best to inform the client about anticipated skin changes before therapy begins and to stress that the red discoloration is only temporary. Although the ionizing radiation used in cancer therapy is a form of energy, it does not produce heat or cause bleeding under the skin. The client's concern is more likely related to his fear of adverse reactions to therapy than about the cosmetic change to his skin; therefore, reassuring him that the redness is hardly noticeable is inappropriate.

Client Needs Category—Health promotion and maintenance
Client Needs Subcategory—None

91. 4. The most important information to give the client with irradiated skin is to protect it from direct sunlight. Advising the client to wear several layers of warm clothing is appropriate if he has poor circulation. For comfort, any individual should avoid becoming chilled or too warm, so this choice is not as important as avoiding sunlight. Wearing a face mask is only warranted if the client has allergies to inhaled substances, has cardiovascular disease in which vasoconstriction causes ischemia, or needs a barrier to infectious microorganisms or environmental pollutants.

> *Client Needs Category—Health promotion and maintenance*
> *Client Needs Subcategory—None*

92. 3. Non-Hodgkin's lymphoma is a malignant disease that primarily affects the lymphatic tissue of older adults. Like Hodgkin's disease, this condition begins with one lymph node and spreads to the rest of the body. Antineoplastic drugs (chemotherapy) can depress bone marrow function and decrease the body's ability to fight infection. If the white blood cell count drops to dangerously low levels, the client becomes susceptible to infection. Then protective isolation is necessary to prevent exposure to microorganisms that can lead to infection. Periodic blood cell counts are monitored to assess for this potential complication. Anorexia, nausea, vomiting, weight loss, and diarrhea are also side effects of cancer treatment, but they are not indications that the client should be placed in protective isolation. Confusion and disorientation suggest that the client is experiencing neurologic problems and should be observed closely to protect his safety, but the symptoms do not justify implementing protective isolation.

> *Client Needs Category—Physiological integrity*
> *Client Needs Subcategory—Safety and infection control*

93. 3. Discussing feelings with another person facilitates grieving. The client should not be left alone immediately after hearing this information. It is important to remain with him until he has processed the information he was just given. The client would also benefit from talking with other supportive individuals, such as a spouse, family member, friend, or clergyman. Reading literature on the subject and thinking in private help some people, but most believe it is more effective to verbalize thoughts and feelings. If the client requests a second opinion, the request should not be denied; however, it would be inappropriate for the nurse to initiate the suggestion. Doing so is considered a form of false reassurance and could prolong the client's denial.

> *Client Needs Category—Psychosocial integrity*
> *Client Needs Subcategory—None*

94. 1, 2, 3, 4, 6. Clients who exhibit the characteristic signs and symptoms of HIV infection will most likely exhibit coughing, fever, fatigue, diarrhea, and swollen lymph nodes. Other signs and symptoms include night sweats, unexplained weight loss, anorexia, and mouth lesions. A ringed lesion on the face is typical of ringworm (a fungal infection) and is not related to HIV infection.

> *Client Needs Category—Physiological integrity*
> *Client Needs Subcategory—Physiological adaptation*

95. 2, 3, 4, 5. Practicing safer sex behaviors includes abstinence and reducing the number of sexual partners to one. The client should be encouraged to notify previous and present partners of his HIV status. Condoms should be used for each sexual encounter, but should be discarded after one use. Anal intercourse should be avoided due to the risk of bleeding from injury to the rectum and anal tissues. Engaging in nonpenetrative sexual activities, such as mutual masturbation or fantasies, demonstrates an understanding of safe sex behavior. Other safe sex behaviors include not sharing needles, razors, toothbrushes, or objects used for sexual activities. Oral intercourse should be avoided, and semen and urine should not be ingested.

> *Client Needs Category—Health promotion and maintenance*
> *Client Needs Subcategory—None*

96. 4. I.V. drug users who share needles, male homosexuals, bisexuals, women who have intercourse with these males, and infants of infected mothers are at greatest risk for developing AIDS. Haitians and Africans also have a high incidence of this disease among their native populations. Vacationing in Africa, drinking alcohol, or having had surgery does not place the client at any greater risk for AIDS than other individuals.

> *Client Needs Category—Physiological integrity*
> *Client Needs Subcategory—Physiological adaptation*

97. 3. ELISA detects the presence of antibodies to viral antigens. A reactive ELISA is generally repeated. If it continues to be reactive, more specific tests for the HIV antibodies, such as the Western blot test or Murex SUDS-HIV-1 test, are performed before making a definitive diagnosis of AIDS. The VDRL test is used as a screening test for syphilis. The Schick test is used to determine if a person has antibodies to the bacterial toxins of the organism causing diphtheria. The Dick test is used to assess the immunologic status of a person to the toxins associated with scarlet fever.

> *Client Needs Category—Physiological integrity*
> *Client Needs Subcategory—Physiological adaptation*

98. 2. Standard precautions are used when a person's infectious status is unknown. Standard precautions involve donning one or more protective garments—depending on the potential for coming into contact with blood or body fluids—and taking precautionary actions to avoid penetrating injuries with objects contaminated with blood or body fluid. In *all* situations, it is important to avoid recapping needles because this will prevent an accidental needle-stick injury.

A face mask provides protection from being splashed with blood or body fluid; however, most dressings absorb liquid drainage, and wearing gloves is more appropriate. Wearing a cover gown is appropriate if there is the potential that blood and body fluid may penetrate clothing; however, this measure is unnecessary when giving most clients a bed bath. Gloves are appropriate when touching areas of the body where there may be contact with blood or body fluids. Wearing gloves while taking vital signs is generally unnecessary.

> *Client Needs Category—Safe, effective care environment*
> *Client Needs Subcategory—Safety and infection control*

99. 1. Setting and reaching realistic daily goals is the most therapeutic approach and can help the client experience a sense of hope. Hope has a powerful influence on a dying person's will to live and can lift a depressed person's spirits. Referring the client to the chaplain is appropriate if he requests contact with a clergyman. Distraction will not help a client deal with his feelings nor will it promote a sense of hope. Contacting the next of kin may be therapeutic, depending on the client's relationship with his family.

> *Client Needs Category—Psychosocial integrity*
> *Client Needs Subcategory—None*

Nursing Care of Clients with Bone Marrow Disorders

100. 1. Polycythemia vera is a life-threatening disorder that results in the concentration of hemoglobin and an increase in the number of red blood cells. Symptoms include weakness, clotting, dizziness, painful extremities, and flushing of the face and extremities. The nurse should observe for thrombus formation. If the client exhibits organ enlargement, sitting upright allows abdominal organs, such as the spleen, liver, and intestines, to fall away from the diaphragm. By reducing crowding of the diaphragm, dyspnea is reduced and the client feels more comfortable. Any other position will cause difficulty breathing.

> *Client Needs Category—Physiological integrity*
> *Client Needs Subcategory—Physiological adaptation*

101. 2. Keeping a client with polycythemia vera well hydrated reduces the blood's viscosity, or thickness. Thrombi are less likely to form if the excessive numbers of blood cells are kept diluted within the plasma. In that way, they move more easily throughout the circulatory system, reducing the possibility of clumping together within a small blood vessel. Diuretics affect fluid balance and can cause dehydration, which may result in clot formation. Restricting dietary sodium and encouraging weight loss are healthful interventions, but they do not have a therapeutic effect on preventing the formation of blood clots.

> *Client Needs Category—Physiological integrity*
> *Client Needs Subcategory—Physiological adaptation*

102. 1. Treatment for polycythemia vera includes measures to remove blood. As much as 500 to 2,000 mL of blood is removed by performing a phlebotomy. This is similar to the technique for donating a unit of blood. Afterward, I.V. fluid is infused to dilute the remaining circulating cells. More aggressive therapy with radiophosphorus and radiation is used in an effort to decrease the bone marrow's cell production. A tourniquet may be used, but this choice does not provide the best evidence that the client understands his treatment. Receiving a blood transfusion will add more blood volume, which is already the cause of the problem. Surgically occluding blood vessels may result in further clot formation.

> *Client Needs Category—Physiological integrity*
> *Client Needs Subcategory—Physiological adaptation*

103. 1. Angina, pain or pressure in the chest, may occur as a result of inadequate blood flow and oxygenation to the heart caused by a thrombus in a coronary artery. Clots are more likely to form due to the thick nature of the circulating blood volume and the increased number of platelets as well as red and white blood cells. Indigestion, burning on urination, and loss of appetite should not be ignored by the nurse, but they are not commonly associated with polycythemia vera.

> *Client Needs Category—Physiological integrity*
> *Client Needs Subcategory—Physiological adaptation*

104. 1. Bone marrow is aspirated from the iliac crest, the curved rim along the upper border of the ileum, felt in the hip area near the level of the waist. The sternum (breastbone), located in the center of the chest, is an alternate site for aspirating a sample of bone marrow. The iliac crest is generally the first choice because it contains more bone marrow than the sternum. The lower spine, upper arm, and groin area are not suitable sites for bone marrow aspiration.

> *Client Needs Category—Physiological integrity*
> *Client Needs Subcategory—Physiological adaptation*

105. 1. The nurse's primary role in assisting with bone marrow aspiration is to help minimize the pain and discomfort the client is likely to experience. Despite the use of local anesthesia, the client typically feels pressure as the needle is driven into the bone, followed by brief but sharp pain as the needle finally enters the bone and marrow is withdrawn. Helpful measures include premedicating the client, providing distraction throughout the procedure, and offering encouragement and support. The physician generally needs no assistance with instruments during the procedure. A suction machine is not used, and oxygen is not usually needed under most conditions.

> *Client Needs Category—Physiological integrity*
> *Client Needs Subcategory—Physiological adaptation*

106. **2.** Bleeding from the puncture site is one of the most common problems after bone marrow aspiration. If bleeding is not controlled, a painful hematoma forms. Firm pressure or an ice pack is used to limit bleeding. Under usual circumstances, bone marrow aspiration does not cause shock. Though the blood pressure and pulse may fluctuate somewhat, any variation is usually due to pain, anxiety, and fear rather than loss of blood volume. The client remains awake and alert throughout and following the procedure.

> *Client Needs Category—Physiological integrity*
> *Client Needs Subcategory—Physiological adaptation*

107. **1.** Aplastic anemia, commonly called bone marrow depression anemia, occurs when the bone marrow fails to produce red blood cells (RBCs). Platelets and white blood cells are also affected. The reduction in the number of circulating RBCs affects the blood's oxygen-carrying capacity. Consequently, clients with this problem have difficulty tolerating activities and may become short of breath with rapid or labored breathing. It is important for the nurse to provide the dyspneic client with frequent rest periods because rest decreases oxygen demands. Nausea is not generally associated with hypoxemia. The pulse rate typically increases with activity and poor oxygenation. Cool, moist skin accompanies a drop in blood pressure or other physical problems. It is not usually a classic sign of fatigue or activity intolerance.

> *Client Needs Category—Physiological integrity*
> *Client Needs Subcategory—Physiological adaptation*

108. **1.** A low number of platelets, also known as *thrombocytes*, increases the risk for bleeding. Bruises indicate bleeding into the skin. Pale skin color is associated with anemia, which is caused by a low red blood cell count. Elevated temperature may be a sign of infection or dehydration. Cool extremities are not associated with thrombocytopenia.

> *Client Needs Category—Physiological integrity*
> *Client Needs Subcategory—Physiological adaptation*

109. **1.** A client with leukopenia, a low number of white blood cells, is at high risk for infection. Hand washing is the best technique for reducing the spread of microorganisms and decreasing infection. Applying direct pressure to puncture wounds is necessary when the client has a low platelet count. Wearing a gown when providing care may help reduce the spread of infection, but it is not as effective as good hand washing. Monitoring baseline vitals signs is important because the red blood cells, white blood cells, and platelets are all affected, but this choice does not address the client's risk for infection.

> *Client Needs Category—Safe, effective care environment*
> *Client Needs Subcategory—Safety and infection control*

110. **3.** After it is collected, all donated blood is tested for HIV antibodies. Donated blood is the safest it has been since early 1985. However, it is still not 100% safe because some blood donors who have the virus in their blood have not produced sufficient antibodies to cause a positive reaction when the blood is tested. All potential blood donors are asked questions about lifestyle behaviors that indicate a risk for HIV infection, but some do not answer the questions honestly. Blood donors are encouraged to call the blood collection agency later and report an identifying number, not their name, if they feel someone is at risk by receiving a unit of their donated blood.

> *Client Needs Category—Health promotion and maintenance*
> *Client Needs Subcategory—None*

111. **1.** A unit of packed blood cells contains a similar number of blood cells found in a regular unit used in transfusions. However, when preparing the unit of packed blood cells, approximately two-thirds of the plasma from a unit of whole blood is removed. The administration of packed cells is preferred for clients who need a blood transfusion but for whom additional fluid in the circulatory system is hazardous. Typically, the candidate for packed cells is someone who is prone to congestive heart failure or who has poor kidney function and does not need the extra fluid. Packed cells pose the same risk for an allergic reaction as whole blood. They do not stimulate the bone marrow to produce blood cells.

> *Client Needs Category—Physiological integrity*
> *Client Needs Subcategory—None*

112. **4.** A person with type A, Rh-positive blood would have a reaction if transfused with type AB, Rh-positive blood. It is always best to administer the same blood type. However, O type blood is referred to as the universal donor. In an emergency, anyone can receive type O blood. People who are Rh-positive can receive compatible blood types that are either Rh-positive or Rh-negative. The reverse is *not* true; in other words, a person who is Rh-negative should never be given Rh-positive blood.

> *Client Needs Category—Physiological integrity*
> *Client Needs Subcategory—Physiological adaptation*

113. **2.** Hypotension is one of the first signs of a serious blood transfusion reaction. In a serious transfusion reaction, urine formation is decreased. Swelling and pale skin at the infusion site are indications that there is a problem with the administration of the blood rather than a reaction to the blood product.

> *Client Needs Category—Physiological integrity*
> *Client Needs Subcategory—Physiological adaptation*

114. **2.** Long-term administration of corticosteroids causes such body changes as moon face and buffalo hump on the back of the neck. These resemble signs of Cushing's syndrome caused by a hyperfunctioning adrenal cortex. The voice is unaffected. Muscle wasting may occur with long-term corticosteroid use. Anabolic steroids cause muscle enlargement. Steroid administration causes the skin to appear thin and transparent, not tanned. Purple striae are found on the abdomen and hips. Due to an inadequately functioning adrenal cortex, bronzed skin is found in individuals who have Addison's disease.
> *Client Needs Category—Physiological integrity*
> *Client Needs Subcategory—Physiological adaptation*

115. **1.** Steroids are known to cause peptic ulcers. For this reason, the physician may also prescribe drugs to protect the gastric mucosa from erosion. Clients who take corticosteroids usually do not experience drowsiness, anorexia, or light-colored urine.
> *Client Needs Category—Physiological integrity*
> *Client Needs Subcategory—Physiological adaptation*

116. **3.** Total body irradiation destroys the client's bone marrow and places the individual at high risk for infection. Medical asepsis is scrupulously followed, prophylactic antibiotics and antifungal medications are administered, and visitors are restricted to prevent the client from acquiring an infection from which she may not recover. The nurse never neglects to promote optimum nutrition and hydration and to help the client cope with fear and depression. However, if these problems occur, they are more easily treated than an infection.
> *Client Needs Category—Safe, effective care environment*
> *Client Needs Subcategory—Safety and infection control*

Nursing Care of Clients with Coagulation Disorders

117. **1.** Small hemorrhages in the skin, mucous membranes, or subcutaneous tissues are referred to as *purpura*. Bleeding also occurs internally when a person has thrombocytopenia. There is no other additional term for dark areas of cyanosis. The term for flushed, red skin is *erythema*. Protruding (distended) veins are referred to as *varicosities*.
> *Client Needs Category—Physiological integrity*
> *Client Needs Subcategory—Physiological adaptation*

118. **4.** Preventing injury is a priority concern when caring for people with thrombocytopenia because they are prone to bleeding. The care plan specifies careful handling of the client, padding the side rails with soft material, using a soft toothbrush for mouth care, and using prolonged pressure when discontinuing I.V. infusions or injections. Activity is restricted to reduce the potential for injury. Generally, clients with thrombocytopenia are not at high risk for infection; therefore, visitors are not restricted. A normal intake of oral fluid is appropriate unless a client experiences a large loss of blood volume.
> *Client Needs Category—Safe, effective care environment*
> *Client Needs Subcategory—Safety and infection control*

119. **2.** Drowsiness, or a change in the level of consciousness, is one of the earliest signs of increased pressure from intracranial bleeding. Other signs include headache, visual problems, vomiting, motor weakness or paralysis, and personality changes. Seizures occur later as the bleeding progresses. Tinnitus, or ringing in the ears, is not commonly associated with active intracranial bleeding. The client should not lose his appetite, but he may vomit with or without nausea.
> *Client Needs Category—Physiological integrity*
> *Client Needs Subcategory—Physiological adaptation*

Nursing Care of Clients with Inflammatory and Obstructive Lymphatic Disorders

120. **2.** When the axillary lymph nodes are removed during a radical mastectomy, lymph circulation is impaired. The lymph collects and pools within the arm on the side of the mastectomy. The condition is generally permanent once it develops. Elevating the affected arm and hand, applying an inflatable pressure sleeve or elasticized bandage, squeezing a rubber ball, and performing active range-of-motion exercises are immediate postoperative interventions designed to prevent, reduce, or eliminate the development of lymphedema. Fractures, pernicious anemia, and smallpox are not associated with lymphedema.
> *Client Needs Category—Physiological integrity*
> *Client Needs Subcategory—Physiological adaptation*

121. **1.** Because circulation in the arm with lymphedema is impaired, certain nursing interventions (administering injections, taking a blood pressure, obtaining blood, or starting an I.V. infusion) are avoided. Prolonged pressure on the affected side during positioning is also avoided, but there is no contraindication to lying on the affected side for brief periods. Appropriate nursing interventions include performing active range-of-motion exercises and maintaining good nail hygiene such as trimming the nails.

Client Needs Category—*Physiological integrity*
Client Needs Subcategory—*Physiological adaptation*

The Nursing Care of Clients with Respiratory Disorders

⇨ *Nursing Care of Clients with Upper Respiratory Tract Infections*
⇨ *Nursing Care of Clients with Inflammatory and Allergic Disorders of the Upper Airways*
⇨ *Nursing Care of Clients with Cancer of the Larynx*
⇨ *Nursing Care of Clients with Inflammatory and Infectious Disorders of the Lower Airways*
⇨ *Nursing Care of Clients with Asthma*
⇨ *Nursing Care of Clients with Chronic Obstructive Pulmonary Disease*
⇨ *Nursing Care of Clients with Lung Cancer*
⇨ *Nursing Care of Clients with Chest Injuries*
⇨ *Nursing Care of Clients with Pulmonary Embolism*
⇨ *Nursing Care of Clients with a Tracheostomy*
⇨ *Nursing Care of Clients with a Sudden Airway Occlusion*
⇨ *Correct Answers and Rationales*

Directions: *With a pencil, blacken the space in front of the option you have chosen for your correct answer.*

Nursing Care of Clients with Upper Respiratory Tract Infections

During a visit to the physician's office, a client complains to the nurse that the physician would not prescribe an antibiotic for a head cold.

1. Which explanation by the nurse regarding the use of antibiotics is best?
[ ] **1.** Antibiotics are ineffective in treating viral infections.
[ ] **2.** Antibiotics are ineffective after cold symptoms develop.
[ ] **3.** Antibiotics only prevent the spread of colds to others.
[ ] **4.** Antibiotics are used only for immunosuppressed individuals.

2. Which symptom reported by the client is the best indicator that complications are developing from his cold?
[ ] **1.** Nasal stuffiness
[ ] **2.** Dry cough
[ ] **3.** High fever
[ ] **4.** Scratchy throat

3. Before recommending the use of a nonprescription decongestant to a client with a cold, the nurse should first determine whether he has which disorder?
[ ] **1.** Arthritis
[ ] **2.** Asthma
[ ] **3.** Hypertension
[ ] **4.** Diabetes

4. When teaching the client about topical nasal decongestants, the nurse should warn him that overuse of such medication is likely to result in which adverse effect?
[ ] **1.** Nasal irritation with rhinorrhea
[ ] **2.** Rebound congestion with nasal stuffiness
[ ] **3.** Ulceration of the nasal mucous membranes
[ ] **4.** Decreased ability to fight microorganisms

5. To prevent the client from developing a secondary ear infection while he has a head cold, which recommendation is most appropriate?
[ ] **1.** Sleeping with the head elevated
[ ] **2.** Blowing the nose very gently
[ ] **3.** Inserting cotton into the ears
[ ] **4.** Massaging the area behind the ears

A woman with a prolonged upper respiratory infection seeks medical attention because she continues to have a low-grade fever, poor appetite, and malaise.

6. If the client has sinusitis in the maxillary sinuses, where is she most likely to report feeling pain?
[ ] **1.** Over her eyes
[ ] **2.** Near her eyebrows
[ ] **3.** In her cheeks
[ ] **4.** Above her ears

7. When teaching a client to self-administer nose drops, which method is most effective?
[ ] **1.** Bending the head forward, then instilling the drops
[ ] **2.** Pushing the nose laterally, then instilling the drops
[ ] **3.** Tilting the head backward, then instilling the drops
[ ] **4.** Turning the head to the side, then instilling the drops

An older woman brings her husband to the physician's office because he has symptoms of a respiratory tract infection. The woman tells the nurse that she has a cool-mist vaporizer at home and plans to use it to help relieve her husband's nasal congestion.

8. Why does the nurse correctly instruct the wife to empty and thoroughly clean the vaporizer after use?
[ ] **1.** Because there is a potential for injury if the vaporizer is accidentally knocked off a nightstand
[ ] **2.** Because water left in the vaporizer can cause a rapid growth of environmental pathogens
[ ] **3.** Because the vaporizer can collect dust, which could affect her husband's breathing
[ ] **4.** Because evaporation of standing water causes accumulation of calcium deposits that will clog the vaporizer the next time it is used

Nursing Care of Clients with Inflammatory and Allergic Disorders of the Upper Airways

The physician orders a throat culture for a client with pharyngitis.

9. Which specimen collection technique is correct for the nurse to use?
[ ] **1.** The nurse asks the client to expectorate sputum into a paper cup.
[ ] **2.** The nurse wipes the inner mouth and tongue with gauze.
[ ] **3.** The nurse swabs the throat with a sterile cotton applicator.
[ ] **4.** The nurse collects saliva in a sterile culture tube.

Laboratory results indicate that the client has an infection caused by group A streptococci. The physician prescribes oral potassium penicillin V (V-Cillin K).

10. The nurse advises the client to make sure he takes his entire antibiotic prescription because an untreated or undertreated strep infection may result in which of the following conditions?
[ ] **1.** Glomerulonephritis
[ ] **2.** Chickenpox
[ ] **3.** Shingles
[ ] **4.** Whooping cough

A male singer calls the physician's office to schedule an appointment regarding his laryngitis.

11. Until the client can be examined later that morning, which advice by the nurse would be most helpful?
[ ] **1.** "Sucking on ice chips should help."
[ ] **2.** "Rest your voice."
[ ] **3.** "Drink plenty of hot liquids."
[ ] **4.** "Massage your throat."

After 2 weeks of symptomatic treatment, the client still complains of hoarseness. The physician schedules him for a direct laryngoscopy.

12. Which statement by the client best indicates that he understands the reason a direct laryngoscopy has been ordered?
[ ] **1.** "The test will tell if my hoarseness is caused by tracheal polyps."
[ ] **2.** "The physician says that hoarseness can lead to bronchitis."
[ ] **3.** "I need to have the test because hoarseness can be caused by laryngeal cancer."
[ ] **4.** "The physician wants to see if my hoarseness is due to enlarged tonsils."

A 23-year-old woman notes that every fall her nasal passages become swollen, she sneezes endlessly, and her eyes become red, itchy, and watery. She makes an appointment with an allergist.

13. When the physician prescribes a first-generation antihistamine for the client's symptomatic relief, the nurse appropriately advises the client that antihistamines are associated with which side effect?
[ ] **1.** Weight loss
[ ] **2.** Constipation
[ ] **3.** Drowsiness
[ ] **4.** Depression

The physician recommends that the client undergo allergy skin testing.

14. When the client asks the nurse why skin testing is beneficial, which explanation is best?
[ ] **1.** The symptoms may be related to more than one substance.
[ ] **2.** Skin testing helps to build up blocking antibodies.
[ ] **3.** Allergic responses vary from person to person.
[ ] **4.** The allergy symptoms could progress to more serious conditions.

15. When the client undergoes scratch skin testing, which sign best indicates that she has a hypersensitivity to the scratched substance?
[ ] **1.** The skin at the test site feels numb.
[ ] **2.** The skin at the test site feels painful.
[ ] **3.** The skin at the test site looks pale.
[ ] **4.** The skin at the test site looks red.

Based on the outcome of the skin tests, the client begins desensitization treatment. She returns for weekly injections of diluted antigens of the substances to which she is allergic.

16. After the client receives her weekly injection, which nursing instruction is essential?
[ ] **1.** Take a couple of aspirin before leaving.
[ ] **2.** Wait at least 20 minutes before going home.
[ ] **3.** Make sure someone else drives the car.
[ ] **4.** Avoid getting the injection site wet.

17. When caring for a client with allergies, which assessment finding is an early indication that the client is developing anaphylaxis?
[ ] **1.** Breathing difficulty
[ ] **2.** Headache
[ ] **3.** Sore throat
[ ] **4.** Cool, pale skin

18. Whenever there is a possibility that a client may develop a severe allergic reaction, which drug should the nurse plan to have available?
[ ] **1.** Codeine sulfate
[ ] **2.** Morphine sulfate (Roxanol)
[ ] **3.** Dopamine (Intropin)
[ ] **4.** Epinephrine (Adrenalin)

19. Which assessment is most important when managing the care of a client experiencing a severe allergic reaction?
[ ] **1.** Urine output
[ ] **2.** Skin color
[ ] **3.** Blood pressure
[ ] **4.** Pupil response

20. If a client experiencing a severe allergic reaction becomes unresponsive, which nursing action becomes the priority?
[ ] **1.** Administering a single blow to the sternum
[ ] **2.** Raising the client's head to 90 degrees
[ ] **3.** Lifting the chin and tilt the head back
[ ] **4.** Administering an epinephrine (Adrenalin) injection

Nursing Care of Clients with Cancer of the Larynx

The nursing team develops a care plan for a male client with cancer of the larynx who is undergoing a total laryngectomy. Following surgery, the client is taken to the recovery room until he stabilizes.

21. Which assessment finding noted upon the client's return to his room is an early indication that his oxygenation status is compromised?
[ ] **1.** The client's dressing is bloody.
[ ] **2.** The client becomes restless.
[ ] **3.** The client's heart rate is irregular.
[ ] **4.** The client indicates he is cold.

22. Because of this client's impaired speech, which nursing action facilitates optimum communication?
[ ] **1.** Lip-read the client's attempts at communication.
[ ] **2.** Inform the client to speak slowly when talking.
[ ] **3.** Listen attentively to the client's vocalizations.
[ ] **4.** Provide the client with paper and pencil.

The nursing team discusses the client's anger and depression related to his cancer diagnosis, the change in his body image, and the loss of speech following a laryngectomy.

23. Which of the following best indicates that the client's grief is beginning to resolve?
[ ] **1.** The client wants only his wife to visit him.
[ ] **2.** The client says his physician made an incorrect diagnosis.
[ ] **3.** The client looks at the tracheostomy tube in a mirror.
[ ] **4.** The client asks the nurse to help him bathe and shave.

Nursing Care of Clients with Inflammatory and Infectious Disorders of the Lower Airways

A client with a persistent upper respiratory infection develops acute bronchitis and is given a prescription for guaifenesin (Robitussin AC), an antitussive that contains codeine.

24. Besides the characteristics of the client's cough, which other pertinent assessment finding should the nurse document?

[ ] **1.** Family history of respiratory disease
[ ] **2.** Current vital signs
[ ] **3.** Presence of respiratory secretions
[ ] **4.** Any self-treatment measures used by the client

25. When the client asks why the physician prescribed this type of cough medicine, the nurse correctly responds that the guaifenesin liquefies mucus while the codeine is responsible for which action?

[ ] **1.** Relieving discomfort
[ ] **2.** Dilating the bronchi
[ ] **3.** Suppressing coughing
[ ] **4.** Reducing inflammation

26. Which instruction regarding the prescribed medication is most appropriate to tell this client?

[ ] **1.** "Do not take the drug more frequently than prescribed."
[ ] **2.** "Avoid taking the medication before going to sleep."
[ ] **3.** "Drink more fluid during the day."
[ ] **4.** "Warm the cough syrup to make it more palatable."

The nurse is caring for a client who must take a liquid cough syrup and several other solid oral tablets at the same time.

27. Which technique is most appropriate when administering both types of medication to this client?

[ ] **1.** Administer the cough syrup, then the solid tablets.
[ ] **2.** Wait 15 minutes after giving the cough syrup before giving the solid tablets.
[ ] **3.** Give the cough syrup between administering the oral tablets.
[ ] **4.** Administer the solid tablets, then the cough syrup.

The prescribed dose of the client's liquid cough syrup is 5 mL.

28. Which household measurement should the nurse use when teaching the client how to self-administer the prescribed amount of liquid cough syrup?

[ ] **1.** One ounce
[ ] **2.** One tablespoon
[ ] **3.** One teaspoon
[ ] **4.** One capful

The client also receives a prescription for aerosol therapy to treat his bronchitis.

29. Which statement by the client best indicates that he understands the purpose of his aerosol therapy?

[ ] **1.** "Aerosal therapy will relieve my tissue irritation."
[ ] **2.** "This therapy will kill infectious organisms."
[ ] **3.** "It's supposed to dry my respiratory passages."
[ ] **4.** "Aerosal therapy will help to slow my respiratory rate."

The physician has written the following order for a client: carbenicillin 500 mg I.M. every 6 hours. The medication requires reconstitution. The label information indicates that the vial contains 2 g of carbenicillin when reconstituted with 5 mL of sterile water to yield 1 g per 3 mL.

30. How many milliliters of the reconstituted solution should the nurse administer to the client?

_____

The nurse is preparing to administer penicillin G to a client. The prescription reads: penicillin G potassium 300,000 units I.M. four times a day. The directions on the label state, "This vial contains 1,000,000 units of penicillin G potassium. Add 9.6 mL sterile water for injection to reconstitute the powder for a concentration of 100,000 units/mL."

31. How many milliliters of the reconstituted medication should the nurse administer to the client?

_____

When an adult male client with a diagnosis of pneumonia is admitted to the unit, the nurse observes that he has shaking chills and a fever of 104.2° F (40.1° C). A chest X-ray and sputum specimens for culture and sensitivity are ordered.

32. Which nursing action is essential before the chest X-ray is taken?

[ ] **1.** Make sure the client does not eat any food.
[ ] **2.** Remove the metal necklace he is wearing.
[ ] **3.** Have the client swallow a contrast medium dye.
[ ] **4.** Administer a parenteral analgesic.

The client has difficulty coughing up his respiratory secretions.

33. Which nursing action is most appropriate when planning to obtain the ordered sputum specimen?
[ ] **1.** Provide the client with a generous fluid intake.
[ ] **2.** Encourage the client to change positions regularly.
[ ] **3.** Ask the dietitian to send the client a clear liquid diet.
[ ] **4.** Administer an antitussive prior to collecting the specimen.

34. Which time of the day is best for the nurse to obtain a sputum specimen from the client?
[ ] **1.** Before bedtime
[ ] **2.** After a meal
[ ] **3.** Between meals
[ ] **4.** Upon awakening

35. Which statement best suggests that the client understands the nurse's instruction on how to handle the sputum specimen container?
[ ] **1.** "I should don gloves before opening the container."
[ ] **2.** "I should wipe the container with an alcohol swab."
[ ] **3.** "I can't touch the outside of the container."
[ ] **4.** "I must not touch the inside of the container."

36. After collecting the sputum specimen, which nursing action is most appropriate?
[ ] **1.** Administer oxygen.
[ ] **2.** Provide mouth care.
[ ] **3.** Offer nourishment.
[ ] **4.** Encourage ambulation.

37. Which assessment finding indicates that the client most likely has also developed pleurisy?
[ ] **1.** Productive cough
[ ] **2.** Pain when breathing
[ ] **3.** Cyanotic nail beds
[ ] **4.** Rapid heart rate

A client with pneumococcal pneumonia receives penicillin (Bicillin) by I.M. injection.

38. When the client asks why the physician chose this particular drug to treat his pneumonia, which response by the nurse is best?
[ ] **1.** "The sensitivity report showed the organism was easily killed by penicillin."
[ ] **2.** "Most viral infections respond well when treated with penicillin drugs."
[ ] **3.** "Penicillin is one of the safest yet most effective antibiotics."
[ ] **4.** "All antibiotics are similar; the choice of drug is not that important."

The nurse chooses to inject the prescribed dose of penicillin (Bicillin) into the dorsogluteal site.

39. If the nurse selects the site correctly, where is the injection administered?
[ ] **1.** The client's hip
[ ] **2.** The client's arm
[ ] **3.** The client's thigh
[ ] **4.** The client's buttock

40. Which instruction should the nurse give to help reduce the client's discomfort when receiving an I.M. injection in the dorsogluteal area?
[ ] **1.** "Point your toes inward."
[ ] **2.** "Tighten your muscles."
[ ] **3.** "Cross your legs."
[ ] **4.** "Flex your knees."

41. If a client is allergic to penicillin, the nurse should anticipate a hypersensitivity response to which other group of antibiotics?
[ ] **1.** Aminoglycosides such as kanamycin sulfate (Kantrex)
[ ] **2.** Tetracyclines such as doxycyline (Vibramycin)
[ ] **3.** Cephalosporins such as ceftriaxone sodium (Rocephin)
[ ] **4.** Fluoroquinolones such as ciprofloxacin (Cipro)

A nurse volunteers to administer influenza vaccines to older adults during a community-wide immunization campaign.

42. Which question is essential for the nurse to ask before administering the influenza vaccine?
[ ] **1.** "Have you had influenza in the past year?"
[ ] **2.** "Did you receive pneumonia vaccine last year?"
[ ] **3.** "Are you allergic to eggs or egg products?"
[ ] **4.** "Do you have a history of respiratory disease?"

43. Other than obtaining a vaccination against influenza, which nursing advice is most helpful to high-risk clients who want to avoid getting influenza?
[ ] **1.** Consume adequate vitamin C.
[ ] **2.** Avoid crowded places.
[ ] **3.** Dress warmly in cold weather.
[ ] **4.** Reduce daily stress and anxiety.

44. When caring for a client with influenza, the nurse would expect to assess for which signs and symptoms of hypoxia? Select all that apply.
[ ] **1.** Cough
[ ] **2.** Restlessness
[ ] **3.** Fever
[ ] **4.** Tachypnea
[ ] **5.** Use of accessory muscles to breathe
[ ] **6.** Cyanosis

A nurse working in an assisted living facility notes that an elderly female client with influenza has a fever of 104.6° F (40.3° C) and a dry cough. The client complains of sore muscles and a headache. The nurse instructs the nursing assistant to encourage the client to consume extra fluids.

45. If the client has normal cardiovascular and renal function, what is an appropriate goal for oral intake in the next 24-hour period?
[ ] **1.** 500 mL
[ ] **2.** 1,000 mL
[ ] **3.** 1,500 mL
[ ] **4.** 3,000 mL

The physician orders the nurse to give two aspirin tablets orally every 4 hours, as needed, if the client has a temperature over 102° F (38.9° C) and to give a tepid sponge bath at the same time.

46. What does the nurse know sponge-bathing the client in this situation will help do?
[ ] **1.** Maintain the client's skin integrity
[ ] **2.** Remove microorganisms
[ ] **3.** Promote heat loss
[ ] **4.** Provide comfort

The nursing assistant helping with the sponge bath asks the nurse to explain what the word tepid *means.*

47. The nurse correctly informs the nursing assistant that *tepid* means lukewarm and instructs her to make sure the water temperature is within what temperature range?
[ ] **1.** 70° to 75° F (21° to 23.9° C)
[ ] **2.** 80° to 93° F (26.7° to 33.9° C)
[ ] **3.** 105° to 110° F (40.6° to 43.3° C)
[ ] **4.** 120° to 130° F (48.9° to 54.4° C)

48. The nurse knows to discontinue the client's sponge bath if the client develops which problem?
[ ] **1.** Nausea
[ ] **2.** Chills
[ ] **3.** Flushing
[ ] **4.** Confusion

49. Which finding best indicates that the sponge bath is having a therapeutic effect on the client?
[ ] **1.** The client states she feels more comfortable.
[ ] **2.** The client begins sweating profusely.
[ ] **3.** The client's temperature is 101° F (38.3° C).
[ ] **4.** The client states that she thinks her fever has broken.

The nurse in a nursing home is required by the state's law to test all newly admitted clients for tuberculosis. The agency's policy is to administer a Mantoux intradermal skin test.

50. The nurse's injection technique is correct if the needle is inserted at which angle?
[ ] **1.** 10-degree angle
[ ] **2.** 30-degree angle
[ ] **3.** 45-degree angle
[ ] **4.** 90-degree angle

51. How long after giving a tuberculin skin test should the nurse inspect the client's injection site?
[ ] **1.** 1 week
[ ] **2.** 1 day
[ ] **3.** 48 hours
[ ] **4.** 5 days

52. What is the significance of a positive tuberculin skin test?
[ ] **1.** The client has an active infection.
[ ] **2.** Antibodies are present in the client's blood.
[ ] **3.** The client is immune to this type of disease.
[ ] **4.** The client needs to be in strict isolation.

53. When a previously negative client has a positive reaction to a tuberculin skin test, which information is most correct?
[ ] **1.** Skin tests will be performed every 6 months.
[ ] **2.** The client will need to quit his job.
[ ] **3.** The client will need to live alone temporarily.
[ ] **4.** An antituberculosis drug will be prescribed.

A homeless client diagnosed with tuberculosis continues to have evidence of the tubercle bacilli in his sputum after 6 weeks of drug therapy.

54. Which question is most important for the nurse to ask at this time?
[ ] **1.** "When did you last take your prescribed medications?"
[ ] **2.** "Have you taken all your medications as prescribed?"
[ ] **3.** "How many drug refills have you obtained?"
[ ] **4.** "Have you experienced any drug side effects?"

Efforts at obtaining a sputum specimen from this client have been unsuccessful. The physician orders a gastric lavage.

55. Which explanation by the nurse is best regarding the reason for performing a gastric lavage?
[ ] **1.** The organism may be found in swallowed sputum.
[ ] **2.** The organism also infects gastrointestinal tissue.
[ ] **3.** The organism migrates from the lungs to the stomach.
[ ] **4.** The organism can be destroyed by instilling fluid.

56. Which health measure is most important to emphasize when instructing the client on ways to prevent transmitting tuberculosis?
[ ] **1.** Eat a nutritious diet.
[ ] **2.** Get adequate sleep.
[ ] **3.** Cover your nose and mouth when coughing.
[ ] **4.** Wash your hands before and after meals.

Aware that the client must manage his nutritional needs on a very low income, the nurse reinforces the dietitian's instructions.

57. If the client identified that his lunches often include the following foods, which meal is the most nutritious?
[ ] **1.** Tossed salad, rice, iced tea
[ ] **2.** Jelly sandwich on whole wheat bread, coffee
[ ] **3.** Meatless chili with beans, corn bread, milk
[ ] **4.** Chicken soup, gelatin, sweetened lemonade

The physician prescribes a combination of rifampin (Rifadin) and isoniazid (INH) to treat this client's tuberculosis.

58. When the client asks the nurse why he is taking two drugs, which response is most accurate?
[ ] **1.** One medication diminishes the side effects of the other.
[ ] **2.** One medication kills the live organism; the other, its spores.
[ ] **3.** Using combined medications can reduce the dosages of both drugs.
[ ] **4.** Using combination medications slows bacterial resistance.

59. If the client complains of gastrointestinal side effects associated with rifampin (Rifadin), which nursing action is best?
[ ] **1.** Administering the drug at night
[ ] **2.** Giving the drug with food or at mealtimes
[ ] **3.** Encouraging the client to drink plenty of water
[ ] **4.** Providing the client with an antacid

Nursing Care of Clients with Asthma

An adult male client who has had asthma since early childhood comes to the emergency department in respiratory distress.

60. Which position is best for the client when the nurse prepares to assess breath sounds?
[ ] **1.** Sitting
[ ] **2.** Standing
[ ] **3.** Lying on the back
[ ] **4.** Lying on the side

61. During auscultation, which adventitious breath sound is most characteristic at the onset of an asthma attack?
[ ] **1.** Wet bubbling
[ ] **2.** Dry crackling
[ ] **3.** Soft blowing
[ ] **4.** Noisy wheezing

The nurse uses pulse oximetry to monitor the asthma client's oxygenation status.

62. Where should the nurse position the sensor of the pulse oximeter to obtain an accurate measurement?
[ ] **1.** Apply it to the client's finger.
[ ] **2.** Apply it to the client's palm.
[ ] **3.** Clip it to the client's earlobe.
[ ] **4.** Wrap it around the client's leg.

63. Which pulse oximetry reading indicates that the client has normal tissue oxygenation?
[ ] **1.** 80 to 90 mm Hg
[ ] **2.** 95 to 100 mm Hg
[ ] **3.** 80% to 85%
[ ] **4.** 95% to 100%

The nurse takes an arterial blood gas (ABG) specimen from the client's radial artery while he is waiting for the physician to examine him.

64. Immediately after the specimen is drawn, which nursing action is most essential?
[ ] **1.** Apply direct pressure to the site for 5 minutes.
[ ] **2.** Warm the blood in the specimen tube for 5 minutes.
[ ] **3.** Assess the client's blood pressure in 5 minutes.
[ ] **4.** Elevate the client's arm for at least 5 minutes.

The physician orders 60% oxygen administration with a partial rebreathing mask and reservoir bag to treat the client's asthma attack.

65. When administering oxygen with a partial rebreathing mask, which observation is most important to report to the respiratory therapy department?
[ ] **1.** Moisture is accumulating inside the mask.
[ ] **2.** The bag collapses during inspiration.
[ ] **3.** The mask covers the client's mouth and nose.
[ ] **4.** The strap around the client's head is snug.

The nurse is aware that oxygen toxicity occurs with oxygen concentrations of more than 50% when oxygen is administered for longer than 48 to 72 hours.

66. Which of the following signs and symptoms would indicate that the client is experiencing oxygen toxicity? Select all that apply.

[ ] **1.** Nonproductive cough
[ ] **2.** Fatigue
[ ] **3.** Hyperventilation
[ ] **4.** Headache
[ ] **5.** Substernal chest pain
[ ] **6.** Nasal stuffiness

The physician also orders 0.1 mg of epinephrine subcutaneously for the client. The label indicates that the epinephrine is a 1:1,000 dilution, which means that 1 g of epinephrine has been mixed with 1,000 mL of liquid.

67. Which is the correct volume needed for the nurse to administer the prescribed dose of 0.1 mg of epinephrine?
[ ] **1.** 0.001 mL
[ ] **2.** 0.1 mL
[ ] **3.** 1.0 mL
[ ] **4.** 10 mL

68. Which nursing measure is most helpful in reducing the client's anxiety during an asthma attack?
[ ] **1.** Close the door to the examination room.
[ ] **2.** Remain within the client's view.
[ ] **3.** Pull the bedside privacy curtain.
[ ] **4.** Notify the client when the respiratory therapist arrives.

Nursing Care of Clients with Chronic Obstructive Pulmonary Disease

The physician orders pulmonary function tests (PFTs) for a male client diagnosed with emphysema. The client has a history of smoking two packs of cigarettes per day for the last 40 years.

69. The best evidence that the client understands the procedure for a PFT is when he states that it involves which action?
[ ] **1.** Having an X-ray taken
[ ] **2.** Drawing a blood specimen
[ ] **3.** Breathing into a mouthpiece
[ ] **4.** Examining expectorated sputum

When the client develops a respiratory infection, his condition worsens and he is admitted to the hospital. An arterial blood gas (ABG) analysis is ordered.

70. The ABG analysis results reveal that the client's partial pressure of arterial carbon dioxide ($Paco_2$) is 65 mm Hg. The nurse recognizes that this is abnormal because normal $Paco_2$ levels fall between which range?
[ ] **1.** 7.35 and 7.45
[ ] **2.** 80 and 100 mm Hg
[ ] **3.** 35 and 45 mm Hg
[ ] **4.** 22 and 26 mm Hg

71. While assisting the client into a hospital gown, the nurse is most likely to find that his chest has which appearance as a result of his emphysema?
[ ] **1.** Funnel-shaped
[ ] **2.** Barrel-shaped
[ ] **3.** Slender
[ ] **4.** Muscular

Based on his ABG results, the client is to receive supplemental oxygen. The nurse prepares to administer oxygen by nasal cannula.

72. Which oxygen flow rate is most appropriate for this client?
[ ] **1.** 2 L/minute
[ ] **2.** 5 L/minute
[ ] **3.** 8 L/minute
[ ] **4.** 10 L/minute

The client receives I.V. fluid containing aminophylline (Truphylline).

73. The nurse accurately explains to the client that which is the primary purpose for using this drug?
[ ] **1.** To relieve persistent coughing
[ ] **2.** To lessen sputum production
[ ] **3.** To dilate the airways
[ ] **4.** To dilute thick secretions

74. Which side effect can the nurse expect when the client receives aminophylline (Truphylline)?
[ ] **1.** Bronchospasm
[ ] **2.** Hypotension
[ ] **3.** Drowsiness
[ ] **4.** Tachycardia

75. The nurse performs postural drainage on the client. Which nursing intervention is most beneficial to loosen secretions?
[ ] **1.** Telling the client to take deep breaths
[ ] **2.** Striking the back with a cupped hand
[ ] **3.** Applying pressure below the diaphragm
[ ] **4.** Placing the client in a sitting position

76. Which nursing observation provides the best evidence that the postural drainage is effective?
[ ] **1.** The client's respiratory rate is increased.
[ ] **2.** The client's heart rate is much improved.
[ ] **3.** The client's sputum culture is negative.
[ ] **4.** The client expels a large volume of sputum.

The physician orders two puffs of albuterol sulfate (Ventolin) four times a day using a metered-dose inhaler.

77. After administering the first puff of aerosol, what does the client do to demonstrate that he is using the inhaler correctly?
[ ]   **1.** He depresses the canister a second time before exhaling.
[ ]   **2.** He holds his breath for up to 10 seconds before exhaling.
[ ]   **3.** He cleans the mouthpiece with a clean paper tissue or cloth.
[ ]   **4.** He bends from the waist to increase the exhaled volume.

Prior to discharge, the client tells the nurse, "This disease makes me a prisoner in my own home."

78. Which is the best response from the nurse?
[ ]   **1.** "Tell me more about how you're feeling."
[ ]   **2.** "There are lots of things you can still do."
[ ]   **3.** "You're just having a bad day today."
[ ]   **4.** "What makes you say that?"

As he prepares to return home, the client verbalizes concern about his continued fatigue and shortness of breath.

79. Which discharge instruction is most appropriate for reducing the client's fatigue and shortness of breath during mealtimes?
[ ]   **1.** "Eat simple carbohydrates for quick energy."
[ ]   **2.** "Eat fatty foods to get maximum caloric intake."
[ ]   **3.** "Eat frequent, small meals to reduce energy use."
[ ]   **4.** "Eat the largest meal late at night before sleep."

Nursing Care of Clients with Lung Cancer

The nurse is caring for an older man who is undergoing several diagnostic tests to determine if he has lung cancer.

80. If the client is typical of most others with cancer of the lung, which early warning sign did he most likely ignore?
[ ]   **1.** Difficulty swallowing
[ ]   **2.** Gradual weight loss
[ ]   **3.** Persistent cough
[ ]   **4.** Coughing up blood

The physician requests a sputum specimen from the client to see if it contains tumor cells.

81. Which nursing action ensures that an appropriate specimen will be collected?

[ ]   **1.** Having the client gargle and expectorate the liquid
[ ]   **2.** Telling the client to provide a large volume of saliva
[ ]   **3.** Explaining to the client that he should attempt a deep, forceful cough
[ ]   **4.** Swabbing the back of the client's throat to stimulate gagging

The client's preliminary diagnostic tests strongly suggest that he has lung cancer. To make a definitive diagnosis, a bronchoscopy is scheduled.

82. Which action is most appropriate for the nurse to take prior to the bronchoscopy?
[ ]   **1.** Keep the client from eating and drinking.
[ ]   **2.** Have the client cough several times.
[ ]   **3.** Ensure that the client gets adequate sleep.
[ ]   **4.** Scrub the client's upper chest with an antiseptic.

83. Following the bronchoscopy, what should the nurse closely monitor?
[ ]   **1.** The client's level of consciousness
[ ]   **2.** The client's mouth status
[ ]   **3.** The client's respiratory effort
[ ]   **4.** The client's ability to speak

After the bronchoscopy, the nurse observes blood when suctioning secretions that have accumulated in the client's mouth.

84. To evaluate the significance of the client's bleeding, which additional assessment is most important for the nurse to make at this time?
[ ]   **1.** Count the pulse rate.
[ ]   **2.** Listen to heart sounds.
[ ]   **3.** Check the pupil response.
[ ]   **4.** Measure the chest expansion.

85. When the nurse empties the secretions from the suction container, which infection control measure is most important to perform?
[ ]   **1.** Wear a mask.
[ ]   **2.** Wear a gown.
[ ]   **3.** Wear goggles.
[ ]   **4.** Wear gloves.

86. Which assessment technique is essential before allowing a client food or fluids following a bronchoscopy?
[ ]   **1.** Touch the arch of the palate with a tongue blade.
[ ]   **2.** Listen to the abdomen for active bowel sounds.
[ ]   **3.** Inspect the oral mucous membranes for integrity.
[ ]   **4.** Palpate the throat while the client swallows.

After the bronchoscopy, the client is diagnosed with advanced lung cancer. Pleural effusion is also discovered. The nurse prepares the client for a thoracentesis.

87. Because of the client's pleural effusion and advanced lung disease, the nurse frequently listens to the client's breath sounds. What would the nurse expect to hear when assessing the breath sounds?
[ ] **1.** Wheezing in the upper lobes
[ ] **2.** A friction rub posterior to the affected area
[ ] **3.** Crackles over the affected area
[ ] **4.** Decreased sounds over the involved area

88. How should the nurse position the client while he is undergoing thoracentesis?
[ ] **1.** Lithotomy position
[ ] **2.** Sitting
[ ] **3.** Prone
[ ] **4.** Supine

After the thoracentesis, the physician tells the client that he will require a pneumonectomy. He explains the surgery and risk factors to the client.

89. Which statement by the client would indicate to the nurse that he has an accurate understanding of the planned surgery?
[ ] **1.** "The surgeon is planning to remove one of my lungs."
[ ] **2.** "Only one lobe of my lung will be removed."
[ ] **3.** "The surgeon will take a sample of my lung tissue to be biopsied during the procedure."
[ ] **4.** "A lung will be opened and examined during surgery."

90. While developing the postoperative care plan for the client, it is essential to stress that he lie in which position?
[ ] **1.** With the healthy lung uppermost
[ ] **2.** With the head lower than his heart
[ ] **3.** With the affected side upward
[ ] **4.** With the arms elevated on pillows

91. For the client who has just had a pneumonectomy, what is a temporary, expected outcome of thoracic surgery?
[ ] **1.** Persistent cough
[ ] **2.** Chest numbness
[ ] **3.** Impaired swallowing
[ ] **4.** Sore throat

The client requests pain medication following his pneumonectomy.

92. After administering morphine sulfate (Roxanol) to the client, which of the following is most important for the nurse to assess?

[ ] **1.** Rate and rhythm of the heart rate
[ ] **2.** Skin color and temperature
[ ] **3.** Presence of bowel sounds
[ ] **4.** Rate and depth of respirations

Nursing Care of Clients with Chest Injuries

A high school football player comes to the emergency department with signs and symptoms suggestive of two fractured ribs.

93. Before discharging a client with fractured ribs from the emergency department, which instruction is most important for the nurse to provide?
[ ] **1.** Breathe deeply several times every hour.
[ ] **2.** Breathe shallowly to avoid discomfort.
[ ] **3.** Breathe rapidly to promote ventilation.
[ ] **4.** Breathe into a paper bag every hour.

While on the way to work one morning, a nurse witnesses a motorcycle accident and stops to assist the victim.

94. When assessing the accident victim, which finding strongly suggests the presence of a flail chest?
[ ] **1.** Sucking air is heard near the chest.
[ ] **2.** The trachea deviates from midline.
[ ] **3.** A portion of the chest moves inward during inspiration.
[ ] **4.** The victim has severe chest pain during expiration.

Upon arrival at the emergency department, it is determined that the victim's lung collapsed during the accident. A hemothorax is diagnosed, and two chest tubes are inserted.

95. Following chest tube insertion, where would the nurse expect to see bloody drainage?
[ ] **1.** From the victim's nose
[ ] **2.** From the victim's mouth
[ ] **3.** From the tube in the upper chest
[ ] **4.** From the tube in the lower chest

Both of the victim's chest tubes are connected to a commercial water-seal drainage system.

96. When the nurse monitors the chamber with the water seal, which finding suggests that the system is functioning correctly?
[ ] **1.** The fluid rises and falls with respirations.
[ ] **2.** The fluid level is lower than when first filled.
[ ] **3.** The fluid bubbles continuously.
[ ] **4.** The fluid looks frothy white.

97. Which assessment finding would best indicate that air is leaking into the tissue around the victim's chest tube insertion site?
[ ] **1.** The tissue appears pale or almost colorless.
[ ] **2.** A hissing sound, like a leaking tire, can be heard.
[ ] **3.** The skin crackles when touched.
[ ] **4.** Air is felt as it escapes.

The victim is transported to another unit for a chest X-ray. His chest tubes and water-seal drainage system are still in place.

98. Which nursing action is most appropriate before transporting the client to have X-rays taken?
[ ] **1.** Clamp the chest tubes before leaving the room.
[ ] **2.** Keep the drainage system below the insertion sites.
[ ] **3.** Attach a portable suction machine to the chest tubes.
[ ] **4.** Provide mechanical ventilation during transport.

99. What is the best method for determining the amount of drainage from a chest tube when a closed water-seal system is used?
[ ] **1.** Empty the collection chamber, and measure the volume.
[ ] **2.** Subtract the client's fluid intake from his output.
[ ] **3.** Instill sterile irrigation solution, and measure the drainage.
[ ] **4.** Subtract the previously marked volume from the current amount.

The nurse is caring for a client who has a chest tube connected to a three-chamber water-seal drainage system.

100. Identify the chamber in which the nurse observes intermittent bubbling until the lung has expanded.

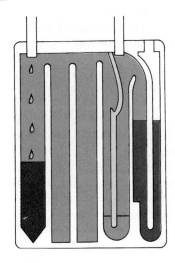

Nursing Care of Clients with Pulmonary Embolism

Following abdominal surgery, a client suddenly experiences severe chest pain and dyspnea. A pulmonary embolism is suspected.

101. Where did the client's embolism most likely originate?
[ ] **1.** The deep veins of the legs
[ ] **2.** The pulmonary artery
[ ] **3.** The superior vena cava
[ ] **4.** The carotid artery

The client suddenly experiences chest pain and dyspnea and tells the nurse, "Nurse, I think I'm dying."

102. Which response by the nurse is most appropriate at this time?
[ ] **1.** "The pain will lessen in a few minutes."
[ ] **2.** "I'll stay with you until the physician comes."
[ ] **3.** "Why would you even think something like that?"
[ ] **4.** "Are your financial affairs in order?"

103. Which nursing intervention is most important at this time?
[ ] **1.** Administering oxygen by face mask
[ ] **2.** Assessing the client's capillary refill
[ ] **3.** Having the client rate the pain on a pain scale
[ ] **4.** Requesting a physician's order for cardiac enzymes

104. Based on the client's clinical presentation, the nurse anticipates which drug will be administered intravenously?
[ ] **1.** Heparin (Hep-Lock)
[ ] **2.** Aminophylline (Truphylline)
[ ] **3.** Nitroglycerin (Nitrodisc)
[ ] **4.** Aspirin (Anacin)

The client becomes unresponsive, stops breathing, and is pulseless. The nurse initiates cardiopulmonary resuscitation (CPR).

105. How many breaths per minute are administered to an adult during CPR?
[ ] **1.** Eight per minute
[ ] **2.** Twelve per minute
[ ] **3.** Fifteen per minute
[ ] **4.** Twenty per minute

Nursing Care of Clients with a Tracheostomy

106. Which assessment finding provides the best indication that the nurse needs to suction the client with a tracheostomy?
[ ] **1.** Respirations are low.
[ ] **2.** Pulse rate is slow.
[ ] **3.** Breath sounds are wet.
[ ] **4.** Blood pressure is elevated.

107. Which nursing action is essential before suctioning the client with a tracheostomy tube?
[ ] **1.** Providing mouth care
[ ] **2.** Moistening the catheter
[ ] **3.** Cleaning around the stoma
[ ] **4.** Removing the inner cannula

108. When suctioning a client with a tracheostomy, when is the best time to occlude the vent on the suction catheter?
[ ] **1.** Before inserting the catheter
[ ] **2.** When inside the inner cannula
[ ] **3.** While withdrawing the catheter
[ ] **4.** When the client begins coughing

109. When suctioning the airway of a client with a tracheostomy, the nurse applies suction for no longer than how many seconds?
[ ] **1.** 5 to 7
[ ] **2.** 10 to 12
[ ] **3.** 15 to 20
[ ] **4.** 25 to 30

110. While withdrawing the suction catheter from a client's tracheostomy tube, which nursing technique is correct?
[ ] **1.** Remove the catheter slowly.
[ ] **2.** Pinch and pull the catheter.
[ ] **3.** Plunge the catheter up and down.
[ ] **4.** Twist and rotate the catheter.

111. What is the best way to determine whether a client with a tracheostomy is becoming hypoxemic during suctioning?
[ ] **1.** Monitoring his level of consciousness
[ ] **2.** Assessing his skin color and temperature
[ ] **3.** Watching his pulse oximetry levels
[ ] **4.** Counting his respiratory rate

112. Which nursing actions are appropriate when monitoring a female client with a finger pulse oximeter? Select all that apply.

[ ] **1.** Remove the client's fingernail polish.
[ ] **2.** Position the sensors so they are directly opposite each other on the client's finger.
[ ] **3.** Connect the cable to the oximeter.
[ ] **4.** Set the SpO_2 alarms between 95% and 100%.
[ ] **5.** Notify the physician each time an alarm sounds.
[ ] **6.** Relocate the spring-loaded sensor periodically.

113. When performing tracheostomy care, which nursing action is correct?
[ ] **1.** Cut a gauze square to fit around the client's stoma.
[ ] **2.** Secure the ties at the back of the client's neck.
[ ] **3.** Attach new ties before removing old ones.
[ ] **4.** Replace the cannula after changing the ties.

114. Which statement best explains the reason for using a cuffed tracheostomy tube?
[ ] **1.** The cuff prevents skin breakdown.
[ ] **2.** The cuff prevents aspiration.
[ ] **3.** The cuff is more comfortable.
[ ] **4.** The cuff reduces infection.

Nursing Care of Clients with a Sudden Airway Occlusion

A nurse working in a physician's office receives a telephone call from a frantic person whose family member is choking on a piece of hard candy.

115. What information does the nurse need to know first before recommending further action?
[ ] **1.** Can the victim walk?
[ ] **2.** Can the victim cough?
[ ] **3.** How is the victim positioned?
[ ] **4.** Can the victim still swallow?

116. The nurse knows that the correct way to position the hands when performing the Heimlich maneuver is with the thumb side of the closed fist on which part of the victim's abdomen?
[ ] **1.** Directly on the manubrium
[ ] **2.** Above the xiphoid process
[ ] **3.** Below the navel
[ ] **4.** Below the sternum

Correct Answers and Rationales

Nursing Care of Clients with Upper Respiratory Tract Infections

1. 1. The common cold, called *rhinitis* or *coryza,* is a viral infection that affects the nasal passages and throat. Colds are spread by inhalation of droplets or direct contact. Antibiotics are only useful in treating bacterial, not viral, infections. No drug cures the common cold. Antibiotics are started only when clients have a secondary bacterial infection; then, most individuals, regardless of their immune status, get a prescription for antibiotics.
    Client Needs Category—Health promotion and maintenance
    Client Needs Subcategory—None

2. 3. A high fever suggests that the client with a common cold has acquired a secondary bacterial infection, such as bronchitis or pneumonia. Viral infections such as the common cold are generally associated with a low-grade fever. Symptoms of the common cold are generally confined to the head and throat. They include nasal congestion and discharge, nose and throat discomfort, sneezing, and watery eyes. The client may also have a headache, chills, fatigue, and loss of appetite. A dry cough is due to irritation from nasal drainage passing into the pharynx. A productive cough indicates that the infection involves the lower respiratory tract.
    Client Needs Category—Physiological integrity
    Client Needs Subcategory—Physiological adaptation

3. 3. Nonprescription decongestants are contraindicated for clients with hypertension and heart disease. Most decongestants contain adrenergic drugs, such as ephedrine sulfate, which stimulate the sympathetic nervous system. Such drugs can cause tachycardia and increased blood pressure, even in normal individuals. Adrenergic drugs are not contraindicated for clients with arthritis, asthma, or diabetes unless they have cardiovascular disease.
    Client Needs Category—Physiological integrity
    Client Needs Subcategory—Pharmacological therapies

4. 2. Nasal decongestants have a vasoconstricting action. Using them more frequently than recommended tends to result in nasal stuffiness from rebound vasodilation. This means that the congestion worsens and recurs in less time after drug use. Decongestants do not cause microbial drug resistance. Ulceration of the nasal mucosa is more likely a consequence of irritation and trauma from blowing and wiping the nose. Most decongestants are adrenergic drugs, which cause vasoconstriction and an increase in heart rate and blood pressure. Decongestants, therefore, do not slow the heart rate. Decongestants do not cause mucosal ulceration; however, they can cause the mucous membranes to sting, burn, or feel dry. The immune system is unaffected by nasal decongestants.
    Client Needs Category—Health promotion and maintenance
    Client Needs Subcategory—None

5. 2. Excessive or forceful nose blowing can propel infectious secretions into the eustachian tube, causing a secondary ear infection. Keeping the head elevated when asleep, placing cotton in the ear canal, or massaging the area behind the ears will not reduce the risk of developing an ear infection.
    Client Needs Category—Health promotion and maintenance
    Client Needs Subcategory—None

6. 3. Sinusitis, an inflammation of the sinuses (hollow cavities in the facial bones), usually follows an upper respiratory infection. The maxillary sinuses are located in the cheeks; therefore, pain from maxillary sinusitis would be felt in the cheek or upper teeth. If the frontal sinuses are infected, the pain would be felt near the eyes. Sinuses are not located above or behind the ears.
    Client Needs Category—Physiological integrity
    Client Needs Subcategory—Physiological adaptation

7. 3. Tilting the head backward enables liquid medication to settle within the nasopharynx by way of gravity. Bending forward would drain the medication from the nasal passages before it had a chance to provide a therapeutic effect. The other positions described would not help to distribute the nasal medication where it is intended for use.
    Client Needs Category—Health promotion and maintenance
    Client Needs Subcategory—None

8. 2. Vaporizers disperse moistened air into the room and are used primarily with clients to help liquefy nasal secretions. Water sitting in a vaporizer for a prolonged time after use is likely to become stagnant, promoting the growth of microorganisms, especially *Pseudomonas* organisms. Vaporizers can disperse cool or warm mist. One that emits warm mist is more likely to cause scalding or injury if it is placed too close to the edge of a nightstand and accidentally knocked over. Although dust can accumulate on the vaporizer if it is left sitting for a prolonged time, this is not as hazardous as the client developing an infection from pathogens. Calcium deposits may form due to the stagnant water, but they will not cause any ill effects.

Client Needs Category—Safe, effective care environment

Client Needs Subcategory—Safety and infection control

Nursing Care of Clients with Inflammatory and Allergic Disorders of the Upper Airways

9. **3.** Pharyngitis, also known as a *sore throat,* can be caused by bacteria (such as streptococci) or by viruses. When obtaining a culture, the nurse swabs the back of the client's throat with a sterile applicator to obtain a sample of infectious organisms in the inflamed tissue of the pharynx. A throat culture is obtained from the posterior pharynx rather than the mouth and tongue. A sputum specimen is obtained by expectoration from the lower respiratory tract. Organisms in saliva would not necessarily indicate the pathogen causing pharyngitis.

Client Needs Category—Physiological integrity

Client Needs Subcategory—Physiological adaptation

10. **1.** Glomerulonephritis, rheumatic fever, and rheumatic heart disease are but a few of the consequences following untreated or undertreated infections caused by the beta-hemolytic *Streptococcus* organism. To ensure that the organism is destroyed, the American Heart Association recommends treating streptococcal infections with a 10-day course of penicillin V (V-Cillin K) or erythromycin (E-Mycin). Chickenpox and shingles are viruses, which are not treated with antibiotics. *Bordetella pertussis* bacteria, not the *Streptococcus* organism, cause whooping cough.

Client Needs Category—Health promotion and maintenance

Client Needs Subcategory—None

11. **2.** Speaking in a normal voice or whispering prolongs laryngitis. Therefore, resting swollen vocal cords allows the local edema to subside and improves hoarseness. Because the larynx is found between the throat and the trachea, sucking on ice chips will not be beneficial but may soothe the sore throat. Likewise, drinking hot liquids may help soothe the throat but will not help the larynx. Massaging the throat provides comfort for some people, but it does not relieve hoarseness.

Client Needs Category—Health promotion and maintenance

Client Needs Subcategory—None

12. **3.** Persistent hoarseness is the earliest symptom of cancer of the larynx. Nagging cough or hoarseness is one of the seven early warning signs of cancer identified by the American Cancer Society. Other symptoms of cancer of the larynx include a lump in the neck, difficulty swallowing, dyspnea, weight loss, and pain radiating to the ear. The other disorders mentioned cause respiratory symptoms but are not associated with hoarseness.

Client Needs Category—Physiological integrity

Client Needs Subcategory—Physiological adpatation

13. **3.** Antihistamines commonly cause people to feel drowsy and fall asleep easily. Anyone taking an antihistamine is warned to use caution if driving or operating machinery. If there is any effect on weight, it is more likely to be weight gain due to a reduction in activity. Gastrointestinal side effects include increased appetite, nausea, and diarrhea, but not constipation.

Client Needs Category—Health promotion and maintenance

Client Needs Subcategory—None

14. **1.** Many hypersensitive people are allergic to more than one substance. Testing does not promote the production of blocking antibodies. Skin testing is considered a standard practice among allergy specialists, and insurance companies partially or completely pay for this service. Allergy symptoms do vary from person to person, but this is not the main reason skin testing is done. Skin testing is not usually performed because of the threat of complications.

Client Needs Category—Health promotion and maintenance

Client Needs Subcategory—None

15. **4.** An area of local erythema (redness) indicates a positive reaction to the antigen applied to the scratched skin. Swelling, known as induration, may also accompany a reaction. A positive reaction does not appear pale or feel especially painful or numb.

Client Needs Category—Physiological integrity

Client Needs Subcategory—Physiological adaptation

16. **2.** The client undergoing desensitization stays in the physician's office for observation for at least 20 minutes following the injection. Occasionally, a person has a severe allergic reaction to even the small amount of antigen used in the desensitization injection. The client's safety is endangered if a severe reaction occurs and medical assistance is not immediately available. Antihistamines may reduce allergic symptoms, but aspirin has no direct effect. If a client waits 20 minutes, driving is not contraindicated. Clients may shower or bathe following such injections.

Client Needs Category—Physiological integrity

Client Needs Subcategory—Reduction of risk potential

17. **1.** An anaphylactic reaction is a systemic hypersensitivity that occurs within seconds to minutes after exposure to certain medications, foods, or insects. Signs of anaphylaxis include labored breathing, hives, and loss of consciousness as blood pressure falls. Other signs and symptoms include itching, chest tightness, flushed and red skin, coughing, tachycardia or bradycardia, and abdominal pain. Headache and sore throat are not associated with an anaphylactic reaction.

> *Client Needs Category—Physiological integrity*
> *Client Needs Subcategory—Physiological adaptation*

18. **4.** Epinephrine (Adrenalin) is the drug of choice when a client experiences a severe allergic reaction. This drug helps raise the blood pressure by constricting blood vessels and dilating the bronchi, thereby facilitating breathing. Without emergency treatment, persons experiencing severe allergic reactions can die in 5 to 10 minutes. Key goals are to establish a patent airway and ventilate the client. Codeine and morphine sulfate (Roxanol) are central nervous system depressants, which potentiate hypotension. Dopamine (Intropin) is an adrenergic drug in the same family as epinephrine (Adrenalin), but it is not the drug of choice during anaphylaxis. It is commonly given later to maintain the blood pressure of individuals in shock.

> *Client Needs Category—Physiological integrity*
> *Client Needs Subcategory—Pharmacological therapies*

19. **3.** Because shock is one of the major problems during a severe allergic reaction, monitoring blood pressure is the most important assessment for evaluating treatment effectiveness. The nurse would expect the client to have increased blood pressure and less labored breathing and to be more alert as a result of treatment. Maintaining adequate urine output indicates that a person's circulatory volume is sufficient, but making this assessment would be difficult unless a urinary catheter is in place. Skin color is not necessarily a valid indicator, but the client's skin color should go from pale to appropriate ethnic color after blood flow is restored to the periphery. As long as the brain is receiving adequate oxygen, the pupils continue to respond by constricting when stimulated with direct light.

> *Client Needs Category—Physiological integrity*
> *Client Needs Subcategory—Physiological adaptation*

20. **3.** Establishing or maintaining an open airway by lifting the chin and tilting back the head is the first step in resuscitation. A precordial thump is not administered in the case of a severe allergic reaction. Raising the head is inappropriate because it interferes with resuscitation efforts and reduces blood flow to the brain. Epinephrine (Adrenalin) is the drug of choice for anaphylactic reactions but should not be given without a physician's order. If the client is unresponsive, emergency rescue interventions are a priority.

> *Client Needs Category—Physiological integrity*
> *Client Needs Subcategory—Physiological adaptation*

Nursing Care of Clients with Cancer of the Larynx

21. **2.** Of the choices provided, restlessness is most indicative of early hypoxia. Other signs of inadequate oxygenation include rapid, shallow breathing, nasal flaring, using accessory muscles for breathing, hypertension, confusion, stupor, coma, and cyanosis of the skin, lips, and nail beds. Blood loss is expected after a laryngectomy; however, profuse or prolonged loss will eventually affect the red blood cells' oxygen-carrying capacity. Clients with compromised oxygenation are more likely to exhibit tachycardia than an irregular heart rhythm. Feelings of being cold are common after surgery and are generally related to the environmental temperature of the operating and recovery rooms.

> *Client Needs Category—Physiological integrity*
> *Client Needs Subcategory—Physiological adaptation*

22. **4.** Until the laryngectomy client learns esophageal speech or the use of a mechanical vibrator, providing paper and pencil or a magic slate is the best alternative for communication. Lipreading is often frustrating for nursing personnel who are unaccustomed to this technique. The client has a permanent loss of natural voice as a result of a total laryngectomy. He may be able to produce random sounds but will have difficulty verbalizing his needs.

> *Client Needs Category—Physiological integrity*
> *Client Needs Subcategory—Physiological adaptation*

23. **3.** Looking at the tracheostomy tube is interpreted as dealing with the reality of the loss. This is a positive step toward acceptance and adaptation. Grieving follows a cycle of denial or disbelief, anger, depression, bargaining, and acceptance. Believing that the physician misdiagnosed his condition is an example of denial. Social isolation indicates a state of depression characterized by withdrawal from human interaction. Asking the nurse to help him bathe and shave suggests that the client perceives himself as helpless.

> *Client Needs Category—Psychosocial integrity*
> *Client Needs Subcategory—None*

Nursing Care of Clients with Inflammatory and Infectious Disorders of the Lower Airways

24. **3.** When assessing a cough, the nurse first determines if the cough is productive or nonproductive. If the cough is productive, the nurse should document the color, odor, amount, and viscosity of sputum that is raised. Other data that may aid the physician in making a diagnosis include the onset, duration, precipitating factors, and relief measures. Although family history is important, it does not relate to the cough itself. The client's vital signs may be affected with persistent coughing, but this does not address the characteristics of the cough. Self-treatment and medications used to control the cough are important things to know, but they are not as pertinent as the presence of secretions.

    Client Needs Category—Physiological integrity
    Client Needs Subcategory—Physiological adaptation

25. **3.** Codeine depresses the cough center in the brain and is used to suppress coughing. Antitussives that contain codeine or a similar synthetic chemical, dextromethorphan, are called *sedative antitussives.* Antitussives are indicated for coughing when a person's lungs are clear or when persistent coughing adversely affects recovery from other conditions. Suppressing a cough is contraindicated if the client needs to expectorate sputum. Bronchodilators open respiratory passages. Salicylates are used to relieve discomfort, while steroids reduce inflammation.

    Client Needs Category—Health promotion and maintenance
    Client Needs Subcategory—None

26. **1.** A patient taking an opioid (codeine) is warned not to exceed the recommended dosage. Extra self-administration leads to sedation and habituation. Opioid antitussives can cause drowsiness but do not interfere with sleep patterns. Many clients take the medication before bed to suppress coughing so they can sleep. Expectorants, not sedative antitussives, are taken with extra fluids to thin mucoid secretions and facilitate their expectoration. Chilling medications, rather than warming them, would help to disguise an unpleasant taste.

    Client Needs Category—Health promotion and maintenance
    Client Needs Subcategory—None

27. **4.** Syrups are given last and are not followed by water or other liquids for a period of time because they are intended to have a soothing effect on the mucosa of the pharynx. Waiting 15 minutes after giving the syrup shortens the time of local effectiveness. The remaining alternatives involve swallowing water immediately after administering the cough syrup and, therefore, are inappropriate.

    Client Needs Category—Safe, effective care environment
    Client Needs Subcategory—Safety and infection control

28. **3.** The approximate equivalent of 5 mL is 1 teaspoon in household measurements. Some manufacturers of nonprescription cough medications include a dosing cup marked with various household equivalents. However, to ensure safety, the nurse should include an explanation of the equivalent during discharge instructions. One ounce equals 30 mL. One tablespoon equals about 15 mL. A capful is not an accurate measure because it can vary depending on the size of the bottle. Also, pouring medication into, then drinking from, the cap is unsanitary and can contaminate the remaining medication.

    Client Needs Category—Health promotion and maintenance
    Client Needs Subcategory—None

29. **1.** Aerosol therapy involves depositing small droplets of moisture onto respiratory tissue. The warmed, moist air soothes the respiratory passages, relieves tissue irritation, and liquefies secretions produced as a result of the inflammation. Other benefits are obtained by adding medications to the vaporized water. Individuals with acute bronchitis are generally bothered initially by a nonproductive cough aggravated by dry air. Oral or parenteral antibiotic therapy, not aerosol therapy, is used to kill infectious organisms. Respiratory mucosa is moist. The respiratory rate is lowered as ventilation is improved. However, this is a secondary benefit of aerosol therapy and not its primary purpose.

    Client Needs Category—Health promotion and maintenance
    Client Needs Subcategory—None

30. **1.5.** To calculate the drug dosage, use the following formula:

$$\frac{\text{Desired dose}}{\text{Dose on hand}} \times \text{Quantity} = X \text{ (amount to administer)}$$

Solve for *X*:

$$\frac{500}{1,000} = \frac{X}{3}$$

$$1,000\,X = 1,500$$
$$X = 1.5 \text{ ml}$$

    Client Needs Category—Physiological integrity
    Client Needs Subcategory—Pharmacological therapies

31. **3.** Desired dose: 300,000 units; dose on hand reconstituted: 100,000 units/ml; correct amount for administration: 3ml.

Client Needs Category— Physiological integrity
Client Needs Subcategory—Pharmacological therapies

32. **2.** Any article containing metal is removed before a chest X-ray is performed. The image of a metal object that remains in place during an X-ray may be misinterpreted as diseased tissue. Fasting is not required before a chest X-ray. No radiopaque dye is given for this test. Analgesia is unnecessary because the client will not have any accompanying discomfort.

Client Needs Category—Safe, effective care environment
Client Needs Subcategory—Coordinated care

33. **1.** Increasing the fluid intake can help thin respiratory secretions that are difficult to expectorate. Increasing moisture in inspired air through humidification also helps. Changing positions improves circulation and prevents pooling of respiratory secretions. Physicians must write an order for dietary changes. A clear liquid diet may thin secretions, but it is not usually ordered when a sputum specimen is needed. Antitussives are cough suppressants. Suppressing the cough will not allow sputum to be coughed up. An expectorant is the drug of choice if the client has a weak cough reflex or his condition warrants its use.

Client Needs Category—Physiological integrity
Client Needs Subcategory—Physiological adaptation

34. **4.** It is easiest to obtain a sputum specimen when the client first awakens in the morning, as secretions tend to accumulate in the respiratory tract during the night. Pooled secretions are more easily raised, especially if the individual is not fatigued from activity. Sputum collection may also be done following an aerosol treatment, which helps to loosen secretions. Forced coughing after a meal can lead to vomiting.

Client Needs Category—Physiological integrity
Client Needs Subcategory—Physiological adaptation

35. **4.** The client must avoid touching the inside of the sputum specimen container or the inside of its lid. The inside of the container must be kept sterile so that no other sources of microorganisms (such as pathogens found on the hands), other than those present in the sputum, are collected. Wearing gloves or wiping the outside of the specimen container is unnecessary because the outside surface is considered unclean anyway.

Client Needs Category—Health promotion and maintenance
Client Needs Subcategory—None

36. **2.** Mouth care is an appropriate hygiene measure after obtaining a sputum specimen. Expectorating sputum often causes a residual foul taste in the mouth or an unpleasant odor to the breath. Oxygen is appropriate if the client is short of breath. Eating is usually delayed until the client is rested and unlikely to become nauseous. Walking may cause further fatigue after the effort of coughing.

Client Needs Category—Physiological integrity
Client Needs Subcategory—Physiological adapation

37. **2.** Pleurisy is an inflammation of the pleural membranes surrounding the lungs. The most classic symptom associated with pleurisy is feeling a sharp, stabbing pain when taking a deep breath. The presence of a cough would be due to some other pulmonary problem. Cyanotic nail beds and tachycardia are caused by any number of cardiopulmonary diseases that interfere with tissue oxygenation.

Client Needs Category—Physiological integrity
Client Needs Subcategory—Reduction of risk potential

38. **1.** Antibiotics are selected on the basis of their effect on the infectious organism, demonstrated by performing a culture and testing drug sensitivity. The organism is first encouraged to grow in the laboratory medium. Then small disks of various drugs are placed in the growing colonies. If growth is inhibited around a certain disk, this indicates that the drug is effective. Antibiotics are ineffective in treating viral infections. Though widely used, penicillin, like any other drug, has dangerous side effects. Various factors (including drug effectiveness, cost, route of administration, and the client's history of drug allergy) affect the physician's choice of which drug to use.

Client Needs Category—Health promotion and maintenance
Client Needs Subcategory—None

39. **4.** The dorsogluteal muscles are located in the buttocks, so the buttock is the correct site for this I.M. injection. The ventrogluteal muscles are in the hips. The deltoid muscles are in the upper arms. The vastus lateralis and rectus femoris muscles are located in the thighs.

Client Needs Category—Safe, effective care environment
Client Needs Subcategory—Safety and infection control

40. **1.** Pointing the toes inward reduces the discomfort of an injection in the dorsogluteal site. Tightening muscles would increase the client's discomfort. Crossing the legs and flexing the knees would be awkward positions to maintain and would not relieve discomfort during an injection.

Client Needs Category—Physiological integrity
Client Needs Subcategory—Physiological adaptation

41. **3.** Cephalosporins are chemically similar to the penicillins. Therefore, the nurse would expect that a client who is allergic to penicillin may also react adversely when given a cephalosporin-type of antibiotic. Before administering a cephalosporin to a client with a penicillin allergy, it is best to consult the physician and observe the client closely if the medical order is not changed. Although allergic reactions occur with the administration of any antibiotic, the other antibiotic groups do not demonstrate the same cross-sensitivity with penicillin.

Client Needs Category—Physiological integrity
Client Needs Subcategory—Pharmacological therapies

42. **3.** The influenza vaccine contains albumin from the eggs in which the virus is cultured. Individuals who are allergic to eggs or egg products may react adversely. Influenza vaccinations, used to prevent flu symptoms caused by a virus, are repeated yearly to provide immunity against viral strains identified during the previous year. Pneumococcal pneumonia vaccine is given to prevent bacterial pneumonia; it is unrelated to the influenza vaccine. Influenza and pneumococcal vaccines are recommended for anyone over age 65 and those with chronic disease. Having a history of a respiratory disease is not an essential criterion for influenza vaccinations.

Client Needs Category—Health promotion and maintenance
Client Needs Subcategory—None

43. **2.** All the options help reduce the potential for infection. However, because respiratory infections are spread primarily by direct contact with another sick individual, avoiding crowds is the best advice. The U.S. Public Health Service Advisory Committee on Immunization recommends annual vaccination against influenza for people over the age of 65 and those with other chronic health problems.

Client Needs Category—Health promotion and maintenance
Client Needs Subcategory—None

44. **2, 4, 5, 6.** Inadequate oxygenation causes the client to initially become restless and anxious. The respiratory rate accelerates in an effort to increase the diffusion of atmospheric oxygen from the lungs to the blood, causing tachypnea. When the increased respiratory rate is insufficient, accessory muscles compensate to increase the inspiratory volume. In the late stages of hypoxia, the client becomes confused as the brain suffers from oxygen deprivation. One of the last signs of hypoxia is cyanosis. Cough and fever may be signs of a respiratory infection that can lead to hypoxia, but they are not manifestations of a hypoxic state.

Client Needs Category—Physiological integrity
Client Needs Subcategory—Physiological adaptation

45. **4.** An intake of 3,000 mL per day is safe in the absence of any preexisting cardiovascular or renal problems. The additional fluid helps to keep the client hydrated and aids in temperature regulation. Less than 3,000 mL is insufficient due to the client's increased metabolic rate secondary to an extremely elevated body temperature.

Client Needs Category—Physiological integrity
Client Needs Subcategory—Reduction of risk potential

46. **3.** A sponge bath enhances loss of body heat by promoting evaporation from the skin's surface. Soap should not be used when giving a sponge bath to a feverish client. Therefore, a sponge bath is not given to remove microorganisms or to maintain skin integrity. For some clients, a sponge bath feels soothing. However, comfort is not the primary purpose for administering the sponge bath to a feverish client.

Client Needs Category—Health promotion and maintenance
Client Needs Subcategory—None

47. **2.** Tepid means a temperature that is cool or lukewarm—usually recognized as within a range of 80° to 93° F. Bath water that is above this temperature would be too hot to reduce a fever. Cold or icy water (between 70° and 75° F) would only be used if the client has severe hyperthermia—for example, from heat stroke.

Client Needs Category—Safe, effective care environment
Client Needs Subcategory—Coordinated care

48. **2.** Chilling is an indication that the body temperature is falling too rapidly. The muscle contraction that accompanies chilling produces heat and interferes with reducing body temperature. When chills occur, it is best to temporarily discontinue the sponge bath, dry the skin, and protect the client from any drafts. Nausea and confusion are not considered adverse effects associated with sponge bathing. A feverish individual is likely to have a flushed appearance that is unrelated to sponge bathing.

Client Needs Category—Physiological integrity
Client Needs Subcategory—Reduction of risk potential

49. 3. A decrease in the client's temperature is the best evidence that the tepid sponge bath is having a therapeutic effect. Sweating may or may not be the result of sponge bathing; it may be an indication of another disease process. Although the client's statements about feeling more comfortable and thinking her fever has broken correlate with fever reduction, such statements reflect subjective data. Objective data, such as taking the client's temperature, are more reliable indicators.

Client Needs Category—Physiological integrity
Client Needs Subcategory—Physiological adaptation

50. 1. When administering an intradermal injection, the needle is inserted between the layers of skin at approximately a 10- to 15-degree angle. Subcutaneous injections are given at either a 45- or 90-degree angle, depending on the size of the client. Intramuscular injections are given at a 90-degree angle.

Client Needs Category—Safe, effective care environment
Client Needs Subcategory—Safety and infection control

51. 3. The standard length of time for reading a tuberculin skin test is 48 to 72 hours after the test is administered. The nurse observes for redness and measures any evidence of an indurated (hard) area of tissue. Some individuals who are immunosuppressed do not always respond positively to the initial skin test, yet they are symptomatic. A second skin test that is more strongly concentrated is administered to immunosuppressed clients and additional diagnostic tests (such as a sputum examination and chest X-ray) are performed to definitively diagnose the disease.

Client Needs Category—Health promotion and maintenance
Client Needs Subcategory—None

52. 2. Tuberculosis is an infectious disease that is transmitted by inhaling moist droplets or dried spores containing the infectious organism. A positive tuberculin skin test indicates that, at some time, the person became infected with the microorganism that causes tuberculosis and developed antibodies. A positive skin test may or may not mean that an active infectious process is occurring. Anyone with a positive tuberculin skin test without any known history of having had the disease must have a subsequent chest X-ray and sputum examinations. Drugs are administered prophylactically to individuals who suddenly test positive after having a history of being negative. A positive skin test does not indicate protective immunity. The U.S. Centers for Disease Control and Prevention recommends following airborne precautions, which require wearing a particulate air filter respirator when caring for hospitalized clients who are actively contagious.

Client Needs Category—Physiological integrity
Client Needs Subcategory—Physiological adaptation

53. 4. Prophylactic drug therapy with isoniazid (INH) is initiated whenever a person with a previously negative skin test demonstrates a positive reaction. INH is combined with other drugs if the disease is confirmed with additional diagnostic tests, such as sputum examinations and chest X-rays. Once a skin test is positive, it remains positive lifelong. Therefore, skin tests every 6 months are not necessary. Most individuals with active tuberculosis become noninfectious within 2 weeks with appropriate drug therapy; therefore, quitting the job is unnecessary. Immediate family members are also tested and treated prophylactically so that living separately is unnecessary.

Client Needs Category—Health promotion and maintenance
Client Needs Subcategory—None

54. 2. Because noncompliance is one of the leading causes of treatment failures, asking the client if he has taken all of the prescribed medication is appropriate. All clients who must take one or more drugs must be informed that their medications should be taken consistently throughout the treatment period. The remaining questions are appropriate but should not be asked until the nurse has determined that the client has been taking the medications appropriately.

Client Needs Category—Health promotion and maintenance
Client Needs Subcategory—None

55. 1. Gastric lavage is the rinsing or irrigating of the stomach to remove irritants or poisons by a nasogastric tube. In this case, it is used to obtain a specimen from a person who swallows respiratory secretions rather than expectorating them. Tuberculosis is spread to other tissues besides the lungs; however, the spread is generally by means of the bloodstream, not the stomach. The gastric secretions tend to destroy organisms and, therefore, do not infect the gastric tissue. The instilled fluid, usually saline, provides sufficient liquid volume in the stomach to aid in removing the desired specimen. Instilling the fluid will not destroy the organism.

Client Needs Category—Physiological integrity
Client Needs Subcategory—Physiological adaptation

56. 3. To prevent the transmission of infectious microorganisms that cause tuberculosis, it is appropriate to instruct the client to cover his nose and mouth when coughing or sneezing, dispose of paper tissues appropriately, and perform frequent hand washing. Although hand washing is important for everyone, there is no logical correlation between preventing tuberculosis, which is spread through droplet secretions, and washing hands before and after meals. Eating nutritiously and getting adequate sleep promote healing and early resolution of the active disease process.

> *Client Needs Category*—*Health promotion and maintenance*
> *Client Needs Subcategory*—*None*

57. 3. Combining beans (chili) and a grain (corn bread) is an economic means of consuming all essential amino acids found in an animal source. Drinking milk also improves the nutrition of this meal choice. The alternative meals are economical. However, because they do not provide adequate sources of protein, they are not considered nutritious choices.

> *Client Needs Category*—*Health promotion and maintenance*
> *Client Needs Subcategory*—*None*

58. 4. Rifampin (Rifadin) and isoniazid (INH) are commonly combined to treat tuberculosis (TB) because resistant strains of TB occur rapidly if either medication is used alone. Side effects are not reduced; they do not act at different periods during the organism's life cycle; and their dosage is not altered when given in combination.

> *Client Needs Category*—*Physiological integrity*
> *Client Needs Subcategory*—*Pharmacological therapies*

59. 2. Giving medication with food protects the stomach from becoming upset. The potential for gastric upset is increased if irritating medications are administered on an empty stomach. Drinking water, providing an antacid, or giving the medication at night will not necessarily reduce gastrointestinal side effects.

> *Client Needs Category*—*Physiological integrity*
> *Client Needs Subcategory*—*Pharmacological therpaies*

Nursing Care of Clients with Asthma

60. 1. A sitting position is preferred when auscultating the chest. This allows the nurse access to the anterior, lateral, and posterior chest areas. Changing positions during auscultation further taxes an already dyspneic client. A client in respiratory distress generally cannot tolerate lying flat or on his side. Standing is unsafe for a client who is having extreme difficulty breathing.

> *Client Needs Category*—*Physiological integrity*
> *Client Needs Subcategory*—*Physiological adaptation*

61. 4. When air passages narrow, as in the onset of an asthmatic attack, the nurse is most likely to hear wheezing. Generally, this is noted during expiration. Wet bubbling sounds indicate accumulated secretions. These sounds are more likely to occur during recovery from the asthmatic attack, when thick secretions are able to move. Dry crackling sounds indicate that air is moving into and opening small airways, such as the terminal bronchioles and alveoli. Soft blowing sounds are normal in open, distal, small airways of the lungs.

> *Client Needs Category*—*Physiological integrity*
> *Client Needs Subcategory*—*Physiological adaptation*

62. 1. Pulse oximetry is a noninvasive method for assessing oxygen saturation in the tissues. In most cases, the sensor of a pulse oximeter is applied to the finger but may also be applied to the earlobe, thumb, toe, or bridge of the nose. The leg is too dense to allow light to transilluminate from tissue to the sensor. Applying the sensor to the thickness of the palm of the hand is inappropriate.

> *Client Needs Category*—*Physiological integrity*
> *Client Needs Subcategory*—*Physiological adaptation*

63. 4. A normal oxygen saturation is 95% to 100%. Supplemental oxygen administration is appropriate if the oxygen saturation is sustained below 90%. The normal level of the partial pressure of oxygen (Pao_2), which is measured by arterial blood gas analysis, is 80 to 100 mm Hg.

> *Client Needs Category*—*Physiological integrity*
> *Client Needs Subcategory*—*Physiological adaptation*

64. 1. To avoid excessive blood loss and a painful hematoma from a punctured arterial site, it is essential to apply direct pressure for a minimum of 3 to 5 minutes. The specimen is cooled in ice after collection. The blood pressure is unlikely to be affected by the loss of a small amount of blood. Elevating the arm is one way to control bleeding from a vein, but it probably would be ineffective in the case of bleeding from an artery.

> *Client Needs Category*—*Safe, effective care environment*
> *Client Needs Subcategory*—*Safety and infection control*

65. 2. The reservoir bag of a partial rebreathing mask remains partially filled during inspiration. If the bag collapses completely, the equipment may be faulty. This information must be reported to the respiratory therapy department. A properly fitting mask should cover the mouth and nose and the strap should fit the head snugly. Moisture is likely to accumulate because the oxygen is humidified; this information does not need to be reported. The nurse can wipe away the moisture and reapply the mask.

Client Needs Category—Safe, effective care environment

Client Needs Subcategory—Coordinated care

66. **1, 2, 4, 5, 6.** Signs and symptoms of oxygen toxicity include a nonproductive cough, substernal chest pain, nasal stuffiness, nausea and vomiting, fatigue, headache, sore throat, and hypoventilation (not hyperventilation).

Client Needs Category—Safe, effective care management

Client Needs Subcategory—Safety and infection control

67. **2.** The volume of epinephrine 1:1,000 needed to administer 0.1 mg is 0.1 mL. To solve the problem using a ratio and proportion method, use the following steps:

$$\frac{1,000 \text{ mg (1 g)}}{1,000 \text{ mL}} = \frac{0.1 \text{ mg}}{X \text{ mL}}$$

$$1,000 \, X = 100$$

$$X = 0.1 \text{ mL}$$

Client Needs Category—Safe, effective care environment

Client Needs Subcategory—Safety and infection control

68. **2.** Remaining with the client in respiratory distress provides support and reassurance that someone is available. This should help to ease the client's anxiety. Closing the door and pulling the privacy curtain are confining actions; they would most likely heighten the client's anxiety and feelings of suffocation. Notifying the client that the respiratory therapist has arrived may decrease his anxiety somewhat but not as much as if the physician had arrived.

Client Needs Category—Psychosocial integrity

Client Needs Subcategory—None

Nursing Care of Clients with Chronic Obstructive Pulmonary Disease

69. **3.** Pulmonary function tests assess the ventilation volume of the lungs by having the client breathe in and out through a mouthpiece. A tube connects the mouthpiece to an air-filled drum. The drum rises and falls with ventilation. A graphic recording of the air volume exchanged during breathing is obtained. X-rays, drawing blood, and analyzing sputum are not associated with pulmonary function tests.

Client Needs Category—Physiological integrity

Client Needs Subcategory—Physiological adaptation

70. **3.** ABG studies indicate the blood pH as well as the amounts of oxygen, carbon dioxide (CO_2), and bicarbonate (HCO_3^-) in the blood. The physician typically orders ABG studies when the client has an acute illness or a history of respiratory disease, or when the client's condition worsens. Normal $Paco_2$ levels are 35 to 45 mm Hg. Clients who have emphysema usually have elevated CO_2 levels related to air trapping. 7.35 to 7.45 is the normal pH of the blood. Normal partial pressure of arterial oxygen (Pao_2) is 80 to 100 mm Hg. Normal HCO_3^- is 22 to 26 mm Hg.

Client Needs Category—Physiological integrity

Client Needs Subcategory—Physiological adaptation

71. **2.** Individuals with long-standing emphysema develop a barrel-shaped appearance to their chests. The physical change is probably due to chronic overdistention of the lungs due to impaired ability to exhale air.

Client Needs Category—Physiological integrity

Client Needs Subcategory—Physiological adaptation

72. **1.** Giving oxygen at greater than 2 L/minute to a client with chronic respiratory disease interferes with the brain's response to the hypoxic drive. In a client with chronic obstructive lung disease, the stimulus to breathe comes from low levels of oxygen rather than higher levels of carbon dioxide. Administering high concentrations of oxygen depresses the respiratory center.

Client Needs Category—Physiological integrity

Client Needs Subcategory—Physiological adaptation

73. **3.** The therapeutic action of aminophylline (Truphylline) is the reduction of respiratory distress. Aminophylline is classified as a bronchodilator. It does not relieve coughing, decrease sputum production, or thin secretions.

Client Needs Category—Physiological integrity

Client Needs Subcategory—Pharmacological therapies

74. **4.** Aminophylline (Truphylline) is likely to cause tachycardia because it affects the sympathetic nervous system. Other side effects include hypertension, insomnia, and restlessness. The therapeutic action of aminophylline is bronchodilation, not bronchospasm.

Client Needs Category—Physiological integrity

Client Needs Subcategory—Pharmacological therapies

75. **2.** Administering rhythmic gentle blows to the back with a cupped hand, known as *percussion*, causes thick secretions to break loose from within the airways. This technique is also combined with vibration. Vibration involves producing wavelike tremors to the chest by making firm, circular movements with open hands.

For draining all but the upper lobes of the lung, the client is positioned so that the lower chest is elevated higher than the head. Sitting does not mobilize the secretions. Deep breathing improves ventilation, but it does not necessarily move secretions. Applying pressure below the diaphragm is an emergency measure for relieving an obstructed airway.

Client Needs Category—Physiological integrity
Client Needs Subcategory—Physiological adaptation

76. **4.** Expectorating a large volume of sputum is the best evidence that postural drainage is effective. The respiratory rate is lowered, not elevated, if hypoxia is relieved. An improved heart rate is not the best evidence that postural drainage is effective. A negative sputum culture only indicates that the client does not have an infection.

Client Needs Category—Physiological integrity
Client Needs Subcategory—Physiological adaptation

77. **2.** To promote maximum distribution of inhaled medication, it is best to hold the breath for up to 10 seconds and then slowly exhale through pursed lips. If a second puff is ordered, the client should wait several minutes before self-administering another dose. The mouthpiece should be cleaned in warm water, rinsed, and allowed to air dry at least once each day. Using pursed-lip breathing rather than bending from the waist is the preferred method for increasing exhaled volume.

Client Needs Category—Health promotion and maintenance
Client Needs Subcategory—None

78. **1.** Encouraging the client to express his feelings is therapeutic. It shows that the nurse has empathy regarding the client's emotional condition and is willing to listen. Disagreeing with the client, belittling feelings, and using a reassuring cliché block the therapeutic effectiveness of communication.

Client Needs Category—Psychosocial integrity
Client Needs Subcategory—None

79. **3.** Eating several small meals each day promotes adequate intake of calories without causing excess tiredness. Simple carbohydrates provide quick energy, but this recommendation is not better than eating a variety of foods at frequent intervals. Dietary fats are higher in calories than carbohydrates and protein, but fat consumption contributes to hyperlipidemia and increases the risk of cardiovascular disease. Most people have more energy early in the day; consequently, eating the largest meal at night is counterproductive.

Client Needs Category—Physiological integrity
Client Needs Subcategory—Reduction of risk potential

Nursing Care of Clients with Lung Cancer

80. **3.** A cough and dyspnea are generally the earliest signs of lung cancer. Most people tend to ignore these signs, rationalizing that they are a consequence of chronic smoking. Therefore, early diagnosis and treatment of lung cancer are often delayed. Later signs of lung cancer include unexplained weight loss, blood-tinged sputum, fatigue, and respiratory distress.

Client Needs Category—Physiological integrity
Client Needs Subcategory—Physiological adaptation

81. **3.** Coughing is the best method for raising sputum. Saliva is not sputum. Gargled solution is not likely to contain adequate secretions or cells from the bronchial or deeper pulmonary structures. Stimulating a gag reflex is more likely to cause the client to vomit.

Client Needs Category—Physiological integrity
Client Needs Subcategory—Physiological adaptation

82. **1.** A bronchoscopy is a diagnostic test that involves the direct visualization of the larynx, trachea, and bronchi. The physician passes a flexible tube through the client's nose or throat. Preparation for a bronchoscopy includes keeping the client from eating or drinking for at least 4 to 8 hours before the procedure. This reduces the risk of aspiration. Coughing several times has no effect on the bronchoscopy. Adequate rest is desirable but not essential. The instrument used for bronchoscopy is introduced through the mouth; therefore, scrubbing the upper chest is unnecessary.

Client Needs Category—Physiological integrity
Client Needs Subcategory—Physiological adaptation

83. **3.** Respiratory effort is the most critical assessment to make following a bronchoscopy because the bronchoscope is passed directly into the larynx, trachea, and bronchi. Respiratory effort is one of the first responses to change if the client experiences edema and trauma in the airway. All of the other assessment alternatives are appropriate but not as likely to indicate life-threatening consequences.

Client Needs Category—Physiological integrity
Client Needs Subcategory—Reduction of risk potential

84. **1.** The pulse rate is the best indication of whether the nurse should be concerned about the presence of blood in the secretions at this time. Slight bleeding is expected following bronchoscopy due to trauma. If hemorrhage or impaired ventilation occurs, the pulse rate is rapid. Pupillary changes are an indication of brain function. Heart sounds indicate how effectively blood is circulating through the heart chambers. Chest expansion is more likely to change if one lung is not filling adequately with air.

Client Needs Category—Physiological integrity
Client Needs Subcategory—Physiological adaptation

85. 4. Gloves are the most important barrier garment in this situation. Gloves are worn whenever there is a possibility of contact with body fluids containing blood. Because the nurse is involved in holding the container, the hands need protection. The nurse may opt to don any or all of the other items, depending on the risk of contact with blood by some other means, such as splashing into the eyes, nose, or mouth or onto the uniform.

Client Needs Category—Safe, effective care environment
Client Needs Subcategory—Safety and infection control

86. 1. The nurse establishes that the gag reflex is present before the client is given food or oral fluids following a bronchoscopy. Stimulating the palatal arch causes the client to gag if the effects of the local anesthetic have worn off. The other choices are techniques of physical assessment but are unlikely to be affected by a bronchoscopy.

Client Needs Category—Physiological integrity
Client Needs Subcategory—Reduction of risk potential

87. 4. Pleural effusion is the accumulation of fluid between the pleural membranes. It is common in clients who have lung cancer, pneumonia, tuberculosis, pulmonary embolism, and heart failure. When auscultating the lungs, the nurse can expect to hear decreased breath sounds over the affected area and dullness when the area is percussed. The changes are related to the amount of fluid displacing the lung tissue. Wheezing is heard in clients with asthma. Crackles are sounds that result from the delayed openings of deflated airways; they sometimes clear when the client is coughing. Friction rubs may result from pleural effusion, but they are heard over the affected area, not posterior to it.

Client Needs Category—Physiological integrity
Client Needs Subcategory—Physiological adaptation

88. 2. Thoracentesis involves draining excess pleural fluid from the pleural space by inserting a needle into the chest wall. A client undergoing this procedure is best placed in a sitting position so that the physician has access to the eighth or ninth rib space. It is helpful for the seated client to rest his head and elevate his arms on the overbed table. If this position is impossible, the nurse may alternatively place the client on his unaffected side. A lithotomy position is used for procedures in which the clinician needs access to genitourinary structures, including the vagina, urinary meatus and, possibly, the rectum. A prone or supine position is inappropriate for a thoracentesis.

Client Needs Category—Physiological integrity
Client Needs Subcategory—Physiological adaptation

89. 1. The prefix *pneumo* refers to lung, and the suffix ectomy means removal; therefore, the client would be correct in understanding that the procedure involves removal of his lung. A lobectomy involves the removal of only a lobe of the lung. Although a pneumonectomy may involve taking a lung sample or opening a lung for examination, these are not the primary reason for performing the surgical procedure.

Client Needs Category—Physiological integrity
Client Needs Subcategory—Physiological adaptation

90. 1. The client with a pneumonectomy lies with the healthy, nonoperative lung uppermost. This position allows for better lung expansion and oxygenation. If the affected side were upward, ventilation would be compromised because of the compression of the remaining healthy lung between the mattress and body weight. Lying with the head lowered interferes with breathing because abdominal contents press against the diaphragm. Elevating the arms on pillows may be an optional position to use if the client's breathing becomes labored.

Client Needs Category—Physiological integrity
Client Needs Subcategory—Reduction of risk potential

91. 2. Removal of the lung is often accompanied by interruption of the intercostal nerves. As a consequence, clients who undergo a pneumonectomy may experience temporary numbness in the operative area. Sore throat and impaired swallowing are related to endotracheal intubation and not the surgery itself. If the client has a persistent cough, it is more likely related to a preexisting disease rather than an expected outcome of the surgical procedure.

Client Needs Category—Physiological integrity
Client Needs Subcategory—Physiological adaptation

92. 4. Morphine sulfate (Roxanol), an opioid analgesic, depresses respiratory rate and depth. If the respiratory rate is severely compromised, the client will have inadequate oxygenation. Morphine indirectly affects heart rate by decreasing the pain that elevates it. Heart rhythm is unaffected. Assessing the skin color and temperature is not related to the use of morphine. Morphine does slow peristalsis, and bowel sounds should be assessed frequently; however, this is not the most important assessment to make.

Client Needs Category—*Physiological integrity*
Client Needs Subcategory—*Pharmacological therapies*

Nursing Care of Clients with Chest Injuries

93. **1.** To prevent the widespread collapse of alveoli known as *atelectasis,* clients with fractured ribs are instructed to breathe deeply several times every hour. People with fractured ribs have a natural tendency to breathe shallowly to avoid discomfort; however, shallow breathing promotes atelectasis. Breathing rapidly leads to respiratory alkalosis. Breathing into a paper bag promotes an increased level of carbon dioxide in the blood, which is appropriate for individuals who are hyperventilating and becoming light-headed.

Client Needs Category—*Health promotion and maintenance*
Client Needs Subcategory—*None*

94. **3.** Flail chest is a condition in which three or more ribs are broken in two or more places, making the chest wall unstable. Paradoxic movement of the unstable section during inspiration and expiration characterizes this condition. In other words, when the client takes a breath, an area of the chest wall moves inward; when the client exhales, the area moves outward. A sucking chest wound and tracheal deviation are associated with a pneumothorax. Chest pain only exhibited during expiration is not a common finding of flail chest.

Client Needs Category—*Physiological integrity*
Client Needs Subcategory—*Physiological adaptation*

95. **4.** When a person experiences a hemothorax, blood collects and drains by gravity through the tube in the lower chest. Air in the chest rises and exits through the tube in the upper chest. It would be unusual to see blood coming from the victim's nose or mouth in this situation. If the client has a productive cough, his sputum may be blood-tinged.

Client Needs Category—*Physiological integrity*
Client Needs Subcategory—*Physiological adaptation*

96. **1.** The fluid in the water-seal chamber should rise and fall in synchrony with respirations or may bubble intermittently immediately after the tube has been inserted. If the lung has expanded, if the drainage system is connected to suction, or if the tubing is kinked or plugged, the rise and fall of fluid and intermittent bubbling would not be seen. If the fluid level falls below the filling line of 2 cm, more fluid should be added. Contin-

uous bubbling indicates a leak in the system. The fluid in the water-seal chamber should be clear.

Client Needs Category—*Physiological integrity*
Client Needs Subcategory—*Physiological adaptation*

97. **3.** Air that is leaking and becoming trapped within the local tissue at the insertion site crackles when touched. The crackling sound, called *crepitus* or *subcutaneous emphysema,* resembles that of crisp rice cereal when mixed with milk. The nurse would not feel puffs of air or hear a hissing sound because the air does not escape into the atmosphere. The air tends to diffuse into the tissue and rise to the upper part of the body. Eventually, the client's face and neck may appear swollen and the tissue around the chest may appear pale; however, this is not a phenomenon directly linked to an air leak.

Client Needs Category—*Physiological integrity*
Client Needs Subcategory—*Physiological adaptation*

98. **2.** When transporting a client to another area of the hospital via stretcher, the water-seal drainage collector is always kept below the tubes' insertion sites to facilitate drainage. As long as the water seal is maintained, the client's lung function should be unaffected. Clamping the chest tubes for an appreciable amount of time would lead to a tension pneumothorax. Suction is not applied directly to the chest tubes. Suction may be added to the water-seal system, but the tube connecting to the suction source is disconnected when the client is ambulated or transported from the room. Mechanical ventilation is necessary only when a client cannot maintain adequate oxygenation even with supplemental oxygen. In that case, a portable X-ray may be ordered and taken to the client's room.

Client Needs Category—*Physiological integrity*
Client Needs Subcategory—*Physiological adaptation*

99. **4.** At the beginning of each shift, the nurse should assess the color, consistency, and amount of drainage present in the water-seal system. The nurse marks the level of drainage on the calibrated collection chamber with the date and time. The drainage volume is calculated by subtracting the previously marked volume from the current total volume. The drainage compartment is never emptied while the chest tube is in place. Subtracting fluid intake from output only helps in evaluating the status of the client's total fluid balance. Chest tubes are not irrigated.

Client Needs Category—*Physiological integrity*
Client Needs Subcategory—*Physiological adaptation*

100.

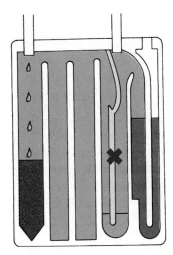

The middle chamber contains the water seal, which bubbles intermittently with the client's respirations until the lung expands. As air exits from the chest tube, it diffuses through the water in the middle compartment and eventually vents into the atmosphere. The water in the middle compartment acts as a seal or barrier, preventing atmospheric air from entering the system and keeping the lung collapsed. The first compartment of multiconnected columns collects bloody drainage. The remaining compartment contains fluid that regulates the amount of suction applied to the system.

Client Needs Category—Physiological integrity
Client Needs Subcategory—Physiological
adaptation

Nursing Care of Clients with Pulmonary Embolism

101. 1. Pulmonary emboli are obstructions (clots) in one or more of the pulmonary vessels. The usual site for clot formation is in the deep veins of the legs or in the pelvis. Conditions that predispose a client to pulmonary emboli include recent surgery, bed rest, immobility, trauma, obesity, and postpartal status. Clots are more likely to form in the veins, where there is venous stasis, although they can form anywhere. They are less likely to form in the pulmonary artery or the carotid artery because the blood pressure is higher in those vessels.

Client Needs Category—Physiological integrity
Client Needs Subcategory—Physiological
adaptation

102. 2. Staying with a frightened client is one of the best methods for relieving or reducing anxiety. Telling the client that symptoms will lessen in a few minutes is nontherapeutic because it offers false reassurance. Asking a "why" question is also nontherapeutic because this demands an explanation from the client rather than acceptance of his feelings. Asking if the client's finances are in order avoids the issue and, therefore, is nontherapeutic.

Client Needs Category—Psychosocial integrity
Client Needs Subcategory—None

103. 1. Administering oxygen is the most significant immediate action for reducing the client's dyspnea and chest pain. The ABCs (airway, breathing, and circulation) are priorities at this point. Assessing capillary refill is a good choice and can be a useful way to monitor tissue perfusion, but it is not the priority action when the client is experiencing chest pain and dyspnea. Having the client rate the pain on a pain scale is another good choice, but not the priority at this time. Cardiac enzymes are ordered for clients suspected of having a myocardial infarction, not a pulmonary embolism.

Client Needs Category—Physiological integrity
Client Needs Subcategory—Physiological
adaptation

104. 1. I.V. heparin (Hep-Lock) is given to treat a pulmonary embolism. This drug prevents further clot development as well as the showering of mini emboli. Through the course of treatment, the client receives I.V. heparin (Hep-Lock) followed by subcutaneous enoxaprin sodium (Lovenox) and heparin, and finally by warfarin (Coumadin), which is given orally. Clotting studies are drawn frequently during anticoagulant therapy. Aminophylline (Truphylline), a bronchodilator, is not used to treat pulmonary embolism. Nitroglycerin (Nitrodisc) is a vasodilator commonly used to treat angina. Aspirin (Anacin), while having anticoagulant properties, is not the drug of choice for this disorder.

Client Needs Category—Physiological integrity
Client Needs Subcategory—Pharmacological
therapies

105. 2. Anyone over the age of 8 is given rescue breaths at a rate of 12 breaths per minute. Infants and children up to the age of 8 are given 20 breaths per minute.

Client Needs Category—Physiological integrity
Client Needs Subcategory—Physiological
adaptation

Nursing Care of Clients with a Tracheostomy

106. 3. Wet breath sounds indicate that secretions are accumulating within the airway. Because a client with a tracheostomy lacks the ability to cough effectively, the nurse protects and maintains an open airway for him. A fast respiratory rate or labored respirations indicate that oxygenation is impaired. A rapid pulse rate is more likely to indicate impaired ventilation.

An elevated blood pressure is unrelated to the need for oxygenation.

Client Needs Category—Physiological integrity
Client Needs Subcategory—Reduction of risk potential

107. **2.** Prior to suctioning the client, the catheter is moistened by immersing it in sterile normal saline solution, then suctioning the solution through the lumen. This tests the function of the suction machine and reduces the surface tension inside the plastic catheter. Although clients with artificial airways need frequent mouth care, this is not essential before performing tracheal suctioning. The stoma is cleaned from time to time, but this does not have to be done before suctioning the airway. The airway is suctioned before removing the inner cannula for cleaning.

Client Needs Category—Physiological integrity
Client Needs Subcategory—Reduction of risk potential

108. **3.** The vent on a suction catheter is occluded after the catheter is fully inserted and being withdrawn. This reduces the potential for hypoxemia. Closing the vent before insertion or when the catheter is just inside the inner cannula prolongs the time that oxygen is removed from the airway. Coughing may or may not coincide with the proper time to occlude the vent; therefore, it is not used as a criterion for this action.

Client Needs Category—Physiological integrity
Client Needs Subcategory—Physiological adaptation

109. **2.** Suctioning should not extend beyond 10 to 12 seconds. Some suggest holding one's own breath during suctioning. This technique promotes awareness of the air hunger the client is experiencing. Suctioning for too little time will not effectively clear the airway. Suctioning longer than 15 seconds causes hypoxemia.

Client Needs Category—Physiological integrity
Client Needs Subcategory—Physiological adaptation

110. **4.** Twisting and rotating the catheter during its withdrawal helps remove secretions located in all directions within the airway. Withdrawing the catheter slowly causes the nurse to exceed the recommended time for suctioning. Neither pinching and pulling the catheter nor plunging it up and down is an acceptable technique during suctioning.

Client Needs Category—Physiological integrity
Client Needs Subcategory—Physiological adaptation

111. **3.** Hypoxemia refers to a decreased amount of oxygen in the blood. Monitoring the pulse oximeter is useful for detecting the saturation of hemoglobin with oxygen. It takes a prolonged state of hypoxemia to alter a client's level of consciousness, skin color, and respiratory rate.

Client Needs Category—Physiological integrity
Client Needs Subcategory—Physiological adaptation

112. **1, 2, 3, 6.** A client's fingernail polish or acrylic nails should be removed before monitoring with a pulse oximeter because they interfere with the transmission of light. The LED and photodetector must be aligned opposite each other on the monitoring site for an accurate reading. A pulse oximeter functions by delivering sensed data to the monitor via a cable. Some pulse oximeters are attached with an adhesive band. Others are spring-loaded; both types must be relocated periodically to avoid injuring the skin.

An arterial oxygen saturation (SpO_2) of at least 95% is clinically acceptable as normal; therefore, the SpO_2 alarm should be set to sound when it detects a level below 95%. (Many agencies suggest setting the alarm for a measurement that is below 85%.) An SpO_2 of 90% is equated with a partial pressure of oxygen of 60 mm Hg, an indication that the client could benefit from the supplemental administration of oxygen. When an alarm sounds, the nurse assesses the client to determine if the sensing device has become loose or has been removed, the client is restless and causing some artifacts that the machine is interpreting as significant changes, or the client is hypoxic. The nurse would notify the physician only if measures to improve the client's oxygenation status, such as administering supplemental oxygen, are ineffective.

Client Needs Category—Physiological integrity
Client Needs Subcategory—Reduction of risk potential

113. **3.** To prevent the possibility that the client may cough the tracheostomy tube out of his airway, the old ties are not removed until the replacement ties are secured. Gauze squares are not cut to fashion a stomal dressing because the cut threads may enter the airway and irritate the tissue. Special drain sponges or tracheostomy dressing materials are used, or gauze is folded rather than cut to fit around the stoma. The inner cannula is replaced as soon as it is cleaned, rinsed, and dried, or within at least 5 minutes. A delay in replacing the inner cannula may cause mucus secretions to accumulate and dry in the outer cannula. This alters the size of the opening and interferes with replacement.

Client Needs Category—Physiological integrity
Client Needs Subcategory—Physiological adaptation

114. **2.** A cuff on a tracheostomy tube forms a tight seal, preventing liquid nasopharyngeal secretions, stomach contents, or tube-feeding formula from entering the lower respiratory passages. If the person is receiving mechanical ventilation, the cuff ensures that the oxygenated air does not escape before it is delivered to the lower areas of the lungs. An inflated cuff may lead to tissue breakdown because the pressure occludes capillary blood flow. Using a cuffed tracheostomy tube does not provide more comfort or reduce infection any better than an uncuffed tracheostomy tube.

> ***Client Needs Category***—*Physiological integrity*
> ***Client Needs Subcategory***—*Physiological adaptation*

Nursing Care of Clients with a Sudden Airway Occlusion

115. **2.** The ability to cough indicates that the foreign object in the airway is not totally obstructing the air passage. As long as the person has only a partial obstruction, he is capable of coughing to clear his own airway. The victim's ability to walk is not important except to verify that the brain is still receiving oxygen and he hasn't lost consciousness. The victim's position is not the most important data to obtain at this time. The ability to swallow will not dislodge an object that is in the victim's airway.

> ***Client Needs Category***—*Physiological integrity*
> ***Client Needs Subcategory***—*Physiological adaptation*

116. **4.** The thumb side of the fist is placed against the abdomen, below the sternum but above the navel. The xiphoid process is the tip of the sternum, and the manubrium is the upper portion of the sternum. Neither location is used when performing the Heimlich maneuver.

> ***Client Needs Category***—*Physiological integrity*
> ***Client Needs Subcategory***—*Physiological adaptation*

TEST 8

The Nursing Care of Clients with Disorders of the Gastrointestinal System and Accessory Organs of Digestion

⇨ **Nursing Care of Clients with Disorders of the Mouth**
⇨ **Nursing Care of Clients with Disorders of the Esophagus**
⇨ **Nursing Care of Clients with Disorders of the Stomach**
⇨ **Nursing Care of Clients with Disorders of the Small Intestine**
⇨ **Nursing Care of Clients with Disorders of the Large Intestine**
⇨ **Nursing Care of Clients with Disorders of the Rectum and Anus**
⇨ **Nursing Care of Clients with Disorders of the Gallbladder**
⇨ **Nursing Care of Clients with Disorders of the Liver**
⇨ **Nursing Care of Clients with Disorders of the Pancreas**
⇨ **Correct Answers and Rationales**

Directions: With a pencil, blacken the space in front of the option you have chosen for your correct answer.

Nursing Care of Clients with Disorders of the Mouth

A client develops mucositis of the oral cavity while receiving chemotherapy for cancer.

1. Which food item is best for the nurse to withhold from the client's dietary tray?
[ ] **1.** Tomato soup
[ ] **2.** Lime gelatin
[ ] **3.** Canned peaches
[ ] **4.** Rice pudding

2. If the nurse plans to assist the client with his oral care, which item should be requisitioned to accomplish the goal?
[ ] **1.** A pediatric toothbrush
[ ] **2.** Waxed dental floss
[ ] **3.** Sponge-tipped swabs
[ ] **4.** Mint-flavored mouthwash

A nurse is assigned to care for several clients, all of whom will receive oral hygiene.

3. The nurse should plan specialized oral care twice a day for which client?
[ ] **1.** The patient who has full dentures
[ ] **2.** The patient who is on fluid restrictions
[ ] **3.** The patient who is on a low-residue diet
[ ] **4.** The patient who sucks on ice chips

4. Which technique is most appropriate when providing oral care for a client's dentures?
[ ] **1.** Using hot water while brushing and rinsing the dentures
[ ] **2.** Holding the dentures over a basin of water or a soft towel
[ ] **3.** Applying solvent to remove the oral adhesive from the dentures
[ ] **4.** Placing the dentures in a clean, dry container after brushing

5. When the nurse is brushing an unconscious client's teeth, how should the client be positioned?
[ ] **1.** Supine with his head elevated
[ ] **2.** Side-lying with his head lowered
[ ] **3.** In Trendelenburg's position with his head slightly raised
[ ] **4.** In a dorsal recumbent position with his head elevated

A male client has been taking a tetracycline antibiotic for the past 2 weeks. A candidal infection is suspected at this time.

6. If the client has candidiasis (thrush), which assessment finding is the nurse most likely to observe when inspecting the oral cavity?

[ ] **1.** Clear, shiny, domed vesicles on the tongue
[ ] **2.** Red, ulcerated patches at the gum margin
[ ] **3.** White, curdlike patches throughout the mouth
[ ] **4.** Dark brown, flat lesions in the oropharynx

The client asks the nurse how he may have acquired this oral infection.

7. The nurse correctly explains that most individuals acquire candidiasis (thrush) by which means?

[ ] **1.** Transferring bacteria from unclean dental instruments
[ ] **2.** Having an unchecked growth of normal mouth organisms
[ ] **3.** Inhaling moist droplets when someone sneezed
[ ] **4.** Drinking or eating using someone's unwashed utensils

The physician prescribes nystatin (Mycostatin) oral suspension to treat the client's candidiasis.

8. Which instruction should the nurse plan to give the client when administering the nystatin (Mycostatin) oral suspension?

[ ] **1.** Drink the medication through a straw.
[ ] **2.** Dilute the medication with cold water.
[ ] **3.** Retain the drug as long as possible in the mouth.
[ ] **4.** Swish the drug in the mouth, but avoid swallowing it.

A 70-year-old man is referred for suspected cancer of the mouth following a routine dental examination.

9. If the client is typical of others with this diagnosis, which etiologic factor is the nurse most likely to find when reading his medical history?

[ ] **1.** The client drinks decaffeinated coffee on a daily basis.
[ ] **2.** The client has used smokeless tobacco most of his life.
[ ] **3.** The client has had a partial dental plate for 5 years.
[ ] **4.** The client has poor dental hygiene with several rotting teeth.

The client's oral cancer is treated with needles containing radioactive cesium that are implanted inside his cheek.

10. Which addition to the care plan is essential for the nurse to make in case the client should vomit after receiving the radioactive implants?

[ ] **1.** Inspect emesis for solid objects before disposing.
[ ] **2.** Rinse the emesis basin with diluted household bleach.
[ ] **3.** Provide a plastic emesis basin rather than a metal one.
[ ] **4.** Cut threads to implanted cesium if vomiting occurs.

11. Assuming the client enjoys all of the following diversional activities, the nurse knows which one is best while he is receiving radiation therapy?

[ ] **1.** Allowing the client's family to visit as long as they like
[ ] **2.** Spending an hour playing cards with the client
[ ] **3.** Providing the client with kits for building miniature airplanes
[ ] **4.** Encouraging the other clients to join him in playing board games

While being prepared for a gynecologic examination, a woman discusses the herpes simplex type 1 lesion on her mouth, which she refers to as a "cold sore."

12. Which statement made by the client indicates that further instruction is needed?

[ ] **1.** "My mouth sore started from a viral infection."
[ ] **2.** "The infection is spread by direct contact."
[ ] **3.** "Emotional stress can trigger a recurrence."
[ ] **4.** "The sores can only form on the lips or in the mouth."

The client tells the nurse that she has been taking acyclovir (Zovirax), which was prescribed by her physician to treat her herpes lesions.

13. Which statement indicates that the client understands the purpose for her drug therapy?

[ ] **1.** "I know that this drug will kill all the virus causing the lesion."
[ ] **2.** "The drug shortens the duration of an outbreak."
[ ] **3.** "The drug prevents future outbreaks from occurring."
[ ] **4.** "I'll need to take the drug daily for the rest of my life."

Nursing Care of Clients with Disorders of the Esophagus

A 60-year-old male client has been experiencing difficulty swallowing. The nurse in the ambulatory surgery department schedules him for an esophagoscopy.

14. Which statement made by the client indicates that he understands the preparations necessary for an esophagoscopy?
[ ] **1.** "I need to eat a light breakfast before the examination."
[ ] **2.** "I should consume a low-residue diet until the test has been completed."
[ ] **3.** "I need to avoid food and fluids after midnight before the test."
[ ] **4.** "I have to drink a quart of liquid before arriving for the test."

The esophagoscopy reveals that the client has a stricture near the end of his esophagus.

15. To help improve the client's ability to swallow, which recommendation made by the nurse is most appropriate?
[ ] **1.** Eat a variety of foods containing a thickener.
[ ] **2.** Thoroughly chew everything that is eaten.
[ ] **3.** Avoid drinking beverages while eating a meal.
[ ] **4.** Refrain from consuming milk and dairy products.

A 38-year-old man is admitted with bleeding esophageal varices. He will have a transfusion.

16. As the nurse reviews the client's medical record, which factor is most likely related to his present condition?
[ ] **1.** The client has attempted suicide by ingesting lye.
[ ] **2.** The client has a history of oral cancer.
[ ] **3.** The client is a known hemophiliac.
[ ] **4.** The client drinks alcohol heavily.

The registered nurse (RN) starts an infusion of whole blood and asks the licensed practical nurse (LPN) to continue monitoring the client during the blood transfusion.

17. According to the National Patient Safety Goals, which nursing action regarding blood administration is most appropriate?
[ ] **1.** Two licensed personnel must review the blood bag and arm bracelet of the client prior to administration.
[ ] **2.** An indwelling (Foley) catheter must be placed during the transfusion.
[ ] **3.** An I.V. using a 22-gauge needle should be started prior to administration.
[ ] **4.** Each unit of blood should be completed within 12 hours of starting it.

18. Which assessment finding provides the best indication that a transfusion reaction is occurring?
[ ] **1.** The client's urine is very dark yellow.
[ ] **2.** The client suddenly becomes dyspneic.
[ ] **3.** The client's skin is pale and cool.
[ ] **4.** The client says he is extremely thirsty.

During a routine home visit, a client describes what the nurse believes may be symptoms related to gastro-esophageal reflux disease (GERD).

19. Which symptom would the nurse expect to be this client's chief complaint?
[ ] **1.** Vomiting
[ ] **2.** Nausea
[ ] **3.** Anorexia
[ ] **4.** Heartburn

20. Until a physician can see the client, which suggestion should the nurse offer to provide some relief from the symptoms?
[ ] **1.** Eat three well-balanced meals a day.
[ ] **2.** Eat foods that are easy to swallow.
[ ] **3.** Avoid lying down after eating.
[ ] **4.** Drink clear liquids at room temperature.

21. Which modification in the client's position is most appropriate to recommend at this time?
[ ] **1.** Have the client remain supine on a mattress that contains a bed board.
[ ] **2.** Advise the client to sleep on a water bed temporarily.
[ ] **3.** Tell the client to elevate his legs on pillows when retiring at night.
[ ] **4.** Have the client raise the head of his bed on 4-inch blocks.

A 75-year-old man with metastatic cancer of the esophagus is undergoing palliative treatment that includes total parenteral nutrition (TPN) through a central subclavian catheter.

22. Which nursing assessment is essential for evaluating the client's response to the TPN?
[ ] **1.** Test the urine's specific gravity.
[ ] **2.** Monitor the capillary blood glucose level.
[ ] **3.** Measure the arterial pulse pressure.
[ ] **4.** Obtain an apical-radial pulse rate.

23. Which finding documented in the client's chart is the best evidence that he is responding favorably to the administration of TPN?
[ ] **1.** The client's electrolytes are in balance.
[ ] **2.** The client is gaining weight.
[ ] **3.** The client's appetite is returning.
[ ] **4.** The client is pain-free.

In anticipation of transferring the client to a nursing home, the physician inserts a gastrostomy tube for nourishment.

24. Immediately after the gastrostomy tube is inserted, which finding should the nurse consider normal when assessing the gastrostomy drainage?
[ ] **1.** Milky drainage
[ ] **2.** Serosanguineous drainage
[ ] **3.** Green-tinged drainage
[ ] **4.** Bright, bloody drainage

25. Which technique is best to determine if the gastrostomy tube has migrated after being inserted?
[ ] **1.** Testing the pH of aspirated secretions
[ ] **2.** Monitoring the results of stomach X-rays
[ ] **3.** Measuring the length of the external tube
[ ] **4.** Palpating the abdomen for distention

The nurse fills a tube-feeding bag with two 8-ounce cans of commercially prepared formula that will infuse continuously through the client's gastrostomy tube via a feeding pump.

26. If the client is to receive 120 mL of formula per hour, the nurse can expect that the entire bag of formula will be empty in how many hours?
[ ] **1.** 2
[ ] **2.** 4
[ ] **3.** 6
[ ] **4.** 8

While the tube-feeding formula is infusing, the client tells the nurse that he is feeling full and nauseated.

27. Which nursing action is most appropriate at this time?
[ ] **1.** Measure the stomach residual.
[ ] **2.** Administer an antiemetic per gastrostomy tube.
[ ] **3.** Stop the infusion temporarily.
[ ] **4.** Add water to dilute the formula.

28. After the tube-feeding formula has infused, which action should the nurse take next?
[ ] **1.** Place the client on his left side.
[ ] **2.** Lower the head of the client's bed.
[ ] **3.** Clamp the opening of the gastrostomy tube.
[ ] **4.** Instill several ounces of plain tap water down the tube.

The client with the gastrostomy is silent and withdrawn as the nurse cares for the insertion site.

29. Which statement made by the nurse is most appropriate for encouraging the client to express his feelings?
[ ] **1.** "Are you feeling angry?"
[ ] **2.** "It must be tough for you."
[ ] **3.** "This may get better soon."
[ ] **4.** "Lots of people eat this way."

Nursing Care of Clients with Disorders of the Stomach

A 46-year-old woman is hospitalized to determine the cause of the intermittent gnawing epigastric pain she is experiencing. The admitting nurse obtains the client's health history and suspects a peptic ulcer.

30. Based on the suspected condition, the nurse would expect the client to report that her epigastric pain decreases with which activity?
[ ] **1.** When she skips a meal
[ ] **2.** When she goes to bed
[ ] **3.** When she eats food
[ ] **4.** When she bends over

31. In addition to the client's clinical presentation, which positive laboratory finding provides further evidence that the client's symptoms are related to a peptic ulcer?
[ ] **1.** Urine that is positive for albumin
[ ] **2.** Blood that is positive for glucose
[ ] **3.** Stool that is positive for blood
[ ] **4.** Emesis that is positive for pepsin

The client is scheduled for an X-ray of the upper gastrointestinal (GI) tract.

32. After the nurse explains the procedure for performing an upper GI X-ray, which statement by the client best indicates that she understands what this test involves?
[ ] **1.** "A flexible tube will be inserted into my stomach."
[ ] **2.** "Dye will be infused into my vein before the test."
[ ] **3.** "My body will be placed within an imaging chamber."
[ ] **4.** "I'll have to swallow a large amount of barium."

Diagnostic tests reveal that the client has a duodenal ulcer. The physician writes an order for a tetracycline antibiotic and for 1 ounce of bismuth subsalicylate (Pepto-Bismol) to be administered every 6 hours.

33. When preparing the client's medication, the nurse correctly administers which equivalent volume?
[ ] **1.** 30 mL
[ ] **2.** 15 mL
[ ] **3.** 10 mL
[ ] **4.** 5 mL

The client asks the nurse why the physician has prescribed an antibiotic for her ulcer.

34. Which explanation by the nurse regarding the use of antibiotics for ulcer therapy is most accurate?
[ ] **1.** Antibiotics heal the irritated mucous membrane of the stomach.
[ ] **2.** Antibiotics eliminate a microorganism that depletes gastric mucus.
[ ] **3.** Antibiotics add a protective coating over the ulcerated mucosa.
[ ] **4.** Antibiotics prevent secondary gastrointestinal infections.

The licensed practical nurse (LPN) assists the team leader in planning the client's discharge teaching. Their goal is to provide the client with information that will help prevent further gastrointestinal irritation.

35. The nurse should instruct the client to follow the label directions when taking which medication to relieve occasional pain and discomfort associated with her ulcer?
[ ] **1.** Acetaminophen (Tylenol)
[ ] **2.** Aspirin (Anacin)
[ ] **3.** Ibuprofen (Advil)
[ ] **4.** Naproxen (Naprosyn)

The nurse prepares a client with a history of recurrent peptic ulcer disease for abdominal surgery.

36. As the nurse performs a head-to-toe physical assessment, which finding best indicates that the client's ulcer has perforated?
[ ] **1.** The client's skin is ecchymotic.
[ ] **2.** The client's abdomen feels boardlike.
[ ] **3.** The client's pupils are widely dilated.
[ ] **4.** The client's respirations are rapid.

The nurse inserts a gastric sump tube in the client with the perforated ulcer and asks an LPN to check its placement.

37. Which is the most appropriate technique for determining if the distal end of the tube is in the stomach?
[ ] **1.** Requesting a portable X-ray of the stomach
[ ] **2.** Listening over the stomach as air is instilled
[ ] **3.** Adding 100 mL of tap water into the tube
[ ] **4.** Feeling for air at the proximal end of the tube

The client with the perforated ulcer senses the critical nature of his condition and asks the nurse, "Am I going to die?"

38. Which response by the nurse is most appropriate?
[ ] **1.** "We are doing everything we can right now to help you."
[ ] **2.** "That is something you'll have to ask your physician."
[ ] **3.** "Now what kind of a silly question is that?"
[ ] **4.** "I've seen patients with similar problems pull through."

A gastrojejunostomy, also called a Billroth II, is performed to treat the client's perforated ulcer. He returns to his room after recovering from the anesthesia.

39. When the client does not adequately cough and deep-breathe postoperatively due to incisional pain, which nursing action is most appropriate at this time?
[ ] **1.** Explain that he is at high risk for developing pneumonia.
[ ] **2.** Have him press a pillow against his incision when coughing.
[ ] **3.** Ask the physician to order some oxygen for him.
[ ] **4.** Keep the head of the bed elevated at all times.

The nurse notes that the nasogastric (NG) tube placed during the client's gastrojejunostomy has stopped draining.

40. Which technique is most appropriate when the nurse irrigates the NG tube?
[ ] **1.** Instilling 30 mL of sterile distilled water into the tube
[ ] **2.** Administering oxygen before the irrigation
[ ] **3.** Recording the volume instilled and removed
[ ] **4.** Asking the client to swallow frequently

The nurse is completing the intake and output for a client with a nursing diagnosis of Risk for deficient fluid volume.

41. Based on the following food intake within the last 8 hours, how many milliliters of intake should the nurse record?

1 cup of thin, cooked cereal
1 8-ounce carton of milk
¼ cup of ice cream
8 ounces of supplemental nutritional drink
6 ounces of creamed soup
½ cup of fruit-flavored gelatin

The nurse creates a teaching plan for a client who develops dumping syndrome following a gastrojejunostomy.

42. After providing the client with dietary instructions for preventing dumping syndrome, which statement by the client indicates that teaching has been effective?
[ ] **1.** "I should drink a large volume of liquid at meals."
[ ] **2.** "I should restrict eating sugary and starchy food."
[ ] **3.** "It would be best to eat large meals during the day."
[ ] **4.** "It would be best to reduce my intake of red meat."

43. Which advice would the nurse offer to a client recovering from a gastrojejunostomy to prevent symptoms associated with dumping syndrome. Select all that apply.
[ ] **1.** Consume a generous intake of fluid during meals.
[ ] **2.** Avoid eating simple carbohydrates.
[ ] **3.** Restrict consumption of raw fruits and vegetables.
[ ] **4.** Eat several small meals throughout the day.
[ ] **5.** Lie down for 30 minutes after a meal.
[ ] **6.** Chew food thoroughly while eating.

A 74-year-old client experiences persistent indigestion, feeling of gastric fullness, and unexplained weight loss.

44. When reviewing the results of the client's diagnostic tests, which finding would strongly suggest to the nurse that the client's symptoms are related to stomach cancer?
[ ] **1.** Gastric analysis showing absence of hydrochloric acid
[ ] **2.** An elevated level of gastrin in the blood
[ ] **3.** Gastric irritation noted during a gastroscopy
[ ] **4.** A decrease in hemoglobin and hematocrit

The client is diagnosed with stomach cancer and scheduled for a total gastrectomy. A single-lumen nasogastric (NG) tube is inserted preoperatively.

45. Which instruction should the nurse give the client when the tube is in the oropharynx?
[ ] **1.** "Breathe deeply as the tube is advanced."
[ ] **2.** "Hold your head in a sniffing position."
[ ] **3.** "Press your chin to your upper chest."
[ ] **4.** "Avoid coughing until the tube is down."

46. Number the following nursing actions in ascending order based on how the nurse would perform an NG tube insertion. Use all the options.

1. Instruct the client to lower his chin to his chest.
2. Have the client sip water through a straw.
3. Secure the tube to the client's nose.
4. Inspect the client's nares.
5. Place the client's head in a sniffing position.
6. Aspirate and check the pH of fluid from the tube.

47. Which setting is most appropriate to use when connecting the client's single-lumen NG tube to suction preoperatively?
[ ] **1.** Low intermittent suction
[ ] **2.** Low continuous suction
[ ] **3.** High intermittent suction
[ ] **4.** High continuous suction

Following surgery, the client informs the nurse that he is very thirsty.

48. In response to the client's statement, which nursing intervention is most appropriate to add to the care plan?
[ ] **1.** Offer fluids at least every 2 hours.
[ ] **2.** Provide crushed ice in sparse amounts.
[ ] **3.** Increase oral liquids on dietary tray.
[ ] **4.** Refill the water pitcher twice each shift.

One year after his gastrectomy, the client develops pernicious anemia. A home health nurse administers 1,000 mcg of vitamin B$_{12}$ intramuscularly every month.

49. If the label on the vial of vitamin B$_{12}$ indicates that there is 1 mg of drug per mL of solution, the nurse is accurate in withdrawing which amount?

[ ] **1.** 0.1 mL
[ ] **2.** 1 mL
[ ] **3.** 10 mL
[ ] **4.** 0.01 mL

The nurse chooses to use the vastus lateralis muscle as the site for the I.M. vitamin B$_{12}$ injection.

50. If the correct technique for administering the injection is followed, the nurse should give the injection in which location?

[ ] **1.** Upper arm at a 45-degree angle
[ ] **2.** Outer thigh at a 90-degree angle
[ ] **3.** Anterior thigh at a 90-degree angle
[ ] **4.** Outer buttock at a 45-degree angle

Nursing Care of Clients with Disorders of the Small Intestine

A 19-year-old female client has been having up to five loose stools per day. She is undergoing diagnostic testing and symptomatic treatment.

51. When the nurse collects a stool specimen for ova and parasites, which action is correct?

[ ] **1.** The nurse holds a specimen container under the client's rectum.
[ ] **2.** The nurse places the collected specimen in a sterile container.
[ ] **3.** The nurse refrigerates the covered specimen after collection.
[ ] **4.** The nurse immediately takes the specimen to the laboratory.

The physician has prescribed diphenoxylate hydrochloride (Lomotil) 5 mg orally q.i.d. for the client's diarrhea.

52. When the nurse checks the medication administration record, which military time schedule for administering this drug is most accurate?

[ ] **1.** 0730, 1130, 0430
[ ] **2.** 0600, 1200, 1800, 0000
[ ] **3.** 0900, 1300, 1700
[ ] **4.** 0400, 0800, 1200, 1600, 2000

The physician restricts the client's diet to include only clear liquids.

53. When the client asks for something to eat, which food is most appropriate for the nurse to provide?

[ ] **1.** Milk
[ ] **2.** Pudding
[ ] **3.** Gelatin
[ ] **4.** Custard

The nurse assesses the client for signs of fluid volume deficit related to the diarrhea.

54. Which assessment finding is most likely to indicate that the client is becoming dehydrated?

[ ] **1.** Elevated blood pressure
[ ] **2.** Irregular heart rate
[ ] **3.** Pink mucous membranes
[ ] **4.** Dark yellow urine

The physician orders a colonoscopy because of the client's persistent diarrhea. The nurse instructs the client to drink 250 mL of an electrolyte solution called GoLYTELY every 15 minutes over a 2-hour period.

55. Which observation by the nurse provides the best evidence that the solution has achieved its primary purpose?

[ ] **1.** The client's serum electrolyte levels are normal.
[ ] **2.** The client's intake approximates her output.
[ ] **3.** The client's stools become clear liquid.
[ ] **4.** The client's bladder fills with urine.

Before the colonoscopy, the client is given moderate sedation using the drug midazolam hydrochloride (Versed).

56. During the colonoscopy and in the immediate recovery period, it is essential that the nurse assess the client closely for which potential undesirable effect of midazolam hydrochloride (Versed)?

[ ] **1.** Unstable blood pressure
[ ] **2.** Cardiac rhythm disturbance
[ ] **3.** Respiratory depression
[ ] **4.** Altered consciousness

The colonoscopy reveals that the client with diarrhea has Crohn's disease. The physician places the client on a fiber-controlled diet.

57. After talking with the dietitian, the client demonstrates an understanding of the therapeutic diet by indicating that fiber refers to which substance?

[ ] **1.** Foods that require chewing
[ ] **2.** The muscle found in red meat
[ ] **3.** The semisolid mass in the stomach
[ ] **4.** The indigestible part of plants

The client eventually develops a draining fistula between a loop of the ileum and the skin. The nursing team meets to revise the client's care plan.

58. Based on this new complication, which problem should the nursing team consider the highest priority when planning the client's care?
[ ] **1.** Pain from complex dressing changes
[ ] **2.** Skin breakdown
[ ] **3.** Body image
[ ] **4.** Containment of the odor from the wound

Nursing Care of Clients with Disorders of the Large Intestine

A 52-year-old man is admitted to the ambulatory surgery department for repair of an inguinal hernia. The nurse takes the operative consent form to the client to obtain his signature. The form states that the surgical procedure will be a right inguinal herniorrhaphy.

59. When the client states to the nurse, "I hope I can get along without that section of my bowel," which action should the nurse take next?
[ ] **1.** Cancel the surgery.
[ ] **2.** Notify the physician.
[ ] **3.** Witness his signature.
[ ] **4.** Shave his right groin.

The client returns from surgery, which was performed under spinal anesthesia.

60. Which postoperative order should the nurse question before carrying it out?
[ ] **1.** Diet as tolerated
[ ] **2.** Fluids as desired
[ ] **3.** Vitals until stable
[ ] **4.** Fowler's position

61. Which postoperative assessment should the nurse consider a priority after the client's herniorrhaphy?
[ ] **1.** Ability to urinate
[ ] **2.** Coughing efforts
[ ] **3.** Level of consciousness
[ ] **4.** Pain tolerance

After surgery, the nurse brings a suspensory (slinglike support) for the client to apply.

62. Which explanation regarding the use of the suspensory is most appropriate?
[ ] **1.** It is used to prevent sexual impotence.
[ ] **2.** It is used to prevent scrotal edema.
[ ] **3.** It is used to prevent strain on the incision.
[ ] **4.** It is used to prevent wound contamination.

The physician orders meperidine hydrochloride (Demerol) 50 mg I.M. every 4 hours as needed to help relieve the client's pain following surgery.

63. If the drug is supplied in ampules of 100 mg/mL, which amount should the nurse administer?
[ ] **1.** 1.0 mL
[ ] **2.** 0.5 mL
[ ] **3.** 2.0 mL
[ ] **4.** 0.2 mL

64. The nurse appropriately documents the administration of meperidine hydrochloride (Demerol) on the client's medical administration record and in which other area?
[ ] **1.** Computer database
[ ] **2.** Opioid control log
[ ] **3.** Drug enforcement form
[ ] **4.** Pharmacy access book

A 31-year-old woman with a long history of ulcerative colitis is admitted to the hospital for a colectomy.

65. Besides the client's report of severe diarrhea, which other characteristic symptom is the nurse most likely to document when admitting this client?
[ ] **1.** Mucus and blood in the stool
[ ] **2.** Hypoactive bowel sounds
[ ] **3.** Striae on the abdomen
[ ] **4.** Shallow ulcerations in the client's mouth

The nurse assesses the client's abdomen for bowel sounds following the sequential anatomic areas of the bowel.

66. Identify the quadrant the nurse auscultates to assess the proximal portion of the ascending colon.

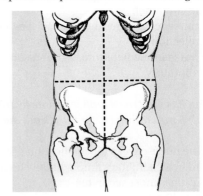

The nursing team includes the nursing diagnosis of Bowel incontinence related to sudden urgency for defecation *on the client's care plan.*

67. Which intervention is most appropriate when managing this nursing diagnosis?

[ ] **1.** Keeping the bedside commode nearby
[ ] **2.** Answering the client's signal for help promptly
[ ] **3.** Putting a disposable diaper on the client
[ ] **4.** Assisting the client to the bathroom frequently

The client tells the nurse that she has been hospitalized several times without much improvement. She is discouraged and states, "I'm sure this surgery will not help either."

68. Which response by the nurse is most appropriate?
[ ] **1.** "You're saying that you doubt that you'll get better."
[ ] **2.** "Do you want to talk to your physician again before surgery?"
[ ] **3.** "I'd recommend a more positive attitude this time around."
[ ] **4.** "Of course surgery will work. Others wish they'd had it done sooner."

69. After giving the client preoperative medications, including meperidine hydrochloride (Demerol), hydroxyzine (Vistaril), and atropine sulfate (Sal-Tropine), what is the most important action for the nurse to perform?
[ ] **1.** Raising the bed side rails
[ ] **2.** Helping the client to the toilet
[ ] **3.** Observing for a dry mouth
[ ] **4.** Placing an emesis basin by the bedside

After recovering from anesthesia following her colectomy, the client is transferred to the nursing unit.

70. When the nurse monitors the client postoperatively, which assessment finding is most indicative of shock?
[ ] **1.** Bounding pulse
[ ] **2.** Slow respirations
[ ] **3.** Low blood pressure
[ ] **4.** High body temperature

The client receives oxygen by nasal cannula at 2 L/minute (28%) postoperatively.

71. If the client is adequately oxygenated, the nurse knows that the pulse oximeter attached to the client's finger should measure oxygen saturation in which range?
[ ] **1.** 25% to 30%
[ ] **2.** 35% to 50%
[ ] **3.** 60% to 80%
[ ] **4.** 95% to 100%

The client's care plan includes providing measures for caring for the ileostomy created at the time of her surgery.

72. Which of the following nursing interventions are appropriate for managing the care of a client with an ileostomy. Select all that apply.
[ ] **1.** Change the faceplate of the appliance and pouch daily.
[ ] **2.** Inspect the size, color, and condition of the stoma.
[ ] **3.** Clean the peristomal area with alcohol or acetone.
[ ] **4.** Attach the opening of the faceplate snugly around the stoma.
[ ] **5.** Empty the pouch of the appliance as soon as stool is expelled.
[ ] **6.** Apply a skin barrier substance to excoriated skin.

73. When implementing the client's care plan, when is the best time of day for the nurse to perform stomal care and to change the appliance?
[ ] **1.** After the client awakens in the morning
[ ] **2.** After the client has showered after breakfast
[ ] **3.** After the client has been ambulating in the hall
[ ] **4.** After the client finishes the evening meal

74. The nurse assesses the stoma of the ileostomy, which, if normal, should be which color?
[ ] **1.** Pale pink
[ ] **2.** Bright red
[ ] **3.** Dark tan
[ ] **4.** Dusky blue

75. When the nurse cleans the skin around the client's stoma, which technique is most appropriate?
[ ] **1.** Cleaning the area with povidone-iodine (Betadine)
[ ] **2.** Swabbing the skin with 70% alcohol
[ ] **3.** Using water and mild soap
[ ] **4.** Scrubbing the skin with peroxide

76. Which technique is most accurate when changing the ileostomy appliance?
[ ] **1.** Placing the faceplate over the opening of the stoma so it occludes it
[ ] **2.** Cutting the appliance opening ⅛″ to ¼″ larger than the stoma
[ ] **3.** Adhering the appliance after the skin has air-dried for 30 minutes
[ ] **4.** Securing the appliance snugly at the waist or belt line

77. Which activity is most unrealistic for a female client with a conventional ileostomy?
[ ] **1.** Swimming
[ ] **2.** Playing tennis
[ ] **3.** Becoming pregnant
[ ] **4.** Controlling defecation

A 20-year-old man comes to the emergency department with pain that is localized on the lower right side of the abdomen, halfway between the umbilicus and the crest of the ileum. The physician suspects appendicitis.

78. Which laboratory test ordered on admission is most important for the nurse to monitor at this time?
[ ] **1.** Bilirubin level
[ ] **2.** Serum potassium level
[ ] **3.** Prothrombin time
[ ] **4.** Leukocyte count

79. If the client is typical of others with appendicitis, the nurse can expect that when the client's abdomen is palpated midway between the umbilicus and right iliac crest, he will experience which adverse effect?
[ ] **1.** More pain when pressure is released
[ ] **2.** A lack of sensation of pain or pressure on palpation
[ ] **3.** Extreme discomfort with the slightest pressure
[ ] **4.** Referred pain in the opposite quadrant

The physician considers removing the client's appendix with laparoscopic surgery.

80. When the client asks the nurse about this type of procedure, which statement is most accurate?
[ ] **1.** The recovery period is shorter.
[ ] **2.** No anesthesia is necessary.
[ ] **3.** There will be no surgical scar.
[ ] **4.** Exercise can be resumed immediately.

When the client's condition worsens, the physician fears that the appendix has ruptured. The client is prepared for an emergency appendectomy. The laparoscopic approach for removing the appendix is no longer an option.

81. Prior to admission, the nurse knows which activity most likely contributed to rupturing the client's appendix?
[ ] **1.** The client stopped eating and drinking.
[ ] **2.** The client continued his usual activities.
[ ] **3.** The client applied a heating pad to his lower abdomen.
[ ] **4.** The client took acetaminophen (Tylenol) for his discomfort.

The client returns from surgery with an open (Penrose) drain extending from his incision. A sterile dressing covers the drain.

82. In which position should the nurse place the client to promote drainage from the wound?
[ ] **1.** Lithotomy
[ ] **2.** Fowler's
[ ] **3.** Recumbent
[ ] **4.** Trendelenburg's

83. When changing the client's dressing, which nursing action is correct?
[ ] **1.** The nurse removes the soiled dressing with sterile gloves.
[ ] **2.** The nurse frees the tape by pulling it away from the incision.
[ ] **3.** The nurse encloses the soiled dressing within the latex glove.
[ ] **4.** The nurse cleans the wound in circles toward the incision.

The client requests medication to relieve his pain from the appendectomy. The physician has ordered meperidine hydrochloride (Demerol) 60 mg I.M. q 4h p.r.n.

84. If the label on the meperidine hydrochloride (Demerol) vial states 50 mg/mL, how much should the nurse administer to the client?

_____

A 68-year-old man has noted blood in his stool for the past 6 months. One possible diagnosis is colorectal cancer.

85. Besides rectal bleeding, which information in the client's medical history strongly suggests that he may have colorectal cancer?
[ ] **1.** He states that his bowel habits have changed.
[ ] **2.** He has insulin-dependent diabetes.
[ ] **3.** He experiences chronic indigestion.
[ ] **4.** He has had a history of hepatitis.

The nurse provides instructions about the client's scheduled sigmoidoscopy. He will prepare himself for the test at home.

86. Which statement by the client indicates that additional teaching is needed before the sigmoidoscopy?
[ ] **1.** "I should sit on the toilet to give myself an enema."
[ ] **2.** "I can eat a light meal the evening before the examination."
[ ] **3.** "A flexible scope will be inserted into my rectum."
[ ] **4.** "I should take my prescribed medications in the morning."

87. The nurse assisting with the sigmoidoscopy correctly places the client in which position?
[ ] **1.** Lithotomy
[ ] **2.** Sims'
[ ] **3.** Orthopneic
[ ] **4.** Fowler's

The client is told that he will need to undergo a bowel resection to remove the cancerous tumor.

88. If a low-residue diet is ordered for the client prior to surgery, which food would be contraindicated?
[ ] **1.** Ground meat
[ ] **2.** Bran cereal
[ ] **3.** Orange juice
[ ] **4.** Baked fish

Before colorectal surgery, the client will receive 1 g of neomycin sulfate (Mycifradin) orally every hour for four doses and then 1 g orally every 4 hours for the balance of the 24 hours.

89. If the neomycin sulfate (Mycifradin) tablets come in a dosage strength of 500 mg per tablet, how many tablets should the nurse administer each time?
[ ] **1.** ½ tablet
[ ] **2.** 1 tablet
[ ] **3.** 2 tablets
[ ] **4.** 4 tablets

90. When the client asks the nurse why he must take the neomycin sulfate (Mycifradin), the most accurate explanation in this case is that the drug is given for which reason?
[ ] **1.** To treat any current infection he may have
[ ] **2.** To suppress the growth of intestinal bacteria
[ ] **3.** To prevent the onset of postoperative diarrhea
[ ] **4.** To reduce the number of bacteria near the incision

During the postoperative period, the client's abdominal incision separates and his bowel protrudes through the opening.

91. What is the first action that the nurse should take at this time?
[ ] **1.** Check the client's vital signs.
[ ] **2.** Call the client's physician.
[ ] **3.** Cover the bowel with moist gauze.
[ ] **4.** Push the bowel back through the opening.

A home health nurse visits a 71-year-old female client and observes that her abdomen is quite distended. The client complains of nausea and reportedly has been vomiting for the past 48 hours.

92. Which question is important for the nurse to ask to determine if the client has a bowel obstruction?
[ ] **1.** "When did you last eat a full meal?"
[ ] **2.** "How much fluid are you vomiting?"
[ ] **3.** "Does the emesis appear to contain feces?"
[ ] **4.** "Has your appetite changed considerably?"

The physician admits the client to the hospital. A nasogastric (NG) tube is inserted.

93. Immediately after the NG tube is inserted, which action should the nurse take next?
[ ] **1.** Request an abdominal X-ray.
[ ] **2.** Secure the tube to the client's nose.
[ ] **3.** Connect the tube to high continuous wall suction.
[ ] **4.** Instill 50 mL of tap water into the tube.

The client's bowel obstruction is unrelieved by gastric decompression. She is scheduled for a laparotomy, possible colon resection, and a temporary colostomy. The client's preoperative orders include giving her meperidine hydrochloride (Demerol) and atropine sulfate (Sal-Tropin) I.M.

94. If the written order for the atropine sulfate (Sal-Tropin) says to administer 5 mg I.M. and the usual adult preoperative dose is 0.4 to 0.6 mg, which action is best for the nurse to take next?
[ ] **1.** Give the usual preoperative dose of atropine.
[ ] **2.** Administer just the meperidine hydrochloride (Demerol) at this time.
[ ] **3.** Withhold all the medication and notify the physician.
[ ] **4.** Consult the pharmacist on the action to take.

A few days after surgery, the physician orders daily colostomy irrigations.

95. Which position is best for the client when irrigating the colostomy?
[ ] **1.** Lying on the left side
[ ] **2.** Sitting on the toilet
[ ] **3.** Standing at the sink
[ ] **4.** Kneeling in the bathtub

During a conversation concerning her feelings about the colostomy, the client suddenly becomes silent and tearful.

96. Which nursing action is most appropriate at this time?
[ ] **1.** Change the subject to something more pleasant.
[ ] **2.** Refrain from interjecting comments or questions.
[ ] **3.** Provide information about colostomy care.
[ ] **4.** Offer a referral for psychological counseling.

The client says to the nurse, "How will I ever adjust to this colostomy?"

97. Which nursing response is most appropriate at this time?
[ ] **1.** Encourage the client to express her concerns.
[ ] **2.** Reassure her that adjustment will come with time.
[ ] **3.** Recommend she investigate care in a nursing home.
[ ] **4.** Say nothing, but quote her statement in the chart.

Nursing Care of Clients with Disorders of the Rectum and Anus

A nurse assesses blood pressures at a senior citizens' community meal site. An 80-year-old man discreetly asks if there are any nonprescription laxatives that he should avoid taking.

98. The nurse correctly explains that, to avoid interfering with the absorption of fat-soluble vitamins, it is best to stay away from frequent use of which laxative?
[ ] **1.** Milk of magnesia
[ ] **2.** Cascara sagrada
[ ] **3.** Mineral oil
[ ] **4.** Castor oil

A nurse who works at a nursing home cares for several clients with bowel elimination problems.

99. When a nursing home resident informs the nurse that he cannot have a bowel movement without taking a daily laxative, which information is essential for the nurse to provide?
[ ] **1.** Long-term use of laxatives impairs natural bowel tone.
[ ] **2.** Stool softeners are likely to be less harsh for him.
[ ] **3.** Daily enemas are more preferable than laxatives.
[ ] **4.** Dilating the anal sphincter may aid bowel elimination.

100. Which of the following strongly indicates that a client has a fecal impaction?
[ ] **1.** The client passes liquid stool frequently.
[ ] **2.** The client has foul-smelling stools.
[ ] **3.** The client requests medication for a stomachache.
[ ] **4.** The client hasn't been eating well lately.

101. Which technique is best for confirming that a client has a fecal impaction?
[ ] **1.** Administering an oil-retention enema
[ ] **2.** Inserting a gloved finger into the rectum
[ ] **3.** Reviewing the results of the client's lower gastrointestinal X-ray
[ ] **4.** Monitoring the client's bowel elimination

102. Before inserting a rectal tube, which nursing measure is most helpful for eliminating a client's intestinal gas?
[ ] **1.** Ambulating the client in the hall
[ ] **2.** Providing a carbonated beverage
[ ] **3.** Restricting the intake of solid food
[ ] **4.** Administering an opioid analgesic

103. If a rectal tube becomes necessary to relieve a client's distention and discomfort, what is the maximum length of time the nurse should plan to leave the tube in place each time it is used?
[ ] **1.** 15 minutes
[ ] **2.** 20 minutes
[ ] **3.** 45 minutes
[ ] **4.** 60 minutes

During the administration of a cleansing soapsuds enema, a client experiences cramping and has the urge to defecate.

104. Which nursing action is most appropriate at this time?
[ ] **1.** Quickly finish instilling the remaining solution.
[ ] **2.** Tell the client to hold his breath and bear down.
[ ] **3.** Briefly stop the administration of the enema solution.
[ ] **4.** Turn the client onto his back and elevate his feet.

105. When the nurse is inserting a rectal suppository to relieve constipation, which nursing action is most appropriate?
[ ] **1.** The nurse dons a sterile glove on the dominant hand.
[ ] **2.** The nurse positions the client on the right side.
[ ] **3.** The nurse inserts the suppository approximately 2″ to 4″ (5 to 10 cm).
[ ] **4.** The nurse instructs the client to retain the suppository for 5 minutes.

106. Which of the following should be planned first before beginning bowel retraining for a client experiencing bowel incontinence?
[ ] **1.** Limit the client's daytime physical activity.
[ ] **2.** Record the time of day when incontinence occurs.
[ ] **3.** Decrease the amount of food eaten at each meal.
[ ] **4.** Empty the client's bowel with a soapsuds enema.

A home health nurse reviews the health history of a female client who has hemorrhoids.

107. Which factor most likely contributed to the development of the client's hemorrhoids?

[ ] **1.** Taking a daily stool softener
[ ] **2.** History of ulcerative colitis
[ ] **3.** Frequent constipation
[ ] **4.** Occupation of a computer programmer

108. Besides increasing her consumption of bulk-forming foods (such as whole grains, fresh fruits, and vegetables), what is the most appropriate dietary instruction the nurse can give the client with hemorrhoids?

[ ] **1.** Eat small meals frequently.
[ ] **2.** Drink eight glasses of fluid per day.
[ ] **3.** Avoid snacking between meals.
[ ] **4.** Reduce the intake of refined sugar.

The client with hemorrhoids eventually has them surgically removed. The nurse assists with giving the client a sitz bath postoperatively.

109. What is the best way to evaluate the effectiveness of the sitz bath for this client?

[ ] **1.** The client says her rectum is less painful.
[ ] **2.** The client has no evidence of body odor.
[ ] **3.** The client indicates that she feels refreshed.
[ ] **4.** The client has no evidence of a hematoma.

The physician prescribes docusate sodium (Colace) for the client. The client asks the nurse to explain why the medication is needed.

110. The nurse correctly explains that which is the purpose of the medication?

[ ] **1.** To ease bowel evacuation and its related discomfort
[ ] **2.** To irritate the bowel and promote stool elimination
[ ] **3.** To stimulate peristalsis to remove wastes after digestion
[ ] **4.** To reduce intestinal activity and decrease stool size

A client is admitted for surgical treatment of a pilonidal cyst.

111. When obtaining the client's health history, which characteristic finding would the admitting nurse expect the client to report?

[ ] **1.** A history of intermittent rectal bleeding
[ ] **2.** An open area near the coccyx that is draining
[ ] **3.** Frequent episodes of diarrhea
[ ] **4.** Very little or baby-fine anorectal hair

Before discharging the client, the nurse teaches him how to apply a nonprescription anesthetic ointment.

112. Which instruction regarding medication administration is essential for promoting the drug's local effect?

[ ] **1.** Use gloves when applying the ointment.
[ ] **2.** Store the ointment in the refrigerator.
[ ] **3.** Apply the ointment just before defecating.
[ ] **4.** Clean the area before applying the drug.

Nursing Care of Clients with Disorders of the Gallbladder

A 45-year-old woman is suspected of having cholecystitis.

113. When the client describes her discomfort to the nurse, she is most likely to indicate that the pain worsens at which time?

[ ] **1.** Shortly after eating
[ ] **2.** When her stomach is empty
[ ] **3.** Following periods of activity
[ ] **4.** Before rising in the morning

114. If this client is typical of others with cholecystitis, besides localized pain, she may describe feeling pain that is referred to which area?

[ ] **1.** Right shoulder
[ ] **2.** Mid-epigastrium
[ ] **3.** Neck or jaw
[ ] **4.** Left upper arm

115. If the cause of the client's inflamed gallbladder is gallstones, the nurse would anticipate the laboratory data to indicate which finding?

[ ] **1.** Low red blood cell count
[ ] **2.** Low hemoglobin level
[ ] **3.** Elevated cholesterol level
[ ] **4.** Elevated serum albumin level

116. If gallstones obstruct the flow of bile, how would the nurse expect the client's stools to appear?

[ ] **1.** Black and tarry
[ ] **2.** Light clay–colored
[ ] **3.** Brown with bloody mucus
[ ] **4.** Greenish yellow

117. When the dietitian has finished instructing the client about a low-fat diet, the nurse knows that the client requires additional teaching based on which statement?

[ ] **1.** "I can eat broiled chicken."
[ ] **2.** "I'll still be able to enjoy my favorite baked meatloaf dish."
[ ] **3.** "Since fish is good for me, I'll still get to have a lot of fried fish."
[ ] **4.** "I guess I'll eat more roasted turkey for dinner."

The client with possible cholecystitis is scheduled for oral cholecystography (an X-ray of the gallbladder). The night before the test, the client receives several oral tablets that will facilitate a sharper X-ray image.

118. Which information is essential for the nurse to know before administering the contrast substance to a client undergoing this type of X-ray?
[ ] **1.** Can the client tolerate holding still?
[ ] **2.** How many X-rays has the client had?
[ ] **3.** Is the client allergic to iodine?
[ ] **4.** Does the client want any anesthesia?

Because the client's gallbladder was unable to concentrate and excrete bile, it could not be visualized by cholecystography. The physician orders an ultrasound of the gallbladder. The nurse explains the scheduled procedure to the client.

119. Which comment indicates that the client has an accurate understanding of the preparation necessary for her procedure?
[ ] **1.** "Preparation involves withholding food for approximately 8 to 12 hours."
[ ] **2.** "I'll need to drink a container of barium just before the X-ray."
[ ] **3.** "I'll be allowed to eat a large test meal the night before the X-ray."
[ ] **4.** "Just before the test, they'll insert a large needle into one of my arm veins."

The physician recommends an open abdominal cholecystectomy to remove the client's gallstones. An I.M. injection of menadiol sodium diphosphate (Synkayvite), a water-soluble derivative of vitamin K, is ordered on the day before surgery.

120. When the client asks the nurse to explain the purpose of the vitamin K injection, which explanation by the nurse is most accurate?
[ ] **1.** It helps promote wound healing.
[ ] **2.** It is used to improve liver function.
[ ] **3.** It promotes general health.
[ ] **4.** It helps promote blood clotting.

The physician prescribes a 10-mg dose of menadiol sodium diphosphate (Synkayvite). The drug is supplied in a dosage strength of 5 mg/mL. The nurse prepares 2 mL of the drug.

121. When planning an appropriate I.M injection site, the nurse knows that the least preferred site for this medication is in which muscle?
[ ] **1.** Dorsogluteal
[ ] **2.** Ventrogluteal
[ ] **3.** Vastus lateralis
[ ] **4.** Deltoid

The client returns from surgery with a nasogastric tube, a T-tube for bile drainage, and a Jackson-Pratt tube for wound drainage in place.

122. Immediately after surgery, the nurse assesses the drainage from the T-tube. Which assessment finding best indicates that the drainage color is normal at this time?
[ ] **1.** The drainage is dark red or pale pink.
[ ] **2.** The drainage is clear or transparent.
[ ] **3.** The drainage is bright red or orange.
[ ] **4.** The drainage is greenish yellow or brown.

123. The nurse is required to take which actions when emptying the drainage receptacle of the client's Jackson-Pratt closed-wound drain? Select all that apply.
[ ] **1.** Empty the drainage into a measuring container.
[ ] **2.** Adjust the suction setting to low continuous suction.
[ ] **3.** Squeeze the receptacle to expel air.
[ ] **4.** Release the roller clamp.
[ ] **5.** Cover the vent.
[ ] **6.** Stabilize the drainage tube.

124. The nurse should anticipate implementing which interventions to manage this client's T-tube? Select all that apply.
[ ] **1.** Record the amount of drainage from the T-tube.
[ ] **2.** Unclamp the T-tube at hourly intervals.
[ ] **3.** Keep the T-tube drainage bag parallel with the incision.
[ ] **4.** Inspect the skin around the tube for irritation.
[ ] **5.** Maintain the client in Fowler's position.
[ ] **6.** Notify the physician if the drainage changes color.

125. When the nurse assesses the T-tube in the early postoperative period, which finding requires immediate action?
[ ] **1.** The drainage bag is hanging below the abdomen.
[ ] **2.** The drainage tubing is currently clamped.
[ ] **3.** The drainage tube is taped to the client's right side.
[ ] **4.** The drainage volume was 100 mL in the last 6 hours.

126. When the client begins to consume food again, which routine for clamping and unclamping the T-tube should the nurse plan to follow?
[ ] **1.** Unclamp the tube during the day.
[ ] **2.** Unclamp the tube during the night.
[ ] **3.** Unclamp the tube for 2 hours after eating.
[ ] **4.** Unclamp the tube for 2 hours before eating.

127. How would the nurse reestablish negative pressure within the Jackson-Pratt tube when emptying the drainage bulb reservoir?
[ ] **1.** By compressing the bulb reservoir and closing the drainage valve
[ ] **2.** By opening the drainage valve, allowing the bulb to fill with air
[ ] **3.** By filling the bulb reservoir with sterile normal saline solution
[ ] **4.** By securing the bulb reservoir to the skin near the wound

Nursing Care of Clients with Disorders of the Liver

A 20-year-old female college student goes to the university health service because she has developed a sudden onset of flulike symptoms.

128. When the health nurse monitors the client's laboratory test results, which elevated level would strongly suggest a possible liver disorder?
[ ] **1.** Serum potassium
[ ] **2.** Serum creatinine
[ ] **3.** Blood urea nitrogen (BUN)
[ ] **4.** Alanine and aspartate aminotransferase (ALT)

The physician determines that the college student has hepatitis A.

129. When the client asks the nurse how she acquired hepatitis A, what is the best answer?
[ ] **1.** A common route of hepatitis A transmission is fecal contamination.
[ ] **2.** A common route of hepatitis A transmission is insect carriers.
[ ] **3.** A common route of hepatitis A transmission is infected blood.
[ ] **4.** A common route of hepatitis A transmission is wound drainage.

An infection control nurse is consulted on measures for reducing the potential transmission of the hepatitis A virus to others.

130. Based on the routes of transmission for this disease, which infection control measure is essential to include in the client's care plan?
[ ] **1.** Wear gloves whenever entering the client's room.
[ ] **2.** Don a mask and gown when providing direct care.
[ ] **3.** Maintain the client in a private room at all times.
[ ] **4.** Perform vigorous hand washing after leaving the room.

Several of the college student's friends call the health service because they are concerned about their own risks for acquiring hepatitis A.

131. To prevent the spread of hepatitis A, the nurse correctly advises that close contacts receive which medication?
[ ] **1.** An antibiotic
[ ] **2.** Serum immunoglobulin
[ ] **3.** Hepatitis vaccine
[ ] **4.** An anti-inflammatory drug

A 23-year-old man develops jaundice and refers himself to the public health department. He tells the nurse that his skin itches terribly.

132. Which suggestion is most appropriate for helping the client manage his discomfort?
[ ] **1.** Discontinue all bathing temporarily.
[ ] **2.** Use only lanolin soap for bathing.
[ ] **3.** Apply rubbing alcohol to the skin.
[ ] **4.** Take showers rather than tub baths.

Testing reveals that the cause of the client's jaundice is hepatitis B. The nurse gathers information regarding the client's social history.

133. Which information from the client's history strongly predisposes him to hepatitis B?
[ ] **1.** The client moved from Europe.
[ ] **2.** The client is an active homosexual.
[ ] **3.** The client abuses alcohol.
[ ] **4.** The client works in a restaurant.

134. Which measure is most appropriate if an unvaccinated nurse experiences a needle-stick injury while caring for this client?
[ ] **1.** Obtain immediate immunization with hepatitis B vaccine.
[ ] **2.** Receive hepatitis B immunoglobulin within 1 week.
[ ] **3.** Take penicillin (Pentam) for a minimum of 10 days.
[ ] **4.** Scrub the puncture site with diluted household bleach.

135. The nurse informs the client that, because of his disease, it is essential for him to avoid which activity for the remainder of his life?
[ ] **1.** Sexual activity
[ ] **2.** Donating blood
[ ] **3.** Drinking excessive amounts of caffeine
[ ] **4.** Traveling to foreign countries

A 60-year-old man seeks medical attention because he has been vomiting blood and passing bloody stools. The tentative diagnosis is cirrhosis of the liver.

136. Which information in the client's health history most likely relates to the development of cirrhosis?
[ ] **1.** He drinks a fifth of whiskey daily.
[ ] **2.** He smokes two packs of cigarettes per day.
[ ] **3.** He has a history of pancreatitis.
[ ] **4.** He has been taking antihypertensive medications for the past 15 years.

137. If the client's cirrhosis is advanced, what will the nurse expect to find during the initial health assessment?
[ ] **1.** Laboratory results that reveal an elevated serum cholesterol level
[ ] **2.** The presence of spiderlike blood vessels on the skin
[ ] **3.** An unusually large and edematous scrotum
[ ] **4.** An abnormally high blood glucose level

138. Which assessment finding indicates that the client is bleeding from somewhere in his upper gastrointestinal tract?
[ ] **1.** He has mid-epigastric pain.
[ ] **2.** He states that he feels nauseated.
[ ] **3.** His stools are black and sticky.
[ ] **4.** His abdomen is distended and shiny.

The care plan indicates that the nurse should monitor the client with cirrhosis each day for signs and symptoms of ascites.

139. To implement this nursing order, which nursing action is most appropriate?
[ ] **1.** Counting the client's apical and radial pulse rates
[ ] **2.** Taking the client's lying and sitting blood pressure
[ ] **3.** Checking the client's urine specific gravity
[ ] **4.** Measuring the client's abdominal circumference

The physician considers performing a liver biopsy to confirm a diagnosis of cirrhosis.

140. If the liver biopsy is performed, the nurse must monitor the client immediately after the procedure for which potential complication?
[ ] **1.** Hemorrhage
[ ] **2.** Infection
[ ] **3.** Blood clots
[ ] **4.** Collapsed lung

141. After a liver biopsy, which nursing order is most appropriate to add to the client's care plan?
[ ] **1.** Ambulate the client twice each shift.
[ ] **2.** Keep the client in high Fowler's position.
[ ] **3.** Position the client on his right side.
[ ] **4.** Elevate the client's legs on two pillows.

The physician orders magnetic resonance imaging (MRI) instead of the liver biopsy to confirm the diagnosis.

142. Before the MRI is performed, which nursing action is essential?
[ ] **1.** Administering a pretest sedative
[ ] **2.** Removing the client's dental bridge
[ ] **3.** Recording the client's body weight
[ ] **4.** Inserting a Foley retention catheter

The MRI confirms the diagnosis of hepatic cirrhosis and reveals a large amount of fluid in the peritoneal cavity. A paracentesis is planned.

143. Which nursing action is most appropriate prior to assisting with the paracentesis?
[ ] **1.** Asking the client to void
[ ] **2.** Withholding food and water
[ ] **3.** Cleaning the client's abdomen with povidone-iodine (Betadine)
[ ] **4.** Placing the crash cart outside the client's room

144. After the paracentesis has been performed, which nursing responsibility is essential?
[ ] **1.** Increasing the client's oral fluid intake
[ ] **2.** Recording the volume of withdrawn fluid
[ ] **3.** Administering a prescribed analgesic
[ ] **4.** Encouraging the client to deep-breathe

145. When administering an I.M. injection to the client with cirrhosis of the liver, which nursing action is essential to perform?
[ ] **1.** Clean the site with povidone-iodine (Betadine).
[ ] **2.** Inject no more than 1 mL at any given site.
[ ] **3.** Obtain a vial of vitamin K to keep at the bedside.
[ ] **4.** Apply prolonged pressure to the injection site.

146. Which laboratory result, if elevated, is most indicative that the client may develop hepatic encephalopathy?
[ ] **1.** Serum creatinine
[ ] **2.** Serum bilirubin
[ ] **3.** Blood ammonia
[ ] **4.** Blood urea nitrogen

147. Which assessment finding best indicates that the cirrhotic client's condition is worsening?

[ ] **1.** He is difficult to arouse.

[ ] **2.** His urine output is 100 mL/hour.

[ ] **3.** He develops pancreatitis.

[ ] **4.** His blood pressure is 122/60 mm Hg.

The seriousness of the client's condition is explained to his wife. She is prepared for the possibility of her husband's death.

148. When the client's wife begins crying as she recalls various significant events she and her husband shared together, which nursing action is most therapeutic at this time?

[ ] **1.** Offer to call a close family member.

[ ] **2.** Listen to her express her thoughts.

[ ] **3.** Suggest that she call the clergy at her church.

[ ] **4.** Ask about her future plans.

Nursing Care of Clients with Disorders of the Pancreas

A 48-year-old man comes to the emergency department because of severe upper abdominal pain. He reports that the pain came on suddenly a few hours ago and nothing so far has relieved it. The nurse observes that the client is curled in a fetal position and is rocking back and forth.

149. Which action would best assist the nurse in further assessing the client's pain?

[ ] **1.** Determining if the client can stop moving

[ ] **2.** Asking the client to rate his pain from 0 to 10

[ ] **3.** Observing whether the client is breathing heavily

[ ] **4.** Giving the client a prescribed pain-relieving drug

150. Which laboratory test, if elevated, provides the best indication that the client's pain is caused by pancreatitis?

[ ] **1.** Serum bilirubin

[ ] **2.** Serum amylase

[ ] **3.** Lactose tolerance

[ ] **4.** Glucose tolerance

The physician orders the insertion of a nasogastric (NG) sump tube.

151. To determine the length of tubing to insert, the nurse correctly places the tip of the tube at the client's nose and measures the distance from there to which area?

[ ] **1.** The jaw and then midway to the sternum

[ ] **2.** The mouth and then between the nipples

[ ] **3.** The midsternum and then to the umbilicus

[ ] **4.** The ear and then to the xiphoid process

152. If the client turns blue and coughs as the NG tube is inserted, which additional sign indicates that the tube has entered the respiratory tract?

[ ] **1.** Inability to speak

[ ] **2.** Inability to swallow

[ ] **3.** Sneezing

[ ] **4.** Vomiting

The client's fluid and nutritional needs are temporarily met by administering I.V. fluid.

153. While assessing the infusion, the nurse should report which finding immediately to the charge nurse?

[ ] **1.** The tubing is coiled on the top of the mattress.

[ ] **2.** The container has approximately 100 mL of fluid left.

[ ] **3.** The fluid is infusing into the client's nondominant hand.

[ ] **4.** Less fluid than ordered has infused at this time.

After the client has been maintained on NPO (nothing by mouth) status for several days, the NG tube is removed and the client is placed on a bland, low-fat diet.

154. Which food should the nurse remove from the client's breakfast tray?

[ ] **1.** Stewed prunes

[ ] **2.** Skim milk

[ ] **3.** Scrambled eggs

[ ] **4.** Whole-wheat toast

155. Before the client is discharged from the hospital, which information is essential for him to receive?

[ ] **1.** He must never donate blood again.

[ ] **2.** He must avoid lifting heavy objects.

[ ] **3.** He must not drink alcohol in any form.

[ ] **4.** He must forgo taking strong laxatives.

A 69-year-old woman is admitted with a diagnosis of cancer of the pancreas.

156. If this client is typical of most others who develop pancreatic cancer, the nurse would expect which early problem to be the one the client sought treatment for?

[ ] **1.** Sharp pain

[ ] **2.** Weight loss

[ ] **3.** Bleeding

[ ] **4.** Fainting

The physician meets with the client to inform her that her pancreatic cancer has metastasized, making aggressive treatment unrealistic. Her condition is terminal.

157. The client asks the nurse, "Am I dying?" What is the best response from the nurse?
[ ] **1.** "Yes, you have little time left."
[ ] **2.** "No, you're not going to die."
[ ] **3.** "Tell me about how you are feeling."
[ ] **4.** "Is there someone you would like me to call?"

The client has an advance directive that requests no aggressive treatment. She is referred for hospice care.

158. If the client has pain medication ordered every 3 to 4 hours as necessary, which action by the hospice nurse is most appropriate to promote maximum comfort at this time?
[ ] **1.** Give the medication immediately at her request.
[ ] **2.** Administer the medication every 3 hours.
[ ] **3.** Ask the physician to prescribe a high dose.
[ ] **4.** Give the medication when the pain is severe.

Correct Answers and Rationales

Nursing Care of Clients with Disorders of the Mouth

1. 1. When the mucous membrane of the oral cavity is inflamed, it is best to eliminate foods that are acidic, salty, spicy, dry, or very hot. Other than tomato soup, none of the other foods have any of these characteristics.
Client Needs Category—Physiological integrity
Client Needs Subcategory—Basic care and comfort

2. 3. Oral swabs can clean plaque from the teeth, promote more comfort, and produce less irritation than a toothbrush—regardless of its size. Even a soft-bristled toothbrush may cause too much trauma. Dental floss alone is not the best choice for mouth care. Normal saline mouth rinse is preferable to one that is flavored. Flavoring may only refresh the breath and irritate the mouth.
Client Needs Category—Physiological integrity
Client Needs Subcategory—Basic care and comfort

3. 2. Clients who are limited in the amount of fluid they may consume need frequent mouth care. Limited hydration can reduce the volume of saliva, which helps keep the teeth clean and inhibits bacterial growth. A client with full dentures has the same oral hygiene needs as a person with natural teeth. A low-residue diet is one that reduces the volume of undigested substances in the bowel; the diet alone does not necessitate specialized oral hygiene. Eating raw fruits or vegetables, such as apples and celery, can act as a dental cleanser. Sucking on ice chips is not an indication for modifying routine measures for oral hygiene.
Client Needs Category—Physiological integrity
Client Needs Subcategory—Basic care and comfort

4. 2. Holding dentures over a basin of water or a soft towel prevents them from breaking if they should slip from the hands. Hot water may warp the plastic from which some dentures are made. Oral adhesives do not require a special solvent for removal. The adhesives usually rinse off easily with water. When not being used, dentures are kept moist to retain their fit and color.
Client Needs Category—Physiological integrity
Client Needs Subcategory—Basic care and comfort

5. 2. When administering oral hygiene to an unconscious client, the nurse should place him on his side with his head slightly lowered. This is the best position for preventing aspiration. Because the unconscious client cannot swallow, this position allows the fluid to run out of the mouth instead of pooling in the back of the throat. Providing mouth care with a client in the prone or face-down position is extremely difficult. Trendelenburg's position, in which the client's legs and feet are higher than the head, is used for treating shock victims; it is inappropriate for oral hygiene. A client in the dorsal recumbent position is placed flat on his back, with the knees bent and feet flat on the mattress. Because the client is flat, the risk for aspiration is greater in this position.

> *Client Needs Category—Safe, effective care environment*
>
> *Client Needs Subcategory—Safety and infection control*

6. 3. Candidiasis (thrush) is a fungal infection that appears as small white patches resembling milk curds on the mucous membranes of the mouth and tongue. Candidiasis often occurs when antibiotic therapy destroys the normal flora of the body. Immunosuppression, such as occurs in clients with acquired immunodeficiency syndrome (AIDS) or cancer, may also result in candidiasis. Red, ulcerated patches near the margin of the teeth and gums are characteristic of gingivitis. Herpes simplex lesions—clear, raised vesicles that transform into shallow ulcers—are not restricted to the tongue. The last option does not describe any particular oral disease.

> *Client Needs Category—Physiological integrity*
>
> *Client Needs Subcategory—Physiological adaptation*

7. 2. An infection with the yeast organism *Candida albicans* is usually acquired from an overgrowth of normal flora found in and on the skin and mucous membranes of the gastrointestinal tract. Candidiasis is considered an opportunistic infection because the source of the infection is usually the client. Antibiotic therapy can upset the balance of organisms in the body, allowing some natural microbes to grow unchecked. It is unlikely that the client would acquire candidiasis from soiled dental instruments because most dentists follow guidelines for sterilizing their equipment between uses. Candidiasis is usually not transmitted by eating or drinking from someone's unclean utensils, especially if the person has a normal immune system. Because the organisms are present in the mouth, it is possible, but highly improbable, that the infection could be acquired by inhaling respiratory droplets from another individual.

> *Client Needs Category—Physiological integrity*
>
> *Client Needs Subcategory—Physiological adaptation*

8. 3. Because nystatin (Mycostatin) is poorly absorbed from the gastrointestinal tract, holding the liquid suspension in the mouth as long as possible facilitates contact of the drug with the organism. The client is allowed to swallow the medication after swishing it

around. There is no need to use a straw or dilute the medication in this instance.

> *Client Needs Category—Physiological integrity*
>
> *Client Needs Subcategory—Pharmacological therapies*

9. 2. Factors that predispose the client to cancer of the mouth include any source of chronic irritation, such as holding a pipe in the mouth, holding chewing or smokeless tobacco in the mouth, alcohol consumption, or prolonged contact with rough dental appliances. Lip cancer is related to prolonged sun or wind exposure. Having a partial dental plate, as long as it fits well, is not as likely to cause cancerous changes. Certain processes for extracting caffeine have been linked with some forms of cancer, but not cancer of the mouth. Poor dental hygiene and decaying teeth are not usually risk factors predisposing the client to cancer of the mouth. However, poor oral and dental hygiene may worsen cancerous lesions.

> *Client Needs Category—Physiological integrity*
>
> *Client Needs Subcategory—Physiological adaptation*

10. 1. All emesis must be inspected to detect the presence of radioactive needles that may have been displaced. Dislodged needles must never be touched with the hands. They should be retrieved with long forceps and placed in a lead container. Bleach is not required for cleaning or disinfecting the emesis basin. There is no reason for using a plastic rather than metal emesis basin. The threads are never cut; they are counted each shift to ensure that the original number inserted is still present.

> *Client Needs Category—Safe, effective care environment*
>
> *Client Needs Subcategory—Safety and infection control*

11. 3. Whenever implanted radiation is used, it is necessary to protect other people by limiting their time with the client and their proximity to him. This may include using physical methods of shielding them from absorbing the radiation. Therefore, a solitary activity is more appropriate than those involving one or more people.

> *Client Needs Category—Safe, effective care environment*
>
> *Client Needs Subcategory—Safety and infection control*

12. 4. The herpes simplex virus causes herpes simplex type 1 infection, and lesions can appear on the face, cheeks, nose, or lips, or in the perioral (mouth) area. Most nonclinicians refer to these lesions as "cold sores" or "fever blisters." The herpes virus remains latent until activated or triggered by stress, sunlight, or fever. The incubation period is usually 2 to 12 days, and transmission is by direct contact. Therefore, hand washing and good personal hygiene are used during the time the virus is replicating and being shed. Usually, herpes type 1 lesions heal within 10 to 14 days.

Client Needs Category—Safe, effective care environment

Client Needs Subcategory—Safety and infection control

13. **2.** Acyclovir (Zovirax) does not cure the infection or prevent future outbreaks. It only shortens the time during which the virus is replicating and being shed. Some of the virus retreats within nerve fibers and escapes detection by the body's immune system, where it remains dormant until stimulated. The drug may be administered orally or topically. Oral acyclovir (Zovirax) is taken when the client first becomes aware of symptoms, such as an area of itching, pain, or tingling on the mucous membrane. Oral doses are generally taken for 10 days.

Client Needs Category—Physiological integrity

Client Needs Subcategory—Pharmacological therapies

Nursing Care of Clients with Disorders of the Esophagus

14. **3.** An esophagoscopy is a diagnostic test that involves passing a flexible fiberoptic tube down the esophagus. Food and fluid are avoided to reduce the potential for aspiration. Therefore, the client should be NPO (nothing by mouth) after midnight. All of the other choices are incorrect because they involve eating or drinking. After the procedure, the nurse should wait for the gag reflex to return before giving the client any food or fluid.

Client Needs Category—Physiological integrity

Client Needs Subcategory—Reduction of risk potential

15. **2.** Taking smaller bites and chewing food thoroughly help the bolus slip through the narrowed stricture. Switching to thickened food and fluid is too drastic at this time. Drinking liquids throughout a meal is beneficial in thinning the bolus of food. Eliminating dairy products will not promote the ability to swallow food.

Client Needs Category—Health promotion and maintenance

Client Needs Subcategory—None

16. **4.** Esophageal varices are dilated, twisted veins found in the lower esophagus. The condition is usually related to portal hypertension from cirrhosis of the liver. Chronic consumption of alcohol can damage the liv-

er and interfere with blood flow from the esophagus and other abdominal organs. Esophageal veins distend and bleed because of the portal hypertension created by the stagnation of blood. Attempted suicide using lye will cause damage to the esophagus, but the damage is not called esophageal varices. Oral cancer has no correlation to esophageal varices. Hemophilia is a hereditary bleeding disorder; however, it is not the cause of the bleeding esophageal varices. Bleeding esophageal varices are life-threatening and can result in shock or death.

Client Needs Category—Physiological integrity

Client Needs Subcategory—Physiological adaptation

17. **1.** The National Patient Safety Goals were developed by the Joint Commission on Accreditation of Healthcare Organizations (JCAHO) as a way of ensuring safe client care in the clinical setting. One of the 11 JCAHO safety goals deals with blood and blood infusions. To be in compliance with the established goals, two licensed personnel must review the blood bag itself for the correct blood type, date, and time, as well as check the client's individual blood tags and arm bracelet before any blood product can be administered. If there is a discrepancy, the blood cannot be given. In most circumstances, the RN is responsible for starting the blood infusion while the LPN monitors the client during the procedure. None of the other options is related to the National Patient Safety Goals. An indwelling (Foley) catheter is not needed during a blood transfusion. Most blood should be infused with an 18- to 20-gauge needle so the blood cells will not be damaged during infusion. Blood should be given within 4 hours of starting, to prevent bacterial growth.

Client Needs Category—Health promotion and maintenance

Client Needs Subcategory—None

18. **2.** Dyspnea, hypotension, chest constriction, tachycardia, and back pain are some of the major symptoms associated with an incompatibility transfusion reaction—a life-threatening reaction. The other assessment findings in this question are signs and symptoms associated with hypovolemia, most likely resulting from the client's blood loss.

Client Needs Category—Physiological integrity

Client Needs Subcategory—Physiological adaptation

19. **4.** GERD results when a weakened area of the diaphragm enables a portion of the stomach to protrude into the esophagus. The acid contents of the stomach reflux into the esophagus, causing irritation and inflammation, which the client describes as heartburn. Other symptoms include belching, epigastric pressure, and pain after eating and when lying down. The other choices in this question are unrelated to the medical diagnosis.

> *Client Needs Category—Physiological integrity*
> *Client Needs Subcategory—Physiological adaptation*

20. **3.** An upright position for at least 2 hours after eating keeps swallowed food and gastric contents within the stomach by means of gravity. The client with a hiatal hernia should also be encouraged to sleep with the head of the bed elevated and to eat small, frequent meals to avoid overdistending the stomach. Drinking room-temperature liquids has no effect on relieving the discomfort associated with this condition.

> *Client Needs Category—Health promotion and maintenance*
> *Client Needs Subcategory—None*

21. **4.** Elevating the head of the bed helps to prevent gastric reflux. The other suggestions are not therapeutic for relieving the client's symptoms.

> *Client Needs Category—Health promotion and maintenance*
> *Client Needs Subcategory—None*

22. **2.** It is essential to monitor the blood glucose level frequently because TPN solutions contain high concentrations of glucose. Insulin coverage may be needed to maintain the blood glucose level within an acceptable range. The specific gravity may become lower if the client begins to excrete large volumes of urine, but it is not generally monitored. Pulse pressure, the difference between the systolic and diastolic arterial pressure measurements, is usually unaffected by TPN. There is no need to monitor apical and radial pulses in relation to the TPN.

> *Client Needs Category—Physiological integrity*
> *Client Needs Subcategory—Physiological adaptation*

23. **2.** Gradual, steady weight gain is one of the best ways to tell that a client is responding favorably to TPN. If laboratory reports are monitored daily, the client's electrolytes should be adjusted based on the results; therefore, they should be in balance. However, a balance in electrolytes does not necessarily indicate that the client is responding favorably to the therapy. Hunger is an emotional and physical phenomenon. Even well-nourished, satiated people can feel hungry when they see, smell, or even think about food. Therefore, return of the client's appetite does not indicate that TPN is successful. The client's pain tolerance may increase with improved nutrition, but this is not the best criterion for determining the effectiveness of TPN.

> *Client Needs Category—Physiological integrity*
> *Client Needs Subcategory—Physiological adaptation*

24. **2.** Slight pinkish (serosanguineous) bleeding or clear serous drainage at the gastrostomy site is a normal finding immediately after a gastrostomy has been performed. Milky drainage suggests an infection; drainage occurring after feedings have been initiated may indicate leakage of formula. Intestinal secretions cause green-tinged drainage, but the gastrostomy is located in the client's stomach, not intestines. Bright, bloody drainage indicates arterial bleeding, which is not a normal finding.

> *Client Needs Category—Physiological integrity*
> *Client Needs Subcategory—Physiological adaptation*

25. **3.** Comparing the measured length of tubing extending from the gastrostomy site is an easy and appropriate technique for determining tube migration. A change in pH from acid to alkaline indicates intestinal migration, but most gastrostomy tubes are too short to reach the small intestine. X-rays are expensive and expose clients to unnecessary radiation. A distended abdomen may indicate many complications, but tube migration is not one of them.

> *Client Needs Category—Safe, effective care environment*
> *Client Needs Subcategory—Safety and infection control*

26. **2.** Each ounce equals 30 mL. Therefore, 8 ounces equals 240 mL. It will take a total of 4 hours to instill 480 mL (two 8-ounce cans) at a rate of 120 mL/hour.

> *Client Needs Category—Safe, effective care environment*
> *Client Needs Subcategory—Safety and infection control*

27. **3.** It is important that the stomach not become overdistended. Therefore, temporarily stopping the infusion will allow the remaining formula in the stomach to be digested. This will decrease the client's feeling of fullness. The stomach residual is checked prior to administering an intermittent feeding. As a rule of thumb, the gastric residual should be no more than 150 mL of the previous intermittent feeding or, if continuous, no more than half of the previous hour's infusion volume. Administering an antiemetic will stop the nausea, but this is not the best choice at this time. Adding water to formula adds more volume and dilutes the nutrients.

> *Client Needs Category—Physiological integrity*
> *Client Needs Subcategory—Physiological adaptation*

28. **4.** The nurse should rinse the feeding tube after each use to maintain its patency and to meet the client's needs for water. To prevent aspiration, the head of the bed should always be elevated during and for at least a half hour after a tube feeding. The client's head should also be turned to the side to allow regurgitated formula and saliva to drain from the mouth. Gastrostomy tubes may be clamped intermittently, but only after they have been rinsed with water.

Client Needs Category—Physiological integrity
Client Needs Subcategory—Physiological adaptation

29. 2. In this case, sharing perceptions or validating the client's statement is the best therapeutic communication technique for encouraging him to discuss his feelings. Most clients tend to deny feeling angry if asked a direct question. Telling the client that his situation may improve offers false reassurance and may cause him to lose trust in the nurse's ability to be supportive. Knowing that many other clients are nourished by tube feedings will not necessarily make it easier for the client to cope with his situation.

Client Needs Category—Physiological integrity
Client Needs Subcategory—None

Nursing Care of Clients with Disorders of the Stomach

30. 3. Clients with peptic ulcers generally find that eating relieves their discomfort. The pain is caused by irritation of the eroded mucosa by hydrochloric acid and pepsin. Food tends to dilute the acid, thereby raising the secretions' pH. This reduces irritation of the ulcerated tissue. Skipping a meal increases the pain because the acid secretions become very concentrated. Many ulcer clients report awakening at night with pain. Bending over does not cause or relieve the discomfort associated with an ulcer.

Client Needs Category—Physiological integrity
Client Needs Subcategory—Physiological adaptation

31. 3. Blood in the stool is a significant finding of peptic ulcer disease. Its presence indicates that bleeding is occurring within the gastrointestinal tract. If bleeding occurs in the upper gastrointestinal tract, the stool appears thick, black, and tarry. This finding is called *melena*. However, blood may be present without an obvious change in the normal color of stool. This finding is referred to as *occult blood*. Although identifying blood in the stool is not proof that the client has a peptic ulcer, it aids in the differential diagnosis. Albumin in the urine is associated with renal disease. An elevated blood glucose level may be due to diabetes mellitus. Emesis is not tested for the presence of pepsin.

Client Needs Category—Physiological integrity
Client Needs Subcategory—Physiological adaptation

32. 4. An upper GI X-ray uses barium as a contrast medium. Once ingested by the client, this opaque substance fills the hollow structures of the esophagus and stomach, improving their image. A gastroscopy involves inserting a flexible tube in the stomach; it is not part of the upper GI procedure. I.V. dye is used in some X-rays of the gallbladder and kidney, but not for an upper GI X-ray. A computerized axial tomography scan involves placing the client within an imaging chamber for testing.

Client Needs Category—Physiological integrity
Client Needs Subcategory—Physiological adaptation

33. 1. There are approximately 30 mL in 1 ounce. Therefore, the nurse should administer 30 mL of medication.

Client Needs Category—Safe, effective care environment
Client Needs Subcategory—Safety and infection control

34. 2. Antibiotics such as tetracycline eliminate *Helicobacter pylori*, the bacterium that depletes gastric mucus and causes the majority of peptic ulcers. Although antibiotics may ultimately heal the irritated mucous membrane of the stomach, this is not the primary reason for giving such drugs. Tetracyclines neither coat the stomach nor are prescribed to prevent secondary infections in the case of ulcers.

Client Needs Category—Physiological integrity
Client Needs Subcategory—Pharmacological therapies

35. 1. Acetaminophen (Tylenol) is not associated with gastritis or ulcer formation; therefore, this drug would be safe to take. However, salicylates such as aspirin (Anacin) and nonsteroidal anti-inflammatory drugs, such as ibuprofen (Advil) and naproxen (Naprosyn), are closely linked to gastric irritation and ulcer formation. This link is well documented.

Client Needs Category—Physiological integrity
Client Needs Subcategory—Pharmacological therapies

36. 2. When the stomach or other gastrointestinal structure perforates, the abdomen becomes very hard, rigid, and tender. The skin becomes pale, not ecchymotic, due to vasoconstriction associated with shock. Dilated pupils are due to a variety of causes and do not necessarily relate to perforation. Rapid respirations are not as significant as a tense abdomen.

Client Needs Category—Physiological integrity
Client Needs Subcategory—Physiological adaptation

37. 2. Hearing a whooshing sound over the stomach as a bolus of air is instilled through the proximal end of the gastric tube is one method for determining placement. If the tube is in the esophagus, the client will belch. Another technique is to aspirate secretions from the tube and test the pH. If the secretions come from the stomach, the pH will be very acidic. A portable X-ray is an accurate method, but the cost and unnecessary radiation exposure make this method inappropriate. Liquids are never instilled through a nasogastric tube until placement has been verified. If the tip is not in the stomach, aspiration could occur. Feeling for air is an unacceptable technique for determining placement.

> *Client Needs Category—Safe, effective care environment*
> *Client Needs Subcategory—Safety and infection control*

38. 1. The nurse offers the client some hope by validating the conscientious efforts being made. The response is objective without giving false reassurance. In the second choice, the client may interpret the nurse's unwillingness to answer as an indication that his worst fear is confirmed. By implying that his serious question is silly or frivolous, as in the third choice, the client may be discouraged from attempting further communication about his fears and feelings. The last choice shows a disregard for the client's unique perception and fears.

> *Client Needs Category—Psychosocial integrity*
> *Client Needs Subcategory—None*

39. 2. Splinting or supporting the incision promotes deeper inhalation and more forceful coughing. Explaining his risks for developing pneumonia is not likely to result in efforts to clear the airway. Oxygen would not be necessary unless ventilation is compromised. A high-Fowler's position facilitates the potential for a larger volume of air, but adequate lung expansion probably will not occur unless the client actively uses his respiratory muscles.

> *Client Needs Category—Physiological integrity*
> *Client Needs Subcategory—Physiological adaptation*

40. 3. Any fluid instilled or removed is recorded to maintain accurate intake and output. An NG tube is usually irrigated with normal saline solution, not water, and the fluid does not have to be sterile. Oxygen is administered prior to tracheobronchial suctioning, not nasogastric irrigation. Swallowing does not affect gastric tube irrigation.

> *Client Needs Category—Physiological integrity*
> *Client Needs Subcategory—Physiological adaptation*

41. 1,080. Fluid intake is the sum of all the following: Liquids the client drinks; the liquid equivalent of melt-ed ice chips; foods that are liquid by the time they are swallowed (such as gelatin, ice cream, and thin, cooked cereal); I.V. infusions; and fluid instillations (such as the fluid used to flush a gastric feeding tube). The fluid volume for this client includes: 1 cup (240 mL) of thin, cooked cereal; 1 carton (8 ounces or 240 mL) of milk; ¼ cup (60 mL) of ice cream; 8 ounces (240 mL) of supplemental nutritional drink; 6 ounces (180 mL) of creamed soup; and ½ cup (120 mL) of fruit-flavored gelatin.

> *Client Needs Category—Physiological integrity*
> *Client Needs Subcategory—Physiological adaptation*

42. 2. Consuming carbohydrates, such as sugar and starch, triggers the release of insulin, causing postprandial hypoglycemia. Therefore, to prevent this component of the dumping syndrome, postgastrectomy clients are instructed to follow a low-carbohydrate diet. The client should not consume fluids with meals because this increases the rapidity with which consumed food is dumped into the small intestine. Eating small meals, not large ones, is recommended for limiting the bolus of food present in the stomach. Reducing the consumption of red meat is a healthy dietary change, but it does not prevent dumping syndrome.

> *Client Needs Category—Physiological integrity*
> *Client Needs Subcategory—Physiological adaptation*

43. 2, 4, 5. Dumping syndrome is the rapid emptying of large amounts of concentrated dietary solids and liquids into the small intestine, resulting in a significant amount of glucose in intrajejunal contents and the consequential release of insulin that causes hypoglycemia. To prevent or manage the symptoms associated with this condition, the nurse teaches the client to limit the consumption of fluid and simple carbohydrates at mealtimes, eat at least six small meals a day, and lie down for 30 minutes after eating to slow gastric emptying.

> *Client Needs Category—Health promotion and maintenance*
> *Client Needs Subcategory—None*

44. 1. Absence of free hydrochloric acid in the stomach is associated with stomach cancer. This finding distinguishes the etiology of the symptoms from other causes such as peptic ulcer. Gastrin is a hormone secreted by the mucosa of the pylorus and stomach that causes hypersecretion of gastric acid. Gastric irritation, or gastritis, and a decrease in hemoglobin and hematocrit are common findings with multiple etiologies; they are not usually related to stomach cancer.

> *Client Needs Category—Physiological integrity*
> *Client Needs Subcategory—Physiological adaptation*

45. 3. Placing the chin to the chest helps to direct the tube into the esophagus rather than the lower airway. The client is given water to sip, which makes breathing deeply difficult. A sniffing position is appropriate when first inserting the tube into a client's nose. Coughing occurs as a reflex if the tube enters the airway; it is a helpful sign that the tube is in the wrong location.

> *Client Needs Category*—*Safe, effective care environment*
>
> *Client Needs Subcategory*—*Reduction of risk potential*

46.

4.	Inspect the client's nares.
5.	Place the client's head in a sniffing position.
1.	Instruct the client to lower his chin to his chest.
2.	Have the client sip water through a straw.
6.	Aspirate and check the pH of fluid from the tube.
3.	Secure the tube to the client's nose.

The nares of the nose are inspected to determine which nostril to use for tube insertion; in most cases, either nostril may be suitable. To minimize trauma to the nasal mucosa, the client's neck is then hyperextended to simulate a sniffing position. Once the tube is visualized in the oropharynx, the client is instructed to lower his chin to his chest to facilitate advancing the tube into the esophagus and stomach rather than into the airway. The client is instructed to sip water as the tube is advanced. To determine if the tube is within the stomach, fluid is aspirated. If the aspirated fluid is acidic (indicating it has been obtained from the stomach), the tube is secured to the nose.

> *Client Needs Category*—*Physiological integrity*
>
> *Client Needs Subcategory*—*Reduction of risk potential*

47. 1. Low intermittent suction is the best setting for a single-lumen NG tube. This setting reduces trauma to the gastric mucosa and reduces the volume of electrolytes that are withdrawn from the client's gastric secretions. Low continuous suction is used for vented, or double-lumen, NG tubes.

> *Client Needs Category*—*Physiological integrity*
>
> *Client Needs Subcategory*—*Physiological adaptation*

48. 2. Clients with NG tubes that are connected to suction are generally placed on NPO (nothing by mouth) status. Providing a few ice chips helps moisten the mouth and quench the thirst. Giving larger amounts of water or other fluids would result in their removal from the stomach because of the suction. Removal of fluids also results in the removal of essential electrolytes.

> *Client Needs Category*—*Physiological integrity*
>
> *Client Needs Subcategory*—*Basic care and comfort*

49. 2. There are 1,000 mcg in 1 mg. The order is for the administration of 1,000 mcg, and there is 1 mg of drug per 1 mL of solution. Therefore, the correct volume in this case is 1 mL.

> *Client Needs Category*—*Safe, effective care environment*
>
> *Client Needs Subcategory*—*Safety and infection control*

50. 2. I.M. injections are given at a 90-degree angle. The vastus lateralis muscle (the site for this injection) is located on the outer aspect of the thigh. The deltoid muscle is in the upper arm. The rectus femoris muscle is located on the anterior thigh, and the dorsogluteal muscle is in the upper outer quadrant of the buttock.

> *Client Needs Category*—*Safe, effective care environment*
>
> *Client Needs Subcategory*—*Safety and infection control*

Nursing Care of Clients with Disorders of the Small Intestine

51. 4. Stool specimens that may contain ova and parasites should be examined when the feces is fresh and warm. Ova and parasites will not survive for long if the feces is kept below body temperature. Drying and cooling destroy the organisms and result in invalid findings. The client can use a bedpan or toilet for bowel elimination and specimen collection. Holding the container under the client's rectum would be inappropriate. Using a tongue blade, the nurse can transfer a portion of stool to a waxed, covered container. The specimen container need not be sterile.

> *Client Needs Category*—*Safe, effective care environment*
>
> *Client Needs Subcategory*—*Safety and infection control*

52. 2. The abbreviation q.i.d. means that the drug is to be administered four times a day. Scheduled hours may differ depending on the predetermined timetable set by the health agency. However, in following the order as it is written, administration can be no less or no more than four times during a 24-hour period. The other choices contain hours that are too few or too many. Military time is based on a 24-hour clock. Each hour is numbered in continuous sequence.

Client Needs Category—Safe, effective care environment
Client Needs Subcategory—Safety and infection control

53. 3. A clear liquid diet includes bouillon, tea or coffee, flavored gelatin, fruit ices, carbonated beverages such as ginger ale, and some clear fruit juices such as apple or grape. Milk or milk products may cause further diarrhea and are not permitted on this type of diet.
Client Needs Category—Physiological integrity
Client Needs Subcategory—Basic care and comfort

54. 4. A dark yellow color indicates that the client's urine is concentrated, a sign of dehydration. Pink mucous membranes are a normal finding. An elevated blood pressure and irregular heart rate are abnormal findings, but these signs are not associated with fluid volume deficit or dehydration.
Client Needs Category—Physiological integrity
Client Needs Subcategory—Physiological adaptation

55. 3. GoLYTELY is given as a colonic lavage. Within 30 minutes of ingesting the first volume of the solution, the client should experience the first of many bowel movements. The bowel must be clear of feces for the colonoscopy to be effective. This solution is preferable to other forms of bowel cleansing because it is less likely to deplete electrolytes or cause water intoxication. The other choices are expected outcomes of administering the colonic lavage solution, but they are not the main reason for its administration.
Client Needs Category—Physiological integrity
Client Needs Subcategory—Pharmacological therapies

56. 3. Respiratory depression is a potential side effect when midazolam hydrochloride (Versed) is administered. This drug allows the client to communicate and cooperate during the procedure, but afterward she will have no memory of doing so. Although many drugs can cause unstable blood pressure and cardiac arrhythmias, these complications are not commonly associated with midazolam hydrochloride (Versed).
Client Needs Category—Physiological integrity
Client Needs Subcategory—Pharmacological therapies

57. 4. Fiber is the undigested portion of fruits, vegetables, grains, and nuts that is not broken down and absorbed during the digestive process. Animal products are not a source of dietary fiber. Food that requires chewing is too limited a definition for fiber, and some foods do not contain fiber. The semisolid mass of food in the stomach is called *chyme*.

Client Needs Category—Health promotion and maintenance
Client Needs Subcategory—None

58. 2. Ileal drainage contains enzymes and bile salts that are very damaging to the skin. Therefore, preserving skin integrity is most important at this time. Intact skin is the first line of defense against microorganisms. The nurse should monitor for fluid and electrolyte imbalances related to wound drainage. Pain management may need to be addressed, especially if dressings are necessary, but this is not as important as maintaining skin integrity. Clients with draining wounds sometimes experience foul-smelling odors, but odor containment also is not the priority at this time. Body image changes are also a complication, especially if the wound is foul smelling and slow to heal; however, body image is a psychological issue and does not take priority over physiological issues such as skin integrity.
Client Needs Category—Physiological integrity
Client Needs Subcategory—Physiological adaptation

Nursing Care of Clients with Disorders of the Large Intestine

59. 2. The client's statement indicates that he does not understand the procedure and, therefore, his consent to undergo the procedure is not valid. In this case, the nurse needs to inform the physician, who is responsible for providing the explanation and obtaining consent. The nurse should never allow a client to sign a contract he does not fully understand. The nurse is responsible for witnessing the client's signature and ensuring that the legal aspects of the contract are upheld. If the client's misinformation is clarified and corrected, the surgery need not be canceled. The nurse does not proceed with skin preparation until the discrepancy is settled.
Client Needs Category—Safe, effective care environment
Client Needs Subcategory—Coordinated care

60. 4. To help prevent headaches after spinal anesthesia, it is customary to keep the client's head flat for 6 to 12 hours postoperatively. Therefore, the nurse should question an order to place the client in Fowler's position. The remaining orders in this question are appropriate and should be implemented.
Client Needs Category—Safe, effective care environment
Client Needs Subcategory—Safety and infection control

61. 1. Although pain is important to assess, the client's safety and welfare are jeopardized if the client experiences undetected urine retention. Coughing is con-

traindicated following this type of surgery. When spinal anesthesia is administered, the client remains alert.
Client Needs Category—Physiological integrity
Client Needs Subcategory—Physiological adaptation

62. **2.** A suspensory is used on a male client following a herniorrhaphy to help prevent scrotal swelling. This device will not prevent impotence, strain on the incision, or wound contamination.
Client Needs Category—Health promotion and maintenance
Client Needs Subcategory—None

63. **2.** The order reads to give the client 50 mg of Demerol. The ampule contains 100 mg/mL. Therefore, the client should receive half of the amount in the vial or 0.5 mL.
Client Needs Category—Safe, effective care environment
Client Needs Subcategory—Safety and infection control

64. **2.** The federal government mandates that the manufacturing, distribution, and dispensing of addictive drugs such as meperidine hydrochloride (Demerol) be controlled. Therefore, an accurate accounting of its administration should be kept in an opioid control log. Some health care facilities may use computerized record keeping or other forms to internally track the use of opioids, but these types of medications still need to be recorded in the opioid log.
Client Needs Category—Safe, effective care environment
Client Needs Subcategory—Safety and infection control

65. **1.** Clients with ulcerative colitis may have 12 or more diarrheal stools per day that contain blood and mucus along with fecal material. Bowel sounds are most likely to be hyperactive related to the frequency of the stools. Striae are red or white streaks on the skin due to stretching. Because the client with ulcerative colitis suffers from weight loss and emaciation, striae do not typically occur. Ulcerated lesions in this disease are confined to the colon, not the mouth.
Client Needs Category—Physiological integrity
Client Needs Subcategory—Physiological adaptation

66.

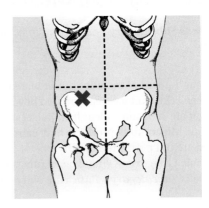

The nurse assesses the right lower quadrant first to listen to bowel sounds in the area of the ascending colon. The right and left upper quadrants of the abdomen are the locations of the transverse colon. The left lower quadrant is the area of the descending colon.
Client Needs Category—Health promotion and maintenance
Client Needs Subcategory—None

67. **1.** According to the scenario, the client is 31 years old. Keeping the commode next to the bedside is the most appropriate intervention because the client will probably be able to get herself in and out of bed with minimal assistance. This intervention would be less appropriate if the client was an older adult or too weak to get up. Answering the client's call light is always appropriate, but may be unnecessary if the client can get up by herself. Using a diaper on a person with fecal incontinence is usually emotionally devastating. It is done only as a last resort, preferably with the client's permission. Assisting the client to the bathroom frequently may or may not be appropriate, depending on the client's last bowel movement.
Client Needs Category—Physiological integrity
Client Needs Subcategory—Physiological adaptation

68. **1.** Reflecting is a response that lets the client know that both the content and the feelings are understood. Offering to contact the physician avoids the chance to provide emotional support and, therefore, is inappropriate. Giving advice and disagreeing with a client are blocks to therapeutic communication.
Client Needs Category—Psychosocial integrity
Client Needs Subcategory—None

69. **1.** After giving the preoperative medication, the nurse should raise the bedside rails and instruct the client to remain in bed because meperidine hydrochloride (Demerol) and hydroxyzine (Vistaril) depress the central nervous system, making it difficult for the client to remain alert. Elimination is accomplished prior to giving the preanesthetic drugs. One of atropine sulfate's

(Sal-Tropin) anticipated side effects is a dry mouth; however, this is not a priority nursing concern. Likewise, nausea is one of the side effects of meperidine hydrochloride (Demerol); placing an emesis basin at the bedside is not as important as ensuring the client's safety.

Client Needs Category—*Safe, effective care environment*
Client Needs Subcategory—*Safety and infection control*

70. 3. A dropping blood pressure is a common indicator that a client is going into shock. A systolic pressure of 90 to 100 mm Hg indicates impending shock; below 80 mm Hg, shock is present. Other signs of shock include a rapid, thready pulse; pale, cold, and clammy skin; rapid respirations; a falling body temperature; restlessness; and a decreased level of consciousness. None of the other choices are associated with the signs or symptoms of shock.

Client Needs Category—*Physiological integrity*
Client Needs Subcategory—*Physiological adaptation*

71. 4. Normal oxygen saturation is between 95% and 100%. The measurements in the other options indicate hypoxemia and should be reported immediately.

Client Needs Category—*Safe, effective care environment*
Client Needs Subcategory—*Safety and infection control*

72. 2, 6. When caring for an ileostomy, the nurse should observe the characteristics of the stoma on a daily basis, making sure to check its size, color, and general condition. A skin protection barrier, such as karaya, should be applied to any excoriated skin. The faceplate of the ileostomy is generally left in place for 3 to 5 days, unless it becomes loose or causes skin discomfort. The pouch is emptied, rinsed, or detached and replaced on an as-needed basis. It is unnecessary to empty the pouch as soon as stool is expelled, but the pouch should be emptied when it is one-third to one-half full to avoid pulling the faceplate from the skin due to the excessive weight of semiliquid stool. The stoma and peristomal area are cleaned with mild soap and water, not alcohol or acetone, which can dry and irritate the tissue. The faceplate should not fit snugly around the stoma; it should be trimmed to allow room for the stoma plus an extra ⅛″ to ¼″ to avoid compromising blood flow to the stoma site.

Client Needs Category—*Physiological integrity*
Client Needs Subcategory—*Basic care and comfort*

73. 1. The best time for changing an appliance and providing stomal care is when the bowel is somewhat inactive. This is usually in the morning before any food has been eaten. Exercise and eating tend to increase bowel activity, making it likely that intestinal contents will spill onto the skin if the procedure is done at that time.

Client Needs Category—*Physiological integrity*
Client Needs Subcategory—*Physiological adaptation*

74. 2. A normal healthy stoma is bright red or pink because of its rich blood supply. If the stoma is light pink or dusky blue, the blood supply to the tissue is compromised. A tan stoma is atypical even in those with a darker complexion; further assessments are necessary to determine the cause.

Client Needs Category—*Physiological integrity*
Client Needs Subcategory—*Physiological adaptation*

75. 3. Mild soap and tepid water are most often recommended for cleaning the skin around the stoma. Povidone-iodine (Betadine) is not recommended because it may irritate the skin. Alcohol is also drying and irritating to the skin. Scrubbing should be avoided because friction is likely to interrupt the skin integrity.

Client Needs Category—*Physiological integrity*
Client Needs Subcategory—*Basic care and comfort*

76. 2. The appliance opening must be large enough to avoid impairing circulation to the stoma but small enough that ileal drainage will not damage the skin. There should be only about a ⅛″ to ¼″ margin of skin exposed around the stoma. This allows room to attach the faceplate to the skin rather than to the stoma. The faceplate needs to cover an adequate amount of skin to prevent excoriation due to contact with enzymes and bile salts in ileal drainage. The stomal opening must not be obstructed, or stool will not pass. Because defecation cannot be controlled and the feces are liquid, it is inappropriate to allow the skin to air-dry for 30 minutes. The appliance must cover the stoma; the bag may or may not be directly at the waist or belt line.

Client Needs Category—*Physiological integrity*
Client Needs Subcategory—*Physiological adaptation*

77. 4. Because there is no sphincter to control the watery discharge from a conventional ileostomy, it is difficult for most clients to gain control of bowel elimination. It is realistic for people with an ileostomy to play tennis, swim, have sexual relations, get pregnant, and generally pursue careers and enjoy all manner of social activities.

Client Needs Category—*Health promotion and maintenance*
Client Needs Subcategory—*None*

78. 4. Appendicitis, the inflammation of the appendix, is often accompanied by infection. White blood cells (leukocytes) increase when infection or inflammation is present and are expected to rise in this case.

These cells fight infection by walling off, destroying, or removing damaged tissues or pathogens. The bilirubin level is typically monitored closely in a client with liver or gallbladder disease. The serum potassium level would be important if the client has anorexia, vomiting, or diarrhea. The prothrombin time is generally monitored when a client is receiving the anticoagulant warfarin sodium (Coumadin).

Client Needs Category—Physiological integrity
Client Needs Subcategory—Physiological adaptation

79. **1.** Appendicitis is typically accompanied by rebound tenderness, which is characterized as more pain after pressure is released than when applied. Although the client may have pain with palpation, the hallmark of appendicitis is the rebound phenomenon. The other options are inconsistent with appendicitis.

Client Needs Category—Physiological integrity
Client Needs Subcategory—Physiological adaptation

80. **1.** A shorter recovery period is only one of the many advantages of laparoscopic surgery. However, some form of anesthesia is used. There is a smaller than usual surgical scar and there are still activity restrictions, which include no lifting for a minimum of 10 to 15 days postoperatively.

Client Needs Category—Physiological integrity
Client Needs Subcategory—Physiological adaptation

81. **3.** Heat applications should be avoided whenever there is a possibility that abdominal discomfort is due to appendicitis. Heat dilates blood vessels, increases swelling, and promotes rupture of the vermiform appendix. Withholding food and fluid is advantageous if the symptoms are due to gastroenteritis or if emergency surgery is necessary. Pain generally limits usual activity. Acetaminophen (Tylenol) is a nonsalicylate that lowers a fever and relieves discomfort but does not predispose to rupturing the appendix.

Client Needs Category—Physiological integrity
Client Needs Subcategory—Physiological adaptation

82. **2.** An open drain relies on gravity to remove secretions absorbed by the dressing. Therefore, Fowler's position is most appropriate for promoting wound drainage. None of the other positions promote the collection of wound drainage near the drain.

Client Needs Category—Physiological integrity
Client Needs Subcategory—Physiological adaptation

83. **3.** Soiled dressings are enclosed in a receptacle or container, such as the nurse's glove, to prevent the transmission of infectious microorganisms. A clean glove is used to remove soiled dressings. Tape is pulled toward the wound to prevent separating the healing edges. Wound cleaning should always carry microorganisms and debris away from, not toward, the incision.

Client Needs Category—Safe, effective care environment
Client Needs Subcategory—Safety and infection control

84. **1.2.** Use the formula:

$$\frac{\text{Desired dose}}{\text{Dose on hand}} \times \text{Quantity} = X \text{ (amount to administer)}$$

Solve for X:
$$\frac{60}{50} \times 1 \text{ mL} = 1.2 \text{ mL}$$

Client Needs Category—Physiological integrity
Client Needs Subcategory—Pharmacological therapies

85. **1.** A change in bowel habits is one of the seven danger signals for cancer identified by the American Cancer Society. The other danger signals include a sore that does not heal, unusual bleeding or discharge, thickening or lump in a breast or elsewhere, indigestion or difficulty swallowing, obvious changes in a wart or mole, and nagging cough or hoarseness. Jaundice is not closely related to colorectal cancer but is related to diseases affecting the liver. Chronic indigestion is more closely related to stomach cancer than colorectal cancer. Being an insulin-dependent diabetic is not a risk factor related to cancer. However, diabetes can cause complications related to healing and recovery.

Client Needs Category—Physiological integrity
Client Needs Subcategory—Physiological adaptation

86. **1.** An enema solution cannot be given very well in a sitting position. Overall, this will result in a less than desirable cleansing effect. Also, because of the pooling of solution within the rectum, the client will need to defecate sooner. The client may eat lightly the evening before a sigmoidoscopy. A flexible scope is more commonly used than a rigid one. Medications are taken before the test and do not interfere with the test findings.

Client Needs Category—Physiological integrity
Client Needs Subcategory—Physiological adaptation

87. **2.** Sims' position, which is a left lateral side-lying position, is commonly preferred when a flexible sigmoidoscope is used. A knee-chest position is used with a rigid sigmoidoscope. A lithotomy position is used for cystoscopy and vaginal examinations. An orthopneic position is helpful for promoting rest in dyspneic individuals. Fowler's position is used for many reasons, including improving ventilation, but not for a sigmoidoscopy.

> ***Client Needs Category***—*Safe, effective care environment*
> ***Client Needs Subcategory***—*Safety and infection control*

88. **2.** A low-residue diet contains no fruits, vegetables, whole-grain breads, or cereals. Fruit and vegetable juices, with the exception of prune juice, are allowed in minimal amounts. Tender or ground meat and refined carbohydrates such as pasta can be eaten.

> ***Client Needs Category***—*Physiological Integrity*
> ***Client Needs Subcategory***—*Physiological adaptation*

89. **3.** There are 1,000 mg in 1 g. The nurse gives the client two 500-mg tablets to administer 1 g of neomycin. A common formula to compute proper dosage is as follows:

$$\frac{\text{Desired dose}}{\text{Dose on hand}} \times \text{Quantity} = \text{Amount to administer}$$

Therefore: $\frac{1,000}{500} \times 1 \text{ tablet} = 2 \text{ tablets}$

> ***Client Needs Category***—*Safe, effective care environment*
> ***Client Needs Subcategory***—*Safety and infection control*

90. **2.** During the operative procedure, the bowel is opened and some contents can leak within the peritoneum. Neomycin sulfate (Mycifradin) destroys intestinal bacteria and reduces the risk of a postoperative infection. Antibiotics commonly cause, rather than prevent, diarrhea. Surgery usually is not performed if the client has an ongoing infection.

> ***Client Needs Category***—*Physiological integrity*
> ***Client Needs Subcategory***—*Physiological adaptation*

91. **3.** The first action to take in the case of evisceration is to cover the bowel with sterile gauze moistened with sterile normal saline solution. The physician would be notified and vital signs taken only after taking emergency action. The bowel should not be manipulated, except by the physician. Evisceration is considered a medical emergency.

> ***Client Needs Category***—*Physiological integrity*
> ***Client Needs Subcategory***—*Physiological adaptation*

92. **3.** When an obstruction interferes with the movement of intestinal contents toward the rectum for elimination, the client begins to experience distention and vomiting. At first, the emesis contains gastric contents. As time passes, the vomitus may contain fecal matter

and have a foul odor. The other questions are appropriate to ask, but they do not necessarily provide information associated with an intestinal obstruction.

> ***Client Needs Category***—*Physiological integrity*
> ***Client Needs Subcategory***—*Physiological adaptation*

93. **2.** Most bowel obstructions are successfully treated by the insertion of an NG tube to decompress the stomach. Prior to insertion, the NG tube is measured from the tip of the nose to the earlobe to the xiphoid process. Then the tube is inserted through the client's nares, nasopharynx, and esophagus into the stomach. After insertion, the next step is to securely tape the tube to the nose, taking care that the tube is not taped so securely to the tip that it causes necrosis of the nares. Requesting an abdominal X-ray is unnecessary because the nurse can check for proper placement by injecting air into the stomach and listening for gurgling. Connecting the NG tube to high continuous wall suction is incorrect. Instead, low intermittent wall suction is usually used to decompress the stomach. Pouring water down the tube is also incorrect because the suction will pull the water back out.

> ***Client Needs Category***—*Physiological integrity*
> ***Client Needs Subcategory***—*Physiological adaptation*

94. **3.** The nurse should always question any written order that is unclear or potentially unsafe. This includes a drug dosage that is higher or lower than the dosages given in approved references. The nurse should never administer a different dosage until consulting a physician about the discrepancy. Written orders for combined preoperative medications indicate that they are given together. Therefore, giving meperidine hydrochloride (Demerol) alone is inappropriate. The pharmacist is a reliable source for obtaining drug information; however, the only person who can revise the order is the physician.

> ***Client Needs Category***—*Safe, effective care environment*
> ***Client Needs Subcategory***—*Coordinated care*

95. **2.** The best position for performing colostomy irrigation is sitting on the toilet. This position and the environment simulate normal bowel elimination. The toilet is also convenient for hanging the distal end of the irrigating sleeve. The stool is easily flushed away along with the drained irrigating solution. Because it takes some time for the bowel evacuation to be complete, clients often appreciate the privacy of the bathroom. If sitting on the toilet is impossible or impractical for the client, ensure privacy by allowing the client to sit in bed with the end of the sleeve placed in a bedpan. Kneeling in the bathtub is not safe. Standing at the sink may be effective, but disposal of the feces and the irrigating solution in the sink would be a problem.

Client Needs Category—Physiological integrity
Client Needs Subcategory—Basic care and comfort

96. 2. Silence, when used appropriately, is a powerful means of communicating without verbalizing. Among other things, silence conveys acceptance, provides the client time to collect her thoughts, allows relief from emotionally charged content, and gives the client the opportunity to proceed when ready. Changing the subject is nontherapeutic. It indicates that the nurse cannot handle the topic of conversation. Switching the discussion to physical care is a form of changing the subject. Active listening, rather than psychological counseling, is sufficient based on the data in the situation.

Client Needs Category—Psychosocial integrity
Client Needs Subcategory—None

97. 1. Encouraging the expression of concerns provides the client with an opportunity to ventilate feelings without fear of retaliation. An open discussion can effectively lower the client's frustration level. Reassurance, in this case, is somewhat premature. The client needs to verbalize and clarify the specific problems she perceives. With the assistance of the nurse and other health care professionals, the client ought to achieve the ability to accomplish self-care. Maintaining the client's independence is preferable to institutionalized care. Saying nothing indicates to the client that the nurse prefers not to become involved with emotional problems. Quoting a client, however, is always appropriate when documenting information.

Client Needs Category—Psychosocial integrity
Client Needs Subcategory—None

Nursing Care of Clients with Disorders of the Rectum and Anus

98. 3. Mineral oil is a petroleum product with lubricating properties. Humans lack the ability to digest and absorb mineral oil. It passes through the digestive system unchanged. Any fat-soluble vitamins present when food is consumed with mineral oil are not absorbed. Occasional use of mineral oil taken at bedtime is not harmful, but frequent use should be avoided. None of the other laxatives interfere with the absorption of fat-soluble vitamins.

Client Needs Category—Physiological integrity
Client Needs Subcategory—Physiological adaptation

99. 1. Long-term use of laxatives causes the bowel to become sluggish because it is repeatedly subjected to artificial stimulation. Stool softeners are less harsh than laxatives. However, it is best to determine the cause of the constipation and treat the etiology with lifestyle changes rather than continue to rely on pharmaceutical interventions. Daily enemas are just as habituating as laxative abuse. Dilating the anal sphincter is not usually a technique for promoting bowel elimination.

Client Needs Category—Physiological integrity
Client Needs Subcategory—Physiological adaptation

100. 1. A client with a fecal impaction tends to expel liquid stool around the hardened mass. Foul-smelling stools are not associated with fecal impactions. A stomachache may be associated with constipation or other conditions, but this is not the main assessment finding associated with fecal impaction. Loss of appetite may be either the cause or the effect of impaired bowel elimination. Its presence is not necessarily an indication of a fecal impaction.

Client Needs Category—Physiological integrity
Client Needs Subcategory—Physiological adaptation

101. 2. By inserting a lubricated, gloved finger within the rectum, it is possible to confirm the presence of a hard mass of stool. An X-ray may confirm the presence of a mass in the rectum but is expensive and relatively unnecessary. An oil-retention enema is a method for relieving the impaction after its presence is confirmed. Monitoring bowel elimination patterns causes unnecessary delay in treating the problem.

Client Needs Category—Physiological integrity
Client Needs Subcategory—Physiological adaptation

102. 1. Activity promotes the movement of gas toward the anal sphincter, where it can be released. Carbonated beverages can increase gas accumulation. Restricting food is inappropriate. It may prevent additional gas from forming, but it will not help eliminate any gas that is already present. Opioid analgesics tend to slow peristalsis and contribute to stool retention and intestinal gas.

Client Needs Category—Physiological integrity
Client Needs Subcategory—Physiological adaptation

103. 2. A rectal tube should remain in place only approximately 20 to 30 minutes at one time to help relieve distention from accumulating gas. Placement for only 5 minutes is unlikely to achieve an optimum effect, yet longer than 30 minutes is unnecessary. The tube is removed and replaced again in 1 to 2 hours if gas continues to accumulate.

Client Needs Category—Physiological integrity
Client Needs Subcategory—Physiological adaptation

104. **3.** Interrupting the instillation of enema solution allows time for the bowel to adjust to the distention. Rapidly instilling the remaining solution may cause the client to lose bowel control and fluid retention. Taking deep breaths or panting rather than holding the breath relieves some discomfort. Placing the client onto his back will not help the client's cramping or the sudden urge to defecate.
Client Needs Category—*Physiological integrity*
Client Needs Subcategory—*Physiological adaptation*

105. **3.** A rectal suppository is inserted approximately 2″ to 4″. For the best effect, the suppository must be beyond the internal sphincter. A clean glove, not a sterile one, is used to avoid contact with organisms in the rectum, stool, or blood. A right lateral position is not the correct anatomic position for suppository placement. Retaining the suppository until the client feels an urge to defecate ensures its effectiveness. Suppositories should be retained for at least 30 minutes.
Client Needs Category—*Physiological integrity*
Client Needs Subcategory—*Physiological adaptation*

106. **2.** Bowel elimination tends to occur in a cyclic pattern. Assessing the bowel elimination pattern precedes other interventions. Limiting activity impairs rather than promotes bowel elimination. The diet should have adequate amounts of water and bulk-forming foods to help the client form soft, rather than dry, hard stool. The regular administration of enemas eventually may help to regulate bowel elimination, but it is not the first step in a bowel-retraining program.
Client Needs Category—*Physiological integrity*
Client Needs Subcategory—*Physiological adaptation*

107. **3.** Chronic constipation, hereditary factors, and conditions that increase venous pressure in the abdomen and pelvic area, such as pregnancy, ascites, and liver disease, foster the development of hemorrhoids. Clients who take daily stool softeners are not usually prone to constipation. Clients diagnosed with ulcerative colitis have diarrhea, not constipation. Sedentary jobs, such as computer programming, may predispose the client to constipation but not necessarily hemorrhoids.
Client Needs Category—*Physiological integrity*
Client Needs Subcategory—*Physiological adaptation*

108. **2.** The cellulose that remains after eating high-fiber foods absorbs water in the bowel, increases bulk, and stimulates peristalsis. This prevents constipation, which can lead to hemorrhoids. Lack of adequate fluid makes constipation more severe. None of the other

recommendations aid in preventing or eliminating constipation.
Client Needs Category—*Health promotion and maintenance*
Client Needs Subcategory—*None*

109. **1.** A sitz bath is primarily a comfort measure because the warm water soothes the discomfort and pain in the surgical area. Secondly, a sitz bath keeps the incisional area clean and promotes healing. Because only the buttocks are submerged in water, evidence of personal hygiene is not an appropriate criterion for effectiveness. The presence of a hematoma has no bearing on the effectiveness of the sitz bath.
Client Needs Category—*Physiological integrity*
Client Needs Subcategory—*Basic care and comfort*

110. **1.** Docusate sodium (Colace) is a stool softener. Retaining water in the stool softens the mass and makes the stool easier and less painful to pass. Some categories of laxatives, including castor oil, stimulate bowel evacuation by irritating the intestinal mucosa. Bulk-forming laxatives such as psyllium (Metamucil) stimulate peristalsis by adding bulk and water to the stool. Drugs that reduce intestinal activity promote constipation rather than stool elimination.
Client Needs Category—*Physiological integrity*
Client Needs Subcategory—*Pharmacological therapies*

111. **2.** The word *pilonidal* means a nest of hair. The growth of stiff body hair in the anorectal area at puberty commonly precipitates irritation within the sinus tract. A pilonidal cyst is actually a sinus with one or more openings onto the skin. Once the integrity of the skin is impaired, microorganisms enter and cause subsequent infection, as evidenced by purulent drainage. Neither rectal bleeding nor diarrhea is associated with a pilonidal cyst.
Client Needs Category—*Physiological integrity*
Client Needs Subcategory—*Physiological adaptation*

112. **4.** Cleaning the area before applying a topical medication ensures that the drug is maximally absorbed. The client may wish to wear gloves for aesthetic and aseptic reasons, but their use will not affect the medication's action. For comfort, an ointment applied to a sensitive area is generally kept at room temperature unless otherwise directed by the manufacturer. It is more appropriate to apply this type of medication immediately following a bowel movement because pain is greater at that time. This drug can also be routinely applied in the morning and evening.
Client Needs Category—*Health promotion and maintenance*
Client Needs Subcategory—*None*

Nursing Care of Clients with Disorders of the Gallbladder

113. **1.** The characteristic upper right quadrant pain of cholecystitis typically occurs after eating. Cholecystitis is especially aggravated when the meal has a high fat content, which impairs bile flow and causes nausea, vomiting, distention, and flatulence. Ulcers are more likely to cause pain when the stomach is empty. Activity is unlikely to influence the discomfort of cholecystitis. The volume and type of foods eaten, rather than the time of day they're consumed, are more significant in the development of gallbladder disease.

Client Needs Category—Physiological integrity
Client Needs Subcategory—Physiological adaptation

114. **1.** The referred pain of cholecystitis is felt either in the right shoulder or in the back at the level of the shoulder blades. Ulcers and esophageal reflux cause pain in the mid-epigastric region. Angina pectoris may be experienced as pain in the neck or jaw or down the left arm.

Client Needs Category—Physiological integrity
Client Needs Subcategory—Physiological adaptation

115. **3.** Evidence suggests that an elevated cholesterol level predisposes certain clients to gallstone formation. The majority of gallstones are thought to form when bile in the gallbladder is thick, high in cholesterol, and low in bile acids. A low red blood cell count or hemoglobin level is commonly found in people with bleeding disorders, nutritional deficiencies, and bone marrow disorders. An elevated serum albumin level is not generally associated with cholecystitis.

Client Needs Category—Physiological integrity
Client Needs Subcategory—Physiological adaptation

116. **2.** Bile pigments cause the normal brown appearance of stool. If bile is prevented from entering the small intestine, the stool is likely to appear clay-colored. Black, tarry stools indicate bleeding high in the gastrointestinal tract; such stools also result from the administration of oral iron therapy. Dark brown stool is normal; the shade may vary depending on the food eaten. Bloody mucus associated with brown stools may indicate hemorrhoids. Greenish yellow stool is more commonly associated with diarrhea.

Client Needs Category—Physiological integrity
Client Needs Subcategory—Physiological adaptation

117. **3.** Greasy fried foods and fatty meats are not allowed on a low-fat diet. Baked fish, poultry, and lean meat are permitted. Leaner cuts of beef, such as round steak, could be ground and used in recipes that call for hamburger. Hard cheese, cream, gravies, salad oil, rich desserts, and nuts are restricted. Whole milk, butter or margarine, and sometimes eggs can be used in limited amounts.

Client Needs Category—Physiological integrity
Client Needs Subcategory—Basic care and comfort

118. **3.** Radiography of the gallbladder involves the use of an oral iodine contrast medium. A client who is allergic to iodine is at increased risk for experiencing an allergic reaction to the radiopaque substance. Because such allergic reactions can be life-threatening, this information is critical to know. Most clients can cooperate by holding still for the brief amount of time required during the gallbladder X-ray. Determining the number of previous X-rays might be appropriate in terms of teaching and preparing a client. However, knowing the precise number would not affect the client's current procedure. No anesthesia is given prior to or during an X-ray of the gallbladder.

Client Needs Category—Physiological integrity
Client Needs Subcategory—Physiological adaptation

119. **1.** The person undergoing an ultrasound of the gallbladder must not eat food for approximately 8 to 12 hours before the test. Restricting food helps to eliminate the presence of gas. Intestinal gas interferes with the transmission of sound waves toward the gallbladder and the scan of the structure's image. Water is permitted. Barium is used as a contrast medium for upper and lower GI X-rays, not a gallbladder ultrasound. Applying a water-soluble lubricant to a hand-held transducer and passing it across the abdomen during ultrasonography produces an image of the gallbladder. Insertion of needles is not part of the procedure.

Client Needs Category—Physiological integrity
Client Needs Subcategory—Physiological adaptation

120. **4.** Biliary obstruction is often accompanied by hypoprothrombinemia. The preoperative administration of vitamin K reduces the risk of hemorrhage. A single dose usually restores the normal prothrombin time within 8 to 24 hours. Vitamins A and C (not K) promote wound healing. Adequate intake of all water- and fat-soluble vitamins is necessary for general health. No specific vitamin promotes liver function.

Client Needs Category—Physiological integrity
Client Needs Subcategory—Pharmacological therapies

121. **4.** Because the deltoid muscle is not capable of absorbing large amounts of solution, I.M. injections into this muscle in adults are limited to 1 mL of solution. The deltoid is avoided in infants and children because the muscle is not sufficiently developed to absorb medication adequately. The dorsogluteal, ventrogluteal, and vastus lateralis muscles are large sites that can absorb greater volumes of injected drugs.

Client Needs Category—Safe, effective care environment

Client Needs Subcategory—Safety and infection control

122. 4. The pigment found in bile is derived from hemoglobin. Depending on the concentration of pigment, the normal appearance of bile drainage is green-yellow to orange-brown. Bile is generally clear, but clear is not a color. Dark red drainage indicates that venous blood is mixed with the biliary drainage. Bright red drainage is a sign of fresh or arterial bleeding.

Client Needs Category—Physiological integrity

Client Needs Subcategory—Physiological adaptation

123. 1, 3, 5, 6. A Jackson-Pratt closed-wound drain removes blood and exudates without using a suction machine. A vacuum or negative pressure is created by expelling air from the receptacle and replacing the cap that covers the vent while still compressing the receptacle. When emptying the receptacle, the cap that covers the vent is opened, the contents of the receptacle are emptied from the open vent and measured, air is expelled from the emptied receptacle, the vent is covered, and the tubing is stabilized to the client's gown or dressing to keep it from tugging at the insertion site. The tubing is kept unclamped at all times to allow fluid to enter the drainage receptacle. Jackson-Pratt drains do not have roller clamps.

Client Needs Category—Physiological integrity

Client Needs Subcategory—Reduction of risk potential

124. 1, 4, 5, 6. A T-tube is inserted to drain bile that is continuously formed by the liver and cannot be stored and concentrated in the gallbladder, which has been surgically removed. The tube is kept unclamped in the immediate postoperative period. The nurse connects the tube to a collection bag and facilitates drainage by keeping the client in Fowler's position with the drainage bag below the site of insertion. The nurse inspects the skin around the tube because bile may leak around the tube insertion site and irritate the skin. The nurse measures and records the volume of drainage from the T-tube. The color of the drainage may be blood-tinged initially, but it should eventually appear greenish brown.

Client Needs Category—Physiological integrity

Client Needs Subcategory—Reduction of risk potential

125. 2. The client's T-tube should remain unclamped until he begins to resume oral feedings. Clamping the tube would cause reflux of bile toward the liver; immediate action is necessary if the nurse finds the tube clamped in the early postoperative period. It would be appropriate to support the tubing to prevent kinking or dislodgement. Placing the drainage bag in a dependent position facilitates drainage by gravity. A volume of up to 500 mL in 24 hours is not unusual.

Client Needs Category—Physiological integrity

Client Needs Subcategory—Physiological adaptation

126. 3. Because bile is essential to digestion, the T–tube is generally unclamped for up to 2 hours after a meal is consumed. As healing takes place and edema is reduced, some bile begins draining into the small intestine even when the tubing is clamped.

Client Needs Category—Physiological integrity

Client Needs Subcategory—Physiological adaptation

127. 1. To establish negative pressure, air and drainage are eliminated from the bulb reservoir and the opening is capped before the squeezed bulb is released. The Jackson-Pratt drain is an example of a closed drainage device. The device could drain by gravity, not negative pressure, if the drainage valve was left open. The bulb reservoir is never filled with normal saline solution. The reservoir is secured to the skin with tape. However, this is done to prevent tension on the tubing and possible dislodgement from the insertion site, not to reestablish negative pressure in the drainage system.

Client Needs Category—Safe, effective care environment

Client Needs Subcategory—Safety and infection control

Nursing Care of Clients with Disorders of the Liver

128. 4. Alanine and aspartate aminotransferase, previously called *transaminase*, are blood tests performed to assess liver function. Liver and other organ diseases result in elevated levels of these particular enzymes. The tests are repeated periodically to evaluate the client's response to treatment. Serum potassium testing is performed to monitor electrolyte balance when a client's nutritional or fluid balance has been altered. Serum creatinine and BUN tests are performed to monitor kidney, not liver, function.

Client Needs Category—Physiological integrity

Client Needs Subcategory—Physiological adaptation

129. **1.** Infectious hepatitis A is generally spread by the oral-fecal route. In other words, the stool contains the virus, and the pathogen is spread to the mouth of a susceptible individual. Transmission is direct following contact with the excrement of an infected person or indirect by ingesting fecally contaminated food or water or food handled by an individual with the virus. This virus is also present in the blood and saliva of infected individuals; however, transmission through these routes is more rare.

> *Client Needs Category—Physiological integrity*
> *Client Needs Subcategory—Physiological adaptation*

130. **4.** Conscientious hand washing is the best defense against disease transmission. Gloves are worn when nursing care involves direct contact with the client, her excrement, or other body fluids. Wearing gloves, though, does not eliminate the need for hand washing. A gown is used if soiling is possible, but a mask is not necessary. Only individuals who cannot be relied on to practice good hand washing are placed in a private room.

> *Client Needs Category—Safe, effective care environment*
> *Client Needs Subcategory—Safety and infection control*

131. **2.** Immunoglobulin, formerly known as *gamma globulin*, is recommended for postexposure to a person infected with the hepatitis A virus. It is most effective if administered within 48 hours to 2 weeks following exposure. Antibiotic therapy is ineffective in preventing or eliminating hepatitis A, which is a viral infection. Hepatitis vaccinations are usually given to clients at risk for contracting hepatitis B. Anti-inflammatory drugs, such as salicylates, nonsalicylates, and steroids, are ineffective in preventing the spread of hepatitis A.

> *Client Needs Category—Health promotion and maintenance*
> *Client Needs Subcategory—None*

132. **2.** Lanolin is an emollient. It softens skin and prevents moisture loss. Dry skin adds to the itching sensation caused by the release of bile salts onto the skin. Bathing is not discontinued altogether. Even in the worst situations, the skin is bathed with tepid water. Alcohol is drying to the skin; its use contributes to itching. There is no advantage to substituting a shower for a tub bath.

> *Client Needs Category—Physiological integrity*
> *Client Needs Subcategory—Basic care and comfort*

133. **2.** Homosexual men are at particularly high risk for acquiring blood-borne infections. The source of the hepatitis B virus is the blood of infected people or carriers. The virus is present in semen, saliva, and blood. It

is transmitted by sexual contact, contaminated blood products, or accidental or intentional puncture with objects or needles that contain traces of infected blood. The client living in Europe has no bearing on the disease. Alcohol abuse compounds, but does not cause, liver damage concurrent with hepatitis. Working in a fast-food restaurant is more of a factor in acquiring hepatitis A than hepatitis B.

> *Client Needs Category—Health promotion and maintenance*
> *Client Needs Subcategory—None*

134. **2.** For anyone who is previously unvaccinated, the best action following exposure to the blood of someone with hepatitis B is to receive the hepatitis B immunoglobulin within 24 hours but no later than 7 days. Vaccination immediately after exposure does not provide sufficient antibody protection. Viruses are unaffected by antibiotics such as penicillin (Pentam). Bleach is an effective antiseptic, but it is not the best prophylaxis to counter exposure to the hepatitis B virus.

> *Client Needs Category—Health promotion and maintenance*
> *Client Needs Subcategory—None*

135. **2.** Donating blood is not recommended for people who have had hepatitis. The virus remains in the blood years after the person has had the acute illness and can be passed to others. Blood collection personnel are taught to screen and reject any potential donor who indicates that he has had jaundice. Safe sex may be practiced, which would include using a latex condom. Convalescence is prolonged following the acute phase of hepatitis, but eventually there are no permanent physical restrictions. Excessive caffeine may have negative effects on the liver, but its use is not necessarily restricted. Individuals with hepatitis antibodies are not barred from foreign travel.

> *Client Needs Category—Health promotion and maintenance*
> *Client Needs Subcategory—None*

136. **1.** The etiology of Laënnec's portal cirrhosis, the most common form of cirrhosis in the United States, is chronic malnutrition and alcoholism. Malnutrition is often a consequence of alcoholism. Smoking is associated with lung cancer, not cirrhosis of the liver. A history of pancreatitis can cause numerous bloody stools daily, but this is not associated with cirrhosis of the liver. The client's hypertension could be secondary to his alcohol abuse.

> *Client Needs Category—Physiological integrity*
> *Client Needs Subcategory—Physiological adaptation*

137. **2.** The skin of a person with cirrhosis usually manifests multiple vascular lesions with a central red body and radiating branches. These are known as *spi-*

der angiomas. They are also referred to as *telangiectasia, spider nevi,* or *vascular spiders.* Clients with cirrhosis also usually have scant body hair. The testes atrophy due to the liver's inability to fully metabolize estrogen. Elevated serum cholesterol levels and hyperglycemia are not usually associated with cirrhosis.
>   ***Client Needs Category****—Physiological integrity*
>   ***Client Needs Subcategory****—Physiological adaptation*

138. 3. In the absence of the client taking an oral iron supplement, a black or tarry stool indicates that a significant amount of blood is being lost from the stomach or somewhere in the proximal end of the intestine. Pain, nausea, and abdominal distention usually do not accompany gastric hemorrhage.
>   ***Client Needs Category****—Physiological integrity*
>   ***Client Needs Subcategory****—Physiological adaptation*

139. 4. Ascites is the collection of fluid within the peritoneal cavity. An appropriate technique for monitoring the increase or decrease in this condition is measuring the abdominal girth. Either the apical or radial pulse measurement is appropriate for a general assessment. The position in which the blood pressure is measured must be consistent, but it may be taken while the client is either lying down or sitting. The urine specific gravity is usually monitored when a client has a problem with intravascular fluid volume or renal disease, not ascites.
>   ***Client Needs Category****—Physiological integrity*
>   ***Client Needs Subcategory****—Physiological adaptation*

140. 1. After a liver biopsy, the client is monitored closely for signs of hemorrhage. The nurse positions the client so that body weight puts pressure on the needle site. A person with cirrhosis is at especially high risk for bleeding or hemorrhage because liver disease results in diminished prothrombin. Prothrombinemia causes a prolonged delay in the time it takes for blood to clot; therefore, blood clots are not usually a problem. Although the client may acquire an infection from the biopsy, an invasive procedure, infection does not usually occur immediately after the procedure. A collapsed lung is not typically an issue unless extremely poor technique was used in the procedure.
>   ***Client Needs Category****—Physiological integrity*
>   ***Client Needs Subcategory****—Physiological adaptation*

141. 3. By positioning the client on the right side, the weight of the body tends to put pressure on the puncture. This compression helps to reduce or prevent bleeding. Ambulation is contraindicated because it promotes bleeding. Neither high-Fowler's position nor elevating the legs is appropriate for controlling bleeding.
>   ***Client Needs Category****—Physiological integrity*
>   ***Client Needs Subcategory****—Physiological adaptation*

142. 2. Metallic objects present a safety hazard during an MRI. Consequently, internal metal objects such as a dental bridge should be removed. Jewelry, chains, and medallions are also removed. Sedation is not usually required except for clients who are severely claustrophobic. There is no relationship between body weight and urinary elimination, although giving the client an opportunity to void is a conscientious comfort measure.
>   ***Client Needs Category****—Safe, effective care environment*
>   ***Client Needs Subcategory****—Safety and infection control*

143. 1. The bladder is emptied just prior to a paracentesis. A full bladder may be punctured as the needle is inserted through the abdominal wall. The client can eat and drink before the test. The physician usually prepares the skin with an antiseptic such as povidone-iodine (Betadine), but this option is not the most appropriate one. There is no need for the crash cart to be outside the client's door because cardiac arrest is not a common occurrence related to this procedure.
>   ***Client Needs Category****—Safe, effective care environment*
>   ***Client Needs Subcategory****—Safety and infection control*

144. 2. Documentation of the total volume of aspirated fluid is essential. Fluid replacement is determined more by the client's urine output and vital signs than by the volume of aspirated fluid. As a rule, clients do not require pain relief after a paracentesis. Ventilation is usually improved after ascitic fluid has been removed; clients generally do not need additional encouragement to deep-breathe.
>   ***Client Needs Category****—Physiological integrity*
>   ***Client Needs Subcategory****—Physiological adaptation*

145. 4. Due to the tendency for the client with cirrhosis to bleed, the nurse applies sustained pressure for a longer period to prevent hematoma formation and bruising. Placing a vial of vitamin K at the bedside is unnecessary, even though vitamin K helps with clotting. There is no scientific rationale for performing any of the other actions.
>   ***Client Needs Category****—Physiological integrity*
>   ***Client Needs Subcategory****—Physiological adaptation*

146. **3.** Rising levels of ammonia in the blood are toxic to the central nervous system and can cause alterations in consciousness. Serum bilirubin is monitored to assess the liver's ability to form bile and transport it to the gallbladder for concentration. Bilirubin is not associated with hepatic encephalopathy. Serum creatinine and blood urea nitrogen are tests used to monitor renal function.

Client Needs Category—Physiological integrity
Client Needs Subcategory—Physiological adaptation

147. **1.** Difficulty in arousing the cirrhotic client indicates a significant neurologic change. It is typically a sign that the client is progressing into hepatic coma. The client's physiological and safety needs become even more important at this time. Jaundice is usually present in clients diagnosed with cirrhosis. Seizures may occur. The urine output and blood pressure are within normal limits. Pancreatitis is not associated with worsening cirrhosis.

Client Needs Category—Physiological integrity
Client Needs Subcategory—Physiological adaptation

148. **2.** Working through grief involves dealing with a loss. Reviewing one's life is often a task that takes place in anticipatory grieving. This is therapeutic and should not be suppressed. Therefore, active listening is the most appropriate nursing measure. Suggesting that a close family member be called is a way of avoiding the situation. Calling the clergy at the church may or may not be appropriate, depending on the client's religious beliefs; however, the nurse can always take this step after listening to the client. It would be unrealistic to expect the client's wife to think about future plans before she has dealt with the reality of her impending loss.

Client Needs Category—Psychosocial integrity
Client Needs Subcategory—None

Nursing Care of Clients with Disorders of the Pancreas

149. **2.** Pain is a subjective experience. Asking the client to rate his pain helps to assess its intensity. A numeric rating scale can be used later to evaluate the effectiveness of the pain-relief techniques used. Noting whether the client is able to stop moving is an invalid assessment technique. A cooperative client may make an effort to stop moving despite the continuation of severe pain. Perspiration is a physiological sign that may accompany pain; however, because many factors can cause perspiration, noting its presence or absence is not the best assessment technique. Administering an analgesic is a nursing intervention, not a form of assessment.

Client Needs Category—Physiological integrity
Client Needs Subcategory—Basic care and comfort

150. **2.** An elevated serum amylase level is the most reliable evidence of pancreatitis. The bilirubin level becomes elevated if the pancreatitis is due to an obstruction of the common bile duct or pancreatic duct. Glucose tolerance test abnormalities indicate dysfunction of the endocrine functions of the pancreas, which is secondary to pancreatitis. Elevated bilirubin and abnormal glucose tolerance tests are not the best indicators of pancreatitis. Lactose tolerance test results have no relationship to pancreatitis.

Client Needs Category—Physiological integrity
Client Needs Subcategory—Physiological adaptation

151. **4.** The distance from the nose (N) to the earlobe (E) to the xiphoid (X) is called the *NEX measurement*. It is commonly used to determine the approximate distance to the stomach. None of the other landmarks is correct for approximating the length for NG tube insertion.

Client Needs Category—Safe, effective care environment
Client Needs Subcategory—Safety and infection control

152. **1.** One indication that the gastric tube has been incorrectly positioned in the respiratory tract is the client's inability to speak. This would occur if the tube was inadvertently located between the folds of the vocal cords, preventing the vibration necessary for speech. The tube would need to be withdrawn to the level of the oropharynx to reestablish the client's ability to breathe and speak. Swallowing would not be affected in this situation. Sneezing and vomiting are not appropriate signs to evaluate whether a gastric tube is in the wrong location.

Client Needs Category—Physiological integrity
Client Needs Subcategory—Safety and infection control

153. **4.** The nurse assigned to care for a client with an I.V. infusion has a responsibility to monitor the infusion to ensure that it is instilling the prescribed volume at the correct rate. Any volume more or less than prescribed must be reported to the nurse in charge. The infusion can flow by gravity with the tubing coiled on the bed. The nondominant hand is preferred for an I.V. infusion. There is ample time, with 100 mL left, to temporarily postpone reporting the information.

Client Needs Category—Safe, effective care environment
Client Needs Subcategory—Safety and infection control

154. **3.** The nurse would be correct to remove scrambled eggs from the dietary tray of a client on a bland, low-fat diet. One scrambled egg made with milk and butter has approximately 8 g of fat. One cup of cooked, unsweetened prunes has only a trace of fat. One cup of nonfat skim milk has a trace of fat. One slice of unbuttered whole-wheat toast has only 1 g of fat.

> *Client Needs Category—Health promotion and maintenance*
> *Client Needs Subcategory—None*

155. **3.** There is an established relationship between the chronic consumption of alcohol and the incidence of pancreatitis. Once an acute attack of pancreatitis has occurred, the client is at risk for chronic pancreatitis. Use of alcohol leads to continued inflammation of the pancreas. It is essential to protect the pancreas from further irritation because serious complications (including destruction of the organ itself, peritonitis, shock, and even death) can occur. Having had pancreatitis does not disqualify a client from donating blood, doing heavy lifting, or taking laxatives.

> *Client Needs Category—Physiological integrity*
> *Client Needs Subcategory—Physiological adaptation*

156. **2.** Anorexia and weight loss appear early in the onset of cancer of the pancreas. Pancreatic cancer, like most other forms of cancer, does not usually cause acute pain in the early stages. If the client with pancreatic cancer experiences pain early on, it is usually dull and more apparent at night. In addition, bleeding is not typically a problem unless the cancer has also affected the liver. Fainting, unless from weight and fluid loss, is not a common sign of pancreatic cancer.

> *Client Needs Category—Physiological integrity*
> *Client Needs Subcategory—Physiological adaptation*

157. **3.** The most therapeutic response in this situation is to encourage the client to talk about her thoughts and feelings. People who are dying often know without being told that they are terminal. It is more important to support a client's hope than to bluntly confirm suspicions. It would be unethical to say that the terminal client's condition will improve. The nurse would be appropriate acting as a liaison in contacting someone who can help the client take care of unfinished business; however, this would not be the first or best nursing response in this case.

> *Client Needs Category—Psychosocial integrity*
> *Client Needs Subcategory—None*

158. **2.** It is better to control pain before it escalates. When pain is intense, relief is more difficult to achieve. Peaks and valleys of pain are reduced by administering pain-relieving drugs on a routine schedule throughout the 24-hour period rather than just when it becomes absolutely necessary to do so. The goal is to keep the client free from pain yet not dull her consciousness or ability to communicate. Asking the physician to order a high dose initially is premature. Tolerance is likely to develop later. It would be more appropriate to consult the physician about changing the medication order when the client's condition warrants it.

> *Client Needs Category—Physiological integrity*
> *Client Needs Subcategory—Basic care and comfort*

The Nursing Care of Clients with Urologic Disorders

⇨ **Nursing Care of Clients with Urinary Incontinence**
⇨ **Nursing Care of Clients with Infectious and Inflammatory Urologic Disorders**
⇨ **Nursing Care of Clients with Renal Failure**
⇨ **Nursing Care of Clients with Urologic Obstructions**
⇨ **Nursing Care of Clients with Urologic Tumors**
⇨ **Nursing Care of Clients with Urinary Diversions**
⇨ **Correct Answers and Rationales**

Directions: With a pencil, blacken the space in front of the option you have chosen for your correct answer.

Nursing Care of Clients with Urinary Incontinence

1. Which nursing assessment is most important before beginning bladder retraining with an incontinent client?
[ ] **1.** Recording the times at which the client is incontinent
[ ] **2.** Checking the specific gravity of the urine
[ ] **3.** Monitoring the extent of bladder distention
[ ] **4.** Observing the color of the client's urine

Postpartum clients who have had vaginal deliveries are taught how to perform Kegel exercises to prevent future problems with urinary stress incontinence.

2. Which instruction by the nurse is correct when teaching a client to perform Kegel exercises?
[ ] **1.** Contract and relax the muscles in the vagina.
[ ] **2.** Stand and rock the pelvis back and forth.
[ ] **3.** Push down with the feet, and elevate the hips.
[ ] **4.** Pull the abdominal muscles inward, then relax.

During bladder retraining, a client tells the nurse that he intends to restrict his fluid intake to remain dry for longer periods of time.

3. Which response by the nurse is best?
[ ] **1.** Encourage the client to restrict his fluid intake because it shows evidence of client cooperation.
[ ] **2.** Encourage the client to restrict his fluid intake because it leads to accomplishing the goal.
[ ] **3.** Discourage the client from restricting his fluid intake because it contributes to constipation.
[ ] **4.** Discourage the client from restricting his fluid intake because it potentiates fluid imbalance.

An elderly nursing home resident who has urinary incontinence says to the nurse, "What's the sense in living? I'm just a baby nowadays."

4. Which comment is the best response the nurse can offer?
[ ] **1.** "You're a very nice gentleman."
[ ] **2.** "Cheer up. You can't be serious."
[ ] **3.** "You should expect this at your age."
[ ] **4.** "You're discouraged right now."

After an incontinent male client has a stroke, the nursing team uses an external catheter to prevent skin breakdown.

5. When applying an external catheter, which action by the nurse is correct?
[ ] **1.** Lubricate the penis before applying the catheter.
[ ] **2.** Measure the length and circumference of the penis.
[ ] **3.** Leave space between the end of the penis and the catheter's drainage end.
[ ] **4.** Retract the foreskin before rolling the catheter sheath over the penis.

6. After inserting an indwelling catheter into a male client, which technique is most appropriate for stabilizing the catheter to avoid a penoscrotal fistula?
[ ] **1.** Tape the catheter to the abdomen.
[ ] **2.** Pass the catheter under the client's leg.
[ ] **3.** Fasten the drainage tubing to the bed with a safety pin.
[ ] **4.** Insert the catheter into the tubing of a collecting bag.

7. When teaching a female client how to catheterize herself, the nurse should instruct her to insert the catheter how far into the urethra?
[ ] **1.** 1″ (2.5 cm)
[ ] **2.** 2″ (5 cm)
[ ] **3.** 3″ (7.5 cm)
[ ] **4.** 4″ (10 cm)

Nursing Care of Clients with Infectious and Inflammatory Urologic Disorders

A woman with type 1 diabetes mellitus consults a physician because she has been experiencing urinary problems.

8. When the nurse interviews the client, which symptom is the client most likely to report if she has a bladder infection?
[ ] **1.** Sharp flank pain
[ ] **2.** Urethral discharge
[ ] **3.** Strong-smelling urine
[ ] **4.** Burning on urination

9. When the nurse instructs the client about the technique for collecting a clean-catch midstream urine specimen for routine urinalysis, which statement is most accurate?
[ ] **1.** Cleanse the urethral area using several circular motions.
[ ] **2.** Void into the plastic liner under the toilet seat.
[ ] **3.** After voiding a small amount, collect a sample of urine.
[ ] **4.** Mix the antiseptic solution with the collected urine specimen.

10. When the nurse reviews the results of the client's urinalysis, which substance in the urine is most suggestive of a bladder infection?
[ ] **1.** Glucose
[ ] **2.** Blood
[ ] **3.** Bilirubin
[ ] **4.** Protein

To relieve the client's symptoms, the physician orders phenazopyridine (Pyridium), a urinary analgesic.

11. It is most appropriate for the nurse to advise the client that taking this medication will have which effect on her urine?
[ ] **1.** The urine will look cloudy.
[ ] **2.** The urine will appear orange.
[ ] **3.** The urine will become scant.
[ ] **4.** The urine will have a strong odor.

12. Which urinary change provides the best evidence that the phenazopyridine (Pyridium) is achieving its intended therapeutic effect?
[ ] **1.** Urinary frequency is decreased.
[ ] **2.** Urinary urgency is decreased.
[ ] **3.** Urinary burning is decreased.
[ ] **4.** Urine output is increased.

A middle-aged woman is involved in a motor vehicle accident. She is to be in traction on bed rest for an extended period of time.

13. Considering the amount of time the client must remain in bed, why is it imperative for the nurse to monitor for a urinary tract infection?
[ ] **1.** The client will not be able to complete her hygiene needs.
[ ] **2.** The client will not be able to fully empty her bladder.
[ ] **3.** The client will not be able to maintain bladder control.
[ ] **4.** The client will not be able to drink sufficient fluids.

14. In evaluating multiple clients with urinary tract infections, the clinic nurse would anticipate which client to be at least risk for developing a urinary tract infection?
[ ] **1.** A client with urethral mucosa damage
[ ] **2.** A client with altered mental conditions
[ ] **3.** A client with altered metabolic states
[ ] **4.** An immunocompromised client

15. When a client asks the clinic nurse why women have more bladder infections than men, which answer is most accurate?

[ ] **1.** The male urethra is straighter, which facilitates elimination of pathogens.

[ ] **2.** The male urethra is lined with a layer of mucous membrane, which traps microorganisms.

[ ] **3.** The female urethra is shorter, and pathogens enter the bladder more easily.

[ ] **4.** The female urethra has a larger diameter and is more easily contaminated.

A nurse at a walk-in clinic near a college campus is caring for a 21-year-old diabetic student who reports that she has frequent urinary tract infections.

16. Which of the following statements made by the student would strongly suggest that she has a urinary tract infection? Select all that apply.

[ ] **1.** "I need to urinate frequently."

[ ] **2.** "I can't hold my urine."

[ ] **3.** "I have a burning sensation when I urinate."

[ ] **4.** "I have itching in my perineal area."

[ ] **5.** "I pass a large quantity of urine."

[ ] **6.** "My urine is foul-smelling."

17. Because the client also has diabetes mellitus, which statement by the nurse best explains why she is at higher risk for acquiring a bladder infection?

[ ] **1.** Glucose in urine supports bacterial growth.

[ ] **2.** Diabetes suppresses white blood cell activity.

[ ] **3.** Dietary therapy may cause a deficiency of nutrients.

[ ] **4.** Having diabetes allows less energy for attending to hygiene.

18. Which recommendation by the nurse is most effective in reducing bacterial growth in the client's bladder?

[ ] **1.** Drink a large quantity of fluid.

[ ] **2.** Change underclothing each day.

[ ] **3.** Avoid the use of public restrooms.

[ ] **4.** Use only white toilet tissue.

19. Which of the following measures performed by the client would offer the best protection against acquiring a urinary tract infection?

[ ] **1.** Wiping away from the urinary meatus after bowel elimination

[ ] **2.** Performing appropriate hand washing after bowel elimination

[ ] **3.** Using a feminine hygiene spray after bowel elimination

[ ] **4.** Drying the perineum thoroughly after bowel elimination

20. When teaching a client with cystitis about urinary tract irritants, the nurse correctly identifies which of the following substances as potential irritants to avoid? Select all that apply.

[ ] **1.** Alcohol

[ ] **2.** Milk

[ ] **3.** Tea

[ ] **4.** Chocolate

[ ] **5.** Coffee

[ ] **6.** Pears

21. When the client with cystitis has difficulty visualizing the urinary tract, the nurse shows her a diagram that includes all the primary structures involved. Identify on the diagram the area of inflammation associated with the client's cystitis.

A female client becomes acutely ill with flank pain, fever, and chills. The physician makes a tentative diagnosis of acute pyelonephritis and orders a catheterized urine specimen for culture.

22. When preparing the client for catheterization, how should the nurse position the client?

[ ] **1.** Lithotomy position

[ ] **2.** Recumbent

[ ] **3.** Knee-chest position

[ ] **4.** Prone

23. When the nurse inserts the catheter into the client's vagina rather than the urinary meatus, which action is best to take next?

[ ] **1.** Wipe the catheter tip with an alcohol swab.

[ ] **2.** Cleanse the catheter tip with povidone-iodine solution (Betadine).

[ ] **3.** Discard the catheter and use another sterile one.

[ ] **4.** Withdraw the catheter and insert it in the urethra.

The physician prescribes a urinary anti-infective combination of trimethoprim (Proloprim) and sulfamethoxazole (Bactrim) twice a day.

24. Which nursing instruction is most appropriate for preventing crystal formation in this client's urine?
[ ] **1.** Eat more acidic citrus fruits.
[ ] **2.** Avoid carbonated soft drinks.
[ ] **3.** Drink 3 quarts of water daily.
[ ] **4.** Take the medication with food.

The client is scheduled for intravenous pyelography (IVP). The nurse prepares to administer a laxative to the client.

25. What is the primary reason for administering a laxative before the procedure?
[ ] **1.** Emptying the bowel aids in examining the lower gastrointestinal tract.
[ ] **2.** Emptying the bowel prevents accidental stool incontinence during the X-ray.
[ ] **3.** Emptying the bowel reduces the potential for constipation or impaction.
[ ] **4.** Emptying the bowel improves the ability to visualize the urinary structures.

26. If the client makes the following statements, which information is most important to report to the physician before the client has IVP?
[ ] **1.** "Strong laxatives give me diarrhea."
[ ] **2.** "I have a low tolerance for pain during procedures."
[ ] **3.** "I had a reaction when my gallbladder was X-rayed before."
[ ] **4.** "My insurance company may require a second opinion."

Despite the fact that a middle-aged woman's symptoms of malaise and headache are rather unremarkable, she is diagnosed with acute glomerulonephritis.

27. Which statement made by the client's spouse most closely correlates with the diagnosis of acute glomerulonephritis?
[ ] **1.** "My wife's face looks rather puffy lately."
[ ] **2.** "Recently my wife has been quite forgetful."
[ ] **3.** "My wife has been salting her food heavily."
[ ] **4.** "It seems that my wife sleeps quite poorly."

28. When the nurse reviews the client's medical history, which finding most likely precipitated her present illness?
[ ] **1.** Trauma to the lower abdomen
[ ] **2.** An upper respiratory infection
[ ] **3.** Treatment with an antibiotic
[ ] **4.** An allergic reaction to X-ray dye

29. If this client is typical of others with glomerulonephritis, which finding would the nurse expect to observe when conducting a head-to-toe physical assessment?
[ ] **1.** Skin hemorrhages
[ ] **2.** Absence of body hair
[ ] **3.** Flushed appearance
[ ] **4.** Peripheral edema

30. If the physician orders all of the following laboratory tests, which one is most important for the nurse to monitor when caring for this client?
[ ] **1.** Serum amylase
[ ] **2.** Blood glucose
[ ] **3.** Blood urea nitrogen (BUN)
[ ] **4.** Complete blood count (CBC)

31. Considering the client's diagnosis, which nursing intervention is the priority at this time?
[ ] **1.** Ambulating the client twice daily
[ ] **2.** Assisting the client with mouth care
[ ] **3.** Monitoring the client's weight daily
[ ] **4.** Encouraging the client to increase her fluid intake

32. When the client complains of a headache, which nursing action should be performed first?
[ ] **1.** Administering a prescribed analgesic
[ ] **2.** Assessing the client's blood pressure
[ ] **3.** Reducing environmental stimuli
[ ] **4.** Changing the client's position

The nurse caring for the client with glomerulonephritis is told during the shift report that a 24-hour urine collection for creatinine clearance is to begin at 8 a.m.

33. Which nursing action is most appropriate in relation to collecting the client's urine specimen?
[ ] **1.** Have the client void at 8 a.m., and refrigerate the specimen.
[ ] **2.** Have the client void at 8 a.m., and dispose of the specimen.
[ ] **3.** Have the client void at 8 a.m., and send the specimen to the laboratory.
[ ] **4.** Have the client void at 8 a.m., and place the specimen in a preservative.

The nurse uses a color reagent strip (dipstick) to test a voided urine specimen.

34. If the reagent strip can detect the following substances, which one would the nurse expect to be present in the urine of a client with glomerulonephritis?
[ ] **1.** Glucose
[ ] **2.** Bilirubin
[ ] **3.** Albumin
[ ] **4.** Acetone

35. When the nurse inspects the client's urine specimen, which finding best indicates that the urine contains red blood cells?

[ ] **1.** The urine appears cloudy.
[ ] **2.** The urine appears smoky.
[ ] **3.** The urine appears bright orange.
[ ] **4.** The urine appears dark yellow.

The client is put on a low-sodium diet.

36. Which menu choice is best for the nurse to recommend?

[ ] **1.** Hot dog with potato salad
[ ] **2.** Beef bouillon and crackers
[ ] **3.** Chicken breast on lettuce
[ ] **4.** Cheese pizza with thin crust

The physician prescribes the steroids methylprednisolone (Medrol) and prednisone (Orasone) on alternate days by oral administration to treat the client's glomerulonephritis.

37. When the client asks the nurse why she should not take the drugs daily, which response is best?

[ ] **1.** The medications are too toxic if taken on a daily basis.
[ ] **2.** This alternating schedule maintains adrenal function.
[ ] **3.** Each medication has a prolonged period of action.
[ ] **4.** Most people cannot tolerate the medications' daily side effects.

Nursing Care of Clients with Renal Failure

A male client who has chronic glomerulonephritis has deteriorated to the early stages of renal failure.

38. Which symptom indicative of renal failure would the nurse expect to note when assessing this client?

[ ] **1.** Anemia
[ ] **2.** Hyperthyroidism
[ ] **3.** Anorexia
[ ] **4.** Diabetes

39. If this client's condition is similar to that of others in the oliguric phase of renal failure, the nurse would anticipate the client's urine output to be within what range?

[ ] **1.** 50 to 100 mL/hour
[ ] **2.** 100 to 150 mL/hour
[ ] **3.** 500 to 1,000 mL/day
[ ] **4.** 100 to 500 mL/day

The nursing team meets to address the client's early renal failure in relation to the care plan.

40. The nurse reports to her colleagues that which diagnostic test, considered a sensitive indicator of advanced kidney disease, will need to be closely monitored by the nursing team?

[ ] **1.** Serum creatinine level
[ ] **2.** Serum sodium level
[ ] **3.** Uric acid level
[ ] **4.** Urea nitrogen level

41. Which nursing assessment is essential to add to the client's care plan?

[ ] **1.** Monitor body temperature.
[ ] **2.** Measure intake and output.
[ ] **3.** Check for urine retention.
[ ] **4.** Listen for bowel sounds.

The physician orders a fluid challenge of 500 mL of I.V. fluid to be infused at a rapid rate, followed by the administration of a loop diuretic I.V. to sustain or improve renal function.

42. While the fluid is being administered, which nursing assessment is most important?

[ ] **1.** Checking for pedal edema
[ ] **2.** Monitoring skin integrity
[ ] **3.** Inspecting the oral mucosa
[ ] **4.** Auscultating for breath sounds

43. Because of the client's impaired urine elimination, which potential skin problem will require additional team planning?

[ ] **1.** Reduced perspiration
[ ] **2.** Extreme oiliness
[ ] **3.** Loss of skin turgor
[ ] **4.** Pronounced itching

The client is placed on a sodium-restricted diet.

44. When the client complains about the bland taste of the food, the nurse appropriately recommends substituting salt with which condiment?

[ ] **1.** Catsup
[ ] **2.** Mustard
[ ] **3.** Soy sauce
[ ] **4.** Lemon juice

45. Which nursing action is most appropriate when the client complains about being thirsty because of his fluid restrictions?

[ ] **1.** Giving the client hard candy to suck
[ ] **2.** Providing the client with ice chips
[ ] **3.** Offering the client an ice cream bar
[ ] **4.** Supplying the client with fresh fruit

The care plan indicates that the client is to be weighed regularly.

46. Which factor is most important for the nurse to consider when planning to weigh the client?
[ ] **1.** When the client was last weighed
[ ] **2.** When the client last took a drink of fluid
[ ] **3.** How much the client has eaten so far today
[ ] **4.** Whether the client feels like being weighed

When it becomes evident that the client will require long-term hemodialysis, an internal arteriovenous fistula is created.

47. Which nursing assessment is most important to perform regularly when a client has an arteriovenous fistula?
[ ] **1.** Checking the color and temperature of the client's hand
[ ] **2.** Monitoring the client's wrist and finger range of motion
[ ] **3.** Observing the tone and coordination of the client's arm muscles
[ ] **4.** Inspecting the client's forearm skin turgor

48. While manually assessing the functioning of the arteriovenous fistula, which sensation would the nurse expect to note over the fistula site?
[ ] **1.** A pulse
[ ] **2.** A bruit
[ ] **3.** A thrill
[ ] **4.** A click

49. Which nursing intervention is most helpful in assisting the client undergoing hemodialysis to cope with his chronic health condition?
[ ] **1.** Giving the client literature to read about renal failure
[ ] **2.** Advising the client's spouse to spend more time with him
[ ] **3.** Keeping the client informed of the latest research findings
[ ] **4.** Exploring with the client how this disorder has affected his life

The nurse is caring for another male client with renal failure who is being treated with peritoneal dialysis.

50. Which assessment taken before and after peritoneal dialysis is most valuable in evaluating the outcome of treatment?
[ ] **1.** Pulse rate
[ ] **2.** Body weight
[ ] **3.** Skin turgor
[ ] **4.** Urine output

51. Before the client is about to begin peritoneal dialysis, the nurse correctly informs him that the procedure involves the movement of urea and creatinine through the peritoneum by means of which force?
[ ] **1.** Osmosis
[ ] **2.** Diffusion
[ ] **3.** Filtration
[ ] **4.** Gravity

52. Immediately after the dialysate solution has been instilled, which nursing action is correct?
[ ] **1.** Clamping the tubing from the infusion
[ ] **2.** Draining the infused dialysate solution
[ ] **3.** Restricting the client's movement as much as possible
[ ] **4.** Encouraging the client to drink fluids

53. Which is the most significant information to report when caring for a client undergoing peritoneal dialysis?
[ ] **1.** Loss of body weight
[ ] **2.** Regular, deep breathing
[ ] **3.** Elevated body temperature
[ ] **4.** Output that exceeds intake

54. Which finding provides the best evidence that peritoneal dialysis is achieving a therapeutic effect?
[ ] **1.** Urine output increases.
[ ] **2.** Appetite improves.
[ ] **3.** Potassium level falls.
[ ] **4.** Red blood cell count is lower.

55. When advising the client about the potential complications associated with peritoneal dialysis, which complication is most important to include?
[ ] **1.** Pulmonary edema
[ ] **2.** Abdominal peritonitis
[ ] **3.** Abdominal hernia
[ ] **4.** Ruptured aorta

A client with renal failure is just informed that he is a candidate for a kidney transplant.

56. When the client asks about the source of donated kidneys, the nurse correctly identifies which of the following as the preferred donor?
[ ] **1.** A recently deceased human
[ ] **2.** A sibling or living relative
[ ] **3.** An unrelated living human
[ ] **4.** A chimpanzee or other primate

57. Which problem is the nurse's immediate concern following kidney transplant surgery?
[ ] **1.** Hypovolemic shock caused by postoperative bleeding
[ ] **2.** Abdominal distention secondary to delayed peristalsis
[ ] **3.** Postoperative paralytic ileus due to colon manipulation
[ ] **4.** Pneumonia secondary to ineffective breathing patterns

Nursing Care of Clients with Urologic Obstructions

58. Which assessment finding strongly suggests that a client's reduced volume of voided urine is due to an obstructive disorder?
[ ] **1.** The client feels a continued need to void.
[ ] **2.** The client's urine appears dark amber.
[ ] **3.** The client's bladder is below the pubis.
[ ] **4.** The client experiences abdominal cramps.

59. If the physician inserts a suprapubic cystostomy tube to drain the accumulating urine, the nurse should assess the characteristics of urine from a catheter that exits from which location?
[ ] **1.** Urethra
[ ] **2.** Abdomen
[ ] **3.** Ureter
[ ] **4.** Flank

60. Which nursing intervention is essential for evaluating the patency of the suprapubic catheter?
[ ] **1.** Inspecting the client's skin around the insertion site
[ ] **2.** Monitoring the client's urine output every 2 hours
[ ] **3.** Attaching the catheter to a leg bag when the client ambulates
[ ] **4.** Encouraging the client to consume 100 mL of oral fluid hourly

A client comes to the emergency department for relief from severe, stabbing, colicky flank pain. The physician makes a tentative diagnosis of urolithiasis.

61. When the nurse examines the voided urine specimen, which finding is most supportive of the diagnosis of urolithiasis?
[ ] **1.** Cloudy pale urine
[ ] **2.** Blood-tinged urine
[ ] **3.** Light yellow urine
[ ] **4.** Strong-smelling urine

A cystoscopy is scheduled to help diagnose the client's suspected condition.

62. If the client asks the nurse to outline the benefits of the cystoscopy procedure, which ones should the nurse list as positive outcomes? Select all that apply.
[ ] **1.** Involves visual examination of the internal structure of the kidney
[ ] **2.** Helps identify the sources of hematuria, incontinence, and urine retention
[ ] **3.** Allows for collection of tissue samples, cell washings, and urine samples
[ ] **4.** Requires no sedation because it is painless
[ ] **5.** Uses a light source to visualize the internal structure
[ ] **6.** Requires no surgical incision because the scope is introduced into the urethra

63. After the cystoscopy, the nurse can expect the client to experience which urinary symptom?
[ ] **1.** Polyuria
[ ] **2.** Dysuria
[ ] **3.** Anuria
[ ] **4.** Pyuria

64. When the client is definitively diagnosed with urolithiasis, which nursing intervention is most appropriate to add to the care plan?
[ ] **1.** Restrict fluids to 1,000 mL/day.
[ ] **2.** Maintain the client in Fowler's position.
[ ] **3.** Limit activity to bed rest.
[ ] **4.** Strain all voided urine.

65. Which nursing intervention is essential for the client at this time?
[ ] **1.** Increasing the client's fluid intake to prevent further stone formation
[ ] **2.** Interrupting the voiding pattern to strengthen the bladder muscles
[ ] **3.** Limiting the client's voiding to allow for releasing a larger stream of urine
[ ] **4.** Increasing the client's dietary calcium to replace losses to renal calculi

The client is scheduled for extracorporeal shock wave lithotripsy (ESWL) to pulverize the stone.

66. After the nurse explains the ESWL procedure to the client, which statement is the best evidence that he understands the scheduled procedure?
[ ] **1.** "I'll be submerged in a tank of water."
[ ] **2.** "Radiation will be focused on my bladder."
[ ] **3.** "A laser beam will be aimed at my kidneys."
[ ] **4.** "I'll experience a tingling sensation."

An older man makes an appointment with a physician concerning urinary symptoms he has been experiencing.

67. When the office nurse obtains the client's history, which statement provides the best indication that the client has benign prostatic hypertrophy (BPH)?
[ ] **1.** "There is some burning when I urinate."
[ ] **2.** "I wake up each night needing to urinate."
[ ] **3.** "I feel pressure in my back before voiding."
[ ] **4.** "My urine is almost colorless, like water."

68. To gather more information about symptoms associated with BPH, which question is most important to ask next?
[ ] **1.** "Have you noticed any changes in sexual function?"
[ ] **2.** "Have you felt any lumps in your scrotum recently?"
[ ] **3.** "Do you have difficulty starting to void?"
[ ] **4.** "Do you have problems controlling urination?"

An older man with a history of BPH has been unable to urinate in 18 hours. The physician instructs the nurse to insert a urethral catheter.

69. Which technique is best for helping the nurse insert the tip of the catheter past the enlarged prostate gland?
[ ] **1.** Angle the penis in the direction of the toes.
[ ] **2.** Massage the tissue below the base of the penis.
[ ] **3.** Push the catheter with additional force.
[ ] **4.** Grasp the penis firmly within the hand.

70. Which catheter is the best choice to use for a client with BPH?
[ ] **1.** A coudé catheter
[ ] **2.** A silicone catheter
[ ] **3.** A rubber catheter
[ ] **4.** A flexible catheter

The client is scheduled to undergo a transurethral resection of the prostate (TURP).

71. Following the TURP, which assessment finding would the nurse expect to observe during the immediate postoperative period?
[ ] **1.** Light pink to clear urine
[ ] **2.** Mucoid sediments in urine
[ ] **3.** Decreased volume of urine
[ ] **4.** Grossly bloody urine

The nurse receives instructions to provide continuous bladder irrigation through a three-way catheter after the client's TURP procedure.

72. What equipment is necessary for the nurse to gather to implement continuous bladder irrigation?
[ ] **1.** An I.V. pole
[ ] **2.** An Asepto (bulb) syringe
[ ] **3.** A round, sterile basin
[ ] **4.** Antiseptic solution

Postoperatively, the client tells the nurse that he is having a great deal of discomfort in his bladder area. The physician has written several analgesic drug orders for the client in anticipation of the pain associated with TURP.

73. Before administering an analgesic to the client, what is important for the nurse to assess?
[ ] **1.** Whether the pulse rate is normal
[ ] **2.** Whether the dressing is dry and intact
[ ] **3.** Whether the catheter is draining urine
[ ] **4.** Whether the client's coughing is adequate

74. Which medication is most appropriate to administer if the client is having bladder spasms?
[ ] **1.** Acetylsalicylic acid (aspirin) by mouth
[ ] **2.** Propoxyphene napsylate (Darvocet) by mouth
[ ] **3.** Meperidine hydrochloride (Demerol) intramuscularly
[ ] **4.** Belladonna and opium (B&O) rectal suppository

A nurse is assigned to care for a client following a suprapubic prostatectomy. The client has one catheter in the urethra and another in an abdominal incision.

75. When documenting the client's urine output in the medical record, which measurement is correct for the nurse to record?
[ ] **1.** Only the output from the urethral catheter
[ ] **2.** Only the output from the wound catheter
[ ] **3.** The outputs from each catheter separately
[ ] **4.** The combined output from both catheters

Several days after the client's procedure, the physician removes the catheter from the abdominal incision.

76. Which nursing intervention is most important to add to the client's care plan following removal of the suprapubic catheter?
[ ] **1.** Reposition the client every 2 hours.
[ ] **2.** Ambulate the client with assistance.
[ ] **3.** Change abdominal dressings when wet.
[ ] **4.** Encourage deep breathing hourly.

Nursing Care of Clients with Urologic Tumors

A physician asks the office nurse to schedule a series of examinations and tests to determine whether a client has cancer of the prostate gland.

77. Which diagnostic test should the nurse schedule before any manipulation of the prostate tissue to avoid erroneous test results?
[ ] **1.** Kidneys, ureters, bladder X-ray
[ ] **2.** Needle biopsy of the prostate gland
[ ] **3.** Prostatic-specific antigen (PSA) test
[ ] **4.** Transrectal ultrasound examination

The client is diagnosed with prostatic cancer and undergoes a radical perineal prostatectomy. Postoperatively, the client has an indwelling (Foley) catheter in place.

78. When managing catheter care, which nursing action is most important for promoting wound healing?
[ ] **1.** Avoid tension on the catheter.
[ ] **2.** Encourage oral fluid intake.
[ ] **3.** Clean the urethral meatus daily.
[ ] **4.** Clamp and release the catheter q2h.

The physician prescribes estradiol (Estrace) for the client following the prostatectomy.

79. Which statement by the client provides the best evidence that he understands the potential side effects associated with his hormonal therapy?
[ ] **1.** "Both of my breasts may enlarge."
[ ] **2.** "I may have spontaneous erections."
[ ] **3.** "My sperm count will be higher."
[ ] **4.** "I'll have strong sexual urges."

A nephrectomy is performed on a client with a kidney tumor.

80. Postoperatively, which assessment finding is most suggestive that the client is hemorrhaging?
[ ] **1.** Acute flank pain
[ ] **2.** Abdominal distention
[ ] **3.** Flushed, warm skin
[ ] **4.** Nausea and vomiting

A nurse is caring for a client with bladder cancer.

81. If this client is typical of others who acquire bladder cancer, which symptom is most likely to have manifested in the early stage of this disease?
[ ] **1.** Difficulty voiding
[ ] **2.** Persistent oliguria
[ ] **3.** Painless hematuria
[ ] **4.** Urethral discharge

82. When asked about factors that are linked to cancerous changes in the bladder, the nurse correctly identifies which factor?
[ ] **1.** Stress incontinence
[ ] **2.** Frequent intercourse
[ ] **3.** Sexual promiscuity
[ ] **4.** Cigarette smoking

The physician recommends that the client's bladder cancer be treated conservatively by instilling an antineoplastic drug within the bladder.

83. When administering the bladder instillation containing the chemotherapeutic drug, which safety precaution is most important?
[ ] **1.** Wear two pairs of latex gloves.
[ ] **2.** Use a glass syringe for the drug.
[ ] **3.** Avoid wearing clothing with long sleeves.
[ ] **4.** Limit contact time with the client.

Nursing Care of Clients with Urinary Diversions

A client whose bladder cancer has been unresponsive to treatment will have his bladder surgically removed. An ileal conduit will be created to facilitate urine elimination.

84. When the client asks the nurse to clarify the surgeon's explanation of the procedure, which statement is most accurate?
[ ] **1.** "Your urine will be deposited in your small intestine."
[ ] **2.** "Urine will be eliminated with stool from the rectum."
[ ] **3.** "Urine will drain from an abdominal opening."
[ ] **4.** "Your urine will empty from a special catheter."

The night nurse reports that the preoperative client scheduled for the cystectomy and ileal conduit was awake much of the night and that, when he slept, he was restless.

85. Which assessment supports the nurse's assumption that the client's sleep disturbance was most likely due to anxiety?
[ ] **1.** Temperature is 98.9° F (37.1° C).
[ ] **2.** Blood pressure is 132/88 mm Hg.
[ ] **3.** Pulse rate is 106 beats/minute at rest.
[ ] **4.** Pulse pressure is 44 mm Hg.

86. To facilitate the client's coping, which statement by the nurse is most therapeutic at this time?

[ ] **1.** "It must be difficult facing this type of surgery."
[ ] **2.** "You have one of the best surgeons at this hospital."
[ ] **3.** "You'll see; everything will turn out OK for you."
[ ] **4.** "Others with your diagnosis have done just fine."

On the morning of surgery, the client tells the nurse, "Imagine not being able to control your urination."

87. Which response by the nurse is most therapeutic?
[ ] **1.** "Tell me what that means to you."
[ ] **2.** "I know just how you're feeling."
[ ] **3.** "Well, it's not quite as bad as that."
[ ] **4.** "You need to think more positively."

Postoperatively, the client wears an appliance that collects his urine. He tells the nurse that his skin feels raw and irritated near the stoma.

88. Which nursing action is most appropriate at this time?
[ ] **1.** Increase the client's oral fluids to dilute the urine.
[ ] **2.** Remove the appliance and inspect the skin.
[ ] **3.** Empty the appliance at more frequent intervals.
[ ] **4.** Leave the appliance off for 1 or 2 days.

89. When providing discharge instructions about the early signs of complications from the ileal conduit, the nurse correctly advises the client to notify the physician immediately if which signs and symptoms develop? Select all that apply.
[ ] **1.** The stoma has a bluish appearance.
[ ] **2.** The urine in the bag is yellow and collects at a rate of 32 mL/hour.
[ ] **3.** The stoma has decreased in size since surgery.
[ ] **4.** The client experiences sharp abdominal pain.
[ ] **5.** The stoma is flush with the skin.
[ ] **6.** The urine has an ammonia odor.

The nurse also teaches the client how to change his ostomy appliance before he is discharged.

90. Which suggestion is most helpful to control leaking urine during the time the appliance is being changed?
[ ] **1.** "When you remove the appliance, let the urine drip into the toilet."
[ ] **2.** "When you remove the appliance, insert a tampon into the stoma."
[ ] **3.** "When you remove the appliance, press a gloved finger over the stoma."
[ ] **4.** "When you remove the appliance, pinch the stoma with two fingers."

Correct Answers and Rationales

Nursing Care of Clients with Urinary Incontinence

1. 1. Keeping a log of incontinence helps the nurse identify patterns in the frequency of urination. The data are then used to schedule toilet activities to correspond to the filling and emptying patterns demonstrated by the client. Checking the urine's specific gravity, monitoring bladder distention, and observing urine color are all appropriate assessments when caring for clients having problems with urinary elimination. However, these assessments are not necessarily as pertinent to planning a successful bladder-retraining program as identifying urinary elimination patterns.
  Client Needs Category—*Physiological integrity*
  Client Needs Subcategory—*Physiological adaptation*

2. 1. By contracting and relaxing the muscles in the vagina, a client can perform Kegel exercises. This technique helps strengthen those muscles so the client is able to control urine elimination from the bladder. Pelvic rocking helps to relieve backache associated with dysmenorrhea and is considered a good conditioning exercise during the prenatal period. The other options describe exercises for improving muscle tone, but they are not specific to the pubococcygeal muscles.
  Client Needs Category—*Health promotion and maintenance*
  Client Needs Subcategory—*None*

3. 4. The nurse should discourage the client from restricting his fluid intake because it can lead to fluid imbalance. In general, fluids are important to flush toxins and infections from the body and to maintain a state of homeostasis. Restricting fluid leads to more concentrated urine, which is more likely to foster stone formation. Inadequate fluid intake does contribute to constipation, but that is not the main reason for discouraging the client from limiting his fluid intake. Although the client is determined to meet his goal, it is unsafe to encourage him in his plan to restrict fluid intake.
  Client Needs Category—*Health promotion and maintenance*
  Client Needs Subcategory—*None*

4. 4. Reflecting feelings is a useful therapeutic communication technique that demonstrates empathy. It lets the client know that the nurse has recognized the emotion underlying the spoken words in the verbal statement. Disagreeing with the client by saying that he is a nice gentleman may block further communication.

Belittling the client's feelings by challenging the seriousness of his statement also interferes with communication. Advising the client to cheer up or to anticipate physical setbacks because of his age are inappropriate, nontherapeutic forms of interaction.

***Client Needs Category**—Psychosocial integrity*
***Client Needs Subcategory**—None*

5. 3. Allowing space between the end of the penis and the drainage end of the catheter helps prevent irritation to the urinary meatus and promotes urine drainage. Lubrication is inappropriate because it would interfere with maintaining the catheter's positioning. External catheters are similar to latex condoms; they stretch to fit; therefore, measuring the penis is unnecessary. The foreskin of an uncircumcised man is never left in a retracted position because it could have a tourniquet effect and interfere with circulation of blood to the tissue.

***Client Needs Category**—Physiological integrity*
***Client Needs Subcategory**—Basic care and comfort*

6. 1. Anchoring the indwelling catheter to the abdomen eliminates pressure and irritation at the penoscrotal angle. Pressure in this area predisposes to fistula formation. The catheter and tubing are passed over a client's leg to prevent obstruction of drainage from body weight. It is appropriate to fasten the drainage tubing to the bed to ensure a straight line from the bed to the collection bag and to insert the catheter into the tubing of the collection bag. However, neither of these nursing actions will prevent a penoscrotal fistula from forming.

***Client Needs Category**—Physiological integrity*
***Client Needs Subcategory**—Reduction of risk potential*

7. 3. The nurse should teach the client to catheterize herself by inserting a catheter 3″ (7.5 cm) into the urinary meatus in a downward and backward direction. At approximately 3″, the client should see urine in the tubing. The catheter may be advanced farther when the balloon is inflated, after the catheter is into the bladder.

***Client Needs Category**—Physiological integrity*
***Client Needs Subcategory**—None*

Nursing Care of Clients with Infectious and Inflammatory Urologic Disorders

8. 4. One of the classic symptoms of a urinary tract infection (cystitis) is pain or burning on urination. Other symptoms include urinary frequency and urgency. People who have pyelonephritis more commonly experience flank pain. The client's urine may contain white blood cells, causing it to appear cloudy, but a purulent discharge is not a common complaint. Concentrated urine has a strong odor, but this usually does not occur among those with cystitis. Although the urine may develop an odor depending on the bacterial growth and amount of urine retained, clients do not commonly report this finding.

***Client Needs Category**—Physiological integrity*
***Client Needs Subcategory**—Physiological adaptation*

9. 3. The initial voided stream is discarded and a portion of what follows is collected as the specimen. Women are instructed to clean the urethral area from front to back; men clean the penis using a circular motion. The specimen is collected in a sterile container. The substance used for cleaning is not mixed with the urine specimen.

***Client Needs Category**—Physiological integrity*
***Client Needs Subcategory**—Reduction of risk potential*

10. 2. Infectious and inflammatory conditions affecting the urinary tract are accompanied by blood and pus in the urine, which may be grossly visible or microscopic. Glucose in the urine may be caused by a metabolic problem such as diabetes mellitus. Liver and gallbladder disorders are evidenced by the presence of bilirubin in the urine. Protein in the urine suggests pathology within the nephrons of the kidneys.

***Client Needs Category**—Physiological integrity*
***Client Needs Subcategory**—Physiological adaptation*

11. 2. Phenazopyridine (Pyridium) changes the color of the urine to orange. It will not cause the urine to look cloudy, decrease in volume, or smell strong.

***Client Needs Category**—Physiological integrity*
***Client Needs Subcategory**—Pharmacological therapies*

12. 3. Phenazopyridine (Pyridium) is a urinary analgesic that rapidly decreases the burning associated with urinary tract infections. Reducing discomfort eventually results in less frequent and urgent urination, but these are secondary effects. Emptying the bladder at less frequent intervals may increase the volume eliminated, but this is also a secondary effect of drug therapy.

***Client Needs Category**—Physiological integrity*
***Client Needs Subcategory**—Pharmacological therapies*

13. 2. The client who must remain on bed rest due to traction has difficulty in fully eliminating urine from the bladder due to the positioning within the bed. This can lead to residual urine in the bladder that prompts bacteria growth. Urinary stagnation can also result in stone formation. Hygiene needs are also important but can be met with regular nursing care. The client should still have bladder control and be able to drink fluids.

Client Needs Category—*Physiological integrity*
Client Needs Subcategory—*Reduction of risk potential*

14. **2.** Altered mental states do not necessarily place a client at higher risk for urinary tract infections, especially if the client can still attend to personal hygiene. A client is at risk for a urinary tract infection if she is immunocompromised and unable to fight bacteria growth, has suffered trauma to the urethral mucosa, or has an altered metabolic state that could change the composition of the urine.

Client Needs Category—*Health promotion and maintenance*
Client Needs Subcategory—*None*

15. **3.** Because the female urethra is shorter, pathogens travel to the bladder at a much faster rate than in a man. Also, the female urethra is more easily contaminated with organisms from the rectum and vagina if hygiene is inadequate. Pathogens have to travel farther in the longer male urethra. Also, the male urethra is more curved, which tends to act as a barrier to the progression of pathogens toward the bladder. Both male and female urethras are lined with mucous membranes. The diameters of the urethras are similar in both sexes.

Client Needs Category—*Physiological integrity*
Client Needs Subcategory—*Reduction of risk potential*

16. **1, 3, 6.** The client with a urinary tract infection typically reports symptoms of urinary frequency, burning upon urination, urinary urgency, and concentrated, foul-smelling urine. The client might also report passing a small amount of urine with each frequent voiding. Urinary incontinence and itching in the perineal area are not symptoms of a urinary tract infection but should be assessed as well.

Client Needs Category—*Physiological integrity*
Client Needs Subcategory—*Physiological adaptation*

17. **1.** Many chronic health states, such as diabetes mellitus, multiple sclerosis, and spinal cord injuries, predispose affected clients to urinary tract infections. Glucose in the urine provides a supportive environment for bacterial growth. Diabetes mellitus does not suppress white blood cell activity. Diet therapy to control diabetes provides sufficient amounts of all essential nutrients needed to maintain health. If diabetes mellitus is controlled, the client should not experience energy reduction.

Client Needs Category—*Physiological integrity*
Client Needs Subcategory—*Physiological adaptation*

18. **1.** A large intake of fluids promotes frequent urinary elimination, which causes pathogens to pass out of the bladder with the urine. Decreasing the number of pathogens present in the urinary tract reduces their growth rate. Changing underclothing regularly is an appropriate hygiene measure; however, it is not the most effective measure for reducing bacteria in the bladder. Personal hygiene measures are more important than the sanitary condition of restrooms in reducing the incidence of bladder infections. The color of toilet tissue does not contribute to or prevent cystitis.

Client Needs Category—*Health promotion and maintenance*
Client Needs Subcategory—*None*

19. **1.** The most important technique for preventing future urinary tract infections is to eliminate the introduction of organisms from the rectum or vagina through improper wiping. Hand washing following elimination assists in reducing the transmission of pathogens to other body structures, such as the eyes and mouth. However, hand washing is not as effective as correct wiping in reducing the risk of cystitis. The use of chemicals, such as those found in feminine hygiene sprays, should be avoided because they commonly contain irritants or substances to which many people are sensitive. Drying the perineum is a comfort measure that also appropriately eliminates moisture that may facilitate bacterial growth; however, it is not as significant as the manner in which the perineum is wiped.

Client Needs Category—*Health promotion and maintenance*
Client Needs Subcategory—*None*

20. **1, 3, 4, 5.** Alcohol, tea, chocolate, and coffee are all urinary irritants. Urinary irritants may exacerbate such conditions as interstitial cystitis. Possible substitutes include apricots, pears, papaya juice, herbal tea, and carob.

Client Needs Category—*Health promotion and maintenance*
Client Needs Subcategory—*None*

21.

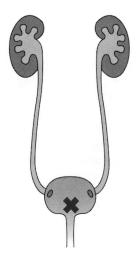

Cystitis is an inflammation of the urinary bladder (as indicated by the X). It is usually caused by a bacterial infection.

> ***Client Needs Category***—*Physiological integrity*
> ***Client Needs Subcategory***—*Physiological adaptation*

22. 2. When it is necessary to insert a catheter, the recumbent position is best for the majority of female clients. This position involves placing the client on the back with the knees flexed and the soles of the feet flat on the bed. For women who have arthritis of the hips or another condition that interferes with recumbent positioning, a side-lying position is used as an alternative. The lithotomy position involves supporting the feet in stirrups. It is used when a woman undergoes a pelvic examination. The knee-chest position is used for rectal or lower bowel examinations. The prone position is used when examining the spine and back.

> ***Client Needs Category***—*Safe, effective care environment*
> ***Client Needs Subcategory***—*Safety and infection control*

23. 3. The urinary tract is a sterile environment; therefore, a contaminated catheter should be discarded and a new one obtained before proceeding with the catheterization. Wiping the contaminated catheter with an alcohol swab or cleaning it with povidone-iodine (Betadine) solution will not ensure sterility. If the catheter contaminated from the vagina is reinserted into the urethra, pathogens may be transferred to the urinary tract.

> ***Client Needs Category***—*Safe, effective care environment*
> ***Client Needs Subcategory***—*Safety and infection control*

24. 3. Clients who take sulfonamides such as sulfamethoxazole (Bactrim) can reduce the risk of developing crystalluria by consuming 3 to 4 quarts of fluid per day. Water is preferred for a diabetic client because it is calorie-free. Sulfonamides are best taken on an empty stomach unless gastric irritation occurs. Carbonated drinks and citrus fruits will not reduce the risk of crystalluria.

> ***Client Needs Category***—*Health promotion and maintenance*
> ***Client Needs Subcategory***—*None*

25. 4. A laxative is given the evening before IVP to empty the bowel of gas and stool, which, if present, could obstruct the view of the urinary structures during the X-ray. IVP is not used to examine the lower gastrointestinal tract. Stool incontinence is not generally a problem with IVP. Laxatives are generally given to treat, not prevent, constipation.

> ***Client Needs Category***—*Physiological integrity*
> ***Client Needs Subcategory***—*Physiological adaptation*

26. 3. A history of a previous allergic reaction to radiopaque dye indicates the client is at risk for a similar episode. The physician may prescribe a corticosteroid or antihistamine prior to the test to reduce the potential for an allergic reaction. The other information has value, but reporting the previous reaction has the greatest potential for ensuring the client's safety.

> ***Client Needs Category***—*Physiological integrity*
> ***Client Needs Subcategory***—*Reduction of risk potential*

27. 1. Family members often notice that the face of a person with glomerulonephritis appears pale and puffy. Mental status is usually unaffected in the early stages of the disease. Salting food and sleeping poorly are atypical signs of glomerulonephritis.

> ***Client Needs Category***—*Physiological integrity*
> ***Client Needs Subcategory***—*Physiological adaptation*

28. 2. Although definite evidence linking a streptococcal infection with glomerulonephritis has not been established, many people identify that they experienced an upper respiratory infection or sore throat 2 to 3 weeks before the onset of glomerulonephritis. There is no correlation between acute glomerulonephritis and trauma, antibiotic therapy, or an allergy specific to X-ray dye.

> ***Client Needs Category***—*Physiological integrity*
> ***Client Needs Subcategory***—*Physiological adaptation*

29. 4. A common sign associated with glomerulo–nephritis is peripheral edema that ranges from slight ankle edema in the evening to generalized fluid retention that may compromise cardiac function. The skin is pale, not flushed. Skin hemorrhages are a common finding in liver disease and blood dyscrasias. The distribution of body hair is not directly related to glomerulonephritis.

Client Needs Category—Physiological integrity
Client Needs Subcategory—Physiological adaptation

30. 3. The results of BUN testing indicate how efficiently the glomeruli are removing nitrogen wastes from the blood. An elevation indicates glomerular dysfunction. Serum amylase levels aid in diagnosing and monitoring pancreatitis. A blood glucose test is used for monitoring diabetes mellitus. A CBC is helpful for baseline information, but it is not as essential in evaluating the course of glomerulonephritis as BUN testing.

Client Needs Category—Physiological integrity
Client Needs Subcategory—Physiological adaptation

31. 3. Because glomerulonephritis impairs renal function, monitoring weight on a daily basis is essential for evaluating how much fluid the person is retaining. Ambulation is not usually impaired; however, if the client is hypertensive or has other circulatory complications, activity may be restricted. Mouth care is important for all who cannot attend to their own self-care; however, it usually is not a problem among those with glomerulonephritis. Many clients with glomerulonephritis are on fluid restrictions; therefore, encouraging fluid intake is an inappropriate nursing action.

Client Needs Category—Physiological integrity
Client Needs Subcategory—Physiological adaptation

32. 2. It is important for the nurse to first assess the client's blood pressure. People with glomerulonephritis are typically hypertensive; hypertension can be accompanied by a headache. Hypertension is also an indication of increased intracranial pressure. If the headache is caused by hypertension, a priority intervention is to reduce the blood pressure and treat the cause. Implementing comfort measures such as reducing environmental stimuli, administering a prescribed analgesic, and changing the client's position are appropriate; however, assessing the client is the nurse's priority in this situation.

Client Needs Category—Physiological integrity
Client Needs Subcategory—Physiological adaptation

33. 2. Urine that formed before the time a 24-hour urine collection starts should not be included with the collected urine. Valid results require that the urine collected be produced within the 24-hour period. Properly collected urine is refrigerated in a large container, or the container is kept in a basin of ice. After all the urine from the 24-hour period is collected, the entire specimen is sent to the laboratory. The nurse should consult the laboratory policy about whether to mix the urine from a 24-hour collection with a preservative or to refrigerate the sample.

Client Needs Category—Physiological integrity
Client Needs Subcategory—Physiological adaptation

34. 3. People with glomerulonephritis generally test positive for albuminuria. Albumin is present in the urine due to the increased permeability of the glomerular membrane. Glucose and acetone are expected in the urine of a person with uncontrolled diabetes mellitus. Bilirubin is present in the urine of a person with liver or gallbladder disease.

Client Needs Category—Physiological integrity
Client Needs Subcategory—Physiological adaptation

35. 2. The presence of blood gives a smoky appearance to urine. Cloudy urine suggests the presence of white blood cells. If the urine appears bright orange, the nurse might investigate whether or not the client has ingested a substance containing a water-soluble dye. Concentrated urine is likely to appear dark yellow.

Client Needs Category—Physiological integrity
Client Needs Subcategory—Physiological adaptation

36. 3. Chicken breast on lettuce is the menu item that contains the least amount of sodium among the options provided. Processed meats are highly salted. Bouillon and other canned soups also generally contain a great deal of salt. Dairy products are high in sodium. Baked goods, such as crackers and pizza crust, also contain sodium bicarbonate or salt.

Client Needs Category—Health promotion and maintenance
Client Needs Subcategory—None

37. 2. Alternate-day therapy is used when administering glucocorticoid drugs to prevent adrenal suppression. By alternating exogenous hormone therapy on one day, it allows the adrenal cortex to produce endogenous hormone as the blood level drops the following day. Steroids have many undesirable side effects, but most are tolerable. Steroids can be and are administered on a daily basis when clients require short-term therapy. The duration of action is generally 24 hours.

Client Needs Category—Physiological integrity
Client Needs Subcategory—Pharmacological therapies

Nursing Care of Clients with Renal Failure

38. 1. Anemia is common in clients with renal failure. The kidney produces erythropoietin, which stimulates the production of red blood cells. If kidney function is diminished, anemia occurs from the decreased red blood cell production. Diabetes, anorexia, and hyperthyroidism may occur in conjunction with renal failure, but they are not caused by it.

> ***Client Needs Category***—*Physiological integrity*
> ***Client Needs Subcategory***—*Physiological adaptation*

39. 4. The first stage of renal failure is generally characterized by oliguria—that is, a urine output of less than 500 mL in 24 hours. The nurse would expect to note a diuretic phase following a period of oliguria or anuria as the client's condition improves.

> ***Client Needs Category***—*Physiological integrity*
> ***Client Needs Subcategory***—*Physiological adaptation*

40. 1. The client's serum creatinine levels should be closely monitored because they are helpful in determining kidney functioning. High serum creatinine levels are commonly noted in conjunction with glomerular damage. Altered levels of serum sodium, uric acid, and blood urea nitrogen may also be seen, but these are not the best indicators of kidney functioning.

> ***Client Needs Category***—*Physiological integrity*
> ***Client Needs Subcategory***—*Physiological adaptation*

41. 2. Measuring intake and output accurately is a priority when planning the care of a client with renal failure. This information aids in evaluating fluid balance and adjusting fluid restrictions. Urine retention is not common in renal failure because the client is not producing much urine. Generally, a urinary catheter is inserted to aid in monitoring the output of a person in renal failure. The body temperature is monitored to assess for signs of infection or other complications; however, it is not likely to be affected by the primary condition. The nurse would not expect to note abnormal bowel sounds in clients with renal failure.

> ***Client Needs Category***—*Physiological integrity*
> ***Client Needs Subcategory***—*Physiological adaptation*

42. 4. It is necessary to assess the client's breath sounds in this situation because administering fluid to someone with oliguria or anuria may lead to heart failure and pulmonary edema. Fluid overload is manifested by pedal edema, but this is not a life-threatening consequence. Although the client's skin integrity becomes impaired due to inactivity, edema, and elimination of nitrogenous wastes through the skin, skin impairment is not considered an immediate problem with fluid therapy. The oral mucosa does not undergo adverse changes with the administration of fluid.

> ***Client Needs Category***—*Physiological integrity*
> ***Client Needs Subcategory***—*Reduction of risk potential*

43. 4. The skin of a client in renal failure becomes dry and intensely itchy due to the excretion and evaporation of nitrogenous wastes through the skin. Skin care involves frequent cleaning with plain, warm water, then patting the skin dry. The client may have increased perspiration due to the excretion process. The skin typically becomes dry, not oily. The nurse may choose to apply a lubricating skin cream or lotion. Edema causes taut, puffy skin, not loss of turgor.

> ***Client Needs Category***—*Physiological integrity*
> ***Client Needs Subcategory***—*Physiological adaptation*

44. 4. Lemon juice is used to enhance the flavor of fish, eggs, and some vegetables. Other recommended seasonings include fresh herbs, such as parsley, dill, and oregano. Fresh onion is also acceptable. Catsup, prepared mustard, and soy sauce are high in sodium and should be avoided.

> ***Client Needs Category***—*Physiological integrity*
> ***Client Needs Subcategory***—*Basic care and comfort*

45. 1. Hard candy, especially if sour or tart-flavored, increases salivation and reduces the sensation of thirst without increasing fluid intake. Clients in renal failure, unless they are diabetic, are not generally restricted in the amount of carbohydrates they may consume. Ice chips, ice cream, and fresh fruit all contain fluid that must be considered in the fluid restriction. Fruit contains potassium, which is also contraindicated for clients with renal failure.

> ***Client Needs Category***—*Physiological integrity*
> ***Client Needs Subcategory***—*Physiological adaptation*

46. 1. To evaluate trends in weight, the nurse weighs the client at the same time daily using the same scale. The amount of clothing is similar at each weighing. If the time of weighing is consistent, the amount of food or liquids the client has been consuming is not likely to vary considerably. It is important to collaborate with the client, but the weighing process should not be omitted or postponed for frivolous reasons.

> ***Client Needs Category***—*Physiological integrity*
> ***Client Needs Subcategory***—*Physiological adaptation*

47. 1. The color and temperature of the hands are assessed regularly for signs of inadequate circulation. Blood clots may form in the joined vessels and occlude tissue perfusion. Joint range of motion, muscle tone and coordination, and skin turgor are not likely to be affected.

> ***Client Needs Category***—*Physiological integrity*
> ***Client Needs Subcategory***—*Reduction of risk potential*

48. **3.** While assessing the arteriovenous fistula, the nurse palpates a thrill, or vibration over the vascular access. The nurse should also expect to note a bruit—a loud sound caused by turbulent blood flow—at the connection site. Both the thrill (vibration) and bruit (sound) must be present. If they are absent, the nurse should postpone further use of the device and notify the physician. The nurse would not expect to note a pulse or a clicking sound in her assessment.

> ***Client Needs Category***—*Physiological integrity*
> ***Client Needs Subcategory***—*Physiological adaptation*

49. **4.** Discussing an actual or potential stressor helps to place the event in more realistic perspective. Giving a client an opportunity for discussion empowers him to confront the issues and acquire support in the process. Although the other options may be explored later, the nurse should focus on the client's feelings about the disorder in relation to his life.

> ***Client Needs Category***—*Psychosocial integrity*
> ***Client Needs Subcategory***—*None*

50. **2.** Along with measuring the volume of infused and drained dialysis solution, comparing the client's weight before and after the procedure provides objective data for evaluating the outcome of peritoneal dialysis.

> ***Client Needs Category***—*Physiological integrity*
> ***Client Needs Subcategory***—*Physiological adaptation*

51. **2.** In peritoneal dialysis, the peritoneum, a serous membrane that covers the abdominal organs and lines the abdominal wall, serves as a semipermeable membrane. Urea and creatinine, metabolic end products normally excreted by the kidney, are cleared from the blood by diffusion as the waste products move from an area of higher concentration (the peritoneal blood supply) to an area of lower concentration (the peritoneal cavity). Osmosis, also helpful in the dialysis process, is the movement of water through the semipermeable membrane. Filtration is movement that occurs according to pressure changes. Gravity is the process by which the dialysate is infused.

> ***Client Needs Category***—*Physiological integrity*
> ***Client Needs Subcategory***—*Physiological adaptation*

52. **1.** The dialysate infusion tubing is clamped, usually for 15 to 45 minutes, to allow osmosis and diffusion to take place between the dialysate and the peritoneum. The peritoneal cavity is then drained after the dwell time. The client is free to ambulate, change positions, or remain in bed during peritoneal dialysis. The amount of activity depends on the client's safety needs. The client may eat and drink during peritoneal dialysis; however, oral fluids continue to be restricted throughout dialysis and for as long as the client is in renal failure.

> ***Client Needs Category***—*Physiological integrity*
> ***Client Needs Subcategory***—*Physiological adaptation*

53. **3.** An elevated temperature is unexpected. Its presence indicates that an infection is occurring, and the nurse should suspect peritonitis. It is expected that a client undergoing peritoneal dialysis will lose weight and have an output that exceeds intake. Regular, deep breathing generally indicates that ventilation is adequate.

> ***Client Needs Category***—*Physiological integrity*
> ***Client Needs Subcategory***—*Physiological adaptation*

54. **3.** One beneficial effect of dialysis is the lowering of the serum potassium level. A goal of dialysis therapy is to maintain a safe concentration of serum electrolytes. A lower red blood cell count is not a desired effect. Most people with renal failure become anemic because the kidney's ability to produce erythropoietin is impaired. Blood transfusions or injections of erythropoietin are commonly necessary. Peritoneal dialysis is not expected to improve urine output. Any improvement in renal function is probably due to accompanying therapy or healing at the cellular level. An improved appetite is far too subjective to be used as an indicator of a therapeutic response to peritoneal dialysis.

> ***Client Needs Category***—*Physiological integrity*
> ***Client Needs Subcategory***—*Physiological adaptation*

55. **2.** Peritonitis is the most serious and common complication in 60% to 80% of clients on long-term peritoneal dialysis. Pulmonary edema is not a common complication. Although cardiovascular disease commonly occurs due to hypertriglyceridemia, a ruptured aorta is not common. An abdominal hernia is common in clients undergoing long-term peritoneal dialysis because of the continuous increased intra-abdominal pressure; however, a hernia is not as common or as serious as peritonitis.

> ***Client Needs Category***—*Physiological integrity*
> ***Client Needs Subcategory***—*Reduction of risk potential*

56. **2.** Relatives, especially siblings who were conceived by the same father and mother, prove to be the most compatible genetic matches for clients who receive transplanted organs. Immunosuppressive drugs make it possible to reduce the potential for rejection regardless of the source of human organs. Kidneys from other species are not successfully transplanted.

Client Needs Category—Physiological integrity
Client Needs Subcategory—Reduction of risk
  potential

57. **1.** Because the kidney is a highly vascular organ, hemorrhage and shock are the most immediate complications of renal surgery. Fluid and blood component replacements are often necessary in the immediate postoperative period. Abdominal distention, paralytic ileus, and pneumonia are fairly common in the postoperative period.

Client Needs Category—Physiological integrity
Client Needs Subcategory—Reduction of risk
  potential

Nursing Care of Clients with Urologic Obstructions

58. **1.** Subjective data that are associated with obstructive urinary disorders include a persistent feeling of needing to void and dull flank pain. Feeling the urge to void is related to urine accumulating in the bladder secondary to incomplete emptying. A palpable bladder above the pubis is an objective sign that urine is being retained. Dark urine is associated with fluid volume deficit. Abdominal cramping is associated with a problem with the bowel.

Client Needs Category—Physiological integrity
Client Needs Subcategory—Physiological
  adaptation

59. **2.** A cystostomy tube is surgically inserted directly into the bladder through the abdominal wall. A ureterostomy tube is inserted into one of the ureters through a flank incision. A retention catheter, such as a Foley catheter, is inserted through the urethra.

Client Needs Category—Physiological integrity
Client Needs Subcategory—Physiological
  adaptation

60. **2.** Ensuring that there is adequate urine output from the suprapubic catheter is the best nursing intervention for evaluating patency of the catheter. Inspecting the skin is essential for detecting breakdown or infection. Attaching the catheter to a leg bag promotes the client's ability to move. Encouraging oral intake promotes urine formation, but increased fluid intake is not a measure of catheter patency.

Client Needs Category—Physiological integrity
Client Needs Subcategory—Reduction of risk
  potential

61. **2.** Gross or microscopic hematuria (blood-tinged urine) is more characteristic of trauma from a moving urinary stone than cloudy, light yellow, or strong-smelling urine.

Client Needs Category—Physiological integrity
Client Needs Subcategory—Physiological
  adaptation

62. **2, 3, 5, 6.** A cystoscopy is the visual examination of the inside of the bladder. The cystoscope consists of a lighted tube with a telescopic lens. It is used to help identify the cause of painless hematuria, urinary incontinence, and urine retention. It also helps to evaluate structural and functional changes of the bladder. The cystoscope is introduced via the urethra while the client is under local, spinal, or general anesthesia; no surgical incision is required. Biopsy samples of tissue, cell washing, and a urine sample may be obtained during the procedure.

Client Needs Category—Physiological integrity
Client Needs Subcategory—Physiological adaptation

63. **2.** Due to the instrumentation and dilation of the urethra, many clients complain of burning when urinating following a cystoscopy. The nurse can reduce or relieve the discomfort by promoting a liberal fluid intake, providing sitz baths, and administering a prescribed mild analgesic. Polyuria, anuria, and pyuria indicate other complications or conditions affecting the renal system.

Client Needs Category—Physiological integrity
Client Needs Subcategory—Physiological
  adaptation

64. **4.** Urine is strained to assess for evidence that the urinary stone or stones have passed. Fluids are encouraged rather than restricted. Activity promotes movement of urinary stones. Fowler's position is unlikely to benefit or interfere with the passage of a urinary stone.

Client Needs Category—Physiological integrity
Client Needs Subcategory—Physiological
  adaptation

65. **1.** Increasing fluid intake helps to move the stone so it may be spontaneously eliminated. The nurse should also encourage the client to increase fluids following stone removal to dilute the urine and prevent further stone production. Strengthening the bladder muscles, voiding a larger stream, and increasing calcium in the diet are not related to urolithiasis.

Client Needs Category—Physiological integrity
Client Needs Subcategory—Physiological adaptation

66. 1. ESWL is a procedure that is performed while the client's lower body is submerged in a tank of water or surrounded by a fluid-filled bag. Ultrasound, not radiation or a laser beam, is the mechanism used to pulverize the stone. Clients are sedated and given preprocedural analgesic medication to reduce the discomfort that is commonly described as a "blow to the body." It is common for bruises to appear as a consequence of the ultrasonic energy.
Client Needs Category—Physiological integrity
Client Needs Subcategory—Physiological adaptation

67. 2. Nocturia, being awakened by a need to urinate, is a common finding among clients with BPH. Burning on urination is more likely a sign of a bladder infection, which could be secondary to BPH. Feeling pressure in the back is more indicative of pathology involving the kidney. Colorless or very light yellow urine indicates that the urine is dilute. This could be caused by an endocrine disturbance, such as diabetes insipidus, or some other dysfunction affecting renal tubular reabsorption.
Client Needs Category—Physiological integrity
Client Needs Subcategory—Physiological adaptation

68. 3. Due to obstruction of the urethra from an enlarging prostate gland, men with BPH often describe hesitancy when initiating urination. In other words, they feel the need to urinate but it takes some time before urine is released. The stream of urine is also diminished. BPH usually does not cause sexual dysfunction or incontinence. The prostate gland is not located in the scrotum; it encircles the urethra and can be palpated by rectal examination.
Client Needs Category—Physiological integrity
Client Needs Subcategory—Physiological adaptation

69. 1. Lowering the penis from an upright position to one in which the penis is pointed in the direction of the toes sometimes helps to pass a catheter beyond the narrowing caused by an enlarged prostate gland. The penis is grasped firmly whenever a catheter is inserted. A catheter is never forced if resistance is met during insertion. Massaging the tissue below the base of the penis does not facilitate the catheter's passage past an enlarged prostate gland.
Client Needs Category—Physiological integrity
Client Needs Subcategory—Physiological adaptation

70. 1. A coudé catheter is used in a client with BPH because it has a curved tip that is able to move around an enlarged prostate. An instillable anesthetic lubricant is commonly used to facilitate the procedure. Silicone,

rubber, and flexible catheters typically meet the resistance of the prostate gland and cannot be advanced.
Client Needs Category—Physiological integrity
Client Needs Subcategory—Reduction of risk potential

71. 4. Hematuria is generally present for at least 24 hours following a TURP. Vital signs are monitored to evaluate if the volume of blood loss is causing shock. It may take 24 to 48 hours for the urine to become light pink and transparent. Following the procedure, the volume of urine is usually within the normal range unless complications, such as hypovolemic shock or obstruction of the catheter, occur. Sediment, if present, is due to the remnants of prostatic tissue; however, the blood that is mixed with the urine initially obscures the nurse's ability to identify the presence of tissue or mucoid debris.
Client Needs Category—Physiological integrity
Client Needs Subcategory—Physiological adaptation

72. 1. Continuous bladder irrigation is performed by instilling normal saline solution hung from an I.V. pole through one lumen of the urinary catheter. The solution flows into the bladder, dilutes the urine and sediment, and drains out the catheter into a gravity drainage bag. An Asepto syringe and sterile container for irrigation solution are used for performing intermittent catheter irrigation. Sterile normal saline, not antiseptic, solution is used for continuous bladder irrigation and intermittent catheter irrigation.
Client Needs Category—Physiological integrity
Client Needs Subcategory—Physiological adaptation

73. 3. The nurse should assess whether the catheter is draining well before administering an analgesic for bladder discomfort. Obstruction of the catheter causes bladder spasms. Restoring patency is more appropriate in the case of catheter obstruction than administering an analgesic. Administering an analgesic is not necessarily contingent upon a normal pulse rate. No dressing is needed following a TURP since the surgery is performed through the urethra. An opioid analgesic may depress the respiratory center, but assessing the client's ability to cough does not affect the decision to withhold or administer an analgesic.
Client Needs Category—Physiological integrity
Client Needs Subcategory—Physiological adaptation

74. 4. Belladonna and opium (B&O) rectal suppositories are considered the most effective drugs for relieving bladder spasms following TURP. Acetylsalicylic acid (aspirin) is avoided because it increases the tendency to bleed. Propoxyphene napsylate (Darvocet) and meperidine hydrochloride (Demerol) are synthetic opioid analgesics. Opioids alone do not lessen the spasms but may decrease the pain.

Client Needs Category—Physiological integrity
Client Needs Subcategory—Pharmacological therapies

75. 3. The best method for recording urine output when a client has more than one catheter is to record the volumes drained from each catheter as separate entries in the medical record. Recording only the output from the urethral catheter or the output from the wound catheter does not provide accurate data on total output. If the two volumes are added and recorded as a single entry, it is difficult to evaluate the status of urine drainage from each catheter.

Client Needs Category—Physiological integrity
Client Needs Subcategory—Physiological adaptation

76. 3. After a suprapubic catheter is removed, urine may leak from the incisional area and saturate the sterile dressing. A wet dressing provides a wicking action by which microorganisms are attracted in the direction of the impaired tissue. A dressing saturated with urine also leads to skin breakdown. If standards of care are followed, the postoperative care plan already indicates nursing orders for repositioning the client, ambulating with assistance, and encouraging deep breathing.

Client Needs Category—Physiological integrity
Client Needs Subcategory—Reduction of risk potential

Nursing Care of Clients with Urologic Tumors

77. 3. A client may have falsely high levels of PSA for up to 12 days after a rectal examination or instrumentation around the prostate gland, such as occurs during a cystoscopy. The other examinations and tests are not influenced by physical manipulation of the prostate gland.

Client Needs Category—Health promotion and maintenance
Client Needs Subcategory—None

78. 1. Tension on the catheter may disrupt healing where the bladder and the urethra have been surgically reconnected following removal of the prostate gland and its capsule. Encouraging oral fluids and cleaning the urinary meatus are appropriate postoperative nursing measures, but they are not likely to have as significant an effect on wound healing. Clients who undergo a radical prostatectomy have a high potential for urinary incontinence as a consequence of the surgical

procedure. Clamping and releasing the catheter is not likely to promote bladder control.

Client Needs Category—Physiological integrity
Client Needs Subcategory—Reduction of risk potential

79. 1. Men who receive estrogen therapy are prone to developing feminizing characteristics, such as breast enlargement, breast tenderness, and testicular atrophy. An alternative approach is to remove both testicles to reduce the production of testosterone. The other effects do not occur as a result of such hormone therapy.

Client Needs Category—Physiological integrity
Client Needs Subcategory—Physiological adaptation

80. 1. The sudden onset of flank pain along with other signs of shock, such as hypotension, restlessness, and tachycardia, is suggestive of hemorrhage. With shock, the skin is generally pale and cool. A distended abdomen is usually caused by the accumulation of intestinal gas. Pain sometimes causes nausea and vomiting, but these signs and symptoms may be due to multiple etiologies.

Client Needs Category—Physiological integrity
Client Needs Subcategory—Physiological adaptation

81. 3. The most common symptom of bladder cancer is painless hematuria. Dysuria, if present, is generally due to a concurrent urinary tract infection secondary to obstruction of urine. Oliguria occurs later as the disease becomes more advanced and obstruction occurs. Bladder cancer that has not spread to adjacent pelvic structures is not usually associated with an unusual discharge from any body orifice.

Client Needs Category—Physiological integrity
Client Needs Subcategory—Physiological adaptation

82. 4. There is a correlation between cigarette smoking, even passive exposure to cigarette smoke, and the development of bladder cancer. Other carcinogenic factors include long-term exposure to chemical solvents and dyes. Neither stress incontinence nor sexual activities are implicated as a causal agent in bladder cancer.

Client Needs Category—Health promotion and maintenance
Client Needs Subcategory—None

83. 1. Recommendations for promoting safety when handling toxic chemotherapeutic agents include wearing two pairs of surgical latex gloves, which are less permeable than polyvinyl gloves. A gown with cuffs and a mask or goggles are also worn to prevent direct contact with the drug. Pregnant nurses should use extreme caution when handling chemotherapeutic agents. There is no particular advantage to using a glass syringe. In fact, there is a greater potential for contamination if a glass syringe is dropped and broken. The uncontained drug is considered a toxic spill. The time spent in contact with the client is not considered a safety hazard with chemotherapy, but it is a factor in radiation therapy involving sealed and unsealed implants.

> *Client Needs Category—Safe, effective care environment*
> *Client Needs Subcategory—Safety and infection control*

Nursing Care of Clients with Urinary Diversions

84. 3. An ileal conduit, or ileal loop procedure, involves implanting the ureters into a section of the ileum that has been removed from the small intestine. The section of ileum is fashioned into a stoma that opens onto the abdomen, from which urine will drain. When ureterosigmoidostomy is performed, the ureters are attached to the sigmoid colon and urine is eliminated with stool by way of the rectum. Currently, there are no procedures in which the ureters are implanted directly into the small intestine. If a Koch pouch, or continent urostomy, is performed, urine is siphoned with a catheter from an internal collection pouch.

> *Client Needs Category—Physiological integrity*
> *Client Needs Subcategory—Physiological adaptation*

85. 3. A pulse rate of more than 100 beats/minute in the absence of activity or some accompanying pathology suggests that the sympathetic nervous system is stimulated. The sympathetic nervous system responds when a person is experiencing a real or perceived threat to his well-being. The data in the other options are generally within normal limits.

> *Client Needs Category—Psychosocial integrity*
> *Client Needs Subcategory—None*

86. 1. Sharing perceptions with the client by stating that it must be difficult shows empathy and allows the client an opportunity to unburden himself. Telling the client that he has one of the best surgeons does not encourage him to verbalize further because it is unlikely that he will disagree. The cliché that everything will turn out OK offers false reassurance. It also communicates that the nurse is uncomfortable discussing the client's feelings. Saying that others have done just fine minimizes and belittles the uniqueness of the situation from the client's perspective.

> *Client Needs Category—Psychosocial integrity*
> *Client Needs Subcategory—None*

87. 1. Encouraging the client to verbalize more and express his feelings is an effective therapeutic communication technique. Because it is impossible for a nurse to know how a client is feeling, stating so diminishes the nurse's credibility. The client may lose faith in the ability of the nurse to be truly empathetic. Minimizing the despair that he is feeling by saying, "It's not as bad as that," is likely to interfere with any further discussion. Advising the client to think more positively is likely to be interpreted as disapproval of the way the client currently feels.

> *Client Needs Category—Psychosocial integrity*
> *Client Needs Subcategory—None*

88. 2. It is important for the nurse to assess the skin's condition to plan appropriate interventions. If the skin is excoriated, it probably will take more than just diluting the urine or emptying the appliance more frequently to restore skin integrity. It would be impossible to leave the appliance off because urine is released constantly.

> *Client Needs Category—Physiological integrity*
> *Client Needs Subcategory—Physiological adaptation*

89. 1, 4. The physician would need to be notified if the stoma became bluish in appearance because this would indicate a diminished blood supply. A healthy stoma appears beefy red and is approximately flush with the skin. The stoma should decrease in size following surgery as the edema around the stoma area resolves. Sharp abdominal pain is an indication of infection or peritonitis; the physician should be notified immediately. Normal urinary findings include a yellow color, output of 30 mL/hour or greater, and an ammonia smell.

> *Client Needs Category—Physiological integrity*
> *Client Needs Subcategory—Reduction of risk potential*

90. 2. Inserting a tampon or gauze square into the stoma momentarily absorbs the urine and keeps the skin dry. Leaning over the toilet puts the client in an awkward position while the appliance is being changed. It generally takes two hands to manipulate the appliance during its application; therefore, pressing a finger over the stoma or pinching the stoma interferes with the coordination needed.

> *Client Needs Category—Health promotion and maintenance*
> *Client Needs Subcategory—None*

The Nursing Care of Clients with Disorders of the Reproductive System

⇨ *Nursing Care of Clients with Breast Disorders*
⇨ *Nursing Care of Clients with Disturbances in Menstruation*
⇨ *Nursing Care of Clients with Infectious and Inflammatory Disorders of the Female Reproductive System*
⇨ *Nursing Care of Clients with Benign and Malignant Disorders of the Uterus and Ovaries*
⇨ *Nursing Care of Clients with Miscellaneous Disorders of the Female Reproductive System*
⇨ *Nursing Care of Clients with Inflammatory Disorders of the Male Reproductive System*
⇨ *Nursing Care of Clients with Structural Disorders of the Male Reproductive System*
⇨ *Nursing Care of Clients with Benign and Malignant Disorders of the Male Reproductive System*
⇨ *Nursing Care of Clients with Sexually Transmitted Diseases*
⇨ *Nursing Care of Clients Practicing Family Planning*
⇨ *Correct Answers and Rationales*

Directions: With a pencil, blacken the space in front of the option you have chosen for your correct answer.

Nursing Care of Clients with Breast Disorders

A 30-year-old woman has an appointment for a routine pelvic examination. She asks the office nurse when she should begin undergoing routine mammography.

1. If the client is asymptomatic and at low risk for breast cancer, the nurse would be correct in advising her to have a baseline mammogram at what age?
[ ] **1.** 25
[ ] **2.** 35
[ ] **3.** 40
[ ] **4.** 50

The nurse asks whether the client currently practices breast self-examination (BSE), then takes the opportunity to show her the proper technique.

2. The client states that she examines her breasts in the shower and while lying down. The nurse recommends that the client should also inspect her breasts from which position?
[ ] **1.** Bending from the waist
[ ] **2.** Standing before a mirror
[ ] **3.** Arching the back
[ ] **4.** Leaning from side-to-side

3. Which breast palpation technique is most correct?
[ ] **1.** Examine the breast while using the heel of the hand.
[ ] **2.** Examine the breast while using the index finger only.
[ ] **3.** Examine the breast while using the index finger and thumb.
[ ] **4.** Examine the breast while using the pads of the fingertips.

4. The nurse correctly informs the client that the BSE techniques that involve making small concentric circles or dividing the breast into wedges, which resemble the spokes of a wheel, should begin from which anatomic point?
[ ] **1.** Beginning with the nipple and extending to the outer margins of the breast
[ ] **2.** Beginning with the outer margins of the breast and extending toward the nipple
[ ] **3.** Beginning with the sternum and extending toward each axilla
[ ] **4.** Beginning with each axilla and extending toward the sternum

5. Which statement made by the client best demonstrates that she understands how frequently to perform a BSE?
[ ] **1.** "I will perform a BSE on a weekly basis."
[ ] **2.** "I will perform a BSE every 6 months."
[ ] **3.** "I will perform a BSE 1 week before each menses."
[ ] **4.** "I will perform a BSE 1 week after each menses."

A 35-year-old woman makes an appointment with her physician because she has felt several lumps in her right breast. She is scheduled for a mammogram.

6. When the office nurse gives the client instructions on how to prepare for the mammogram, which is most accurate?
[ ] **1.** "You will need to shave all of your underarm hair the morning of the test."
[ ] **2.** "Do not wear any underarm deodorant the day of the test."
[ ] **3.** "Wipe each breast with an antiseptic pad before the test."
[ ] **4.** "Do not wear a bra to the test."

7. Which assessment finding recorded by the nurse before the mammogram indicates a high risk factor for developing breast cancer?
[ ] **1.** Menses beginning before age 16
[ ] **2.** Three full-term pregnancies
[ ] **3.** Sister with breast cancer
[ ] **4.** History of breast-feeding

The radiologist interprets the findings on the mammogram as benign fibrocystic disease.

8. The nurse correctly informs the client that fibrocystic lesions may become larger and more tender at what time?
[ ] **1.** After the menstrual cycle
[ ] **2.** Following sexual intercourse
[ ] **3.** Nearer to beginning menopause
[ ] **4.** Just before menstruation

9. Although it has not been conclusively proven, the nurse explains that some women with fibrocystic disease get relief from their symptoms by eliminating which substance from their diet?
[ ] **1.** Alcohol
[ ] **2.** Caffeine
[ ] **3.** Saturated fat
[ ] **4.** Refined sugar

A home health nurse visits a postpartum client with a breast abscess. The client has purulent drainage from one breast and is receiving antibiotic therapy.

10. Which information is most appropriate to give the client to help prevent the spread of the infectious microorganisms elsewhere?
[ ] **1.** "Eat a balanced diet and include more sources of protein."
[ ] **2.** "Keep your breasts supported in a tight brassiere."
[ ] **3.** "Shower daily and wash your hands frequently."
[ ] **4.** "Apply warm compresses at least four times a day."

During a presurgical assessment, a 67-year-old woman tells the nurse that she has felt a lump in her left breast for the past 6 months.

11. If the lump has the following characteristics when the nurse palpates the breast tissue, which one is most suggestive that the lump may be cancerous?
[ ] **1.** The lump can be easily moved about.
[ ] **2.** The lump is about ½″ (1 cm).
[ ] **3.** The lump is irregularly shaped.
[ ] **4.** The lump is near the areola.

The physician recommends an excisional biopsy followed by an immediate modified radical mastectomy if the biopsy shows malignant cells.

12. If the client tells the nurse that she would prefer to postpone the mastectomy until the biopsy has been more thoroughly examined, which is the most appropriate initial nursing action?
[ ] **1.** Explain that most biopsies are accurate.
[ ] **2.** Advocate her choice of treatment.
[ ] **3.** Discourage her from opposing the physician.
[ ] **4.** Recommend that she seek a second opinion.

The client's breast tumor is malignant and she undergoes a left modified radical mastectomy.

13. Which nursing order is most appropriate to add to the client's immediate postoperative care plan?
[ ] **1.** Maintain the client in a dorsal recumbent position.
[ ] **2.** Limit oral fluid intake to no more than 2,000 mL/day.
[ ] **3.** Use the right arm when assessing blood pressures.
[ ] **4.** Inspect the incision at least once each shift.

14. Based on the location and extent of this client's surgery, it is most appropriate for the nurse to closely assess for which postoperative complication?
[ ] **1.** Shallow breathing
[ ] **2.** Inadequate nutrition
[ ] **3.** Impaired bowel motility
[ ] **4.** Signs of skin breakdown

15. Which activity of daily living is most therapeutic for the nurse to recommend for preserving the client's muscle strength and joint flexibility in the arm on the operative side?
[ ] **1.** Feeding herself
[ ] **2.** Brushing her hair
[ ] **3.** Writing letters
[ ] **4.** Washing her chest

16. When modifying the postoperative care plan, the nurse should plan to include which nursing measure to prevent arm swelling on the client's operative side?
[ ] **1.** Applying an ice pack to the site
[ ] **2.** Applying warm compresses to the site
[ ] **3.** Keeping the arm elevated
[ ] **4.** Ambulating the client frequently

17. If the client asks for information on special bras and other aspects of life following her mastectomy, which organization is the best resource to recommend?
[ ] **1.** American Garment Industry
[ ] **2.** American Cancer Society
[ ] **3.** Breast Prosthetics Association
[ ] **4.** Organization for Mammary Cosmetics

18. Before discharging the mastectomy client, which instruction concerning BSE is most correct?
[ ] **1.** Examine your breast upon awakening from sleep.
[ ] **2.** Examine your breast on the first day of the month.
[ ] **3.** Examine your breast after you finish your shower.
[ ] **4.** Examine your breast before your yearly mammogram.

19. The physician prescribes tamoxifen (Nolvadex) 10 mg P.O. b.i.d. for a client who underwent a modified radical mastectomy to treat her estrogen-sensitive breast cancer. The drug label indicates that there are 20 mg in each tablet. How many tablets should the nurse administer to the client?

_____

20. Identify the area where breast cancer is most likely to metastasize initially.

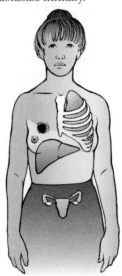

Nursing Care of Clients with Disturbances in Menstruation

21. A nurse has been asked to teach ovulation and menstruation to a class of secondary school students. Place the events listed below in ascending chronological order in the way that they occur during the menstrual cycle. Use all the options.

1. Ovum is released	
2. Progesterone decreases	
3. Endometrium begins to thicken	
4. Ovarian follicle matures	
5. Endometrium is shed	
6. Corpus luteum forms	

A nurse obtains a history from a 20-year-old client who says she does not menstruate.

22. Which question is most important for the nurse to ask next?
[ ] **1.** "Have you ever had any menstrual periods?"
[ ] **2.** "Do you have any pubic hair growth?"
[ ] **3.** "Have you ever been sexually attracted to males?"
[ ] **4.** "Are there any siblings with a similar problem?"

An 18-year-old female client confides to the nurse that she has cramps that accompany the onset of menstruation.

23. Besides a mild analgesic such as ibuprofen (Motrin), which therapeutic intervention is most appropriate for the nurse to recommend?
[ ] **1.** Obtaining a prescription for an oral contraceptive
[ ] **2.** Switching from menstrual pads to tampons
[ ] **3.** Using local applications of heat
[ ] **4.** Reducing physical activity

A 34-year-old woman makes an appointment with a physician concerning her pattern of heavy menstrual bleeding. A pelvic examination is scheduled.

24. Which instruction is most appropriate if a Papanicolaou (Pap) smear will be obtained at the time of the pelvic examination?
[ ] **1.** Avoid douching for several days before your appointment.
[ ] **2.** Stop using any and all forms of contraception temporarily.
[ ] **3.** Drink at least 1 quart of liquid an hour before your appointment.
[ ] **4.** Take a mild laxative the night before your scheduled appointment.

25. Before taking the client to the room where the pelvic examination will be performed, which nursing action is most appropriate?
[ ] **1.** Ask the client to sign a consent form.
[ ] **2.** Give the client an opportunity to void.
[ ] **3.** Offer the client a mild analgesic.
[ ] **4.** Help the client instill a vaginal lubricant.

26. Which question is most important to ask to ensure valid analysis of the vaginal specimen?
[ ] **1.** "When did you last have sexual intercourse?"
[ ] **2.** "How old were you when you had your first pregnancy?"
[ ] **3.** "What was the date of your last menstrual period?"

[ ] **4.** "Have you ever used oral contraceptives?"

27. The nurse correctly places the client in which position when the physician is ready to perform the pelvic examination?
[ ] **1.** Sims' position
[ ] **2.** Trendelenburg's position
[ ] **3.** Fowler's position
[ ] **4.** Lithotomy position

28. Before the physician performs the vaginal examination, which nursing intervention is most important?
[ ] **1.** Arrange to have a female nurse present during the examination.
[ ] **2.** Instruct the client on the dangers of cervical cancer.
[ ] **3.** Palpate the internal organs to obtain a baseline assessment.
[ ] **4.** Encourage the client to instill a personal vaginal lubricant.

A 22-year-old woman calls her physician's office and reports to the nurse that she is bleeding vaginally at a time other than her expected menses.

29. If the client reports all of the following data, which factor is most likely contributing to the bleeding?
[ ] **1.** The client has been taking an oral contraceptive for 2 months.
[ ] **2.** The client has just changed employment and is under unusual stress.
[ ] **3.** The client's sexual partner is uncircumcised.
[ ] **4.** The client has been constipated for 2 days.

Nursing Care of Clients with Infectious and Inflammatory Disorders of the Female Reproductive System

A 25-year-old woman has repeated vaginal infections. The symptoms suggest that the client has candidiasis caused by the yeast-like microorganism Candida albicans.

30. After *Candida albicans* is identified as the causative organism, the nurse would expect the physician to prescribe which treatment?
[ ] **1.** A nonprescription antifungal medication
[ ] **2.** A prescription oral penicillin
[ ] **3.** A prescription broad-spectrum antibiotic

[ ]   **4.** A vaginal douche with a vinegar solution

31. Which instruction is best when teaching the client about inserting vaginal medication?
[ ]   **1.** Place the applicator just inside the vaginal opening.
[ ]   **2.** Insert the applicator while sitting on the toilet.
[ ]   **3.** Instill the medication just before retiring for sleep.
[ ]   **4.** Put on disposable latex gloves before applying the drug.

32. Which health practice is most appropriate for the nurse to teach this client?
[ ]   **1.** Take showers rather than tub baths if possible.
[ ]   **2.** Wipe away from the vagina following a bowel movement.
[ ]   **3.** Use a lanolin-based soap for genital cleansing.
[ ]   **4.** Avoid sexual intercourse more than once a week.

33. What information provided by the nurse is most appropriate for the client who plans on douching twice a week?
[ ]   **1.** Use a concentrated solution of vinegar and water.
[ ]   **2.** Avoid frequent douching because it removes helpful microorganisms.
[ ]   **3.** Instill no more than 8 to 16 oz of irrigant solution with each douching.
[ ]   **4.** Discontinue the instillation if cramping occurs.

34. To reduce the potential for toxic shock syndrome, which nursing instruction is most appropriate when teaching menstruating women?
[ ]   **1.** Avoid using superabsorbent brands of tampons.
[ ]   **2.** Use a nondeodorant type of sanitary product.
[ ]   **3.** Refrain from taking tub baths while menstruating.
[ ]   **4.** Report menses that last longer than 7 days.

A 21-year-old client is recovering from acute pelvic inflammatory disease (PID).

35. When assigning a nursing assistant to this client's care, which instruction for disposing of soiled drainage pads is correct?
[ ]   **1.** Flush all perineal pads down the toilet.
[ ]   **2.** Double wrap the pads in infectious waste bags.
[ ]   **3.** Place the pads in the client's wastebasket.
[ ]   **4.** Enclose the soiled pads in a clean paper bag.

36. If the client asks what, if any, long-term consequences are associated with this disorder, the nurse accurately identifies which reproductive sequela?
[ ]   **1.** Cancer of the cervix
[ ]   **2.** Premature labors

[ ]   **3.** Spontaneous abortions
[ ]   **4.** Prolonged infertility

A 24-year-old woman is being treated for endometriosis. A laparoscope will be used to remove ectopic tissue.

37. When the client asks where the laparoscope will be inserted, the nurse correctly identifies which structure?
[ ]   **1.** Abdomen
[ ]   **2.** Vagina
[ ]   **3.** Uterine cervix
[ ]   **4.** Uterine fundus

38. If the client experiences all of the following signs and symptoms following the laparoscopy, which one can the nurse attribute directly to the endoscopic procedure?
[ ]   **1.** Nausea and vomiting
[ ]   **2.** Shoulder discomfort
[ ]   **3.** Urinary frequency
[ ]   **4.** Leg cramps

A 68-year-old woman experiences painful intercourse and is concerned about possible reproductive disease.

39. Based on this client's age, which statement by the nurse best explains the reason for the client's discomfort?
[ ]   **1.** The pelvic muscles are more sensitive to pressure after menopause.
[ ]   **2.** The clitoris is less responsive to sexual foreplay as women age.
[ ]   **3.** The vagina atrophies if intercourse is infrequent.
[ ]   **4.** The mucus-producing glands decrease with aging.

Nursing Care of Clients with Benign and Malignant Disorders of the Uterus and Ovaries

The physician sees a 42-year-old woman for suspected fibroid tumors (myomas).

40. In addition to pressure in the pelvic region, which sign or symptom is the client most likely to reveal during a nursing history?
[ ]   **1.** Heavy menstrual bleeding
[ ]   **2.** Light menstrual bleeding
[ ]   **3.** Abdominal pain at the time of ovulation
[ ]   **4.** Breast tenderness during menstruation

A pelvic ultrasound (sonogram) using a transabdominal approach is scheduled for the client.

41. When preparing the client for the sonogram, which instruction is most important for the nurse to emphasize?

[ ] **1.** Do not void for several hours before the test.

[ ] **2.** Begin fasting at midnight before the test.

[ ] **3.** Take a mild analgesic such as aspirin before the test.

[ ] **4.** Use an antiseptic soap when showering before the test.

After the diagnosis of fibroid tumors is confirmed, the client is scheduled for a dilation and curettage in the ambulatory surgery department.

42. Before the client is discharged, which nursing observation is most important for the nurse to document?

[ ] **1.** The client can eat without nausea.

[ ] **2.** The client can empty her bladder.

[ ] **3.** The client's pelvic pain is relieved.

[ ] **4.** The client's perineal pad has been changed.

A client with an abnormal Pap smear has a colposcopy performed in her physician's office.

43. Before the client leaves the office, the nurse correctly instructs her to report which unusual problem associated with this procedure?

[ ] **1.** Excessive bleeding

[ ] **2.** Inability to void

[ ] **3.** Pressure during bowel elimination

[ ] **4.** Pain in the right lower quadrant

A client makes an appointment with her gynecologist because she has been having vaginal bleeding between her regular menstrual periods. Based on the client's history and physical examination, the physician suspects cervical cancer and orders further diagnostic tests.

44. To determine the extent of the client's symptomatic bleeding, which question is most important for the nurse to ask?

[ ] **1.** "Has your energy level changed remarkably?"

[ ] **2.** "Do you have intercourse more than once a week?"

[ ] **3.** "How many sanitary pads do you use?"

[ ] **4.** "Is the bleeding light or dark red?"

45. Based on her knowledge of and experience with gynecologic disorders, the nurse would expect bleeding in which client to indicate a serious problem that requires further evaluation?

[ ] **1.** A client taking oral contraceptives

[ ] **2.** A client on hormone replacement therapy

[ ] **3.** A perimenopausal client

[ ] **4.** An adolescent who recently began menstruating

The client is scheduled to undergo electrocauterization after the diagnostic tests confirm that she has an early stage of cervical cancer.

46. After the electrocauterization procedure, which discharge instruction is most appropriate?

[ ] **1.** "Douche in 24 hours to remove debris and blood clots."

[ ] **2.** "Avoid heavy lifting until you have had a surgical follow-up exam."

[ ] **3.** "Remain in bed as much as possible over the next 5 days."

[ ] **4.** "Avoid any sexual activity for 1 week."

Internal radiation therapy is used to treat a 54-year-old client with cervical cancer. An applicator containing radioactive material is inserted into the client's vagina.

47. Because the client is receiving this type of radiation therapy, the nurse should plan to include which nursing intervention in the care plan?

[ ] **1.** Elevate the head of the bed to 90 degrees.

[ ] **2.** Maintain the client on strict bed rest.

[ ] **3.** Offer nourishment every 2 hours.

[ ] **4.** Weigh the client daily before breakfast.

48. If the nurse finds the radioactive insert in the client's bed, which nursing action is most appropriate?

[ ] **1.** Return it to the nuclear medicine department.

[ ] **2.** Discard it in the infectious waste receptacle.

[ ] **3.** Reinsert it immediately.

[ ] **4.** Place it in a lead container.

49. If the nurse must handle the radioactive implant, which action best protects her?

[ ] **1.** Putting on sterile vinyl gloves

[ ] **2.** Washing the hands thoroughly before putting on vinyl gloves

[ ] **3.** Using long-handled forceps to handle the implant

[ ] **4.** Enclosing the implant in a glass jar

50. Which staff nurse is best suited to care for a client with a radioactive implant?

[ ] **1.** A male nurse with oncology nursing experience

[ ] **2.** A female nurse who has had a hysterectomy

[ ] **3.** A female nurse who has survived cancer herself

[ ] **4.** A male nurse whose mother died of cancer

A 64-year-old client with uterine cancer is scheduled to undergo an abdominal hysterectomy under general anesthesia. The nurse will insert a retention catheter prior to surgery.

51. How far into the client's urinary meatus should the nurse insert the catheter?

[ ] **1.** ½" (1 cm)

[ ] **2.** 1″ (2.5 cm)
[ ] **3.** 2″ to 3″ (5 to 8 cm)
[ ] **4.** 5″ to 6″ (13 to 15 cm)

Before the client returns from the postanesthesia care unit, the registered nurse asks the practical nurse to help revise the hysterectomy client's care plan.

52. Which nursing diagnosis is most appropriate for the nurse to add to the client's care plan at this time?
[ ] **1.** *Risk for ineffective airway clearance*
[ ] **2.** *Risk for imbalanced nutrition*
[ ] **3.** *Ineffective coping*
[ ] **4.** *Impaired verbal communication*

Postoperative orders call for applying antiembolism stockings to the client's legs following her hysterectomy.

53. Which intervention for applying antiembolism stockings is most appropriate to include in the client's care plan?
[ ] **1.** Have the client wear the stockings continuously, but remove and reapply them at least twice a day
[ ] **2.** Have the client wear the stockings continuously during the day hours, and remove them at night
[ ] **3.** Have the client wear the stockings only when getting up to ambulate
[ ] **4.** Have the client wear the stockings only while in bed

54. The licensed practical nurse realizes that the nursing assistant requires further instruction when observing her performing which action following the client's hysterectomy?
[ ] **1.** Offering the client a variety of oral fluids frequently
[ ] **2.** Helping the client ambulate in the hall
[ ] **3.** Raising the knee-gatch on the hospital bed
[ ] **4.** Helping the client with menu selections

55. After the physician indicates that the client's retention catheter can be removed, which action is most important for the nurse to perform first?
[ ] **1.** Clean the client's labia with soap and water.
[ ] **2.** Measure the urine in the drainage bag.
[ ] **3.** Remove the fluid from the balloon.
[ ] **4.** Disconnect the client's catheter and drainage bag.

The client's bladder is distended after the catheter is removed even though she is urinating approximately 100 mL with each voiding. The physician instructs the nurse to catheterize the client and measure the residual urine.

56. Which nursing action is most appropriate to carry out the medical order?

[ ] **1.** Catheterize the client as soon as possible.
[ ] **2.** Catheterize the client after her next voiding.
[ ] **3.** Connect the catheter to gravity drainage.
[ ] **4.** Use a small-gauge catheter to drain the bladder.

A 59-year-old client with ovarian cancer is receiving antineoplastic chemotherapy following a total hysterectomy.

57. To accurately determine the dosage of antineoplastic drugs, which information is essential to obtain from the client's chart?
[ ] **1.** Blood pressure and pulse
[ ] **2.** Body weight and height
[ ] **3.** Age and date of surgery
[ ] **4.** Food and drug allergies

58. Because many antineoplastic drugs affect bone marrow function, which laboratory test is most important to monitor for client safety?
[ ] **1.** Mean cell volume
[ ] **2.** Total leukocyte count
[ ] **3.** Differential cell count
[ ] **4.** Complete blood count

59. When the nurse administers the parenteral form of the antineoplastic drug, which nursing action is best for preventing accidental self-absorption of the drug?
[ ] **1.** Use only prefilled syringes.
[ ] **2.** Wear disposable examination gloves.
[ ] **3.** Dilute the drug with saline solution.
[ ] **4.** Mix the drug in a closed vial.

The client experiences almost total hair loss as antineoplastic drug therapy progresses.

60. Which statement is most accurate when discussing hair loss with the client?
[ ] **1.** The hair loss is permanent, but attractive wigs are available.
[ ] **2.** The hair loss is permanent, but hair transplantation is a possible solution.
[ ] **3.** The hair loss is temporary; hair may grow back in several years.
[ ] **4.** The hair loss is temporary; hair will regrow after chemotherapy is finished.

Nursing Care of Clients with Miscellaneous Disorders of the Female Reproductive System

The transfer form for a 72-year-old woman being admitted to a nursing home indicates that she has a prolapsed uterus.

61. When the nurse does a physical assessment, which technique is best for determining the extent of the prolapse?

[ ] **1.** Examine the perineum when the client rolls from side to side.

[ ] **2.** Examine the perineum as the client stands and bears down.

[ ] **3.** Examine the perineum with the client in a dorsal recumbent position.

[ ] **4.** Examine the perineum with a lubricated speculum and flashlight.

A 53-year-old woman becomes symptomatic as a result of a cystocele.

62. If this client is typical of others with this condition, she will most likely report to the nurse that she experiences urinary incontinence during which time?

[ ] **1.** When she awakens

[ ] **2.** As she walks

[ ] **3.** During sleep

[ ] **4.** Upon sneezing

63. If the cystocele is not severe, which suggestion by the nurse can best aid the client's incontinence?

[ ] **1.** Recommend the purchase of absorbent underwear.

[ ] **2.** Show her how to apply an external catheter.

[ ] **3.** Teach her to exercise her perineal muscles.

[ ] **4.** Instruct her to limit her fluid intake.

Because of her persistent symptoms, the client chooses to undergo surgery to correct the cystocele. She is instructed to catheterize herself for approximately 1 week after being discharged.

64. Which outcome best demonstrates that the client is performing self-catheterization appropriately?

[ ] **1.** She empties 50 mL of urine from her bladder each time.

[ ] **2.** She is free of signs of a urinary tract infection.

[ ] **3.** She inserts the catheter for 30 minutes each time.

[ ] **4.** She maintains a urinary record of time and amount.

65. A postmenopausal woman receives a prescription for alendronate (Fosamax). What health teaching information should the nurse provide? Select all that apply.

[ ] **1.** Take the medication with a full glass of water.

[ ] **2.** Refrain from eating for 30 minutes after taking the medication.

[ ] **3.** This medication helps relieve hot flashes and irritability.

[ ] **4.** Take the medication upon awakening.

[ ] **5.** Do not lie down after taking the medication.

[ ] **6.** Take the medication with food or a full glass of milk.

Nursing Care of Clients with Inflammatory Disorders of the Male Reproductive System

A physician prescribes an oral antibiotic for a client with prostatitis.

66. Which instruction by the nurse about the client's antibiotic use is a priority?

[ ] **1.** Drink a glass of milk when taking the medication.

[ ] **2.** Report if your urine becomes a lighter color.

[ ] **3.** Take the medication until it is completely gone.

[ ] **4.** Monitor your body temperature on a daily basis.

In addition to a mild analgesic, the physician also recommends that the client use sitz baths as a comfort measure for the prostatitis.

67. Which instruction by the nurse is correct concerning sitz bath regimen?

[ ] **1.** Use cool tepid water.

[ ] **2.** Soak for 20 minutes.

[ ] **3.** Add mild liquid soap to the water.

[ ] **4.** Massage the scrotum while bathing.

The physician examines a 22-year-old client who has a swollen, painful scrotum. The physician suspects epididymitis and orders a clean-catch urine specimen for a culture and sensitivity test.

68. When the nurse asks the client to repeat the instructions for collecting a clean-catch urine specimen, which statement indicates the client needs further clarification?

[ ] **1.** "I must clean my penis."

[ ] **2.** "I must collect all the urine."

[ ] **3.** "I must retract the foreskin."

[ ] **4.** "I must use a sterile container."

69. Which suggestion by the nurse will best promote the client's comfort?

[ ] **1.** Using a scrotal support

[ ] **2.** Wearing cotton briefs

[ ] **3.** Buying larger underwear

[ ] **4.** Applying a hot compress

A middle-age client with inflamed testes is being seen at a local clinic. The physician diagnoses orchitis.

70. When the nurse gathers the client data, which information is most suggestive as the cause of the client's condition?
[ ] **1.** The client has multiple sexual partners.
[ ] **2.** The client is an active homosexual.
[ ] **3.** The client was never immunized for mumps.
[ ] **4.** The client is a military veteran.

During a subsequent visit, when the client has recovered from the orchitis, the nurse uses the opportunity to teach him how to perform testicular self-examination.

71. Which statement by the nurse accurately explains the technique for testicular self-examination?
[ ] **1.** Palpate each testicle simultaneously.
[ ] **2.** Roll each testicle between the thumb and fingers.
[ ] **3.** Examine your testicles at least once yearly.
[ ] **4.** Perform the self-examination in a cool room.

Nursing Care of Clients with Structural Disorders of the Male Reproductive System

During a physical examination, the nurse notes that a 25-year-old male client has an undescended testicle.

72. When the client asks how this condition affects his masculinity, which response by the nurse is most appropriate?
[ ] **1.** "It most likely has little effect on your masculinity."
[ ] **2.** "It means that you are probably impotent."
[ ] **3.** "You may notice that your breasts will enlarge later."
[ ] **4.** "Your libido is probably reduced."

A 56-year-old client has had difficulty retracting the foreskin over the glans of his penis. He is scheduled for a circumcision.

73. Besides assessing the dressing for signs of bleeding, which other postoperative nursing assessment is a priority following this surgical procedure?
[ ] **1.** Checking the client's deep-breathing efforts
[ ] **2.** Assessing the client's ability to achieve an erection
[ ] **3.** Monitoring the volume of urine output
[ ] **4.** Monitoring the pattern of bowel elimination

A client with a hydrocele has the fluid aspirated from his scrotum. The physician orders a cold application to the area.

74. When carrying out this intervention, which action is most appropriate?
[ ] **1.** Apply ice to the site in a sealed plastic bag.
[ ] **2.** Place a covered ice pack to the scrotum.
[ ] **3.** Position the client on a hypothermia blanket.
[ ] **4.** Seat the client on an ice-filled ring.

Nursing Care of Clients with Benign and Malignant Disorders of the Male Reproductive System

A 65-year-old client makes an appointment for a routine physical examination.

75. When the physician asks the nurse to prepare the client for a prostate gland examination, which position is preferred?
[ ] **1.** Lithotomy
[ ] **2.** Modified standing
[ ] **3.** Dorsal recumbent
[ ] **4.** Fowler's

A 72-year-old client with a history of benign prostatic hypertrophy (BPH) phones the nurse at his physician's office, stating that he has not been able to urinate in the past 16 hours.

76. In the early stages of BPH, the nurse expects the physician to monitor the progression of disease with which diagnostic test?
[ ] **1.** A semi-annual prostate-specific antigen (PSA) test
[ ] **2.** An annual cystoscopy
[ ] **3.** A digital rectal examination
[ ] **4.** A retrograde pyelogram

The physician advises the client to go to the emergency department for catheterization.

77. Unless the physician specifies otherwise, what is the maximum volume of urine the nurse should withdraw at this time?
[ ] **1.** 500 mL
[ ] **2.** 1,000 mL
[ ] **3.** 1,500 mL
[ ] **4.** 2,000 mL

The client is scheduled for a sonogram of his prostate.

78. When the nurse provides the client with pretest instructions, which statement is most correct?
[ ] **1.** "You'll need to fast from midnight the night before the test."
[ ] **2.** "You'll need to empty your bladder just before the test begins."

[ ] **3.** "You'll need to consume at least a quart of water an hour before the test."

[ ] **4.** "You'll need to self-administer an enema 1 hour before the test."

The client undergoes a transurethral resection of the prostate (TURP) and is returned to the nursing unit with a 3-way catheter for administering intermittent bladder irrigations.

79. When the client's spouse asks about the catheter drainage, the nurse correctly explains that immediately after a TURP, the urine will most likely be which color?

[ ] **1.** Light pink

[ ] **2.** Dark amber

[ ] **3.** Dark red

[ ] **4.** Light yellow

80. To calculate the client's urine output during bladder irrigations, which technique is correct?

[ ] **1.** Measure the total volume in the urinary drainage bag.

[ ] **2.** Add together the volume of irrigant and the urinary drainage.

[ ] **3.** Divide the urinary drainage by the volume of irrigant.

[ ] **4.** Subtract the volume of irrigant from the urine drainage.

81. To promote patency of the urinary catheter, which nursing order is most appropriate to add to the client's care plan?

[ ] **1.** Milk the urinary catheter every hour and p.r.n.

[ ] **2.** Deflate the catheter balloon once each shift.

[ ] **3.** Empty the drainage container every 4 hours.

[ ] **4.** Maintain an oral fluid intake of at least 2 L/day.

82. When a client with a TURP complains of bladder discomfort and a feeling of urgency to void, which nursing action is best to take first?

[ ] **1.** Check that the urinary drainage catheter is patent.

[ ] **2.** Administer a prescribed analgesic as soon as possible.

[ ] **3.** Change the client to semi-Fowler's position.

[ ] **4.** Get the client out of bed to ambulate for a while.

83. The client's discharge plan should include which measure for reducing episodes of urinary incontinence?

[ ] **1.** Void at least every 2 hours when awake.

[ ] **2.** Start and stop the urinary stream when voiding.

[ ] **3.** Avoid drinking caffeinated beverages.

[ ] **4.** Sit rather than stand when attempting to void.

A 68-year-old client with prostate cancer undergoes a suprapubic prostatectomy. He returns to the nursing unit with an indwelling catheter in his urethra and a cystostomy tube in his abdomen.

84. Which nursing order is most appropriate to add to the client's initial postoperative care plan?

[ ] **1.** Connect the cystostomy tube to a leg bag for drainage.

[ ] **2.** Secure the cystostomy tube to the client's thigh.

[ ] **3.** Ensure that the cystostomy tube is unclamped at all times.

[ ] **4.** Clamp the indwelling catheter when the cystostomy tube is irrigated.

85. What special instruction concerning the technique for taking vital signs is most important when assigning this task to a nursing assistant?

[ ] **1.** Count the client's respirations while he is resting.

[ ] **2.** Assess the client's pulse at the radial artery.

[ ] **3.** Measure the client's blood pressure with an aneroid manometer.

[ ] **4.** Avoid taking a rectal temperature.

A radical inguinal orchiectomy is performed on a 22-year-old client with testicular cancer.

86. Which comment by the patient indicates that he has misinterpreted the consequences of his surgery?

[ ] **1.** "My beard will continue to grow."

[ ] **2.** "My voice will sound higher."

[ ] **3.** "My sperm count will be raised."

[ ] **4.** "My sex drive will be unaffected."

Nursing Care of Clients with Sexually Transmitted Diseases

A nurse makes an office appointment for a male client who describes having a slight tickling sensation during urination and a urethral discharge.

87. To facilitate obtaining truthful information regarding this client's sexual history, which attitude is most important for the nurse to convey?

[ ] **1.** Sympathetic

[ ] **2.** Nonjudgmental

[ ] **3.** Encouraging

[ ] **4.** Optimistic

88. When obtaining a sexual history from this client, which question is most important for the nurse to ask?

[ ] **1.** "Have you ever had a painless sore on your penis?"

[ ] **2.** "Does any sexual partner have similar symptoms?"

[ ] **3.** "At what age did you first have sexual intercourse?"

[ ] **4.** "When did you last have sexual intercourse?"

The physician informs the nurse that, during the examination, a culture of urethral secretions will be needed.

89. Besides furnishing a sterile swab and culture tube, it is most important for the nurse to provide the physician with which other piece of equipment during the examination?

[ ] **1.** An antiseptic swab

[ ] **2.** A tube of lubricant

[ ] **3.** A common mask

[ ] **4.** A pair of gloves

90. The school nurse who discusses healthy sexual behaviors with a 16-year-old should stress which risk factor as predisposing the client to acquiring a sexually transmitted disease?

[ ] **1.** Experiencing early puberty

[ ] **2.** Finding sex information on the Internet

[ ] **3.** Having multiple sex partners

[ ] **4.** Receiving limited sex education

A male client reports symptoms that are suggestive of gonorrhea.

91. If a culture is ordered to detect the causative organism, which body substance will the nurse collect?

[ ] **1.** Venous blood

[ ] **2.** Sterile urine

[ ] **3.** Ejaculated semen

[ ] **4.** Urethral drainage

92. When collecting a specimen from the client who may have gonorrhea, which nursing action is correct?

[ ] **1.** Wearing latex gloves

[ ] **2.** Using a disinfectant

[ ] **3.** Asking the client to provide the specimen

[ ] **4.** Refrigerating the specimen immediately

93. When counseling a female client with a new diagnosis of genital herpes, which statement by the nurse is accurate?

[ ] **1.** "Have a Pap test done at least every 6 months."

[ ] **2.** "Avoid having vaginal intercourse for at least 6 months."

[ ] **3.** "If you take your medicine, you will not infect anyone else."

[ ] **4.** "Your infection provides immunity for any future children."

94. While assessing a male client with tertiary syphilis, which finding is most characteristic of this stage of the disease?

[ ] **1.** Sharp leg pains

[ ] **2.** Red rash

[ ] **3.** Penile ulcer

[ ] **4.** Patchy hair loss

95. Which comment indicates that the client lacks a clear understanding of this disease?

[ ] **1.** "I can be cured using antibiotic therapy."

[ ] **2.** "My sexual partner should be tested for the disease."

[ ] **3.** "Syphilitic lesions may be present in my partner's vagina."

[ ] **4.** "One infection provides lifelong immunity."

A culture indicates that a client has nonspecific urethritis from a nongonococcal organism, Chlamydia trachomatis. *The physician prescribes doxycycline (Vibramycin) 100 mg b.i.d. with a sufficient number of capsules for 7 days of treatment.*

96. Which information given by the nurse is most appropriate to provide to the client?

[ ] **1.** Take the medication until the symptoms clear.

[ ] **2.** Refill the prescription if symptoms persist.

[ ] **3.** Take the medication for the full amount of time.

[ ] **4.** Treatment of the infection is likely to be lifelong.

97. Which nursing instruction is best to prevent a recurrence of a chlamydial infection?

[ ] **1.** Shower or bathe after intercourse.

[ ] **2.** Wash your hands well using an antiseptic soap.

[ ] **3.** Encourage your sexual partners to be tested and treated.

[ ] **4.** Make sure you receive adequate nutrition and fluid intake.

98. When the nurse teaches a client who has been diagnosed with a chlamydial infection, which statement is accurate?

[ ] **1.** "Your sexual partner needs simultaneous treatment."

[ ] **2.** "There's no known cure for this kind of infection."

[ ] **3.** "This is a rare type of sexually transmitted disease."

[ ] **4.** "Men manifest symptoms, but infected women do not."

99. Which gynecologic symptom reported by a female client is most suggestive of trichomoniasis?
[ ] **1.** A series of fluid-filled vesicles on the vagina
[ ] **2.** Vaginal drainage that causes intense itching
[ ] **3.** Vaginal drainage that resembles milk curds
[ ] **4.** Tenderness and pressure in the lower abdomen

The client with trichomoniasis is treated with oral metronidazole (Flagyl).

100. Which nursing instruction is essential for preventing a drug-food interaction while the client is taking metronidazole (Flagyl)?
[ ] **1.** Use plain salt rather than the iodized type.
[ ] **2.** Stop eating anything with aspartame (NutraSweet).
[ ] **3.** Eliminate sources of monosodium glutamate (MSG).
[ ] **4.** Avoid consuming alcohol in any form.

A nurse refers a client with genital warts to a gynecologist, who confirms that they are caused by human papillomavirus.

101. When the client asks if there is any danger associated with this condition, which response by the nurse is best?
[ ] **1.** "The condition can be treated with an antibiotic, such as penicillin or tetracycline."
[ ] **2.** "The condition appears to increase the risk of cancer of the vulva, vagina, and cervix."
[ ] **3.** "The condition can be prevented by taking birth control pills."
[ ] **4.** "The condition is not dangerous and requires no treatment at this time."

To prevent infection with the human immunodeficiency virus (HIV), a client says he uses a condom when having intercourse.

102. Which technique can the nurse suggest to provide additional protection from HIV?
[ ] **1.** Remove the condom immediately after intercourse.
[ ] **2.** Wash the penis with a dilute vinegar solution.
[ ] **3.** Use a spermicide containing nonoxynol-9.
[ ] **4.** Apply copious amounts of vaginal lubricant.

103. When managing the care of a client with acquired immunodeficiency syndrome (AIDS), which method best evaluates the effectiveness of zidovudine (AZT) therapy?
[ ] **1.** Assessing the client's vital signs
[ ] **2.** Assessing the client's blood counts
[ ] **3.** Monitoring the client's blood culture reports
[ ] **4.** Monitoring the client's viral load tests

Nursing Care of Clients Practicing Family Planning

A female client receives a 6-month supply of oral contraceptives.

104. Which instruction is appropriate to include when providing the client with oral contraceptive teaching?
[ ] **1.** Take oral contraceptives at the same time each day.
[ ] **2.** Take oral contraceptives on an empty stomach.
[ ] **3.** Take oral contraceptives on the first day of menses.
[ ] **4.** Take oral contraceptives in the morning with food.

105. Which recommendation by the nurse is most appropriate to reduce the risk of blood clots while the client is taking hormonal contraceptives?
[ ] **1.** Stop smoking while taking hormonal contraceptives.
[ ] **2.** Drink a high volume of fluid to dilute the blood.
[ ] **3.** Keep the legs elevated while sitting in a chair.
[ ] **4.** Eat more garlic and onions on a weekly basis.

A pregnant client is considering a tubal ligation after the birth of her child.

106. Which statement indicates that the client is misinformed?
[ ] **1.** "I will have a small abdominal incision."
[ ] **2.** "This procedure is not easily reversed."
[ ] **3.** "I will no longer menstruate afterward."
[ ] **4.** "Recovery should occur in a brief time."

107. If a female client with an intrauterine device describes the following symptoms, which one is most likely related to her birth control device?
[ ] **1.** Breast tenderness
[ ] **2.** Heavy menstrual flow
[ ] **3.** Steady weight gain
[ ] **4.** Chronic acne

108. The nurse correctly teaches a couple that immediately after a vasectomy, it is best to continue using an alternative birth control method for which time period?
[ ] **1.** 1 week
[ ] **2.** 1 month
[ ] **3.** 6 weeks
[ ] **4.** 6 months

109. When teaching a male client about how to use a condom, which instruction is correct?

[ ] **1.** "Wait until your penis becomes limp before removing it from the vagina."

[ ] **2.** "You can reuse a condom as long as you wash it between uses."

[ ] **3.** "Leave a small space between the end of the condom and the penis."

[ ] **4.** "Apply the condom before your penis is in an erect state."

110. The physician prescribes medroxyprogesterone acetate (Depo-Provera) 150 mg I.M. for contraception for a 28-year-old woman. What actions are appropriate when administering this medication? Select all that apply.

[ ] **1.** Confirm that the client is not pregnant.

[ ] **2.** Give the injection deeply into the dorsogluteal site.

[ ] **3.** Schedule administration of the first injection to coincide with the time of ovulation.

[ ] **4.** Inform the client to return every 3 months for another injection.

[ ] **5.** Inform the client to use an additional form of contraception for the first week after an injection.

[ ] **6.** Apply ice to the injection site for 2 to 3 minutes before administering the drug.

A 16-year-old student comes to the local public health department requesting information about birth control. She tells the nurse that she "wants something" so that she does not get pregnant.

111. Which information should be gathered before the nurse can advise the student appropriately regarding methods of birth control? Select all that apply.

[ ] **1.** The adolescent's lifestyle

[ ] **2.** Whether she is currently sexually active

[ ] **3.** Whether she has had a Pap smear in the past year

[ ] **4.** The date of her last menstrual period

[ ] **5.** Where she is currently working

After discussing various birth control methods with the client, the nurse advises her about safe sex practices.

112. Which information regarding safe sex practices should the nurse include in the client's teaching plan? Select all that apply.

[ ] **1.** "Be selective in choosing sexual partners."

[ ] **2.** "Do not share vibrators or other sexual equipment."

[ ] **3.** "Avoid intercourse if you have signs of a sexually transmitted disease."

[ ] **4.** "Urinate after having intercourse."

[ ] **5.** "Store condoms away from excessive heat."

[ ] **6.** "Keep birth control patches in the refrigerator."

The nurse is assigned to discuss family planning and various methods of contraception with a group of women who have expressed an interest in this topic. One participant asks the nurse, "How do oral contraceptives prevent pregnancy?"

113. The nurse correctly explains that the combination oral contraceptives prevent pregnancy by interfering with the sperm reaching the ovum and by which other method?

[ ] **1.** Preventing ovulation

[ ] **2.** Depressing progesterone secretion

[ ] **3.** Depressing formation of the corpus luteum

[ ] **4.** Thickening the uterine lining

Another participant asks the nurse to explain the difference between oral contraceptive packages that have 21 pills and those that have 28 pills.

114. Which statement correctly describes oral contraceptive packages that contain 28 pills?

[ ] **1.** Packages containing 28 pills are biphasic and release a constant amount of estrogen and an increasing amount of progesterone throughout the cycle.

[ ] **2.** Packages containing 28 pills have 7 placebo pills and allow a woman to maintain a routine of taking a pill a day without missing a dose.

[ ] **3.** Packages containing 28 pills have 21 pills that contain estrogen and 7 pills that contain progesterone and are called combination oral contraceptives.

[ ] **4.** Packages containing 28 pills are prescribed for women who have a 28-day menstrual cycle instead of a 21-day menstrual cycle.

115. Which statement by a participant indicates a need for additional teaching regarding safe and effective use of oral contraceptives?

[ ] **1.** "An alternative form of contraceptive is used if more than one dose of the oral contraceptive has been missed."

[ ] **2.** "Oral contraceptives are not taken by women who have a history of primary dysmenorrhea."

[ ] **3.** "Oral contraceptives should be discontinued 3 to 4 months before a planned pregnancy."

[ ] **4.** "Oral contraceptives cause breakthrough bleeding when used concurrently with some antibiotics and antihistamines."

A participant asks the nurse about the use of the birth control patch that some of her friends have started to use. The nurse explains about the use of the patch and reviews the side effects of this type of birth control.

116. Which side effects should the nurse cover in the explanation? Select all that apply.
- [ ] 1. Skin irritation
- [ ] 2. Irregular vaginal bleeding
- [ ] 3. Fluid retention
- [ ] 4. Increased blood pressure
- [ ] 5. Nausea and vomiting
- [ ] 6. Hepatitis

At the family planning class, the nurse describes to the participants the various barrier methods of contraception.

117. Which statement made by a participant indicates the need for additional teaching about barrier methods of contraception?
- [ ] 1. "A diaphragm is refitted or replaced if there is a weight gain or loss of 10 lb or more."
- [ ] 2. "Use of the intrauterine device is not recommended for women who have never been pregnant."
- [ ] 3. "Toxic shock syndrome is a potential side effect associated with the use of the cervical cap."
- [ ] 4. "Use of the female condom is not recommended for women who are allergic to latex."

One participant states that she is considering using the basal body temperature method of natural family planning and asks the nurse the correct way to use this method.

118. Which statement is correct concerning the proper use of the basal body temperature method of natural family planning?
- [ ] 1. The client should record the pattern of her menstrual cycle for 6 to 8 months before actually using the method.
- [ ] 2. The client should regularly monitor the consistency of vaginal secretions along with body temperature.
- [ ] 3. The client should take her temperature every morning before rising for 6 months before using the method.
- [ ] 4. The client should have her sex partner withdraw his penis from the vagina just before ejaculation.

Correct Answers and Rationales

Nursing Care of Clients with Breast Disorders

1. 3. The American Cancer Society recommends that all women have an initial baseline mammogram beginning at age 40. Between the ages of 20 and 30, women should have a clinical breast examination by a health care professional every 3 years. Between ages 40 and 49, women should have mammograms every 1 to 2 years and a clinical breast examination by a health care professional on a yearly basis. Yearly mammograms should begin at age 50. Several studies suggest that screening for high-risk women with a family history of breast cancer should begin approximately 10 years before the age of diagnosis of the family member with breast cancer.
Client Needs Category—Health promotion and maintenance
Client Needs Subcategory—None

2. 2. Women should begin conducting breast self-examinations (BSEs) in their twenties and having a breast examination by a health care professional every 3 years. When conducting BSE, the client should inspect her breasts during a shower, when lying down, and while standing before a mirror. Ominous signs include a change in the size of one breast, dimpling of the skin, or an altered nipple appearance.
Client Needs Category—Health promotion and maintenance
Client Needs Subcategory—None

3. 4. The pads of the four fingertips are used to feel for breast abnormalities during BSE. The pads of the fingers are especially sensitive and can note lumps or changes in breast tissue. Commercial products are available to increase the ability to slide the pads of the fingers over the skin surface.
Client Needs Category—Health promotion and maintenance
Client Needs Subcategory—None

4. 2. Although there is more than one method of performing BSE, all include palpating from the outer margins toward the nipple. The client should develop a specific pattern for examination to follow on a monthly basis.
Client Needs Category—Health promotion and maintenance
Client Needs Subcategory—None

5. **4.** Premenopausal women should perform a BSE every month, 1 week after the menses begin. When a client is past menopause, a BSE should be performed on a selected date each month, for example, the first day of the month.

> ***Client Needs Category***—*Health promotion and maintenance*
> ***Client Needs Subcategory***—*None*

6. **2.** Underarm deodorant, body powder, or ointments on the breast can produce artifacts on the mammogram film. The artifacts may be misinterpreted as pathologic findings. The client may wear a bra before and after the test, but not during a mammogram. Shaving underarm hair is a cultural choice; it is not a test requirement. Normal hygiene measures are appropriate, but wiping the breasts with an antiseptic before the test is unnecessary.

> ***Client Needs Category***—*Health promotion and maintenance*
> ***Client Needs Subcategory***—*None*

7. **3.** Having a close blood relative with breast cancer places the client at high risk for developing this disease. The risk factor increases twofold if the relative is a first-degree female, such as a sister, mother, or daughter. Menstruating before age 12 and being nulliparous are additional predisposing factors. Breast-feeding has many advantages, but protection against breast cancer is not one of them.

> ***Client Needs Category***—*Health promotion and maintenance*
> ***Client Needs Subcategory***—*None*

8. **4.** Fibrocystic lesions cause more discomfort before menstruation because the lesions are affected by increasing levels of estrogen. Estrogen appears to be a factor because cysts usually disappear after menopause. Many women experience relief of symptoms when menstruation occurs. Symptoms do not commonly increase with aging. Fibrocystic lesions are not affected by sexual activity.

> ***Client Needs Category***—*Health promotion and maintenance*
> ***Client Needs Subcategory***—*None*

9. **2.** Some women report that eliminating coffee, tea, cola, and chocolate reduces their breast discomfort. Limiting sodium intake, taking a warm bath, or administering an anti-inflammatory such as ibuprofen (Motrin) also helps. Objectively, however, there is no evidence that the fibrocystic lesions become smaller or disappear with any particular diet modification. Consuming a high-fat diet seems to have a relationship in developing breast cancer. Refined sugar and alcohol are not linked to breast disease.

> ***Client Needs Category***—*Health promotion and maintenance*
> ***Client Needs Subcategory***—*None*

10. **3.** Cleaning with soap and water is one of the best methods for reducing transmission of microorganisms. Eating more sources of protein is a healthful measure, but it is not as specific as maintaining intact skin. Supporting the breasts and applying warm compresses provide comfort but have no effect on preventing the transmission of microorganisms elsewhere.

> ***Client Needs Category***—*Safe, effective care environment*
> ***Client Needs Subcategory***—*Safety and infection control*

11. **3.** Cancerous tumors tend to be irregularly shaped and attached firmly to surrounding tissue. Benign breast tumors tend to have a well-defined border and to be freely movable. Neither the lump's size nor the location can necessarily predict if the lump is benign or malignant. However, cancerous tumors in nulliparous women or those who have not breast-fed infants are more commonly located in the upper outer quadrant of the breast.

> ***Client Needs Category***—*Physiological integrity*
> ***Client Needs Subcategory***—*Physiological adaptation*

12. **2.** Competent adult clients have the right to self-determination once they have all the pertinent information to make a decision. When that occurs, nurses have a duty to facilitate whatever choices the clients make. Discouraging the client from opposing the physician's recommendation promotes passivity. Even if most biopsies are accurate, some are not. Even though a second opinion may eventually prove to be appropriate, the nurse should try to facilitate communication between the client and physician; in most cases, the treatment plan can be modified to suit the client's wishes.

> ***Client Needs Category***—*Safe, effective care environment*
> ***Client Needs Subcategory***—*Coordinated care*

13. **3.** Because this surgery compromises the client's vascular and lymphatic circulation, blood pressures and any other invasive procedures involving an arm are performed on the opposite upper extremity. Postmastectomy clients generally are not restricted to any one particular position; however, a sitting position tends to promote incisional drainage. Fluids usually are not restricted. It is appropriate to assess the dressing and drainage, but the incisional wound is inspected only at the time of a dressing change, which may take place several days later.

14. **1.** Following a mastectomy, the client's breathing may be compromised due to the thoracic incision and restrictive (pressure) dressing. This type of dressing prevents movement of the chest muscles and thus reduces lung capacity until the dressing is removed. Having the client take deep breaths and encouraging coughing every 2 hours is critical to prevent such respiratory problems as atelectasis and hypostatic pneumonia. The client should be encouraged to assume her regular diet soon after surgery; therefore, her nutrition should not be compromised. The client should also begin ambulating while decreasing her pain medication, thereby helping to increase bowel motility. Her risk of pressure sores should also decrease when she begins moving.

Client Needs Category—Physiological integrity
Client Needs Subcategory—Reduction of risk potential

15. **2.** Most mastectomy clients tend to avoid raising the arm on the operative side following surgery. If this practice is prolonged, they tend to lose their full range of motion. Using the affected arm for hair brushing requires using muscles that elevate the arm and extend the chest muscles. Although self-feeding, writing, and washing the chest are good activities, they are not as likely to exercise the muscle groups to the same extent as brushing the hair.

Client Needs Category—Physiological integrity
Client Needs Subcategory—Reduction of risk potential

16. **3.** In postmastectomy clients, the standard practice is to elevate the affected arm on pillows while the client is in bed, to raise the client's arm and exercise the hand muscles, and to support the client's arm in a sling while she is ambulating. Applying ice reduces swelling, and warm compresses dilate blood vessels; however, because this surgery tends to compromise the client's circulation and sensory perception, these two measures are not the most appropriate to use. Frequent ambulation of the client would be contraindicated.

Client Needs Category—Physiological integrity
Client Needs Subcategory—Reduction of risk potential

17. **2.** The American Cancer Society includes a group of trained volunteers who offer personal support and printed materials for postmastectomy clients in its program called Reach to Recovery. None of the other associations or organizations in the remaining options exists.

Client Needs Category—Health promotion and maintenance
Client Needs Subcategory—None

18. **2.** Clients who have had breast cancer are at risk for cancer in the opposite breast. Therefore, they must be conscientious about performing monthly BSEs. Postmenopausal women pick an arbitrary date and perform BSE on that date each month. The time of day is not pertinent. Breasts are examined during a shower, not afterward, when it is easier for the fingers to glide over the breast tissue. BSEs are performed monthly, not once a year.

Client Needs Category—Health promotion and maintenance
Client Needs Subcategory—None

19. **0.5.** To calculate the drug dosage, use the formula:

$$\frac{\text{Desired dose}}{\text{Dose on hand}} \times \text{Total quantity} = \text{Desired dose}$$

In this case, $\frac{10}{20} \times 1 \text{ tablet} = 0.5 \text{ tablet}$

Client Needs Category—Physiological integrity
Client Needs Subcategory—Pharmacological therapies

20.

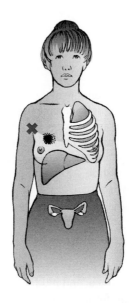

Breast cancer usually spreads first to the axillary lymph nodes, the structures closest to the primary site. Distant metastasis in advanced stages of breast cancer may be found in the bones, liver, lungs, and brain.

Client Needs Category—Physiological integrity
Client Needs Subcategory—Physiological adaptation

Nursing Care of Clients with Disturbances in Menstruation

21.

4. Ovarian follicle matures

3. Endometrium begins to thicken

1. Ovum is released

6. Corpus luteum forms

2. Progesterone decreases

5. Endometrium is shed

The ovarian follicle matures when the anterior pituitary gland secretes follicle-stimulating hormone. This is accompanied by an increase in estrogen, which promotes thickening of the endometrium. At about midcycle, the anterior pituitary gland releases luteinizing hormone, which causes the follicle to rupture and release an ovum. The ruptured follicle is transformed into the corpus luteum and secretes progesterone. If fertilization fails to occur, the progesterone level decreases and the endometrium is shed.

Client Needs Category—Physiological integrity
Client Needs Subcategory—Physiological adaptation

22. **1.** It is important to differentiate between primary amenorrhea, a condition in which a female has never menstruated, and secondary amenorrhea, in which menstruation has occurred but has been absent for more than 3 months. This differentiation can provide important diagnostic information. Although the other questions may be pertinent, they are not as important to know at this time.

Client Needs Category—Health promotion and maintenance
Client Needs Subcategory—None

23. **3.** Local applications of heat and mild analgesics are the first line of treatment for minor symptoms of dysmenorrhea. It would be premature to seek a prescription for an oral contraceptive at this time, although oral contraception is effective in certain cases for relieving dysmenorrhea. There is no correlation between hygiene products chosen and dysmenorrhea.

Client Needs Category—Health promotion and maintenance
Client Needs Subcategory—None

24. **1.** Douching in the days preceding a Pap smear interferes with accurate test results because it removes exfoliated cells. None of the other instructions are necessary when preparing a client for a pelvic examination.

Client Needs Category—Physiological integrity
Client Needs Subcategory—Reduction of risk potential

25. **2.** If the bladder is empty, pelvic organs are more easily palpated and the client experiences less discomfort. It is inappropriate to instill a vaginal lubricant before the examination. Analgesia is generally unnecessary. No special consent form is required for the examination.

Client Needs Category—Physiological integrity
Client Needs Subcategory—Reduction of risk potential

26. **3.** It is best to document the date of a client's last menstrual period to assist the pathologist in determining if the microscopic cells are appropriate for the current stage in the menstrual cycle. Answers to the other questions are immaterial to the results of the Pap smear.

Client Needs Category—Health promotion and maintenance
Client Needs Subcategory—None

27. **4.** A supine lithotomy position is preferred for a pelvic examination; however, an upright lithotomy position is also used. In unusual circumstances, Sims' position may be used. Neither Trendelenburg's nor Fowler's position facilitates access to the vagina.

Client Needs Category—Physiological integrity
Client Needs Subcategory—Reduction of risk potential

28. **1.** To reduce the claim of sexual impropriety and to make the client feel more comfortable, an important nursing consideration is to have a female nurse present during the pelvic examination. Instructing on the dangers of cervical cancer is good general information; however, it is not known if the client has cervical cancer. The physician usually completes the internal examination and documents the findings. A personal vaginal lubricant is not instilled prior to the examination, although the physician may use a lubricant on the fingers during the internal examination.

Client Needs Category—Safe, effective care environment
Client Needs Subcategory—Coordinated care

29. **1.** Breakthrough bleeding or spotting may occur among clients who take oral contraceptives with low dosages of estrogen or progesterone. Stress has been implicated in delaying menses or causing irregularity in a previously regular cycle, but it is uncommon for stress to cause midcycle bleeding. Having sexual intercourse with an uncircumcised partner is not a common cause of vaginal bleeding. Straining to have a stool is not a common cause of vaginal bleeding except when the client has had recent vaginal surgery or a vaginal birth.

Client Needs Category—*Health promotion and maintenance*
Client Needs Subcategory—*None*

Nursing Care of Clients with Infectious and Inflammatory Disorders of the Female Reproductive System

30. 1. *Candida albicans,* a common cause of vaginitis, is usually treated with an antifungal medication. Several former antifungal prescription drugs are now available without a prescription. Over-the-counter drugs, such as miconazole (Monistat) and clotrimazole (Gyne-Lotrimin), are available in various forms, including vaginal tablets, creams, and suppositories. Oral antibiotics are not used to treat *Candida albicans* and, in fact, are frequently the cause of the vaginitis. Irritating vaginal douches are not recommended for treatment.

Client Needs Category—*Physiological integrity*
Client Needs Subcategory—*Pharmacological therapies*

31. 3. Instilling the drug before bedtime aids in retaining the medication within the vagina for a substantial period of time. When this is not possible, the client is instructed to recline for 10 to 30 minutes after insertion. The applicator is inserted approximately 2″ to 4″ (5 to 10 cm) within the vagina. The best position for instilling the drug is reclining in a dorsal recumbent position. Latex gloves are a matter of personal choice when self-administering vaginal medication; however, they are required when instilling the drug into someone else. Good hand washing is important in either case.

Client Needs Category—*Physiological integrity*
Client Needs Subcategory—*Pharmacological therapies*

32. 2. Yeasts are present in the intestinal tract and introduced into the vagina if stool is wiped across rather than away from the vaginal opening. This is often a common etiologic factor in urinary tract infections as well. Showers versus tub baths are a matter of personal preference as long as the tub is cleaned on a routine basis. Some types of vaginal infections are spread from infected sexual partners, but limiting intercourse to once a week is not likely to prevent them. Lanolin soap is no more effective than antiseptic body soaps for reducing microorganism growth.

Client Needs Category—*Health promotion and maintenance*
Client Needs Subcategory—*None*

33. 2. Douching for the purpose of hygiene is unnecessary and can be harmful because it depletes helpful microorganisms that tend to prevent vaginal infections. A vinegar solution alters the pH of the vagina and makes it an inhospitable environment for microbial growth, but it is better to use a dilute solution rather than one that is concentrated. The volume of douche solutions can be more than 16 oz. The solution drains out by gravity when the vaginal capacity is reached. Cramping is not common with douching.

Client Needs Category—*Health promotion and maintenance*
Client Needs Subcategory—*None*

34. 1. Toxic shock syndrome is caused by *Staphylococcus aureus.* The use of superabsorbent tampons tends to result in less frequent changing of tampons. Retaining the organism in a confined area with access to a rich blood supply promotes its growth and proliferation. It is appropriate to report prolonged menses because this can lead to anemia from blood loss; however, this is unrelated to toxic shock syndrome. A woman should never neglect her hygiene because she is menstruating. Some individuals are sensitive to scents used in sanitary products, but they have no relationship to toxic shock syndrome.

Client Needs Category—*Health promotion and maintenance*
Client Needs Subcategory—*None*

35. 2. It is essential to contain any and all infectious drainage from a client with PID within specially marked infectious waste bags. Double wrapping soiled items prior to disposal or terminal cleaning protects other health care workers from accidental contamination with infectious microorganisms. Flushing absorbent pads down the toilet could cause plumbing problems. Neither an open wastebasket nor paper bags are sufficient barriers for containing the infectious microorganisms.

Client Needs Category—*Safe, effective care environment*
Client Needs Subcategory—*Safety and infection control*

36. 4. Infertility is a common consequence of PID. Infertility results from the scarring of fallopian tubes, which subsequently blocks passage for both sperm and ovum. With early and aggressive treatment, the sequela may be prevented or minimized. Cancer of the cervix, premature labor, and spontaneous abortion are not directly related to a prior incidence of PID.

Client Needs Category—*Physiological integrity*
Client Needs Subcategory—*Physiological adaptation*

37. **1.** A laparoscope is inserted through the abdominal wall. Once inserted, the instrument is used to visualize the intra-abdominal and pelvic organs, obtain biopsies of tissue, and perform therapeutic treatment procedures.

> *Client Needs Category—Physiological integrity*
> *Client Needs Subcategory—Physiological integrity*

38. **2.** Shoulder or abdominal discomfort may be experienced for 1 to 2 days after a laparoscopy. The discomfort is caused by the bolus of carbon dioxide instilled to distend the abdominal cavity. Nausea and leg cramps are unrelated to the laparoscopic procedure. Urinary urgency may occur following removal of the retention catheter used to keep the bladder empty during the laparoscopy, but it is not a direct effect of the procedure.

> *Client Needs Category—Physiological integrity*
> *Client Needs Subcategory—Reduction of risk potential*

39. **4.** Decreased estrogen production after menopause reduces the potential for vaginal lubrication. A dry vaginal mucous membrane is a common etiologic factor in painful intercourse after menopause. Pelvic muscles usually do not become more sensitive to pressure with age. The amount of foreplay, no matter how long it continues, cannot stimulate mucus secretion if mucus cannot be produced. The vagina atrophies from age-related changes and has no relationship to the frequency of intercourse.

> *Client Needs Category—Physiological integrity*
> *Client Needs Subcategory—Physiological adaptation*

Nursing Care of Clients with Benign and Malignant Disorders of the Uterus and Ovaries

40. **1.** Fibroid tumors respond to estrogen stimulation. Heavy menstrual bleeding is a common complaint of clients with myomas. Myomas arise from muscle tissue in the uterus and are usually benign. If pain occurs, it usually accompanies menstruation. Irregular light menses and breast tenderness, if present, are not associated with fibroid tumors.

> *Client Needs Category—Physiological integrity*
> *Client Needs Subcategory—Physiological adaptation*

41. **1.** A full bladder is essential when performing a pelvic sonogram. Clients must consume at least a quart of water 1 hour before the examination and refrain from urinating until the examination is completed. Fasting is unnecessary. The examination is not painful, so an analgesic is unnecessary. No special skin preparation is required prior to the examination.

> *Client Needs Category—Physiological integrity*
> *Client Needs Subcategory—Reduction of risk potential*

42. **2.** All the data described are valid facts to document. However, documenting that this client has voided a sufficient amount to empty her bladder is most pertinent to the client's safety after discharge.

> *Client Needs Category—Physiological integrity*
> *Client Needs Subcategory—Reduction of risk potential*

43. **1.** It is common to have slight vaginal bleeding after a colposcopy; however, excessive bleeding is unusual and should be reported. None of the other options describes a common problem following colposcopy.

> *Client Needs Category—Physiological integrity*
> *Client Needs Subcategory—Physiological adaptation*

44. **3.** Identifying the number of sanitary pads used helps to quantify the extent of bleeding. It provides more information than asking how often the client has sexual intercourse or if her energy level has changed. The color of the blood provides a characteristic of the blood loss, but it does not indicate the extent of bleeding.

> *Client Needs Category—Physiological integrity*
> *Client Needs Subcategory—Physiological adaptation*

45. **2.** Metrorrhagia, vaginal bleeding between regular menstrual periods, is significant in a woman who is receiving hormonal replacement therapy because it may signal cancer, tumors of the uterus, or other gynecologic problems that require further evaluation. Bleeding between menstrual periods by a woman taking oral contraceptives is not usually serious. Dysfunctional irregular bleeding may also occur in individuals at the opposite ends of the reproductive lifespan, such as adolescents and perimenopausal women, and usually is not as much of a concern.

> *Client Needs Category—Physiological integrity*
> *Client Needs Subcategory—Physiological adaptation*

46. **2.** Following electrocauterization, the client is told to avoid straining and heavy lifting because these activities may cause bleeding from the cauterized site. The physician usually reexamines the client in 2 to 4 weeks. Absolute bed rest is unnecessary, but the client should rest more than usual. Neither douching nor sexual intercourse is permitted until the physician indicates it is safe to do so.

Client Needs Category—Health promotion and maintenance
Client Needs Subcategory—None

47. **2.** Bed rest must be maintained to retain the applicator within the vagina. In fact, the head of the bed should not be raised more than 45 degrees while the radioactive applicator is in place. Nourishment is important, but it is related more to the client's nutritional status than to radiation therapy. Weighing the client is postponed while the radioactive applicator is in place.

Client Needs Category—Safe, effective care environment
Client Needs Subcategory—Safety and infection control

48. **4.** Displaced radioactive materials are placed in a lead container as soon as they are discovered. The nurse should avoid contact with the radioactive materials if at all possible and should call the radiation safety department or nuclear medicine department. The lead container blocks the transmission of radioactivity. The nuclear medicine department then manages the substance appropriately. Radioactive substances are never discarded. The physician, not the nurse, is responsible for reinserting the implant.

Client Needs Category—Safe, effective care environment
Client Needs Subcategory—Safety and infection control

49. **3.** Distance is one measure used to reduce exposure to radiation. Therefore, radioactive substances are never held with the hands. A long-handled forceps and lead container should be in the room of a client who has a radioactive implant in a body orifice. Neither washing the hands nor using a glass jar will control exposure to radiation. Rubber gloves rather than vinyl gloves provide better protection, but the radioactive substance should never be touched with the hands.

Client Needs Category—Safe, effective care environment
Client Needs Subcategory—Safety and infection control

50. **2.** All the described nurses have strengths that may be helpful to this client. However, because exposure to radiation can affect male and female gametes, it is best that a nurse for whom pregnancy is unlikely or a male nurse who has had a vasectomy should care for the client.

Client Needs Category—Safe, effective care environment
Client Needs Subcategory—Safety and infection control

51. **3.** The female urethra is approximately 1½″ to 2″ (3.8 to 5 cm) long. Inserting the catheter 2″ to 3″ (5 to 8 cm) places the tip of the catheter into the bladder, which should allow urine to flow. Once urine flows, the catheter is advanced another ½″ to 1″ to ensure that the balloon of the indwelling catheter is well past the bladder neck.

Client Needs Category—Physiological integrity
Client Needs Subcategory—Reduction of risk potential

52. **1.** All clients who receive general anesthesia are prone to respiratory complications. Because a clear airway and breathing are higher priorities than nutrition to maintain immediately postoperatively, *Risk for ineffective airway clearance* is the most appropriate addition at this time. It is too early to make the diagnosis of *Ineffective coping.* The client should have no difficulty communicating verbally when she is returned from the postanesthesia recovery room.

Client Needs Category—Physiological integrity
Client Needs Subcategory—Reduction of risk potential

53. **1.** Antiembolism stockings are frequently ordered for postoperative clients and those unable to ambulate to circulate their blood. These clients are at high risk for developing a blood clot. Antiembolism stockings should be worn continuously except when removed for assessment and hygiene.

Client Needs Category—Physiological integrity
Client Needs Subcategory—Reduction of risk potential

54. **3.** Clients who have had abdominal surgery are prone to developing blood clots in their lower extremities. Therefore, the knees should not be elevated because doing so promotes stasis of blood flow. All the other activities are appropriate for a client recovering from a hysterectomy.

Client Needs Category—Safe, effective care environment
Client Needs Subcategory—Coordinated Care

55. **3.** It is important to deflate the balloon first so that the catheter can be removed from the urethra. Not deflating the balloon can lead to urethral trauma and damage. Cleaning the client's perineum and measuring her urine output are essential actions, but they can be postponed until after the catheter has been removed. It is unnecessary to separate the catheter from the drainage bag. After the bag is emptied, both can be disposed of in an appropriate waste receptacle.

Client Needs Category—*Physiological integrity*
Client Needs Subcategory—*Reduction of risk potential*

56. 2. To measure the volume of urine retained in the bladder, it is important to catheterize the client within 10 minutes after voiding. The size of the catheter is relative to the size of the client. However, the size is not pertinent to the purpose of the procedure. The catheter is connected to gravity drainage only if the physician orders a retention catheter based on a certain retained volume.

Client Needs Category—*Physiological integrity*
Client Needs Subcategory—*Reduction of risk potential*

57. 2. The dosages of many toxic drugs administered to adults, as well as drugs administered to children, are calculated on the basis of the client's body surface area. Body surface area is calculated by using both body weight and height. The other data are important to obtain but have no relationship to the dosage of the drug that will be administered.

Client Needs Category—*Physiological integrity*
Client Needs Subcategory—*Pharmacological therapies*

58. 4. Antineoplastic medications can affect the function of bone marrow, which produces the blood cells. A complete blood count provides information about all the cells that the bone marrow produces. The mean cell volume, total leukocyte count, and differential cell count are all important, but none is as comprehensively informative as a complete blood cell count.

Client Needs Category—*Physiological integrity*
Client Needs Subcategory—*Pharmacological therapies*

59. 2. Examination gloves act as a barrier against contact between the drug and the nurse's skin. Regardless of the drug manufacturer's directions for preparing the drug, such as using only prefilled syringes, diluting the drug with saline solution, or mixing the drug in a closed vial, wearing gloves reduces the risk of accidentally absorbing the medication.

Client Needs Category—*Safe, effective care environment*
Client Needs Subcategory—*Safety and infection control*

60. 4. The hair lost with some antineoplastic drugs returns after chemotherapy is terminated. The return of hair growth varies from client to client, but in all cases it is restored in less than 2 years. However, the hair growth may be different in color or texture from the past hair type of the individual.

Client Needs Category—*Health promotion and maintenance*
Client Needs Subcategory—*None*

Nursing Care of Clients with Miscellaneous Disorders of the Female Reproductive System

61. 2. Standing and bearing down is the best technique for determining the extent of uterine prolapse. Using this technique, the nurse can evaluate the effect of gravity in relation to the relaxed pelvic muscles. The other assessment techniques are used if the client is unable to stand.

Client Needs Category—*Physiological integrity*
Client Needs Subcategory—*Physiological adaptation*

62. 4. The majority of clients with a cystocele experience stress incontinence. Stress incontinence is manifested by a slight loss of urine when abdominal pressure increases as with sneezing, coughing, laughing, and lifting heavy objects. Awakening in the morning, walking, and sleeping do not promote stress incontinence.

Client Needs Category—*Physiological integrity*
Client Needs Subcategory—*Physiological adaptation*

63. 3. Perineal exercises, also known as *Kegel exercises*, strengthen the muscles that help suspend the bladder. Purchasing absorbent underwear is an option if the cystocele is more serious or if the client chooses not to proceed with a surgical repair. Applying an external catheter is an option, but not a very effective or popular one. It is inappropriate to limit oral fluid intake as a means of controlling adult incontinence.

Client Needs Category—*Health promotion and maintenance*
Client Needs Subcategory—*None*

64. 2. Absence of a urinary tract infection is the best indication that the client is following appropriate aseptic principles when performing self-catheterization. The volume of urine should be more than 50 mL if the bladder is being emptied completely. The catheter should be removed immediately after the bladder is emptied. The frequency of catheterization depends on the client's rate of urine formation and sensation of a need to void. Frequency of catheterization is not an indication of appropriate technique.

Client Needs Category—*Health promotion and maintenance*
Client Needs Subcategory—*None*

65. **1, 2, 4, 5.** Alendronate (Fosamax) may be prescribed to help increase bone mass when bone resorption exceeds bone formation—a condition that occurs among women as they age, especially during the postmenopausal years when estrogen levels decrease significantly. Alendronate (Fosamax) may cause esophageal irritation; therefore, measures to promote gastric emptying are encouraged. This includes taking the medication upon awakening with 6 to 8 ounces of water (not food or milk) and remaining upright for at least 30 minutes. Alendronate (Fosamax) neither relieves hot flashes or irritability nor any other discomforts commonly associated with menopause.

> *Client Needs Category—Physiological integrity*
> *Client Needs Subcategory—Pharmacological therapies*

Nursing Care of Clients with Inflammatory Disorders of the Male Reproductive System

66. **3.** Inadequate treatment leads to the development of a chronic condition. Whenever an antibiotic is prescribed, it is important to stress that the client take all the medication prescribed. Taking only a portion of the medication may not be sufficient to destroy the infectious microorganism; it can also contribute to the development of resistant strains. Drinking milk, reporting significant information, and monitoring body temperature may be important in some cases. The latter recommendations are based more on such factors as the side effects of the drug, the condition for which the drug is prescribed, and the client's physical condition.

> *Client Needs Category—Physiological integrity*
> *Client Needs Subcategory—Pharmacological therapies*

67. **2.** The prostate surrounds the urethra and can induce discomfort and difficulty passing urine due to a stricture. A sitz bath soothes the area, relieving pain and possible inflammation. It is more effective if it lasts approximately 20 minutes. The water should be about 110° F (37.8° C), which is considered warm, not tepid. Soap is omitted with a sitz bath; the bath's purpose is to apply heat and relieve discomfort, not clean the area. Massaging the scrotum has no direct benefit in relieving the client's symptoms.

> *Client Needs Category—Physiological integrity*
> *Client Needs Subcategory—Physiological adaptation*

68. **2.** Only a small portion of urine voided in midstream (after the first release of urine is wasted) is collected in a clean-catch specimen. The procedure does require cleaning the penis, retracting the foreskin if the client is uncircumcised, and depositing the urine directly into a sterile container.

> *Client Needs Category—Safe, effective care environment*
> *Client Needs Subcategory—Safety and infection control*

69. **1.** Elevating and supporting the scrotum helps to relieve the discomfort of epididymitis. Analgesics are also prescribed. Wearing larger underwear or cotton briefs is a personal choice and does not inherently relieve the client's symptoms. Heat is contraindicated because it can damage sperm.

> *Client Needs Category—Physiological integrity*
> *Client Needs Subcategory—Physiological adaptation*

70. **3.** The mumps virus can infect the testes of males who have not been adequately immunized before puberty. A sexually transmitted disease would be likely if the client's testes and epididymis are co-infected, but that is not the case in this situation. Although many conditions have been documented among military veterans, orchitis is not commonly reported.

> *Client Needs Category—Physiological integrity*
> *Client Needs Subcategory—Physiological adaptation*

71. **2.** When performing a testicular self-examination, the client should examine each testicle separately, rolling it between the thumb and fingers. It is easier to palpate the testes when the scrotum is warm, such as during or after a shower. Testicular self-examination should be performed monthly.

> *Client Needs Category—Health promotion and maintenance*
> *Client Needs Subcategory—None*

Nursing Care of Clients with Structural Disorders of the Male Reproductive System

72. **1.** As long as one testicle is descended, the testicle most likely produces sufficient testosterone for normal secondary sexual characteristics, adequate sperm for conception, and a healthy sex drive. Impotence, the inability to achieve an erection, is not generally compromised.

> *Client Needs Category—Physiological integrity*
> *Client Needs Subcategory—Physiological adaptation*

73. **3.** The priority nursing assessments following a circumcision include checking the amount of local bleeding and the client's ability to void. Swelling can obstruct the urethra and interfere with the urine release. Deep breathing and bowel patterns are routine assessments for surgical clients who have received general anesthesia. It would be inappropriate to assess the client's erectile function at this time.

> ***Client Needs Category***—*Physiological integrity*
> ***Client Needs Subcategory***—*Physiological adaptation*

74. 2. Whenever a cold or warm device is placed on a client's body, the device is placed within some type of fabric cover. A plastic bag is not an appropriate cover. A hypothermia blanket is too large for the local effect desired. An ice-filled ring would not cover the area sufficiently to produce a local effect.

> ***Client Needs Category***—*Safe, effective care environment*
> ***Client Needs Subcategory***—*Safety and infection control*

Nursing Care of Clients with Benign and Malignant Disorders of the Male Reproductive System

75. 2. The best position for assessing the characteristics of the prostate gland is one in which the client leans forward from the waist while standing, bracing his body against the examination table for support. The rectum can be examined with the client in the lithotomy and dorsal recumbent positions, but these are not the preferred positions. A Fowler's position does not facilitate a rectal examination.

> ***Client Needs Category***—*Physiological integrity*
> ***Client Needs Subcategory***—*Physiological adaptation*

76. 3. In the early stages of BPH, the progression of prostatic enlargement is monitored with periodic digital rectal examinations. A PSA test is typically done on a yearly basis; the frequency of testing does not usually increase unless the digital rectal examination indicates a need. As the disease progresses, the physician may use cystoscopy to expose the extent of the infringement on the urethra and the effects on the bladder. A retrograde pyelogram is a diagnostic test commonly used to provide information about the possible damage to the upper urinary tract due to urine retention.

> ***Client Needs Category***—*Health promotion and maintenance*
> ***Client Needs Subcategory***—*None*

77. 2. After draining 1,000 mL of urine, the client should feel relief. Withdrawing any more than 1,000 mL in a short amount of time can contribute to rupture of mucosal blood vessels. More urine is drained after waiting a period of time. The physician may override this rule of thumb in special circumstances.

> ***Client Needs Category***—*Physiological integrity*
> ***Client Needs Subcategory***—*Reduction of risk potential*

78. 4. When a prostate sonogram is performed, a rectal probe is inserted. The presence of stool can interfere with imaging the prostate as well as contribute to discomfort. Therefore, it is important to empty the rectum completely. The client may wish to empty his bladder as well, but that is not necessary with this test. The test does not require fasting. Water may be instilled within the sheath surrounding the rectal probe; the client is not required to consume a large volume of water.

> ***Client Needs Category***—*Physiological integrity*
> ***Client Needs Subcategory***—*Physiological adaptation*

79. 3. Dark red urine is expected after a TURP due to bleeding that occurred during the procedure and in the immediate postoperative period. The color becomes lighter and clearer during or after bladder irrigations and as the postoperative time progresses.

> ***Client Needs Category***—*Physiological integrity*
> ***Client Needs Subcategory***—*Physiological adaptation*

80. 4. The irrigation solution is a part of the volume that collects in the drainage bag. Therefore, to find the true urine output, the amount of instilled irrigant is subtracted from the volume in the drainage bag.

> ***Client Needs Category***—*Physiological integrity*
> ***Client Needs Subcategory***—*Physiological adaptation*

81. 4. In the absence of fluid precautions, increasing the oral fluid intake helps to dilute the urine and reduce the potential for obstruction. Milking the tubing helps to dislodge clots, but it is not as effective as keeping the urine dilute. It is inappropriate to deflate the balloon. Emptying the drainage container does not maintain catheter patency.

> ***Client Needs Category***—*Physiological integrity*
> ***Client Needs Subcategory***—*Physiological adaptation*

82. 1. Obstructions in the drainage catheter are the chief cause of bladder discomfort following TURP. Therefore, the nurse should check for patency of the drainage catheter. A belladonna and opium suppository may be helpful, but this option is not the first course of action. Sitting can increase intra-abdominal pressure and contribute to more bleeding. Ambulating may or may not improve drainage through the catheter, but it is not the first choice of actions.

Client Needs Category—Physiological integrity
Client Needs Subcategory—Reduction of risk potential

83. 2. The tendency to dribble urine is reduced or prevented by alternately stopping the flow of urine and resuming urination during voiding. Caffeine is a bladder irritant, but eliminating it is not the best measure for promoting urinary control. Standing is the most natural position for men when voiding. Sitting does not promote urinary control.
Client Needs Category—Health promotion and maintenance
Client Needs Subcategory—None

84. 3. In the immediate postoperative period, all urinary drainage catheters, including the cystostomy tube, are unclamped to facilitate drainage. The suprapubic cystostomy tube is clamped later when bladder retraining is begun. A cystostomy catheter is too short to attach to the thigh or a leg bag.
Client Needs Category—Physiological integrity
Client Needs Subcategory—Physiological adaptation

85. 4. The temperature should be taken by any route other than rectal for the first postoperative week following prostatic surgery. Inserting a rectal thermometer can result in perforation of the rectal mucosa and damage to the prostatic capsule that was left behind when the prostate was removed. All the other instructions are correct, but they are not the most important instruction to give the nursing assistant.
Client Needs Category—Safe, effective care environment
Client Needs Subcategory—Coordinated care

86. 3. One functioning testis ought to produce enough testosterone to sustain all a man's secondary sex characteristics and his libido. However, after this surgery, the sperm count is reduced and their mobility is impaired.
Client Needs Category—Physiological integrity
Client Needs Subcategory—Physiological adaptation

Nursing Care of Clients with Sexually Transmitted Diseases

87. 2. Conveying a nonjudgmental attitude facilitates obtaining truthful information from the person who feels uncomfortable discussing sexual information. Being sympathetic, encouraging, and optimistic are all positive attributes, but none of these is as important as being nonjudgmental.

Client Needs Category—Psychosocial integrity
Client Needs Subcategory—None

88. 2. Asking a person if any sexual partner has similar symptoms helps to determine if the cause is due to a sexually transmitted disease. A painless sore is more likely a symptom of syphilis, which does not commonly cause the symptoms this client has described. The age at which a person first had sexual intercourse is unrelated to the present symptoms. Incubation periods vary among sexually transmitted diseases; identifying the most recent date of sexual intercourse will not provide significant information.
Client Needs Category—Physiological integrity
Client Needs Subcategory—Reduction of risk potential

89. 4. Because body secretions potentially contain microorganisms that can be transmitted to caregivers, it is important to wear gloves as a barrier against direct contact with infectious material. The use of an antiseptic swab or lubricant interferes with obtaining an adequate specimen. Wearing a mask is not as important as wearing gloves because the urethral secretions are unlikely to splash or spray such areas as the nose or mouth. Sexually transmitted diseases are spread by direct contact rather than droplet or air transmission.
Client Needs Category—Safe, effective care environment
Client Needs Subcategory—Safety and infection control

90. 3. Intimate sexual contact with one or more sexual partners is the highest risk factor among the options listed for acquiring a sexually transmitted disease. Developing sexually at an early age does not necessarily affect a person's sexual choices. Internet access for children and adolescents can be informative if the site is reputable. Sex education is important and too little accurate information does predispose individuals to making poor sexual choices. However, it is not as great a risk factor as having multiple sexual partners.
Client Needs Category—Health promotion and maintenance
Client Needs Subcategory—None

91. 4. The most likely substance to be cultured if a client has gonorrhea is urethral drainage. However, the organism might also be cultured from swabs taken from other areas, including the rectum, pharynx, and vagina (in women). The organism causing gonorrhea is not generally found in blood or urine. It is found in semen; however, collection is complicated because producing the specimen requires masturbation and ejaculation.
Client Needs Category—Physiological integrity
Client Needs Subcategory—Reduction of risk potential

92. **1.** Gloves are worn as a standard precaution when collecting body substances from any client regardless of the tentative diagnosis. The hands should also be washed after glove removal. Using a disinfectant is not appropriate for any specimen collection. As long as gloves are worn, the nurse can touch the client. Cultures for the gonorrhea organism are inoculated onto a culture medium as soon as possible; therefore, refrigeration is undesirable.

> *Client Needs Category—Safe, effective care environment*
> *Client Needs Subcategory—Safety and infection control*

93. **1.** Women infected with the herpes simplex type 2 virus are at greater risk for developing cervical cancer. Therefore, frequent Pap smears are necessary. Men infected with the virus are at greater risk for developing prostatic cancer. Clients may have vaginal intercourse, but a condom should be used and all sexual partners should be informed of the potential for infection. Drugs may decrease the frequency of outbreaks and reduce the length of time when symptoms are manifested. However, taking medication does not provide protection for others. Spontaneous abortions increase among infected pregnant women. Infants can acquire the herpes virus at the time of vaginal delivery.

> *Client Needs Category—Health promotion and maintenance*
> *Client Needs Subcategory—None*

94. **1.** Tertiary syphilis is the final stage in the natural course of the disease. In this stage, syphilis presents as a slow, progressive inflammatory disease. One of the manifestations of tertiary syphilis is sharp, stabbing leg pains. The client may also have other organ system damage involving the heart, brain, liver, bones, and eyes. A painless ulcer is a characteristic of primary-stage syphilis. The secondary stage of syphilis is accompanied by a red rash and patchy hair loss.

> *Client Needs Category—Physiological integrity*
> *Client Needs Subcategory—Physiological adaptation*

95. **4.** There is no lifelong immunity to syphilis. Each new incident is treated with antibiotic therapy. Antibiotic therapy destroys the microorganism and prevents further consequences from the disease. Sexual partners are tested and treated if they are infected. Syphilitic lesions can appear on the penis, outside and inside the vagina, around the mouth, and even on the nipple.

> *Client Needs Category—Physiological integrity*
> *Client Needs Subcategory—Reduction of risk potential*

96. **3.** To ensure adequate treatment, the client with a sexually transmitted disease is told to continue taking the prescribed medication for the full amount of time. Symptoms may clear in a short time after initial treatment, but the organisms might not be totally destroyed. The infection may persist without adequate treatment. The need for a refill is at the discretion of the health care professional. Long-term or repeated use of an antibiotic can cause an organism to develop resistance. Aggressive and appropriate short-term treatment is adequate for the present infection. Further treatment is not required unless reinfection occurs.

> *Client Needs Category—Physiological integrity*
> *Client Needs Subcategory—Physiological adaptation*

97. **3.** Although all of the measures listed are important health practices for preventing infections, the most important method for preventing the recurrence of a sexually transmitted disease is to eliminate the infection in other sex partners. Unless this occurs, the pathogenic organism can be transmitted again.

> *Client Needs Category—Health promotion and maintenance*
> *Client Needs Subcategory—None*

98. **1.** To avoid a continuous cycle of reinfection, the client's sexual partners must be simultaneously treated with the same drug therapy. Appropriate treatment can cure this sexually transmitted disease, but it will not prevent reinfection. Chlamydial infections are extremely common. A large proportion of both men and women are asymptomatic and go undiagnosed until a complication of the infection is manifested.

> *Client Needs Category—Physiological integrity*
> *Client Needs Subcategory—Reduction of risk potential*

99. **2.** Vaginal pruritus (itching) is a common problem experienced by women infected with *Trichomonas vaginalis*. Other clinical manifestations include yellow-brown malodorous vaginal discharge and thin vaginal secretions. Fluid-filled vesicles are associated with herpetic lesions. Vaginal drainage that seems to contain flecks of milk is characteristic of candidiasis (moniliasis). Women with gonorrhea or chlamydial infections commonly experience abdominal discomfort among other symptoms.

> *Client Needs Category—Physiological integrity*
> *Client Needs Subcategory—Physiological adaptation*

100. **4.** Consuming alcohol while taking metronidazole (Flagyl) can cause disorientation, headache, cramps, vomiting, and convulsions. There are no known food-drug interactions with this drug and iodized salt, aspartame, or MSG.

Client Needs Category—Physiological integrity
Client Needs Subcategory—Pharmacological therapies

101. **2.** There is a relationship between genital warts and an increased risk of cancer of the vulva, vagina, and cervix. Genital warts are treated with topical applications of chemicals or surgical removal. If sexual partners are not treated, the virus can be retransmitted. The use of a condom is recommended until the warts disappear.

Client Needs Category—Health promotion and maintenance
Client Needs Subcategory—None

102. **3.** Nonoxynol-9 has been shown to inhibit HIV and reduce the potential for infection. Removing the condom immediately, washing with a dilute solution of vinegar, and using vaginal lubricant are not recommended techniques for preventing an HIV infection.

Client Needs Category—Safe, effective care environment
Client Needs Subcategory—Safety and infection control

103. **4.** Viral load tests are considered to be the best marker of disease progression in AIDS, even surpassing T4 cell counts. Blood counts reveal if the cell counts are increasing, decreasing, or staying the same, but they are not as effective as the newer viral load tests. Assessing for changes in vital signs can help signal complications such as infection; however, this is not the best method for monitoring drug effectiveness. Viruses can only be cultured in living tissue. Consequently, this approach is not used except in research.

Client Needs Category—Physiological integrity
Client Needs Subcategory—Pharmacological therapies

Nursing Care of Clients Practicing Family Planning

104. **1.** Oral contraceptives should be taken at approximately the same time each day, preferably in the evening. They do not need to be taken on an empty stomach. An oral contraceptive is started on the fifth day of menstruation and, depending on the type used, is taken for 20 or 21 days.

Client Needs Category—Health promotion and maintenance
Client Needs Subcategory—None

105. **1.** Smoking increases the risk of developing blood clots in women who take hormonal contraceptives. Maintaining a high fluid volume and elevating the legs are ways of preventing venous stasis, but they are not directly related to the cause-and-effect nature of this question. There are claims that garlic and onions have an anticoagulant effect, but these claims have not been thoroughly documented in scientific research.

Client Needs Category—Health promotion and maintenance
Client Needs Subcategory—None

106. **3.** Menstruation continues because the ovarian hormones are circulated in the blood, not through the fallopian tubes. A tubal ligation performed through the abdomen leaves only a small incisional scar. Hospitalization is brief. Although tubal ligations have been reversed, they are still considered a permanent form of contraception.

Client Needs Category—Health promotion and maintenance
Client Needs Subcategory—None

107. **2.** After an intrauterine device is inserted, many women experience menstrual cramps, an increase in blood loss, and longer duration of menstrual periods. Breast tenderness, weight gain, and acne are more common with hormonal methods of birth control.

Client Needs Category—Health promotion and maintenance
Client Needs Subcategory—None

108. **3.** Having a vasectomy does not ensure sterility immediately. A sperm count is done at 6 weeks, 6 months, and yearly thereafter. When the sperm count is zero for 6 weeks, the chances for conception are almost impossible.

Client Needs Category—Health promotion and maintenance
Client Needs Subcategory—None

109. **3.** Leaving a space between the tip of the condom and the penis allows an area where the ejaculate can be contained. Condoms are designed for one use only. A new condom is applied with each new erection. To prevent semen leakage, the condom is grasped as the erect penis is withdrawn from the vagina. Condoms are applied as the penis becomes erect.

Client Needs Category—Health promotion and maintenance
Client Needs Subcategory—None

110. **1, 2, 4.** Before administering medroxyprogesterone (Depo-Provera), the physician should validate that the client is not currently pregnant. Medroxyprogesterone (Depo-Provera) is administered deeply into the gluteal or deltoid muscle within the first 7 days of the menstrual cycle and thereafter every 3 months. The injection is effective within 24 hours. Since ovulation is unlikely during days 1 through 7 of the menstrual cycle, any additional contraception is unnecessary. There is no reason to apply ice to the injection site before administration.

> *Client Needs Category—Physiological integrity*
> *Client Needs Subcategory—Pharmacological therapies*

111. **1, 2, 4.** Before advising the client about methods of birth control, the nurse needs to gather more information. Knowing about the client's lifestyle is important because it can provide clues about the need to exclude certain types of birth control. For example, birth control pills may be inadvisable if the client does not like to take pills or cannot remember to take medicine. Also, smoking is contraindicated with some forms of birth control. The nurse needs to ascertain whether the client is currently sexually active and whether she is practicing safe sex. Both answers can provide additional teaching opportunities regarding the avoidance of pregnancy and sexually transmitted diseases. The nurse also needs to explore when the client had her last menstrual period because this will help determine whether or not she is currently pregnant. Information about the client's last Pap smear and workplace is irrelevant to helping her choose an appropriate birth control method.

> *Client Needs Category—Health promotion and maintenance*
> *Client Needs Subcategory—None*

112. **1, 2, 3, 4, 5.** Safe sex practices include being selective in choosing sexual partners. Sex with a partner who has had numerous casual encounters with bisexual or same-sex partners or with someone who is an I.V. drug user increases the chance of acquiring a sexually transmitted disease. Sharing vibrators or other sexual equipment can lead to the transfer of diseases and should be avoided. Avoiding intercourse if either partner has signs of a sexually transmitted disease is safe practice in preventing the spread of disease. Sexual partners must always be notified when a sexually transmitted disease has been diagnosed. Urinating after intercourse can help prevent urinary tract infections; it also washes away contaminates on the labia. Storing condoms away from excessive heat helps prevent deterioration of the latex. Storing birth control patches in the refrigerator is inappropriate; they should be kept at room temperature.

> *Client Needs Category—Health promotion and maintenance*
> *Client Needs Subcategory—None*

113. **1.** Combination oral contraceptives contain estrogen and progesterone. The estrogen is thought to prevent follicle maturation and thus prevent ovulation. The progesterone is thought to inhibit thickening of the uterine lining. The other two options do not reflect correct functions of the combination oral contraceptive.

> *Client Needs Category—Health promotion and maintenance*
> *Client Needs Subcategory—None*

114. **2.** The 28-pill package has 7 placebo pills that allow the woman to maintain a routine of taking the pills daily. This reduces the possibility of the client forgetting to take a pill. The menstrual cycle's length has nothing to do with the number of pills dispensed in the package. Monophasic, biphasic, and triphasic are categories of combination pills that refer to how the estrogen and progesterone are released over the course of the menstrual cycle. All combination oral contraceptives have estrogen and progesterone in each pill.

> *Client Needs Category—Health promotion and maintenance*
> *Client Needs Subcategory—None*

115. **2.** Oral contraceptives are sometimes prescribed for women who have primary dysmenorrhea because the oral contraceptive is thought to create a better hormonal balance and may help decrease the client's discomfort related to menstrual cramping. All of the other statements are accurate regarding oral contraceptives.

> *Client Needs Category—Health promotion and maintenance*
> *Client Needs Subcategory—None*

116. **1, 2, 3, 4, 5.** Hormonal contraceptives such as the patch are used to prevent pregnancy. The patch transfers hormones through the skin and must stick securely in order to work properly. The patch is applied once a week for 3 weeks to the abdomen, buttocks, upper outer arm, or upper torso, but not on the breasts. Major side effects include skin irritation or rash at the site of application, irregular vaginal bleeding or spotting (which is temporary), fluid retention that causes edema of the fingers and ankles, a rise in blood pressure (due to fluid retention), and nausea and vomiting. Hepatitis is not a common side effect of the patch. Women with a history of hepatitis, smoking, breast cancer, or liver, gall bladder, kidney or heart disease should refrain from using the patch.

> *Client Needs Category—Health promotion and maintenance*
> *Client Needs Subcategory—None*

117. **4.** The female condom is made of polyurethane, not latex; thus, the client who has an allergy to latex can use a female condom without experiencing an allergic reaction. All other statements include accurate information about barrier forms of contraception.

> *Client Needs Category—Health promotion and maintenance*
> *Client Needs Subcategory—None*

118. 3. The client who wishes to use the basal body temperature method of natural family planning should take her temperature every morning before rising for 6 months with a special thermometer. Recording the pattern of the menstrual cycle for 6 to 8 months is used for the rhythm or calendar method of natural family planning. Monitoring the consistency of vaginal secretions is used with the Billings or ovulation method of natural family planning. Having the male sex partner withdraw his penis from the vagina before ejaculation is called coitus interruptus and is not an effective birth control method because semen contains sperm.

Client Needs Category—*Health promotion and maintenance*
Client Needs Subcategory—*None*

UNIT II

The Nursing Care of the Childbearing Family

The Nursing Care of Clients During the Antepartum Period

⇨ **Anatomy and Physiology of the Male and Female Reproductive Systems**
⇨ **Signs and Symptoms of Pregnancy**
⇨ **Assessing the Pregnant Client**
⇨ **Nutritional Needs During Pregnancy**
⇨ **Teaching the Pregnant Client**
⇨ **Common Discomforts of Pregnancy**
⇨ **High-Risk Factors and Pregnancy**
⇨ **Complications of Pregnancy**
⇨ **Elective Abortion**
⇨ **Correct Answers and Rationales**

Directions: With a pencil, blacken the space in front of the option you have chosen for your correct answer.

Anatomy and Physiology of the Male and Female Reproductive Systems

A 30-year-old woman and her husband attend an infertility clinic. They have no children and have had several appointments with the physician regarding their infertility problems. After receiving information about reproduction, the client asks the nurse where fertilization takes place.

1. The nurse correctly explains that fertilization usually takes place in which structure?
[ ] **1.** Outer third of the fallopian tube
[ ] **2.** Ovary
[ ] **3.** Fundus of the uterus
[ ] **4.** Vagina

2. When the client asks the nurse about the viability of the ovum after she ovulates, the nurse correctly explains that, after ovulation, the ovum remains alive for how many hours?
[ ] **1.** 2 hours
[ ] **2.** 24 hours
[ ] **3.** 48 hours
[ ] **4.** 72 hours

3. To improve sperm production, the nurse should instruct the client's husband to avoid which activity?
[ ] **1.** Swimming in chlorinated water
[ ] **2.** Sitting in hot tubs
[ ] **3.** Wearing boxer shorts
[ ] **4.** Wearing colored underwear

The client tells the nurse that she desperately wants to have a baby but is concerned about a vaginal birth because of her small hips.

4. Which response by the nurse is most appropriate when addressing the client's concerns?
[ ] **1.** "Your hips are measured to make an accurate determination of whether or not the baby can be delivered vaginally."
[ ] **2.** "The size of your true pelvis, not the size of your hips, determines whether or not you can deliver a baby vaginally."
[ ] **3.** "It doesn't really matter whether you deliver vaginally or by cesarean birth because the risk for both types of delivery is the same."
[ ] **4.** "The size of the baby's head is the only factor that determines whether the infant can be delivered vaginally."

After discussing various options regarding the correction of their infertility problems, the client's husband asks the nurse when the sex of the baby is determined.

5. The nurse accurately explains that the sex of a baby is determined at which point?

[ ] **1.** During maturation of the ovum in the ovaries

[ ] **2.** During maturation of the sperm in the epididymis

[ ] **3.** When the fertilized ovum implants in the uterine lining

[ ] **4.** When the sperm fertilizes the ovum in the fallopian tube

During a discussion regarding menstruation, the client asks the nurse, "Where does the blood flow come from when a woman has her monthly period?"

6. The nurse correctly explains that the bleeding is the result of sloughing of which structure?

[ ] **1.** Endometrium

[ ] **2.** Perimetrium

[ ] **3.** Myometrium

[ ] **4.** Epimetrium

Signs and Symptoms of Pregnancy

A 22-year-old woman visits the prenatal clinic for the first time. During the health history assessment, the client reveals to the nurse that she thinks she may be 2 months pregnant.

7. Based on the health history data, how should the nurse record the client's pregnancy status on the prenatal records?

[ ] **1.** Multipara

[ ] **2.** Primipara

[ ] **3.** Primigravida

[ ] **4.** Multigravida

The client informs the nurse that twins "run" in her family. The client asks the nurse why some women have identical twins and others have twins that do not look alike.

8. Which explanation by the nurse correctly describes the occurrence of identical twins?

[ ] **1.** Two separate ova are fertilized by identical sperm.

[ ] **2.** The mother releases two identical ova.

[ ] **3.** One fertilized ovum divides into two identical halves.

[ ] **4.** Two identical ova are fertilized by two identical sperm.

9. If the client reports the following signs and symptoms, which one represents a probable sign of pregnancy?

[ ] **1.** Absence of monthly periods

[ ] **2.** Abdominal enlargement

[ ] **3.** Nausea and vomiting

[ ] **4.** Frequent urination

The physician examines the client and orders a pregnancy test.

10. The nurse correctly sends a requisition and specimen for which laboratory test?

[ ] **1.** Alpha-fetoprotein (AFP)

[ ] **2.** Corticotropin-releasing hormone (CRH)

[ ] **3.** Human chorionic gonadotropin (HCG)

[ ] **4.** Follicle-stimulating hormone (FSH)

The client asks the nurse if an ultrasound could confirm her pregnancy if she is in her second month of pregnancy.

11. Which statement by the nurse regarding an ultrasound is most accurate?

[ ] **1.** "Transvaginal ultrasound is used to diagnose pregnancy as early as 2½ to 3 weeks."

[ ] **2.** "Ultrasounds aren't usually performed during the first trimester because of the risk to the baby."

[ ] **3.** "An X-ray is just as reliable as an ultrasound and poses less of a risk to the baby."

[ ] **4.** "Ultrasounds aren't used until the uterus ascends out of the pelvis into the abdomen."

The physician informs the client that her pregnancy test is positive and tells her that during the pelvic examination she had a positive Chadwick's sign. After the physician leaves, the client asks the nurse to explain the significance of a positive Chadwick's sign?

12. Which response by the nurse about Chadwick's sign is most accurate?

[ ] **1.** "It's the spontaneous occurrence of intermittent painless contractions that begin early in pregnancy and continue throughout the entire period of gestation."

[ ] **2.** "It's a bluish discoloration of the cervix, vagina, and vulva that occurs as a result of the presence of an increased number of blood vessels."

[ ] **3.** "It's a softening of the cervix that occurs because of an increased amount of blood flowing to the reproductive organs."

[ ] **4.** "It's a dark brown line extending from the umbilicus to the symphysis pubis that occurs as a result of hormonal changes."

When reviewing the client's medical record, the nurse notes that the physician documented the presence of ballottement.

13. Based on this finding, the nurse can assume that the client is at least how many months' pregnant?
[ ] **1.** 5 months
[ ] **2.** 6 months
[ ] **3.** 7 months
[ ] **4.** 8 months

The physician also documented that the client had a positive sign of pregnancy.

14. Which assessment finding best represents a positive sign of pregnancy?
[ ] **1.** Palpable fetal outline
[ ] **2.** Blotchy tan facial skin
[ ] **3.** Positive pregnancy test
[ ] **4.** Fetal heartbeat

The client asks the nurse when she should be able to feel the baby move.

15. In the primigravid client, when is fetal movement typically felt for the first time?
[ ] **1.** Between 10 and 14 weeks
[ ] **2.** Between 16 and 20 weeks
[ ] **3.** Between 22 and 26 weeks
[ ] **4.** Between 28 and 32 weeks

Assessing the Pregnant Client

A 32-year-old multigravid client visits the prenatal clinic for the first time during this pregnancy and states to the nurse that she knows she is pregnant and has already felt her baby move.

16. Based on the client's statement, what can the nurse conclude?
[ ] **1.** The client is having twins.
[ ] **2.** The client is between 14 and 18 weeks' gestation.
[ ] **3.** The client is in the first trimester.
[ ] **4.** The client's due date will be difficult to calculate.

During the interview, the client informs the nurse that she has three children—a son and twin daughters. She states that she has not had any abortions or stillbirths.

17. According to the TPAL method, which of the following accurately records the client's obstetric history?
[ ] **1.** T-III, P-0, A-0, L-III.
[ ] **2.** T-III, P-III, A-0, L-0.
[ ] **3.** T-III, P-II, A-0, L-II.
[ ] **4.** T-II, P-0, A-0, L-III.

The client informs the nurse that her last menstrual period began on March 13. She asks when her baby is due.

18. Using Nägele's rule, the nurse can assume the client's expected delivery date to be approximately which date?
[ ] **1.** November 13
[ ] **2.** November 23
[ ] **3.** December 3
[ ] **4.** December 20

The physician asks the nurse to prepare the client for a pelvic examination.

19. The nurse correctly assists the client into which position?
[ ] **1.** Lithotomy
[ ] **2.** Prone
[ ] **3.** Sims'
[ ] **4.** Trendelenburg's

20. Prior to the pelvic examination, which intervention by the nurse is most appropriate?
[ ] **1.** Give the client an enema.
[ ] **2.** Instruct the client to empty her bladder.
[ ] **3.** Shave the client's perineum.
[ ] **4.** Give the client a mild sedative.

21. Which method best promotes client comfort during the pelvic examination?
[ ] **1.** Have the client lift her head off the table.
[ ] **2.** Have the client press her back into the examination table.
[ ] **3.** Have the client tighten her buttocks.
[ ] **4.** Tell the client to let her knees fall outward.

The physician determines that the client is in her 15th week of pregnancy. The client asks if it is too early to hear the baby's heartbeat.

22. How early in a pregnancy can the fetal heartbeat be heard using a Doppler device?
[ ] **1.** 4 to 6 weeks
[ ] **2.** 8 to 10 weeks
[ ] **3.** 12 to 14 weeks
[ ] **4.** 16 to 18 weeks

23. Which action by the nurse best ensures that an accurate fetal heart rate is obtained?
[ ] **1.** Assess the fetal heart rate when the client is lying on her right side.
[ ] **2.** Assess the fetal heart rate when the client reports fetal movement.
[ ] **3.** Assess the fetal heart rate between Braxton Hicks contractions.
[ ] **4.** Assess the maternal pulse and fetal heart rate, and compare the two.

24. Which fetal heart rate must the nurse report immediately to the physician?
[ ] **1.** 100 beats/minute
[ ] **2.** 120 beats/minute
[ ] **3.** 140 beats/minute
[ ] **4.** 160 beats/minute

The client tells the nurse that her cousin's baby was born with spina bifida. She asks if it is possible to detect the presence of this condition during her pregnancy.

25. Which response by the nurse is most accurate?
[ ] **1.** FTA-ABS test can detect this type of defect.
[ ] **2.** HBsAg test can detect this type of defect.
[ ] **3.** MSAFP test can detect this type of defect.
[ ] **4.** VDRL test can detect this type of defect.

Prior to leaving the clinic, the client asks the nurse about the schedule for her next few perinatal visits.

26. The nurse responds that, for clients with uncomplicated pregnancies, it is usually best to plan monthly visits for the first 28 weeks and then more frequent visits following which schedule?
[ ] **1.** Weekly for the remainder of the pregnancy
[ ] **2.** Every 2 weeks for the remainder of the pregnancy
[ ] **3.** Every 2 weeks up to 36 weeks, then weekly for the last month
[ ] **4.** Weekly up to 36 weeks, then twice weekly for the last month

The client also asks the nurse whether she can continue to exercise routinely throughout the pregnancy.

27. Which nursing instructions concerning exercise during pregnancy are accurate? Select all that apply.
[ ] **1.** Avoid exercising during hot, humid weather.
[ ] **2.** Avoid any jerking, bouncing, or jumping movements.
[ ] **3.** Drink plenty of fluids before and after exercising.
[ ] **4.** Limit strenuous activity to no more than 60 minutes a session.
[ ] **5.** Perform exercises only in the supine position.
[ ] **6.** Limit exercising to once per week.

The client returns for follow-up visits on a regular basis, following the prearranged schedule. According to the client's most recent examination, she is estimated to be at 20 weeks' gestation.

28. Where can the nurse expect to palpate the fundus at this time?
[ ] **1.** Just above the symphysis pubis
[ ] **2.** Just below the xiphoid process
[ ] **3.** Near the level of the umbilicus
[ ] **4.** Just below the symphysis pubis

29. At 24 weeks' gestation, the nurse prepares the client for which routine test?
[ ] **1.** Coombs' test
[ ] **2.** Glucose tolerance test
[ ] **3.** Papanicolaou (Pap) smear
[ ] **4.** Rubella titer

The client has progressed to her last month of pregnancy. The physician orders a nonstress test.

30. When planning for this test, the nurse should have which of the following available?
[ ] **1.** I.V. magnesium sulfate
[ ] **2.** A cardiac monitor
[ ] **3.** I.V. oxytocin (Pitocin)
[ ] **4.** A fetal monitor

A physician recommends amniocentesis to a pregnant woman whose first child has Down syndrome.

31. The nurse advises the client that this test is typically performed at which time during the pregnancy?
[ ] **1.** Just after the pregnancy has been confirmed
[ ] **2.** Early in the second trimester
[ ] **3.** Prior to delivery
[ ] **4.** Just after the client feels the first fetal movements

Nutritional Needs During Pregnancy

During a routine prenatal visit, the physician determines that a client in her fourth month of pregnancy is not eating an appropriate diet and asks her if she has been taking her prenatal vitamins, folic acid, and iron supplements that had previously been prescribed. The physician asks the nurse to instruct the client about nutritional needs during pregnancy.

32. Prior to teaching the client about the nutritional needs during pregnancy, what should the nurse do?
[ ] **1.** Determine if the client needs to gain or lose weight.
[ ] **2.** Assess the client's current eating pattern and preferences.
[ ] **3.** Determine if the client knows how to accurately count calories.
[ ] **4.** Develop a sample menu that includes the required nutrients.

While discussing her prepregnancy eating habits with the nurse, the client asks, "What's the normal weight gain during pregnancy?"

33. Which explanation by the nurse accurately identifies the recommended weight gain for a woman who has a normal prepregnancy weight?
[ ] **1.** Less than 15 lb (6.8 kg)
[ ] **2.** 15 to 20 lb (6.8 to 9 kg)
[ ] **3.** 25 to 35 lb (11 to 15.8 kg)
[ ] **4.** No more than 40 lb (18 kg)

After interviewing the client, the nurse determines that the client is not getting an adequate intake of calcium.

34. The nurse correctly instructs the client to drink how many glasses of milk per day to meet her calcium requirements?
[ ] **1.** 1 to 2
[ ] **2.** 3 to 4
[ ] **3.** 5 to 6
[ ] **4.** 7 to 8

The client tells the nurse that it is hard for her to get the calcium she needs because she does not like milk.

35. Which food provides the best alternative source of calcium?
[ ] **1.** Organ meats
[ ] **2.** White bread
[ ] **3.** Leafy green vegetables
[ ] **4.** Dark turkey meat

The nurse asks the client if she is taking her daily iron supplement. The client states that she has not been taking the iron routinely because she experiences constipation.

36. When providing information about iron supplements, which instruction by the nurse is most appropriate?
[ ] **1.** "Take the supplement with meals."
[ ] **2.** "Be aware that iron can cause abdominal pain."
[ ] **3.** "Make sure you drink plenty of fluids."
[ ] **4.** "You can substitute dietary sources of iron for this medication."

37. The nurse should also include which information about the side effects of iron supplements during her instruction?
[ ] **1.** "You may notice that your stools will be black."
[ ] **2.** "Your teeth will become stained."
[ ] **3.** "Vomiting is likely to occur."
[ ] **4.** "You may have diarrhea several times per day."

During the visit, the nurse also asks the client if she has been taking her prescribed folic acid.

38. When the client asks why folic acid is important, which response by the nurse is most accurate?
[ ] **1.** "Folic acid helps prevent your baby from developing neural tube defects such as spina bifida."
[ ] **2.** "Folic acid helps build strong bones for your baby."
[ ] **3.** "Folic acid helps your baby become resistant to infections."
[ ] **4.** "Folic acid prevents your baby from becoming anemic."

A 17-year-old primigravid client is seen at the health clinic for the first time. The nurse assesses the teenager's nutritional status and provides nutritional guidance.

39. Which dietary adjustment is most appropriate for a pregnant teenager?
[ ] **1.** Increase caloric intake to 2,500 calories/day.
[ ] **2.** Drink presweetened lemonade instead of carbonated beverages.
[ ] **3.** Eat foods that are low in carbohydrates and fats.
[ ] **4.** Choose soft foods that are easy to digest.

After interviewing the client, the nurse determines that the client lives with her boyfriend and works several hours per week. She frequently skips meals or eats at fast-food restaurants. The client drinks beer or wine when she is with her friends. She is constantly concerned about her appearance and weight gain.

40. How many factors in this scenario place the client at risk for nutritional deficiencies and the need for dietary guidance and counseling?
[ ] **1.** Three
[ ] **2.** Four
[ ] **3.** Five
[ ] **4.** Six

During a subsequent visit, the nurse notes that the client is eating a bag of potato chips and drinking a diet cola. The nurse revises the client's care plan accordingly.

41. Which expected outcome should the nurse include based on the client's eating habits?
[ ] **1.** The client will eat three balanced meals and two snacks daily while pregnant.
[ ] **2.** The client will gain a total of 12 pounds during the pregnancy.
[ ] **3.** The client will take two prenatal vitamins daily.
[ ] **4.** The client will report that she eats about 2,000 calories per day.

During the visit, the client expresses concern about her increased weight gain over the past month. She explains to the nurse that her boyfriend thinks she is getting fat.

42. Which response by the nurse is most appropriate?
[ ] **1.** "A weight gain of about 10 pounds is recommended during pregnancy."
[ ] **2.** "Your weight gain depends on the amount of food that you eat."
[ ] **3.** "It's normal for adolescent girls to be worried about weight gain."
[ ] **4.** "The average weight gain during pregnancy is between 25 and 35 pounds."

The nurse helps the client to compile lists of healthy and unhealthy foods as a guide for the remainder of her pregnancy.

43. Which of the following beverages should be included in the list of unhealthy drinks to avoid? Select all that apply.
[ ] **1.** Alcohol
[ ] **2.** Coffee
[ ] **3.** Tea
[ ] **4.** Cola beverages
[ ] **5.** Sports drinks
[ ] **6.** Orange juice

At a subsequent prenatal visit, the client complains of edema in her lower extremities.

44. After gathering further information about the client's complaint, the nurse advises her to limit her intake of which substance?
[ ] **1.** Sodium
[ ] **2.** Potassium
[ ] **3.** Vitamin C
[ ] **4.** Magnesium

A nurse conducts a nutrition class for newly pregnant women at a local public health department. During the class, the nurse collects information about each woman's nutritional status and assesses the group for nutritional risk factors during pregnancy.

45. Which of the following clients are at risk for nutritional problems during pregnancy? Select all that apply.
[ ] **1.** A 17-year-old primigravid client
[ ] **2.** A 25-year-old woman who weighs 250 lb at conception
[ ] **3.** A 19-year-old woman who admits that she smokes cigarettes and drinks alcohol
[ ] **4.** A 30-year-old woman who is unemployed and uses food stamps
[ ] **5.** A 25-year-old woman whose prepregnancy hemoglobin level is 13 g/100 mL
[ ] **6.** A 30-year-old woman who drinks four glasses of milk per day

Teaching the Pregnant Client

A 26-year-old primigravid client visits her obstetrician for her first prenatal visit. The physician confirms that she is in the ninth week of her pregnancy. The nurse and client discuss general health needs during pregnancy.

46. Which client statement regarding bathing indicates a need for additional teaching?
[ ] **1.** "I should avoid taking tub baths if my membranes rupture."
[ ] **2.** "I should avoid taking tub baths at any time during my pregnancy."
[ ] **3.** "I shouldn't sit in a hot tub because the heat could affect my baby."
[ ] **4.** "I should use safety mats and handrails so that I don't fall while getting into the tub."

The client asks the nurse if she can have sexual intercourse during pregnancy.

47. The nurse correctly explains that sexual intercourse should be avoided at what time?
[ ] **1.** Throughout pregnancy
[ ] **2.** Until the baby is fully developed
[ ] **3.** Once the abdomen starts to enlarge
[ ] **4.** Once the membranes rupture

The client informs the nurse that she and her husband plan to take a vacation next month before she gets too "big." The client asks if there are any special instructions regarding traveling.

48. Which response by the nurse regarding travel is most appropriate?
[ ] **1.** "Carry a copy of your medical record with you when traveling."
[ ] **2.** "Refrain from traveling until after the baby is born."
[ ] **3.** "Plan to travel no farther than 100 miles from home."
[ ] **4.** "Avoid using a seatbelt for extended periods of time."

The client informs the nurse that she had some spotting during the first week of her pregnancy. She asks if she should report this fact to the physician.

49. The nurse correctly explains that the spotting the client experienced is probably normal and the result of what occurrence?
[ ] **1.** The baby implanting in the lining of the uterus
[ ] **2.** Increased blood circulation to the vaginal area
[ ] **3.** Hormonal changes that occur during pregnancy
[ ] **4.** The cervical opening enlarging and thinning out

At nine weeks' gestation, the client asks the nurse, "What does my baby look like now?"

50. The nurse explains that between 8 and 12 weeks' gestation, the baby has what characteristics?
[ ]   **1.** The zygote looks like a bumpy ball.
[ ]   **2.** The embryo has a well-defined head.
[ ]   **3.** The embryo's sex is distinguishable.
[ ]   **4.** The fetus has fully developed arms and legs.

In a discussion regarding body changes, the nurse informs the client that as the fetus grows, the amount of amniotic fluid increases. The client asks the nurse to explain the purpose of the amniotic fluid.

51. Which response given by the nurse is most appropriate regarding the purpose of amniotic fluid?
[ ]   **1.** It provides the fetus with antibodies from the mother.
[ ]   **2.** It helps protect the fetus from external injury.
[ ]   **3.** It provides oxygen for the fetus.
[ ]   **4.** It helps lower the mother's body temperature.

52. In a discussion about hormonal changes, the nurse informs the client that the placenta produces which hormone?
[ ]   **1.** Estrogen
[ ]   **2.** Testosterone
[ ]   **3.** Oxytocin
[ ]   **4.** Follicle-stimulating hormone

Common Discomforts of Pregnancy

The nurse conducts a prenatal class on common discomforts of pregnancy. One woman attending the class asks the nurse how to relieve constipation.

53. Which response by the nurse is most appropriate?
[ ]   **1.** "Resting helps to relieve constipation."
[ ]   **2.** "Exercising can help relieve constipation."
[ ]   **3.** "A low-fat diet helps to relieve constipation."
[ ]   **4.** "Prenatal vitamins help to relieve constipation."

Several women attending the prenatal class ask the nurse to discuss the causes of varicose veins and how to relieve the discomfort associated with them.

54. The nurse explains that, in addition to increased blood volume, which condition causes varicose veins during pregnancy?
[ ]   **1.** Impaired venous return
[ ]   **2.** Decreased cardiac output
[ ]   **3.** Changes in the body's center of gravity
[ ]   **4.** Impaired kidney function

55. The nurse correctly explains to the group that the discomfort associated with varicose veins is relieved by which activity?
[ ]   **1.** Resting with the feet in a dependent position
[ ]   **2.** Sitting when possible
[ ]   **3.** Putting on calf-length, elastic-top hose
[ ]   **4.** Moving around when standing in one position

56. When teaching the class about varicose veins, which symptom should the clients be instructed to report immediately?
[ ]   **1.** The appearance of additional varicose veins
[ ]   **2.** Varicose veins that are purple in color
[ ]   **3.** Legs that begin to ache and feel heavy
[ ]   **4.** Calves that become red, tender, and warm

One of the participants in the prenatal class tells the nurse, "My skin itches so much. What can I do about it?"

57. Which nursing instruction is most appropriate regarding the relief of itchy skin during pregnancy?
[ ]   **1.** Take a hot bath daily.
[ ]   **2.** Increase fluid intake.
[ ]   **3.** Add a daily vitamin C tablet to the diet.
[ ]   **4.** Take diphenhydramine (Benadryl) twice per day.

One participant who is in her third trimester states that she has started to experience shortness of breath. She asks the nurse if she should be concerned.

58. Which information about shortness of breath during pregnancy is correct?
[ ]   **1.** It is not a common complaint during pregnancy and may be the result of a blood clot in the lungs.
[ ]   **2.** It is probably the result of anxiety about the baby's impending delivery.
[ ]   **3.** It is probably caused by the enlarged uterus pressing against the diaphragm.
[ ]   **4.** It is probably caused by decreased oxygen secondary to slow venous circulation.

59. Which nursing instruction given to the client complaining about shortness of breath is most appropriate?
[ ]   **1.** "Contact your health care provider immediately."
[ ]   **2.** "Decrease your activity level to conserve oxygen."
[ ]   **3.** "Ask your physician for a mild sedative."
[ ]   **4.** "Sleep with your upper body elevated on pillows."

Several participants in the prenatal class complain of frequent urination.

60. The nurse explains to the group that frequent urination during early pregnancy usually subsides when what occurs?
[ ] **1.** The placenta is fully developed
[ ] **2.** Fetal kidneys begin to function
[ ] **3.** The uterus rises into the abdominal cavity
[ ] **4.** The hormonal balance is reestablished

61. The nurse correctly explains to the group that the most probable cause of frequent urination late in pregnancy is related to what factor?
[ ] **1.** Loss of bladder tone in the mother
[ ] **2.** The presence of a urinary tract infection
[ ] **3.** The enlarging uterus exerting pressure on the bladder
[ ] **4.** The growing fetus excreting increased amounts of waste

62. Which statement made by a participant indicates the need for additional teaching regarding management of urinary frequency?
[ ] **1.** "Limiting my fluid intake will help me control this problem."
[ ] **2.** "I should report a burning sensation during urination."
[ ] **3.** "Urinating before going to bed may help control my problem."
[ ] **4.** "Avoiding highly caffeinated beverages may help control this problem."

One participant who is 5 months' pregnant complains of annoying backaches.

63. Which advice can the nurse give to relieve the client's backache?
[ ] **1.** Avoid tight-fitting clothing around the waist.
[ ] **2.** Sleep on a heating pad.
[ ] **3.** Take a nonopioid pain reliever regularly.
[ ] **4.** Wear low-heeled shoes.

The nurse advises the class about ways to minimize the occurrence of heartburn and nausea.

64. Which statement made by a participant regarding remedies for heartburn and nausea indicates that teaching has been effective?
[ ] **1.** "I should eat frequent, small meals."
[ ] **2.** "I should take an antacid after eating."
[ ] **3.** "I should eat my largest meal of the day after 7 p.m."
[ ] **4.** "I should drink extra water with my meals."

65. When one participant asks the nurse what she can do to relieve leg cramps, which instruction by the nurse would be correct?
[ ] **1.** Increase her protein intake to five to six servings per day.
[ ] **2.** Place a heating pad on the affected leg.
[ ] **3.** Stretch the legs frequently by pointing the toes to the floor.
[ ] **4.** Massage the leg when a cramp occurs.

66. Which response by the nurse is most appropriate when another participant states that she is concerned about having frequent mood swings?
[ ] **1.** "You should try to avoid fatigue and decrease your stress."
[ ] **2.** "You should avoid interactions with people who upset you."
[ ] **3.** "Have you asked the physician about your wide mood swings?"
[ ] **4.** "I'm concerned about your mood swings, too."

The nurse leads a discussion with the group about distinguishing between danger signs and common discomforts of pregnancy.

67. The nurse considers her teaching successful when the class correctly identifies which of the following as a danger sign of pregnancy?
[ ] **1.** Headache and swelling of the face and fingers
[ ] **2.** Constipation and flatulence
[ ] **3.** Lower extremity muscle cramping and varicosities
[ ] **4.** Large amounts of odorless, colorless vaginal secretions

High-Risk Factors and Pregnancy

A nurse discusses high-risk complications with a group of women at a prenatal clinic.

68. Which client would the nurse identify as being at highest risk for developing complications during pregnancy?
[ ] **1.** A 25-year-old gravida I client
[ ] **2.** A client with the placenta implanted on the fundus of the uterus
[ ] **3.** A client who has nausea and vomiting during the first trimester
[ ] **4.** A 35-year-old gravida V client

One participant tells the nurse that she drinks a beer every night before going to bed. She asks the nurse if occasional alcohol consumption will harm her unborn baby.

69. Which response by the nurse is best?
[ ] **1.** "Any alcohol consumption during pregnancy will cause the infant to have complications at birth."
[ ] **2.** "The minimal safe amount of alcohol consumption during pregnancy has not yet been determined."
[ ] **3.** "Alcohol consumption has a harmful effect on the baby only if consumed during the first trimester of pregnancy."
[ ] **4.** "Occasional intake of a small amount of alcohol during pregnancy will not adversely affect the unborn baby."

Another participant informs the nurse that she smokes about a pack of cigarettes a day.

70. The nurse correctly informs the participants that women who smoke during pregnancy have a greater risk of which problem?
[ ] **1.** Having a premature delivery
[ ] **2.** Having a cesarean birth
[ ] **3.** Having a large overweight baby
[ ] **4.** Developing a prenatal infection

A 40-year-old participant, a gravida V para I in her 10th week of pregnancy, tells the nurse that she is concerned about how her age may affect the health of her baby. She asks the nurse if there is a test that can identify any genetic disorders that the baby may have.

71. At this point in the client's pregnancy, which test is typically used to detect genetic disorders?
[ ] **1.** Amniocentesis
[ ] **2.** Chorionic villi sampling
[ ] **3.** Rapid plasma reagin
[ ] **4.** Ultrasound

At the clinic, an 18-year-old primigravid client is seen for the first time. The physician determines that the client is 3 months' pregnant and diagnoses a sexually transmitted disease, chlamydia.

72. Which assessment finding best indicates the presence of this condition?
[ ] **1.** Painful blisters on the labia
[ ] **2.** Heavy, grayish white discharge
[ ] **3.** Milky white discharge that smells like fish
[ ] **4.** Thick, white, curdlike vaginal discharge

73. Which statement by the client indicates a need for additional teaching regarding chlamydial infection?
[ ] **1.** "My sex partner should be treated also."
[ ] **2.** "I will have to have a cesarean birth to protect my baby."
[ ] **3.** "The physician will probably give me some antibiotics."
[ ] **4.** "My Pap smear results may show abnormal cells."

Before the client leaves the clinic, the nurse teaches her about danger signs of the infection that should be reported immediately to the physician.

74. The nurse correctly instructs the client to contact the physician immediately under which circumstances?
[ ] **1.** When she feels the first fetal movement
[ ] **2.** If her breasts become tender
[ ] **3.** If she experiences vaginal bleeding
[ ] **4.** When she experiences frequent urination

A 30-year-old client comes to the clinic complaining of severe nausea and vomiting. She tells the nurse she has had these symptoms for the past 7 days. The physician determines that the client has hyperemesis gravidarum and is moderately dehydrated.

75. Which equipment should the nurse plan to have available to treat this client?
[ ] **1.** I.V. start kit
[ ] **2.** Warmed speculum
[ ] **3.** Oxygen and face mask
[ ] **4.** Cardiac monitor

Complications of Pregnancy

A nurse on the obstetrics unit cares for several pregnant clients.

76. Which client is most likely to be identified as being at high risk for pregnancy complications?
[ ] **1.** A client who is pregnant for the third time
[ ] **2.** A client who has gained 30 pounds during the pregnancy
[ ] **3.** A client who has a history of twins in the family
[ ] **4.** A client who has primary hypertensive disease

At a routine clinic visit, a pregnant factory worker in her seventh month of pregnancy verbalizes concern about her work schedule.

77. What can the nurse advise the client to do to avoid complications during the last part of her pregnancy?
[ ] **1.** Avoid standing in one place for prolonged periods of time.
[ ] **2.** Only lift heavy objects by bending at the waist.
[ ] **3.** Ask the employer for bathroom breaks every hour.
[ ] **4.** Reduce her work schedule to 20 hours per week until after delivery.

The obstetrician sees a 31-year-old multipara client in her first trimester of pregnancy. When sharing her health history, the client tells the nurse that her last pregnancy ended in a spontaneous abortion because of an incompetent cervix. She asks the nurse to clarify what is meant by an incompetent cervix.

78. Which statement by the nurse best explains what occurs with an incompetent cervix?
[ ] **1.** The cervix is not large enough for passage of the fetus.
[ ] **2.** The cervix cannot support the weight of the fetus.
[ ] **3.** The cervix has an external opening but not an internal opening.
[ ] **4.** The cervix has an internal opening but not an external opening.

At the end of the first trimester, the physician puts a cerclage in the client's cervix. The client asks the nurse how long the cerclage will remain in place.

79. The nurse correctly explains to the client that the physician will probably leave the cerclage in place until what occurs?
[ ] **1.** The client goes into labor.
[ ] **2.** The client's baby is delivered.
[ ] **3.** The second trimester ends.
[ ] **4.** The client is near term.

A 29-year-old primigravid client is in her 22nd week of pregnancy. The physician informs the client that she has pregnancy-induced hypertension (PIH).

80. When assessing a client with a history of PIH, the nurse should thoroughly explore which finding at each visit?
[ ] **1.** A decrease in urine protein level
[ ] **2.** An increase in urine output
[ ] **3.** A decrease in pulse rate
[ ] **4.** Any sudden weight gain

81. Which assessment finding is most indicative of mild PIH?
[ ] **1.** A 15 mm Hg rise in the baseline systolic blood pressure
[ ] **2.** A weight gain of 1 pound per week in the second trimester
[ ] **3.** A +1 protein reading on the urine reagent test strip
[ ] **4.** The presence of frequent ankle edema

The physician decides that the client can manage her PIH at home and requests that the nurse provide instructions for home care.

82. Which instruction regarding the home care of PIH is most appropriate?
[ ] **1.** Decrease fluid intake.
[ ] **2.** Return for bimonthly checkups.
[ ] **3.** Eat high-protein foods.
[ ] **4.** Limit activity to light housework.

The client's condition worsens and she is admitted to the hospital. The physician orders magnesium sulfate.

83. While the client is receiving magnesium sulfate, the nurse should routinely assess the client's vital signs and what else?
[ ] **1.** Urine for glucose
[ ] **2.** Deep tendon reflexes
[ ] **3.** Stool for blood
[ ] **4.** Pupils for constriction

84. Which medication should the nurse have on hand when the client is receiving magnesium sulfate?
[ ] **1.** Hydralazine (Apresoline)
[ ] **2.** Oxytocin (Pitocin)
[ ] **3.** Methylergonovine (Methergine)
[ ] **4.** Calcium gluconate (Kalcinate)

85. Which assessment finding best indicates the presence of magnesium sulfate toxicity?
[ ] **1.** Brisk deep tendon reflexes
[ ] **2.** Respiratory rate less than 14 breaths/minute
[ ] **3.** Protein in the urine
[ ] **4.** Magnesium blood level of 5 mg/dL

The nurse frequently assesses the client and finds that her condition has progressed to eclampsia.

86. The nurse knows to notify the physician immediately when the client has which assessment finding?
[ ] **1.** Seizures
[ ] **2.** Long periods of sleep
[ ] **3.** Fetal heart rate greater than 100 beats/minute
[ ] **4.** Vomiting

A 28-year-old multipara client is admitted to the hospital for observation during her 10th week of pregnancy. She has a history of spontaneous abortions and is spotting.

87. Which finding reported by the client best suggests a spontaneous abortion?
[ ] **1.** Cold, clammy skin
[ ] **2.** Severe headache
[ ] **3.** Persistent tachycardia
[ ] **4.** Abdominal cramping

The physician examines the client and determines that her cervix is dilated but the fetus and placenta are still in the uterus.

88. Which nursing intervention is most appropriate when a spontaneous abortion is inevitable?
[ ] **1.** Prepare the client for dilation and curettage (D&C).
[ ] **2.** Place the client in Trendelenburg's position.
[ ] **3.** Prepare the client for placement of a purse-string stitch.
[ ] **4.** Place the client in the side-lying position.

The client comments to the nurse, "This is like a recurring nightmare. This same thing happened last year. I don't want to lose another baby."

89. Which response by the nurse is most appropriate at this time?
[ ] **1.** "I know this is painful for you. Would you like to talk about how you are feeling about this?"
[ ] **2.** "Be positive. It's too early to know whether or not you will lose your baby."
[ ] **3.** "I know you are scared, but you must try to stay calm. Stress will make the situation worse."
[ ] **4.** "I know things seem really bad, but trust me. Everything will work out for the best in the end."

A 22-year-old woman, gravida I, para 0, has insulin-dependent diabetes mellitus and is being seen by the obstetrician for the first time. She was diagnosed with diabetes at age 6. Her diabetes has been well controlled since her initial diagnosis. While waiting to see the physician, the client asks the nurse if the pregnancy will increase the need for insulin.

90. Which explanation by the nurse is correct concerning the client's need for insulin during pregnancy?
[ ] **1.** Insulin level will most likely increase.
[ ] **2.** Insulin level will most likely decrease.
[ ] **3.** Insulin level will most likely fluctuate.
[ ] **4.** Insulin level will most likely not change.

The client also asks the nurse what kinds of diabetes-related complications she should expect during her pregnancy.

91. The nurse correctly informs the client that she is at risk for developing which condition?
[ ] **1.** Hyperemesis gravidarum
[ ] **2.** Pregnancy-induced hypertension
[ ] **3.** Placenta previa
[ ] **4.** Toxoplasmosis

The client is in her last trimester of pregnancy and her diabetes has been well controlled. She tells the nurse that she is excited but also scared that something could be wrong with her baby because of her diabetes.

92. Which response by the nurse is most appropriate?
[ ] **1.** "Your baby may be large and initially will need blood glucose monitoring."
[ ] **2.** "Your baby may be small but otherwise healthy."
[ ] **3.** "Your baby will be diabetic."
[ ] **4.** "Your baby will have a minor birth defect."

A 21-year-old multigravid client who is 8 months' pregnant is admitted to the obstetric unit for observation. The admission diagnosis is partial placenta previa. The client's partner asks the nurse, "What is placenta previa?"

93. Which response by the nurse provides the best explanation regarding placenta previa?
[ ] **1.** "The placenta is implanted over or close to the internal cervical opening."
[ ] **2.** "The placenta isn't producing the hormones needed to maintain the pregnancy."
[ ] **3.** "The placenta is invaded by polyps that cause premature uterine contractions."
[ ] **4.** "The placenta is producing antibodies that are destroying the baby's red blood cells."

The client's partner verbalizes concern about how placenta previa is treated.

94. The nurse correctly states that the physician is most likely to do which of the following if the client's condition remains stable?
[ ] **1.** Induce labor
[ ] **2.** Perform an emergency cesarean birth
[ ] **3.** Require the client to be on bed rest until she is at full term
[ ] **4.** Start the client on ritodrine (Yutopar)

After a short observation period, the client with placenta previa is sent home. One week later, the client reports to the hospital with complications.

95. Based on the client's earlier diagnosis, the admitting nurse would expect the client to report which finding?
[ ] **1.** Sudden, sharp abdominal pain
[ ] **2.** Painless bleeding from the vagina
[ ] **3.** Persistent headache
[ ] **4.** Continuous, painless contractions

96. Based on the client's clinical presentation, which admission information should the nurse obtain first?
[ ] **1.** Height and weight
[ ] **2.** Blood pressure and pulse rate
[ ] **3.** Pregnancy and prior delivery history
[ ] **4.** General health and drug history

A 30-year-old multigravid client who is in her last trimester of pregnancy is diagnosed with abruptio placentae.

97. Which assessment finding is considered a predisposing factor for the development of abruptio placentae?
[ ] **1.** Gestational diabetes
[ ] **2.** Hyperemesis gravidarum
[ ] **3.** Oligohydramnios
[ ] **4.** Pregnancy-induced hypertension

98. Which finding is most indicative of abruptio placentae and should be reported to the physician immediately?
[ ] **1.** Rigid, boardlike, tender abdomen
[ ] **2.** Severe nausea and vomiting
[ ] **3.** Fetal heart rate of 110 beats/minute
[ ] **4.** Painless vaginal bleeding

99. If the client develops a complete abruption, which nursing action is most appropriate?
[ ] **1.** Obtain a written consent for an immediate cesarean birth.
[ ] **2.** Give the client an enema and prep her abdomen.
[ ] **3.** Place the client in Trendelenburg's position.
[ ] **4.** Prepare the client for a contraction stress test.

A client, gravida I, para 0, who is 3 months' pregnant, tells the nurse that she had rubella (German measles) 2 months ago.

100. Which possible complication should the nurse discuss with the client?
[ ] **1.** Premature labor
[ ] **2.** Fetal deformities
[ ] **3.** Severe preeclampsia
[ ] **4.** Hydatidiform mole formation

101. Which of the following is most indicative of the presence of hydatidiform mole?
[ ] **1.** A blotchy brown discoloration on the face
[ ] **2.** A positive Chadwick's sign
[ ] **3.** The presence of ballottement
[ ] **4.** A uterus that is larger than expected

102. Which pregnant client should the nurse encourage to undergo hepatitis B testing?
[ ] **1.** A client with a history of cigarette smoking
[ ] **2.** A client who is single and pregnant for the first time
[ ] **3.** A client who emigrated from Haiti
[ ] **4.** A client who was recently exposed to *Haemophilus influenzae*

Elective Abortion

An 18-year-old primigravid client is considering terminating her pregnancy. She tells the nurse that she needs more information before making her decision. She asks the nurse, "At what point during pregnancy can a baby live outside the mother?"

103. Which response by the nurse concerning the legal threshold of viability is correct?
[ ] **1.** It is usually estimated to be 36 to 40 weeks.
[ ] **2.** It is usually estimated to be 30 to 35 weeks.
[ ] **3.** It is usually estimated to be 20 to 24 weeks.
[ ] **4.** It is usually estimated to be 10 to 15 weeks.

Correct Answers and Rationales

Anatomy and Physiology of the Male and Female Reproductive Systems

1. 1. The ovum is released from the ovary and enters the outer third of the fallopian tube, where the sperm fertilizes it. After fertilization, the fertilized ovum travels through the remainder of the fallopian tube and enters the uterus, where it implants and remains throughout pregnancy.
Client Needs Category—Health promotion and maintenance
Client Needs Subcategory—None

2. 2. The ovum remains viable for 24 hours after being released from the ovary. If fertilization does not occur within this time frame, conception cannot take place.
Client Needs Category—Health promotion and maintenance
Client Needs Subcategory—None

3. 2. Because heat can damage or kill sperm, men should avoid hot tubs or taking hot baths if attempting to prevent infertility. Tight-fitting clothing, such as jeans or briefs, may also have the same effect by trapping body heat and elevating the temperature of the testes. Swimming does not affect the viability of sperm.
Client Needs Category—Health promotion and maintenance
Client Needs Subcategory—None

4. 2. The true pelvis is the part of the pelvis that influences the woman's ability to deliver vaginally. The false pelvis, which is formed by the iliac portion of the innominate bone, is what accounts for hip measurements. The fetus must be in an appropriate position and small enough to pass through the true pelvis for a successful vaginal delivery.
Client Needs Category—Health promotion and maintenance
Client Needs Subcategory—None

5. 4. The sex of the baby is determined at fertilization, which occurs in the outer third of the fallopian tube. Each parent contributes one sex chromosome. The mother always contributes an X chromosome. The father contributes an X or a Y chromosome. If a sperm containing an X chromosome fertilizes the ovum, the offspring is a female. If a sperm containing a Y chromosome fertilizes the ovum, the offspring is a male.
Client Needs Category—Health promotion and maintenance
Client Needs Subcategory—None

6. 1. Vaginal discharge, often called "menstrual flow" or "menses," consists of endometrial cells sloughed from the thickened uterine lining formed to prepare for pregnancy. When fertilization does not occur, the lining is sloughed. The discharge contains mucus, tissue, and blood. The first day of blood flow is considered the first day of the monthly cycle, which lasts about 28 days. The bleeding continues for 3 to 7 days and may be dark red, bright red, or rust-colored. The perimetrium is the thin outer layer of the uterus. The myometrium is the muscle layer of the uterus. The epimetrium is part of the peritoneum.
Client Needs Category—Health promotion and maintenance
Client Needs Subcategory—None

Signs and Symptoms of Pregnancy

7. 3. Primigravida describes a woman who is pregnant for the first time. Multipara describes a woman who has delivered more than one viable infant. A primipara is a woman who has delivered her first viable infant. Multigravida describes a woman who has been pregnant more than once.
Client Needs Category—Health promotion and maintenance
Client Needs Subcategory—None

8. 3. Identical twins result when one fertilized ovum divides into two identical halves that develop into two individuals with the same appearance and same gender. Fraternal twins are the result of two separate ova fertilized by two different sperm at the same time. They may or may not resemble each other and may or may not be of the same gender.
Client Needs Category—Health promotion and maintenance
Client Needs Subcategory—None

9. 2. Abdominal enlargement is considered a probable sign of pregnancy. Amenorrhea (absence of monthly periods), nausea, vomiting, and frequent urination are all considered to be presumptive signs of pregnancy because they can also be indications of conditions other than pregnancy.
Client Needs Category—Health promotion and maintenance
Client Needs Subcategory—None

10. 3. Levels of HCG rise significantly shortly after implantation of the ovum. Blood and urine testing for HCG is the basis for most pregnancy tests. The AFP test

is performed during pregnancy to determine the presence of neural tube defects such as spina bifida. FSH is not associated with pregnancy but is related to the maturation of the ovum prior to ovulation.
Client Needs Category—*Health promotion and maintenance*
Client Needs Subcategory—*None*

11. **1.** A transvaginal ultrasound can detect pregnancy as early as 2½ to 3 weeks. An abdominal ultrasound can detect pregnancy as early as 5 to 6 weeks, well before the uterus ascends out of the pelvis. The ultrasound has replaced the X-ray as a diagnostic tool for pregnancy, eliminating the risks associated with fetal radiation exposure.
Client Needs Category—*Health promotion and maintenance*
Client Needs Subcategory—*None*

12. **2.** Chadwick's sign is a bluish discoloration of the cervix, vagina, and vulva caused by increased vascularization of the reproductive organs. Braxton Hicks contractions are spontaneous intermittent contractions that occur during pregnancy. Goodell's sign is the softening of the cervix, and linea nigra is the dark brown line extending from the umbilicus to the symphysis pubis that appears on the skin of many pregnant women.
Client Needs Category—*Health promotion and maintenance*
Client Needs Subcategory—*None*

13. **1.** Ballottement is observed when the fetus rises (or bounces) in the amniotic fluid, then returns to its normal position after a gentle push or tapping of the lower portion of the uterus by the examiner. Ballottement is usually first observed during the fourth or fifth month of pregnancy.
Client Needs Category—*Health promotion and maintenance*
Client Needs Subcategory—*None*

14. **4.** The health care provider's detection of the fetal heartbeat confirms pregnancy. A palpable fetal outline and positive pregnancy test are probable signs of pregnancy but are not conclusive evidence. A blotchy tan discoloration of the face is known as chloasma and is a presumptive sign of pregnancy.
Client Needs Category—*Health promotion and maintenance*
Client Needs Subcategory—*None*

15. **2.** The first fetal movement felt by the mother is referred to as quickening. If this is the woman's first pregnancy, quickening is usually experienced between 16 and 20 weeks' gestation.
Client Needs Category—*Health promotion and maintenance*
Client Needs Subcategory—*None*

Assessing the Pregnant Client

16. **2.** Quickening, the term attributed to the mother's first feeling of fetal movement, is often described as a fluttering sensation. In a primigravid client, quickening usually occurs in the second trimester, between the 16th and 20th weeks of gestation. In a multipara client, it typically occurs earlier, at about 14 to 18 weeks' gestation. Due dates are calculated based on the first day of the last menstrual period, not on fetal movement. Quickening occurs at about the same time regardless of whether a woman is carrying one or two fetuses.
Client Needs Category—*Health promotion and maintenance*
Client Needs Subcategory—*None*

17. **4.** TPAL is an acronym used when documenting the client's obstetrical history. T represents the number of term pregnancies; P represents the number of premature infants delivered; A represents the number of abortions or miscarriages; and L represents the number of living children. The client in this situation has had two term pregnancies, no premature deliveries, no abortions, and has three living children. Therefore, the correct TPAL is T-II, P-0, A-0, L-III.
Client Needs Category—*Health promotion and maintenance*
Client Needs Subcategory—*None*

18. **4.** Nägele's rule is one method of determining the estimated date of delivery. When using Nägele's rule, add 7 days to the first day of the last menstrual period, and count back 3 months. In this situation, the estimated delivery date is December 20.
Client Needs Category—*Health promotion and maintenance*
Client Needs Subcategory—*None*

19. **1.** When preparing the client for a pelvic examination, the nurse assists her into the lithotomy position. In this position, the client lies on her back with the knees bent and feet resting flat on the table or placed in stirrups. Her buttocks should extend slightly beyond the edge of the examination table. All of the other positions (prone, Sims', and Trendelenburg's) do not accommodate this type of examination.
Client Needs Category—*Health promotion and maintenance*
Client Needs Subcategory—*None*

20. 2. Prior to the pelvic examination, the client should be encouraged to empty her bladder. This action increases the client's comfort during the examination and facilitates a more accurate assessment of the pelvic structures. It is not necessary nor is it routine for the client to receive an enema, sedative, or shave and prep prior to having a pelvic examination.
Client Needs Category—Health promotion and maintenance
Client Needs Subcategory—None

21. 4. The nurse instructs the client to let her knees fall outward and to relax during the examination; this increases the client's comfort level. The client should have a pillow under her head and should not lift her head off the pillow during the examination, Raising the head tightens the abdominal muscles, making the examination more difficult. Having the client press her back into the examination table and tighten her buttocks will not promote relaxation because these actions cause increased tension in the muscles of the perineum.
Client Needs Category—Health promotion and maintenance
Client Needs Subcategory—None

22. 2. With the use of a Doppler device, the examiner can detect fetal heart tones as early as 8 to 10 weeks' gestation. The fetal heartbeat is audible with a standard fetoscope between 18 and 20 weeks' gestation.
Client Needs Category—Health promotion and maintenance
Client Needs Subcategory—None

23. 4. When auscultating for the fetal heart rate, the nurse may also hear the uterine souffle (a soft whirling sound produced by the maternal blood moving through the uterine vessels). To differentiate between fetal heart tones and the uterine souffle, the nurse should count the maternal pulse rate and compare it to the rate obtained when listening for the fetal heart tones. Placing the client on her right side, counting during fetal movement, and counting between Braxton Hicks contractions will not ensure an accurate fetal heart rate.
Client Needs Category—Health promotion and maintenance
Client Needs Subcategory—None

24. 1. The fetal heart rate is normally between 120 and 160 beats/minute. A fetal heart rate less than 120 beats/minute or greater than 160 beats/minute may indicate fetal distress and should be immediately reported.
Client Needs Category—Health promotion and maintenance
Client Needs Subcategory—None

25. 3. The maternal serum alpha-fetoprotein (MSAFP) test is used to screen for neural tube defects such as spina bifida. This test should be performed between 14 and 16 weeks' gestation. The HBsAg test is used to detect hepatitis B. The VDRL (Venereal Disease Research Laboratory) and FTA-ABS (fluorescent treponemal antibody absorption) tests are used to screen for syphilis.
Client Needs Category—Health promotion and maintenance
Client Needs Subcategory—None

26. 3. A pregnant woman who is experiencing no complications usually visits the health care provider every 4 weeks for the first 28 weeks of pregnancy, then every 2 weeks from 28 to 36 weeks' gestation, and then weekly from the 37th week to delivery.
Client Needs Category—Health promotion and maintenance
Client Needs Subcategory—None

27. 1, 2, 3. Exercise raises body temperature and speeds the metabolism and heart rate. For these reasons, exercising during pregnancy should be carefully monitored so that no harm comes to the mother or baby. The nurse should advise the client to avoid exercising in hot, humid weather to ensure that her core body temperature does not rise and possibly affect the baby. Likewise, she should avoid any jerking, bouncing, or jumping movements that could harm the growing fetus. It is important for the client to drink plenty of fluids before and after exercising to prevent dehydration, which can alter her electrolyte balance and temperature as well as those of the fetus. She should also exercise only during the cooler part of the day or in an air-conditioned environment.

Although the client should be able to tolerate exercising at least three times per week (not just once weekly), she should limit any strenuous workouts to no more than 15 minutes per session. Exercises should never be done in the supine position, especially after the fourth month, to avoid supine hypotension and insufficient blood flow to the baby.
Client Needs Category—Health promotion and maintenance
Client Needs Subcategory—None

28. 3. At 20 weeks' gestation, the fundus of the uterus can be palpated near the level of the umbilicus. At 16 weeks' gestation, the fundus is located halfway between the top of the symphysis pubis and the umbilicus. Close to term (38 to 40 weeks), the uterus can be palpated just below the xiphoid process.
Client Needs Category—Health promotion and maintenance
Client Needs Subcategory—None

29. 2. The glucose tolerance test is a routine test performed between 24 and 28 weeks' gestation as a screening tool for gestational diabetes. A Pap smear and rubella titer are usually performed at the first prenatal visit. Coombs' test is not routinely performed during pregnancy; it is used to determine the possibility of Rh incompatibility between the mother and fetus or neonate.

> *Client Needs Category—Health promotion and maintenance*
> *Client Needs Subcategory—None*

30. 4. To perform the nonstress test, the nurse attaches a fetal monitor to the client's abdomen and monitors the response of the fetal heart rate to fetal movement. I.V. magnesium sulfate is given to the client experiencing severe preeclampsia. I.V. oxytocin (Pitocin) may be given for several reasons, including augmentation of labor and control of postpartum hemorrhage. A cardiac monitor is not used during a nonstress test.

> *Client Needs Category—Health promotion and maintenance*
> *Client Needs Subcategory—None*

31. 2. Amniocentesis is an invasive procedure in which a sterile needle is inserted through the uterine wall and a small sample of amniotic fluid is withdrawn and used for analysis. This test is usually performed in the second trimester to rule out congenital abnormalities, such as Down syndrome or spinal cord defects. It may also be used during the third trimester to assess fetal lung maturity, postmaturity of the fetus, or fetal death. An amniocentesis is usually performed after the 14th week of gestation, when there is sufficient fluid to sample.

> *Client Needs Category—Health promotion and maintenance*
> *Client Needs Subcategory—None*

Nutritional Needs During Pregnancy

32. 2. The client's current eating pattern and preferences should be assessed before a teaching plan can be formulated and implemented. Once this information is obtained, the nurse can show the client what foods to add or delete to ensure a balanced, nutritious diet. The nurse should include the client in the planning process to ensure her cooperation with the choices made and to advise her on calorie recommendations, nutritional requirements, and food equivalencies (such as 1 cup of milk equaling 10 mg of calcium). After initiating this teaching, the nurse can work with the client to develop sample menus to meet her nutritional needs during the pregnancy. Regardless of her prepregnancy weight, a pregnant client should gain sufficient weight to meet the needs of her baby.

> *Client Needs Category—Health promotion and maintenance*
> *Client Needs Subcategory—None*

33. 3. The weight gain recommended during pregnancy is individualized, and the client's prepregnancy weight must be taken into consideration. The guidelines for weight gain for the client with a normal prepregnant weight is between 25 and 35 pounds. A weight gain of 28 to 40 pounds is generally recommended for a client who is underweight. Clients who are moderately overweight can gain between 15 and 25 pounds. Clients who are very overweight can gain approximately 15 pounds.

> *Client Needs Category—Health promotion and maintenance*
> *Client Needs Subcategory—None*

34. 2. During pregnancy, the recommended intake of milk is 3 to 4 servings (3 to 4 cups) daily. Milk is an excellent source of calcium and protein, both of which are essential for the proper development of strong bones, healthy teeth, healthy nerves and muscles, and normal blood clotting for the client and her fetus.

> *Client Needs Category—Health promotion and maintenance*
> *Client Needs Subcategory—None*

35. 3. Of the foods listed in this question, leafy green vegetables contain the highest amount of calcium. Examples of such vegetables include lettuce, kale, and spinach.

> *Client Needs Category—Health promotion and maintenance*
> *Client Needs Subcategory—None*

36. 3. A client receiving iron supplements may complain of constipation or an upset stomach. The nurse should encourage the client to increase her fiber and fluid intake to help prevent or control this problem. Iron requirements double during pregnancy, and the demand for iron usually exceeds the amount that can be provided from dietary sources. Therefore, if the physician orders an iron supplement, the client should not attempt to substitute dietary sources of iron for the prescribed iron supplement. Iron supplements are best absorbed when taken between meals. Iron usually does not cause abdominal pain unless it is associated with constipation.

> *Client Needs Category—Health promotion and maintenance*
> *Client Needs Subcategory—None*

37. 1. Because the client's iron requirements will increase during pregnancy, constipation may become a problem. The nurse should advise the client that her stools may become greenish black, hard, and dry and offer instructions on how to prevent constipation. Diarrhea is not a side effect of iron supplements and vomiting is unlikely to occur, although gastric upset is possible. The teeth are not likely to become stained unless the iron preparation is in liquid form. Most prenatal iron supplements, however, come in tablet form.

Client Needs Category—Health promotion and maintenance
Client Needs Subcategory—None

38. 1. Folic acid, a B vitamin, is thought to prevent neural tube defects. Neural tube deficits occur in embryonic development when the spinal column fails to close. In general, good sources of folic acid and B vitamins include eggs, beans, whole grains, and dark, leafy green vegetables. The recommended amount of folic acid for pregnant women is 0.4 mg/day. Calcium is needed for fetal bone formation. Vitamin A helps build fetal resistance to infection. Iron is needed to build the fetus's hemoglobin and blood supply.

Client Needs Category—Health promotion and maintenance
Client Needs Subcategory—None

39. 1. To meet the pregnant teenager's energy needs, a diet of 2,500 calories/day is necessary. Adequate nutrition is a problem for pregnant teens because of their own growth coupled with the demands of pregnancy. Pregnant teenagers are often deficient in calcium, iron, folic acid, and calories. In their search for independence and identity, pregnant adolescents often refuse to eat foods suggested by their parents; instead, they eat fast food and junk food, and they snack throughout the day. Eating centers on social gatherings and peer pressure. Lemonade contains sugar and empty calories, so substituting that in place of soft drinks is not appropriate. Milk is a better choice. Carbohydrates and fats are needed every day to meet the teenager's energy needs. Limiting them does not ensure adequate nutrition. Digestion is not affected in the pregnant teenager, so easy to digest foods are not necessary.

Client Needs Category—Health promotion/maintenance
Client Needs Subcategory—None

40. 3. Adolescent girls frequently exhibit poor food choices and irregular eating habits related to their active schedules and busy lifestyles. Other risk factors related to poor nutritional intake include frequently omitting meals or eating fast food. Fast food is usually cheap, easily accessible, high in fat and sodium, and low in nutrition. Adolescent girls are usually social and spend large amounts of time with peers. They often worry about body shape and weight gain. Living with a boyfriend is not necessarily a risk factor for nutritional deficiencies.

Client Needs Category—Health promotion and maintenance
Client Needs Subcategory—None

41. 1. An acceptable expected outcome for a pregnant adolescent client is that she will eat three balanced meals and two nutritious snacks each day. Normal weight gain during pregnancy is between 25 and 35 pounds. Therefore, a total weight gain of 12 pounds is an inappropriate outcome. Only one prenatal vitamin is required per day. Normal caloric intake should increase to about 2,300 to 2,500 calories during pregnancy to support fetal growth.

Client Needs Category—Health promotion and maintenance
Client Needs Subcategory—None

42. 4. The average recommended weight gain during pregnancy is between 25 and 35 pounds. Therefore, a weight gain of 10 pounds is inadequate to maintain fetal growth. Although weight gain is affected by food intake, this is not the most appropriate response. The nurse needs to point out the normalcy of gaining weight during pregnancy. Likewise, even though it may be normal for adolescents to be concerned about body image and appearances, pregnant adolescents need to be counseled and carefully monitored to ensure they gain adequate weight.

Client Needs Category—Health promotion and maintenance
Client Needs Subcategory—None

43. 1, 2, 3, 4, 5. Alcohol should be avoided during pregnancy because of the numerous documented psychophysiologic effects it has on the developing fetus. Coffee, tea, and cola beverages contain caffeine, a central nervous system stimulant that increases the heart rate of both the mother and fetus. Sports drinks such as Gatorade should be limited because the effects on the fetus are not yet known. Orange juice is recommended because it is a good source of vitamin C, an essential vitamin that also helps with iron absorption.

Client Needs Category—Health promotion and maintenance
Client Needs Subcategory—None

44. 1. Edema is affected by sodium retention. Therefore, omitting or limiting salt from the diet will help alleviate lower extremity edema. Some edema is normal during the latter stages of pregnancy. However, a client with edema of the hands and face may have pregnancy-induced hypertension, a serious complication. Vitamin C, magnesium, and potassium are not associated with fluid retention and edema.

Client Needs Category—Health promotion and maintenance
Client Needs Subcategory—None

45. **1, 2, 3, 4.** Because of their rapid growth and development, adolescents normally have a variety of nutritional concerns, including the need for additional calories and increased levels of vitamins and minerals. Being pregnant adds to their nutritional requirements and puts them at increased risk for nutritional deficiencies. Women who are overweight or underweight at the time of conception are also at risk for nutritional deficits based on their prepregnancy eating patterns. Women who consume alcohol or smoke cigarettes during pregnancy are robbing their bodies and their growing fetuses of valuable nutritional intake; they are also placing their fetuses at risk for fetal alcohol syndrome. Those with a low income are at risk for nutritional problems because they may not have the financial resources to eat well-balanced meals or buy prenatal vitamins. Women who have a prepregnancy hemoglobin level of 13 g/100 mL are within normal limits and are not at risk for nutritional problems related to anemia. Drinking four glasses of milk is the recommended daily requirement for pregnant women.

Client Needs Category—Health promotion and maintenance
Client Needs Subcategory—None

Teaching the Pregnant Client

46. **2.** Daily tub baths or showers are recommended for the client during pregnancy because women usually perspire more heavily and have a heavier vaginal discharge at this time. However, tub baths during the latter part of pregnancy increase the risk for falls because the protruding abdomen shifts the client's center of gravity. Safety mats, handgrips, and other safety precautions are recommended to prevent falls. Hot tubs should be avoided because an elevated maternal core body temperature can produce harmful effects on the fetus. Once the membranes rupture, tub baths should be avoided because of the increased risk of developing an infection.

Client Needs Category—Health promotion and maintenance
Client Needs Subcategory—None

47. **4.** If the client has a healthy pregnancy, no restrictions are placed on sexual intercourse. However, sexual intercourse is contraindicated if the client experiences vaginal bleeding, if the physician has diagnosed placenta previa, or if the membranes have ruptured. Also, a client with a history of premature labor should be cautioned about the danger of premature labor when experiencing orgasms after 32 weeks' gestation.

Client Needs Category—Health promotion and maintenance
Client Needs Subcategory—None

48. **1.** Travel restrictions during pregnancy are indicated only when the client is unhealthy or experiencing complications. The optimal time for travel is during the second trimester of pregnancy, when the client is typically most comfortable. The client should be encouraged to carry a copy of her medical record whenever she travels. Wearing a seatbelt is the law in most states. When traveling, the pregnant woman should avoid sitting for prolonged periods and should walk every couple of hours to avoid complications related to venous stasis.

Client Needs Category—Health promotion and maintenance
Client Needs Subcategory—None

49. **1.** Once fertilized, the ovum travels through the fallopian tube to the uterus, where it will be implanted, usually within 7 days. At the time of implantation there may be a small amount of bleeding similar to menstrual spotting. Such spotting is unrelated to increased circulation to the vagina or to hormonal changes. Dilation and effacement (enlargement and thinning of the cervix) occur during labor; they are not associated with spotting during the early stages of pregnancy.

Client Needs Category—Health promotion and maintenance
Client Needs Subcategory—None

50. **4.** By the 8th week of gestation, the embryo has developed enough to be called a fetus. The fetal stage of development, which lasts from the 8th week until term (40 weeks), mostly involves growth and maturation of structures begun during the embryonic stage. At 8 weeks, the extremities are developed; by the 12th week, the fetus has not only arms and legs, but also fingers and toes. A zygote is the term used to identify the newly formed cell that develops when the sperm penetrates the ovum and fertilization occurs. During this stage, which lasts from fertilization to implantation in the uterus (usually 3 to 4 days), the zygote cell divides and grows, resembling a bumpy ball. During the embryonic stage, which marks the time from implantation to about 8 weeks' gestation, the body begins forming and the sex is distinguishable.

Client Needs Category—Health promotion and maintenance
Client Needs Subcategory—None

51. **2.** The amniotic fluid primarily serves as a medium to protect the fetus. It allows the fetus to move while keeping the fetal environment at a constant temperature. It also provides some nourishment for the fetus and prevents the amnion from adhering to the fetus. The amniotic fluid does not provide the fetus with antibodies or oxygen, and it does not lower the mother's body temperature.

Client Needs Category—Health promotion and maintenance
Client Needs Subcategory—None

52. 1. During pregnancy, the placenta is considered a temporary endocrine gland. It secretes estrogen as well as progesterone and human chorionic gonadotropin. Testosterone is a male hormone. Oxytocin, a hormone secreted by the posterior pituitary gland, is normally released near the time of delivery to begin and maintain uterine contractions during labor. It is also administered in some cases to augment labor and prevent postpartal hemorrhage. Oxytocin also causes the release of breast milk. Follicle-stimulating hormone is excreted by the anterior pituitary gland prior to pregnancy and matures the follicle in the ovary prior to ovulation.
Client Needs Category—Health promotion and maintenance
Client Needs Subcategory—None

Common Discomforts of Pregnancy

53. 2. Constipation may occur because of hormonal changes, increased uterine size, and decreased peristalsis later in pregnancy. Exercise, not rest, may assist with the control or relief of this discomfort. Also, a diet containing fresh fruit and vegetables, whole grains, and increased fluids will assist with controlling or relieving constipation. Prenatal vitamins will not relieve constipation and may even contribute to it due to the large amount of iron in each tablet. A low-fat diet is not associated with constipation or its relief.
Client Needs Category—Health promotion and maintenance
Client Needs Subcategory—None

54. 1. During pregnancy, the client may develop varicose veins, especially in the lower extremities and rectal area (hemorrhoids). Varicose veins occur during pregnancy primarily because of impaired venous return, which is caused by the pressure of the enlarged uterus on venous circulation and the increased blood volume normally associated with pregnancy. Decreased cardiac output and changes in the body's center of gravity are not associated with the occurrence of varicose veins. Kidney function is not normally impaired during pregnancy.
Client Needs Category—Health promotion and maintenance
Client Needs Subcategory—None

55. 4. It is recommended that pregnant women with varicose veins move around when standing for extended time periods. This prevents stasis of blood in the lower extremities. Clients with varicose veins should be instructed to rest with their feet elevated, not in a dependent position. They should avoid wearing garters or knee- or calf-length elastic-top hose because of the risk of impaired circulation.
Client Needs Category—Health promotion and maintenance
Client Needs Subcategory—None

56. 4. A client with varicose veins whose calves are red, tender, or warm to the touch should report this finding immediately because it could signal thrombophlebitis, a more serious problem. The presence of additional varicose veins is not a condition that needs immediate attention from the physician but should be addressed at the next routine visit. Varicose veins are normally purple in color. The client with varicose veins may complain of her legs feeling achy, tired, and heavy.
Client Needs Category—Health promotion and maintenance
Client Needs Subcategory—None

57. 2. Itching of the skin is a common and annoying discomfort of pregnancy. It may occur during pregnancy because the enlarging uterus causes the abdominal skin to stretch. Drying agents, such as soaps and alcohol, as well as hot baths, may also increase itching. Increasing fluid intake may improve skin elasticity and decrease the occurrence of itching. There is no correlation between vitamin C intake and decreased itching. Benadryl is used for itching, but it is contraindicated for frequent use during pregnancy because of the risk of fetal damage.
Client Needs Category—Health promotion and maintenance
Client Needs Subcategory—None

58. 3. The uterus rising in the abdomen exerts pressure on the diaphragm, thereby decreasing the client's lung capacity and causing her to feel short of breath. This problem is common during the third trimester of pregnancy and is considered normal. Shortness of breath during the third trimester is not related to anxiety about the impending delivery, nor is it associated with a decreased oxygen supply secondary to slow venous circulation or clots in the lungs.
Client Needs Category—Health promotion and maintenance
Client Needs Subcategory—None

59. 4. Elevating the upper body on pillows while resting may help to relieve shortness of breath. Maintaining an erect posture when sitting or standing may also help to relieve this problem by increasing oxygen intake. It is unnecessary for the client to notify the physician immediately, but the physician should be made aware of any difficulty in breathing to rule out the presence of a serious problem. A mild sedative is not indicated for clients who exhibit shortness of breath. Decreasing activity may reduce the shortness of breath, but only temporarily.

Client Needs Category—*Health promotion and maintenance*
Client Needs Subcategory—*None*

60. **3.** Frequent urination is common early in pregnancy because the enlarging uterus causes pressure on the urinary bladder. When the uterus rises into the abdominal cavity, urinary frequency subsides. Placental maturity, fetal kidney function, and hormonal balance are not usually causes of urinary frequency during early pregnancy.

Client Needs Category—*Health promotion and maintenance*
Client Needs Subcategory—*None*

61. **3.** Frequent urination is common in late pregnancy because the enlarged uterus descends into the pelvis, causing pressure on the urinary bladder. Frequency is unrelated to increased fetal waste. A urinary tract infection could cause frequency, but this is not the most probable cause late in pregnancy. A urinary tract infection is likely to cause additional symptoms, such as burning and painful urination. During the late stages of pregnancy, loss of bladder tone resulting in urinary frequency does not commonly occur.

Client Needs Category—*Health promotion and maintenance*
Client Needs Subcategory—*None*

62. **1.** Although limiting fluid intake prior to going to bed at night may help to manage nighttime urinary frequency, the patient should be advised to maintain adequate intake during the day to help prevent dehydration. Reducing the intake of high-caffeine fluids and voiding before going to bed are both acceptable means of controlling urinary frequency. The client should also be taught to recognize and report signs of a urinary tract infection.

Client Needs Category—*Health promotion and maintenance*
Client Needs Subcategory—*None*

63. **4.** Wearing low-heeled shoes helps maintain the back in a more proper alignment and may relieve backaches associated with pregnancy. A firm mattress may also help to relieve backaches by providing increased support to the lower back. Sleeping on a heating pad is likely to cause burns and may increase the maternal core temperature, which could harm the fetus. Regular use of pain relievers is contraindicated during pregnancy. Tight-fitting clothes do not usually cause backaches in pregnancy.

Client Needs Category—*Health promotion and maintenance*
Client Needs Subcategory—*None*

64. **1.** Nausea and heartburn, which are common discomforts during pregnancy, are believed to occur because of hormonal changes, decreased gastric motility, and displacement of the stomach and duodenum by the enlarging uterus. Eating frequent small meals, avoiding liquids during meals, and avoiding lying down after meals can prevent or limit nausea and heartburn. Antacid preparations may relieve these discomforts, but they should be taken only under a physician's direction. Fluid and electrolyte imbalances and decreased iron absorption may occur with prolonged use of antacids.

Client Needs Category—*Health promotion and maintenance*
Client Needs Subcategory—*None*

65. **2.** Decreased calcium levels and normal stretching of muscles and tendons cause leg cramps during pregnancy. Stress may also cause muscle cramping. Placing a heating pad on the affected area may help to prevent or relieve the client's leg cramps. Elevating the legs or pointing the toes to the knee (rather than the floor) may also help to relieve leg cramps. Increasing milk rather than protein intake will increase calcium levels. The client should be instructed not to massage her legs because of the danger of clot formation.

Client Needs Category—*Health promotion and maintenance*
Client Needs Subcategory—*None*

66. **1.** Mood swings are common during pregnancy and are related to the hormonal and psychological changes that accompany pregnancy. Mood changes are often unpredictable and can cause tension with the client's partner and within the family. Fatigue and stress decrease normal defenses and may cause or contribute to unpredictable behavior. The nurse should advise the client to avoid becoming fatigued and stressed and to get plenty of sleep. Mood swings produce erratic behavior; a situation that may appear acceptable one minute may be unacceptable the next. Therefore, it is unrealistic to advise the client to avoid interactions as a means of controlling her mood. Asking the client if she has discussed mood swings with her physician and stating concern about her emotional lability implies that there is something abnormal or wrong with the client; therefore, these responses are inappropriate.

Client Needs Category—*Psychosocial integrity*
Client Needs Subcategory—*None*

67. **1.** The nurse is responsible for teaching pregnant clients about signs and symptoms of potentially serious problems or complications associated with pregnancy or delivery. Headache and swelling of the face and fingers are signs of pregnancy-induced hypertension and need to be reported immediately. Constipation, flatulence, muscle cramping, varicosities, and an increase in colorless, odorless vaginal secretions are all uncomfortable during pregnancy; however, they are not generally considered a cause for alarm.

> ***Client Needs Category***—*Health promotion and maintenance*
> ***Client Needs Subcategory***—*None*

High-Risk Factors and Pregnancy

68. 4. A client who is older than age 35 or younger than age 18 is considered at the highest risk for complications during pregnancy. A client who has had more than 4 pregnancies is also considered at risk for complications. A 25-year-old client experiencing her first pregnancy is not typically at an increased risk for complications. Nausea and vomiting are common in the first trimester, and placental attachment to the fundus is normal.

> ***Client Needs Category***—*Physiological integrity*
> ***Client Needs Subcategory***—*Physiological adaptation*

69. 2. There is no known safe amount of alcohol that can be consumed by the mother during pregnancy. The effects of a mother's occasional alcohol consumption on the fetus are unknown. Harmful effects of alcoholism can occur throughout pregnancy, not just in the first trimester. The pregnant woman is encouraged to stop drinking all alcoholic beverages during her pregnancy. Women with alcohol abuse problems are referred to rehabilitation programs.

> ***Client Needs Category***—*Health promotion and maintenance*
> ***Client Needs Subcategory***—*None*

70. 1. A woman who smokes during pregnancy increases the risk of complications for herself and her unborn child. Smoking constricts the blood vessels; during pregnancy, it is linked to premature births, low-birth-weight infants (not overweight ones), spontaneous abortions, and delayed mental and physical development of the child. There is no known association between cigarette smoking and prenatal infections or increased incidence of cesarean births.

> ***Client Needs Category***—*Health promotion and maintenance*
> ***Client Needs Subcategory***—*None*

71. 2. Chorionic villi sampling (CVS) is the preferred procedure for the client because CVS can be done as early as 8 to 11 weeks' gestation. An additional advantage of CVS is that the results are obtained within 1 to 7 days of the procedure. Amniocentesis cannot be performed until the client is between 14 and 20 weeks' gestation, and the results usually are not available for 1½ to 4 weeks. Ultrasound can detect some congenital anomalies, but it is more useful as an adjunct to other tests such as amniocentesis. The rapid plasma reagin test is designed to screen for syphilis and does not detect genetic defects in the fetus.

> ***Client Needs Category***—*Health promotion and maintenance*
> ***Client Needs Subcategory***—*None*

72. 2. Chlamydia is a sexually transmitted disease caused by the bacterium *Chlamydia trachomatis*. A female client with this infection usually presents with a heavy, grayish white discharge and a complaint of intense itching. Pain during urination and intercourse also occurs. Diagnosis is made by culture of the organism; treatment involves administering antibiotics. Erythromycin is the drug of choice during pregnancy. Painful blisters are associated with herpes simplex type 2 virus. A white, curdlike vaginal discharge is associated with candidiasis (yeast infection), while a milky discharge that smells like fish is characteristic of bacterial vaginosis.

> ***Client Needs Category***—*Physiological integrity*
> ***Client Needs Subcategory***—*Physiological adaptation*

73. 2. The pregnant woman with a chlamydial infection requires further teaching if she states that she will need to deliver her baby by cesarean birth. This procedure is unnecessary because antibiotics easily treat the condition. Erythromycin is the drug of choice for pregnant clients, whereas tetracycline is used for nonpregnant clients (tetracycline is harmful to the fetus). Sexual partners of the client with *Chlamydia trachomatis* infection should be treated because this is a sexually transmitted disease. Atypical cells may show up on the Pap smear results.

> ***Client Needs Category***—*Physiological integrity*
> ***Client Needs Subcategory***—*Reduction of risk potential*

74. 3. Bleeding from the vagina may indicate a complication of pregnancy, such as abruptio placentae, spontaneous abortion, or placenta previa. This problem must be brought to the physician's attention immediately. Breast tenderness, fetal movement, and frequent urination are usually normal occurrences during pregnancy and can be discussed with the physician during a routine visit.

> ***Client Needs Category***—*Health promotion and maintenance*
> ***Client Needs Subcategory***—*None*

75. 1. Hyperemesis gravidarum is a serious condition characterized by persistent vomiting. It can result in dehydration and electrolyte imbalances. Severe cases of hyperemesis gravidarum require hospitalization for I.V. therapy to correct the dehydration and electrolyte imbalances. The other equipment identified in this question may be ordered for various other reasons, but it is not routinely used in the care of the client hospitalized for hyperemesis gravidarum.

> **Client Needs Category**—*Physiological integrity*
> **Client Needs Subcategory**—*Pharmacological therapies*

Complications of Pregnancy

76. 4. Pregnant clients with a preexisting disease such as hypertensive disease have an increased risk of developing complications during pregnancy. Pregnant clients who have more than 4 pregnancies are also considered to be at increased risk for complications. A family history of twins does not increase the client's risk of complications. Normal weight gain during pregnancy is between 25 and 35 pounds.

> **Client Needs Category**—*Health promotion and maintenance*
> **Client Needs Subcategory**—*None*

77. 1. Most women work throughout their pregnancy. Therefore, it is important to include work-related guidelines in the pregnant client's care plan, when appropriate. To avoid such complications as venous stasis, advise the client to avoid standing in one place for a prolonged period of time. Also advise her to avoid exposure to toxic substances, working overtime hours, and lifting heavy objects. Teach her to empty her bladder every 2 to 3 hours, wear support stockings, take extra care around equipment that requires balance (such as ladders), and use her lunch hour to rest. All of these measures can help prevent pregnancy-related complications while working.

> **Client Needs Category**—*Health promotion and maintenance*
> **Client Needs Subcategory**—*None*

78. 2. An incompetent cervix dilates prematurely because it is unable to support the weight of the growing fetus. This complication usually occurs during the second trimester of pregnancy. If untreated, an incompetent cervix may result in a spontaneous abortion. None of the remaining options describe this complication.

> **Client Needs Category**—*Health promotion and maintenance*
> **Client Needs Subcategory**—*None*

79. 4. The treatment of choice for a client with an incompetent cervix who is not experiencing labor contractions is the placement of a purse-string suture (cerclage) in the cervix to close the cervical opening. The suture is left in place until the client is near term, when the client may go into labor spontaneously or be a candidate for a cesarean birth.

> **Client Needs Category**—*Physiological integrity*
> **Client Needs Subcategory**—*Reduction of risk potential*

80. 4. The nurse should suspect PIH when a client has any sudden weight gain. Other signs include proteinuria, decreased urine output, and a rise in blood pressure (over 140/90 mm Hg).

> **Client Needs Category**—*Physiological integrity*
> **Client Needs Subcategory**—*Physiological adaptation*

81. 3. Clients experiencing mild PIH will have proteinuria, with a +1 or +2 reading on the urine reagent test strip. Other findings include a 30 mm Hg rise in the baseline systolic blood pressure or a 15 mm Hg rise in the baseline diastolic blood pressure, and a weight gain of 2 or more pounds per week during the second trimester. Edema may be present, but it is usually noted in the face and hands. Ankle edema may be present during pregnancy for reasons other than PIH.

> **Client Needs Category**—*Physiological integrity*
> **Client Needs Subcategory**—*Physiological adaptation*

82. 3. The care of the client with mild PIH can usually be managed at home; however, it is important for the client to return to the physician on a weekly basis. The client also needs to eat a diet high in protein and ensure that she is consuming adequate fluids because of protein loss during urination. She should also be instructed to remain on bed rest. The nurse should teach the client about danger signs, such as seizures, that must be reported to the physician immediately.

> **Client Needs Category**—*Physiological integrity*
> **Client Needs Subcategory**—*Reduction of risk potential*

83. 2. Magnesium sulfate is the drug of choice for treating PIH. In addition to assessing the vital signs, the nurse should check the client's deep tendon reflexes, urine output, fetal heart tones, and serum magnesium blood level. Close monitoring of these measures is necessary to detect the presence of or potential for magnesium toxicity. Glucose in the urine, blood in the stool, and constricted pupils are unrelated to magnesium toxicity.

> **Client Needs Category**—*Physiological integrity*
> **Client Needs Subcategory**—*Pharmacalogical therapies*

84. 4. The antidote for magnesium toxicity is a 10% solution of calcium gluconate (Kalcinate). The medication is usually given I.V. and is injected over 3 or more minutes to prevent the occurrence of ventricular fibrillation. Hydralazine (Apresoline) is an antihypertensive; methylergonovine (Methergine) is usually given to control postpartum bleeding; and oxytocin (Pitocin) is used to augment labor and to control postpartum bleeding.

Client Needs Category—Physiological integrity
Client Needs Subcategory—Pharmacological therapies

85. 2. A respiratory rate of less than 14 breaths/minute is associated with magnesium toxicity. Additional indications of magnesium toxicity include diminished deep tendon reflexes, urine output of less than 100 mL in 4 hours, signs of fetal distress, and a magnesium serum level above 10 mg/dL. If any of these occur, magnesium sulfate should be discontinued and the physician notified immediately.

Client Needs Category—Physiological integrity
Client Needs Subcategory—Physiological adaptation

86. 1. The client with PIH is said to have developed eclampsia if she begins to have seizures. Severe headache, abdominal pain, muscle hyperirritability, apprehension, and twitching often precede seizures associated with eclampsia. The other signs and symptoms listed are not manifestations of eclampsia.

Client Needs Category—Physiological integrity
Client Needs Subcategory—Physiological adaptation

87. 4. Vaginal bleeding and abdominal cramping or backaches are typical symptoms that clients report with the occurrence of a spontaneous abortion. Severe headaches and persistent tachycardia are not normal and should be reported to the health care provider, but someone experiencing a spontaneous abortion does not usually manifest these symptoms. Cold, clammy skin is also not associated with spontaneous abortion.

Client Needs Category—Physiological integrity
Client Needs Subcategory—Physiological adaptation

88. 1. When the cervix is dilated but the fetus and placenta remain in the uterus, spontaneous abortion is inevitable and the client will more than likely require a D&C to remove the remaining products of conception. The client should be prepared physically and emotionally for the procedure. The other options are not usually included in the care of the client experiencing an inevitable spontaneous abortion.

Client Needs Category—Physiological integrity
Client Needs Subcategory—Physiological adaptation

89. 1. An inevitable spontaneous abortion means that there is no hope of saving the fetus. The nurse must be honest with the client and provide much-needed emotional support. The client and family members are encouraged to verbalize their feelings to facilitate their abilities to cope with the situation. Telling the client that the outcome is uncertain at this point is untrue. Suggesting that the client remain calm and to avoid stress does not facilitate expression of her feelings and hinders her ability to cope with the situation. Telling the client that things will work out for the best does not acknowledge the justifiable sorrow that the client is experiencing. It also does not show much-needed emotional support.

Client Needs Category—Psychosocial integrity
Client Needs Subcategory—None

90. 3. The insulin requirement for the pregnant diabetic client will fluctuate during pregnancy. During the first 18 weeks of pregnancy, the need for insulin decreases because the mother is transporting increased amounts of glucose to the growing fetus. Later in pregnancy, the need for insulin usually increases because increasing amounts of hormones cause insulin resistance in the client. During the postpartum period, the hormone levels drop, thereby decreasing the need for insulin.

Client Needs Category—Physiological integrity
Client Needs Subcategory—Pharmacological therapies

91. 2. The pregnant diabetic client has an increased risk of developing pregnancy-induced hypertension. Some other complications that may occur secondary to diabetes during pregnancy include infection, hydramnios, possible birth trauma related to the size of the fetus, and postpartum hemorrhage. Hyperemesis gravidarum, placenta previa, and toxoplasmosis are not associated with diabetes during pregnancy.

Client Needs Category—Physiological integrity
Client Needs Subcategory—Physiological adaptation

92. 1. The pregnant diabetic client is at greatest risk for having a baby that is larger than average in both size and weight. Because hypoglycemia is a complication, the baby will require frequent blood glucose testing for the first several hours. Other fetal effects of diabetes include congenital anomalies, prematurity, and respiratory distress syndrome. However, a client whose diabetes is well controlled during pregnancy rarely experiences the other fetal effects listed here.

Client Needs Category—Health promotion and maintenance
Client Needs Subcategory—None

93. **1.** Placenta previa is a condition in which the placenta totally (complete or total placenta previa) or partially (partial placenta previa) covers the cervical os (opening) or the placenta is implanted low in the uterus (marginal placenta previa) without covering any part of the os. The painless bleeding associated with placenta previa is due to a separation of the placenta from the uterus in the area that is near or covers the cervical os. The separation is caused by normal cervical changes that occur in preparation for labor. Placenta previa is unrelated to the development of polyps, hormonal deficiencies, or antibody production.

> *Client Needs Category*—*Physiological integrity*
> *Client Needs Subcategory*—*Physiological adaptation*

94. **3.** The preferred course of treatment is to maintain the pregnancy as close to term as possible. If the client is stable, the physician usually orders bed rest and continuous client observation. With marginal or partial placenta previa, vaginal birth is possible. Uncontrolled hemorrhaging, fetal distress, or complete placenta previa requires immediate delivery of the baby, usually by cesarean birth. Ritodrine (Yutopar) is indicated for premature labor; however, this medication is not routinely used for clients with placenta previa.

> *Client Needs Category*—*Physiological integrity*
> *Client Needs Subcategory*—*Reduction of risk potential*

95. **2.** Because of changes in the cervix during the second and third trimesters, the placenta begins to detach from the uterine wall, resulting in painless vaginal bleeding. Placenta previa is the most common cause of bleeding during the second and third trimesters of pregnancy. Sharp abdominal pain, persistent headache, and continuous, painless contractions are not associated with placenta previa.

> *Client Needs Category*—*Physiological integrity*
> *Client Needs Subcategory*—*Physiological adaptation*

96. **2.** The client with placenta previa is at risk for hemorrhaging and shock. Therefore, a baseline blood pressure measurement and a pulse rate should be obtained so that those involved in the client's care can evaluate further changes. Significant findings can also be reported to the physician in a timely manner. When a client is admitted to the hospital, the client's height and weight as well as her obstetric, general health, and drug histories are obtained. In this situation, obtaining the client's blood pressure and pulse takes priority over admittance information.

> *Client Needs Category*—*Physiological integrity*
> *Client Needs Subcategory*—*Physiological adaptation*

97. **4.** The client with pregnancy-induced hypertension is at risk for developing abruptio placentae. Other factors associated with the occurrence of abruptio placentae include essential hypertension, previous history of placenta previa, dietary deficiencies, trauma to the abdomen, multiparity, and a history of alcohol or drug abuse. Gestational diabetes, hyperemesis gravidarum, and oligohydramnios are not associated with abruptio placentae.

> *Client Needs Category*—*Physiological integrity*
> *Client Needs Subcategory*—*Physiological adaptation*

98. **1.** Abruptio placentae is characterized by premature detachment of the placenta from the uterus. The bleeding associated with the detachment may be obvious or concealed. A rigid, boardlike abdomen is commonly observed in clients with concealed hemorrhaging. Other signs and symptoms of abruptio placentae include severe abdominal pain, dark red vaginal bleeding, maternal shock, and fetal distress with a heart rate less than 100 beats/minute. Severe nausea and vomiting and painless vaginal bleeding are not manifestations of abruptio placentae.

> *Client Needs Category*—*Physiological integrity*
> *Client Needs Subcategory*—*Physiological adaptation*

99. **1.** A complete abruption requires emergency cesarean birth. Written consent should be obtained immediately from the client or a family member. A client with vaginal bleeding is not given an enema. A client with a complete abruption is not usually placed in Trendelenburg's position. A contraction stress test is inappropriate for a client with any type of abruption.

> *Client Needs Category*—*Safe, effective care environment*
> *Client Needs Subcategory*—*None*

100. **2.** Exposure to rubella (German measles) during the first trimester of pregnancy increases the risk of the fetus developing congenital rubella syndrome. Major manifestations of this congenital condition include blindness, deafness, heart defects, mental retardation, cleft lip, and cleft palate. Premature labor, severe preeclampsia, and hydatidiform moles are not associated with rubella exposure.

> *Client Needs Category*—*Health promotion and maintenance*
> *Client Needs Subcategory*—*None*

101. **4.** A hydatidiform mole occurs when the chorionic membrane starts to deteriorate. This results in numerous clear vesicles resembling grapes. A hydatidiform mole is suspected when there is abnormally rapid uterine growth resulting in a uterus that is larger than expected for the woman's gestational dates. This condition is also suspected when fetal heart tones and fetal movement are not detected, when there is excessive or persistent nausea and vomiting, and when pregnancy-induced hypertension develops prior to 20 to 24 weeks' gestation. Vaginal bleeding may be continuous or intermittent and the human chorionic gonadotropin level is greatly elevated. A blotchy brown discoloration to the face (chloasma) is not associated with this condition. A positive Chadwick's sign refers to the purple coloring of the vulva and vagina early in pregnancy; this is a normal finding. Ballottement is a normal indication of pregnancy occurring between the 16th and 20th week of gestation; it is elicited when the examiner taps the uterus and the fetus floats to the top of the uterus, then back down.

> ***Client Needs Category***—*Physiological integrity*
> ***Client Needs Subcategory***—*Physiological adaptation*

102. 3. The U.S. Centers for Disease Control and Prevention recommends that pregnant women who are at risk for hepatitis B virus be tested during pregnancy. High-risk groups include women of Asian, Pacific Island, Alaskan Eskimo, and Haitian descent; recipients of repeated blood transfusions; I.V. drug users or partners of I.V. drug users; women who have been exposed to hepatitis B; and women who have multiple sex partners. Hepatitis B testing is not necessary for clients who smoke, who are single and pregnant for the first time, or who have been exposed to *H. influenzae*.

> ***Client Needs Category***—*Health promotion and maintenance*
> ***Client Needs Subcategory***—*None*

Elective Abortion

103. 3. During the first trimester of pregnancy, a woman has the right to have an abortion without legal restraints. During the second trimester, states can regulate the conditions under which an abortion is performed but cannot prohibit abortion. After viability, which according to legal guidelines is considered after 20 to 24 weeks' gestation, the state may, and usually does, prohibit abortion except in a situation that is perceived as a threat to the life or health of the pregnant woman.

> ***Client Needs Category***—*Health promotion and maintenance*
> ***Client Needs Subcategory***—*None*

The Nursing Care of Clients During the Intrapartum and Postpartum Periods

⇨ Admission of the Client to a Labor and Delivery Facility
⇨ Nursing Care of Clients During the First Stage of Labor
⇨ Nursing Care of Clients During the Second Stage of Labor
⇨ Nursing Care of Clients During the Third Stage of Labor
⇨ Nursing Care of Clients During the Fourth Stage of Labor
⇨ Nursing Care of Clients Having a Cesarean Birth
⇨ Nursing Care of Clients Having an Emergency Delivery
⇨ Nursing Care of Clients Having a Stillborn Baby
⇨ Nursing Care of Clients During the Postpartum Period
⇨ Nursing Care of the Newborn Client
⇨ Nursing Care of Newborns with Complications
⇨ Correct Answers and Rationales

Directions: *With a pencil, blacken the space in front of the option you have chosen for your correct answer.*

Admission of the Client to a Labor and Delivery Facility

A 25-year-old primigravid client in her last trimester of pregnancy calls the physician's office and tells the nurse that she thinks she is in labor.

1. Which finding would warrant instructing the client to notify the physician and report to the hospital's labor and delivery unit immediately?
[ ] **1.** The client is having contractions every 10 minutes.
[ ] **2.** The client feels a sudden burst of energy.
[ ] **3.** The client experiences a sudden gush of fluid from her vagina.
[ ] **4.** The client experiences urinary frequency.

The client arrives at the hospital and is admitted to the labor, delivery, recovery, and postpartum (LDRP) unit. The nurse obtains the client's health and pregnancy history.

2. As the nurse collects the client's history, which question has the lowest priority?
[ ] **1.** "When did you last eat?"
[ ] **2.** "Have you ever had an enema?"
[ ] **3.** "When did your contractions start?"
[ ] **4.** "When is your baby due?"

The client informs the nurse that she was admitted to the unit 3 days ago but that turned out to be a "false labor."

3. Which statement made by the client indicates an understanding of Braxton Hicks contractions?
[ ] **1.** "The contractions are less strong when I walk."
[ ] **2.** "The contractions are regular and I can time them."
[ ] **3.** "The contractions get stronger no matter what I am doing."
[ ] **4.** "The contractions start in my lower back."

During the admission process, the nurse obtains the client's vital signs.

4. When is the most appropriate time to take the client's vital signs?
[ ]   **1.** At the peak of a contraction, with the client positioned on her left side
[ ]   **2.** At the peak of a contraction, with the client positioned on her right side
[ ]   **3.** Between contractions, with the client positioned on her right side
[ ]   **4.** Between contractions, with the client positioned on her left side

Nursing Care of Clients During the First Stage of Labor

A 30-year-old primigravid client is admitted to the LDRP unit of a local hospital. The physician plans to perform a vaginal examination to determine the status of her labor.

5. How can the nurse best prepare to assist with the vaginal examination?
[ ]   **1.** By having sterile gloves available for the examiner
[ ]   **2.** By placing the client in the left side-lying position
[ ]   **3.** By instructing the client to hold her breath during the examination
[ ]   **4.** By giving the client an enema before the examination is performed

After the vaginal examination, the physician indicates that the client is in the latent phase of the first stage of labor. A progress note is written in the client's admission records.

6. When the nurse reviews the client's admission records, which assessment finding is the most reliable indicator that the client is in true labor?
[ ]   **1.** Contractions are regular and increasing in duration and intensity
[ ]   **2.** Contractions radiate from the lower back to the lower abdomen
[ ]   **3.** Bloody show is present
[ ]   **4.** The cervix is dilating

7. During the latent phase, which finding can the nurse expect when assessing the client?
[ ]   **1.** Contractions occurring every 3 to 5 minutes
[ ]   **2.** Fetal heart rate of 120 to 160 beats/minute
[ ]   **3.** Bulging perineum
[ ]   **4.** Early decelerations

8. During the latent phase of labor, which instruction given by the nurse to the client is most appropriate?

[ ]   **1.** "Remain in bed on your left side."
[ ]   **2.** "Keep drinking clear fluids."
[ ]   **3.** "Pant when you experience a contraction."
[ ]   **4.** "Avoid bathing until after the delivery."

9. During the latent phase of the first stage of labor, how often should the nurse plan to assess the fetal heart rate?
[ ]   **1.** Every 5 minutes
[ ]   **2.** Every 15 minutes
[ ]   **3.** Every 30 minutes
[ ]   **4.** Every 60 minutes

The client tells the nurse that she plans to have an epidural for pain management and asks the nurse when she can expect to receive it.

10. An epidural is best performed when the client is how many centimeters dilated?
[ ]   **1.** 3 to 4
[ ]   **2.** 5 to 6
[ ]   **3.** 7 to 8
[ ]   **4.** 9 to 10

The registered nurse performs a vaginal examination of the client. The nurse determines that the labor is progressing and the cervix is dilated 6 centimeters.

11. When assessing the frequency and duration of the client's contractions during this phase of labor, the nurse expects to find that the contractions are occurring every 3 to 5 minutes and lasting up to how many seconds?
[ ]   **1.** 30
[ ]   **2.** 40
[ ]   **3.** 60
[ ]   **4.** 90

Labor has progressed, and the client enters the transition phase of the first stage of labor.

12. Which assessment finding can the nurse expect to observe during this phase?
[ ]   **1.** Cervix dilated to 10 centimeters
[ ]   **2.** Crowning of the presenting part
[ ]   **3.** Increased bloody show
[ ]   **4.** Contractions lasting up to 60 seconds

13. Which nursing action best meets the client's needs during the transition phase?
[ ]   **1.** Encouraging the client to ambulate
[ ]   **2.** Praising the client frequently
[ ]   **3.** Instructing the client to push with each contraction
[ ]   **4.** Massaging the client's back between contractions

A 29-year-old multiparous client who has had an uneventful healthy pregnancy is admitted to the hospital. The physician informs the client that she is in the active phase of the first stage of labor. The records also show that the full-term baby is in the left occipitoposterior (LOP) position.

14. When the fetus is in the LOP position, which nursing intervention is most appropriate?
[ ] **1.** Assisting the client to the knee-chest position to relieve her back pain
[ ] **2.** Placing the client in Trendelenburg's position to prevent cord prolapse
[ ] **3.** Assisting with preparation of equipment for a precipitous delivery
[ ] **4.** Having the client void frequently to minimize displacement of the uterus

15. To prevent distention of the client's bladder during the active phase of labor, which nursing intervention is most appropriate?
[ ] **1.** Instructing the client to limit her fluid intake
[ ] **2.** Decreasing the rate of the I.V. infusion
[ ] **3.** Offering solid foods instead of liquids
[ ] **4.** Encouraging the client to void every 2 hours

16. To correctly assess the duration of a contraction, the nurse counts the time between which intervals?
[ ] **1.** The beginning of one contraction and the end of the same contraction
[ ] **2.** The end of one contraction and the beginning of the next contraction
[ ] **3.** The beginning of one contraction and the end of the next contraction
[ ] **4.** The beginning of one contraction and the beginning of the next contraction

17. Which method is most accurate when assessing the client's contractions?
[ ] **1.** Place the hand over the fundus of the uterus, which is located just above the umbilicus.
[ ] **2.** Place the hand over the corpus of the uterus, which is located just above the umbilicus.
[ ] **3.** Place the hand over the fundus of the uterus, which is located midway between the umbilicus and the symphysis pubis.
[ ] **4.** Place the hand over the corpus of the uterus, which is located midway between the umbilicus and the symphysis pubis.

18. How often should the nurse assess fetal heart rate during the active phase of labor?
[ ] **1.** Every 5 minutes
[ ] **2.** Every 10 minutes
[ ] **3.** Every 15 minutes
[ ] **4.** Every 30 minutes

The client tells the nurse that she thinks her membranes have ruptured. The nurse performs a nitrazine test and confirms that the membranes have ruptured.

19. Which test result indicates that the membranes have ruptured?
[ ] **1.** The test strip turns blue.
[ ] **2.** The test strip turns yellow.
[ ] **3.** The test strip turns red.
[ ] **4.** The test strip turns green.

20. Which action should the nurse perform immediately after the membranes are ruptured?
[ ] **1.** Check the client's pulse.
[ ] **2.** Insert an indwelling catheter.
[ ] **3.** Perform a vaginal examination.
[ ] **4.** Check the fetal heart rate.

21. After the membranes have ruptured, how often should the nurse take the client's temperature?
[ ] **1.** Every hour
[ ] **2.** Every 2 hours
[ ] **3.** Every 3 hours
[ ] **4.** Every 4 hours

Because the nitrazine test results indicate that the membranes have ruptured, the physician orders internal electronic fetal monitoring. The client asks the nurse, "Is there any danger of this procedure causing harm to my baby?"

22. Which response by the nurse provides the best explanation of internal electronic fetal monitoring?
[ ] **1.** "The procedure requires attachment of a small spiral electrode to the fetal scalp and poses a slight risk of soft-tissue injury and infection."
[ ] **2.** "The procedure requires insertion of a soft, water-filled catheter into the uterus and poses no risk of injury to you or your baby."
[ ] **3.** "The procedure requires placement of an ultrasound transducer over your abdomen and poses no risk to you or your baby."
[ ] **4.** "The procedure requires application of a suction cup to the fetal scalp and poses a slight risk for the development of a hematoma."

23. Which assessment finding is most indicative of fetal distress?
[ ] **1.** Fetal heart rate of 140 beats/minute
[ ] **2.** Presence of fetal heart rate accelerations
[ ] **3.** Presence of green amniotic fluid
[ ] **4.** Increased amount of bloody show

The client continues in active labor and tells the nurse that she has not had anything to eat for 24 hours and would like something to eat now.

24. Which response by the nurse best explains why solid food is not given at this time?
[ ] **1.** "It may alter the absorption of regional anesthetics."
[ ] **2.** "It may alter the duration and frequency of contractions."
[ ] **3.** "It may cause fetal distress."
[ ] **4.** "It may cause nausea and vomiting."

After a sterile vaginal examination is performed, the client tells the nurse she heard the physician say that her baby is in the vertex position. The client asks the nurse what this means.

25. Which response by the nurse provides the best explanation regarding vertex positioning?
[ ] **1.** "The head is entering the birth canal first."
[ ] **2.** "The feet are entering the birth canal first."
[ ] **3.** "The buttocks are entering the birth canal first."
[ ] **4.** "The shoulder is entering the birth canal first."

26. During evaluation of the client's contractions during the active phase of the first stage of labor, when is it important for the nurse to notify the physician?
[ ] **1.** When the contractions occur every 3 to 5 minutes
[ ] **2.** When the contractions last longer than 45 seconds
[ ] **3.** When the uterus relaxes between contractions
[ ] **4.** When the fetal heart rate drops after the acme of a contraction

The nurse is caring for a client in preterm labor. The physician writes an order for terbutaline sulfate (Brethine).

27. When is it necessary for the nurse to withhold the terbutaline sulfate (Brethine) and notify the physician?
[ ] **1.** When the electronic monitor reveals that the client is having mild contractions
[ ] **2.** When the cervix is dilated 4 centimeters or greater or effaced 50% or more
[ ] **3.** When the electronic monitor reveals the presence of fetal heart rate variability
[ ] **4.** When the client states that the contractions are milder and occurring less frequently

Nursing Care of Clients During the Second Stage of Labor

The nurse cares for a 30-year-old multiparous client who is in the transition phase of the first stage of labor.

28. Which assessment finding best indicates that the client has entered the second stage of labor?
[ ] **1.** The perineum is bulging.
[ ] **2.** Contractions are lasting 30 to 60 seconds.
[ ] **3.** The cervix is dilated to 8 centimeters.
[ ] **4.** The uterus is at the level of the umbilicus.

29. When should the nurse begin delivery preparations for this client?
[ ] **1.** When the client is about 7 centimeters dilated
[ ] **2.** When the fetal head begins to crown
[ ] **3.** When the physician or midwife arrives
[ ] **4.** When the client is completely dilated

The client tells the nurse that she feels the urge to push.

30. Which action should the nurse take initially?
[ ] **1.** Instruct the client to push when she feels the next contraction.
[ ] **2.** Ensure that the client is in semi-Fowler's position.
[ ] **3.** Ensure that the client's cervix is fully dilated.
[ ] **4.** Instruct the client to take a cleansing breath before pushing.

The client complains of pain and asks the nurse, "Can I have some more Nubain?"

31. The nurse correctly explains that nalbuphine hydrochloride (Nubain) is not given at this time because opioid analgesics during this stage of labor may have which effect?
[ ] **1.** Decrease the effectiveness of the contractions
[ ] **2.** Cause the uterus to rupture
[ ] **3.** Result in respiratory depression in the newborn
[ ] **4.** Cause increased fetal activity

The obstetrician prepares for delivery and requests that the client be prepared for a saddle (subarachnoid) block.

32. The nurse is aware that, with this type of medication, the anesthetic will take how long to become effective?
[ ] **1.** Immediately
[ ] **2.** In 10 to 20 minutes
[ ] **3.** In 30 to 40 minutes
[ ] **4.** In approximately 1 hour

33. The nurse assesses for which complication during the immediate postprocedural period?
[ ] **1.** Maternal hypotension
[ ] **2.** Fetal tachycardia
[ ] **3.** Spinal headache
[ ] **4.** Lower extremity paralysis

34. Which modification to the client's care plan is required after the client has undergone the saddle block?
[ ] **1.** Oxygen is administered.
[ ] **2.** The nurse instructs the client when to push.
[ ] **3.** Oxytocin (Pitocin) is administered to augment labor.
[ ] **4.** The client is catheterized.

35. Which sequence should the nurse follow when cleaning the client's perineum in preparation for delivery of the baby?
[ ] **1.** Pubic bone to lower abdomen, both inner thighs, right and left labia, vagina to anus
[ ] **2.** Vagina to anus, right and left labia, both inner thighs, pubic bone to lower abdomen
[ ] **3.** Both inner thighs, right and left labia, vagina to anus, pubic bone to lower abdomen
[ ] **4.** Left and right labia, vagina to anus, both inner thighs, pubic bone to lower abdomen

The physician informs the client that she needs to have an episiotomy. The client begins to cry and asks the nurse, "Why do I have to have an episiotomy?"

36. Which response by the nurse best explains the need for an episiotomy?
[ ] **1.** "An episiotomy is necessary to prevent uterine rupture."
[ ] **2.** "An episiotomy is necessary to prevent postpartum infection."
[ ] **3.** "An episiotomy is necessary to prevent perineal laceration."
[ ] **4.** "An episiotomy is necessary to prevent bowel trauma."

Nursing Care of Clients During the Third Stage of Labor

A 31-year-old client just delivered a healthy baby girl. The nurse tells the father that the infant will receive an injection of vitamin K (AquaMEPHYTON) and erythromycin (Ilotycin) eye ointment.

37. To meet the infant's priority needs immediately after delivery, which of the following equipment should the nurse have ready?
[ ] **1.** Cord clamp
[ ] **2.** Warm blanket
[ ] **3.** Bulb syringe
[ ] **4.** Oxygen supply

The newborn is assigned an Apgar score of 7 at 5 minutes.

38. Based on the baby's Apgar score, the nurse anticipates providing care for a newborn in what condition?
[ ] **1.** Severely distressed
[ ] **2.** Moderately distressed
[ ] **3.** Stable but requiring close monitoring
[ ] **4.** Vigorous with no signs of distress

39. To best facilitate mother-infant attachment and prevent the newborn from developing distress, what should the nurse do initially?
[ ] **1.** Give the newborn to the mother immediately after initial care is given in the delivery room.
[ ] **2.** Immediately dry the newborn, then place her skin-to-skin on the mother's abdomen.
[ ] **3.** Place the newborn in a radiant warmer for 5 minutes, then wrap her and give her to the mother.
[ ] **4.** Place the newborn in the radiant warmer, and position the warmer so the mother can see her.

40. When preparing to administer the vitamin K (AquaMEPHYTON), the nurse chooses which site for injection?
[ ] **1.** Ventrogluteal muscle
[ ] **2.** Deltoid muscle
[ ] **3.** Vastus lateralis muscle
[ ] **4.** Gluteus maximus muscle

41. The nurse correctly explains to the father that vitamin K (AquaMEPHYTON) is given for what reason?
[ ] **1.** To stimulate respirations
[ ] **2.** To start peristaltic movements
[ ] **3.** To decrease the risk for hemorrhage
[ ] **4.** To increase calcium absorption

42. The nurse explains to the father that erythromycin (Ilotycin) is given to protect the infant from neonatal blindness, which can occur if the infant develops an eye infection caused by which organisms?
[ ] **1.** Gonococcal and chlamydial organisms
[ ] **2.** Gonococcal and streptococcal organisms
[ ] **3.** Gonococcal organisms and *Candida albicans*
[ ] **4.** Gonococcal organisms and *Pneumocystis carinii*

43. After instillation of the eye ointment, the nurse informs the father that his baby may experience which of the following?
[ ] **1.** Swelling of the eyes
[ ] **2.** Temporary blurred vision
[ ] **3.** Purulent eye drainage
[ ] **4.** Conjunctival hemorrhage

The patient care technician weighs the newborn.

44. Which action by the technician indicates a need for additional teaching regarding accurate and safe assessment of the newborn's weight?
[ ] **1.** The technician undresses the newborn before obtaining the weight.
[ ] **2.** The technician places a diaper or paper barrier on the scale before balancing it.
[ ] **3.** The technician keeps one hand on the newborn while obtaining the weight.
[ ] **4.** The technician cleans the scale with an antiseptic before using it.

45. Which intervention is most important for the nurse to implement before transporting the newborn from the delivery area to the nursery?
[ ] **1.** Placing matching identification bracelets on mother and baby
[ ] **2.** Administering prophylactic eye medication
[ ] **3.** Giving I.M. vitamin K (AquaMEPHYTON)
[ ] **4.** Obtaining a blood sample for phenylketonuria (PKU) testing

Nursing Care of Clients During the Fourth Stage of Labor

The nurse observes the client for signs of impending delivery of the placenta.

46. To facilitate delivery of the placenta, what should the nurse instruct the client to do?
[ ] **1.** Turn on her right or left side.
[ ] **2.** Breathe slowly and deeply.
[ ] **3.** Tighten and relax the perineum intermittently.
[ ] **4.** Push when she feels a contraction occurring.

47. Which observation regarding the delivery of the placenta should the nurse report to the physician?
[ ] **1.** Bulging perineum
[ ] **2.** Shortening of the umbilical cord
[ ] **3.** Rise of the fundus in the abdomen
[ ] **4.** Decreased vaginal discharge

Just after the delivery of the placenta, the client complains of uncontrollable shaking and of being cold.

48. Which action by the nurse is most appropriate at this time?
[ ] **1.** Explaining that the shaking is normal
[ ] **2.** Placing a warmed blanket over the client
[ ] **3.** Suggesting that the client try not to think about the shaking
[ ] **4.** Notifying the physician or nurse-midwife

49. At which location can the nurse expect to palpate the fundus of the uterus immediately after delivery?
[ ] **1.** At or just below the level of the umbilicus
[ ] **2.** Just above the level of the umbilicus
[ ] **3.** Just above the level of the symphysis pubis
[ ] **4.** Midway between the umbilicus and symphysis pubis

50. When performing postpartal checks just after delivery, which assessment finding should the nurse report immediately?
[ ] **1.** A pulse rate between 70 and 80 beats/minute
[ ] **2.** Presence of dark red, fleshy-smelling lochia
[ ] **3.** Saturation of one perineal pad per hour
[ ] **4.** A systolic blood pressure less than 90 mm Hg

The placenta is delivered and the physician sutures the episiotomy. The physician instructs the nurse to add oxytocin (Pitocin) to the client's I.V. fluids. The client asks the nurse why she has to have this drug.

51. The nurse explains that oxytocin (Pitocin) is given after delivery of the baby and placenta for which purpose?
[ ] **1.** To increase the blood pressure
[ ] **2.** To prevent the uterus from inverting
[ ] **3.** To decrease the likelihood of hemorrhage
[ ] **4.** To prevent rupture of the uterus

Nursing Care of Clients Having a Cesarean Birth

A 26-year-old gravida I client is admitted to the hospital in active labor. The physician examines the client and determines that she has cephalopelvic disproportion. A cesarean birth using epidural anesthesia is scheduled. The physician orders the insertion of an indwelling urinary catheter before surgery. The client asks the nurse why she needs a urinary catheter.

52. Which response by the nurse regarding the placement of the indwelling catheter is most accurate?
[ ] **1.** "It will prevent the development of postpartum hemorrhaging."
[ ] **2.** "It needs to be inserted to keep the bladder empty during the surgical procedure."
[ ] **3.** "It's used as a landmark for the physician during surgery."
[ ] **4.** "It's inserted to provide a safe way of collecting urine specimens."

The client asks the nurse if she will feel any pain while the surgery is performed.

53. Which response by the nurse regarding the client's pain is most appropriate?
[ ] **1.** "You may experience pressure, but you will not feel any pain during the procedure."
[ ] **2.** "You may experience a brief sting when the first incision is made."
[ ] **3.** "You won't remember anything about the procedure because you will be asleep."
[ ] **4.** "You won't feel any pain once the anesthesia takes effect."

The client's husband asks the nurse if he can remain with his wife during the cesarean birth.

54. Which statement by the nurse is most appropriate in response to the husband's request?
[ ] **1.** "Only your wife and surgical personnel are allowed in the operating room because of the need to maintain a sterile environment."
[ ] **2.** "You'll be allowed to join your wife in the operating room only after the baby has been delivered and your wife and baby are stable."
[ ] **3.** "You'll be allowed to join your wife in the operating room after you change into the appropriate attire."
[ ] **4.** "You'll be allowed to join your wife when she is transferred to the recovery area and she is no longer under the influence of the anesthesia."

The client is transferred to the operating room. The physician plans to perform a lower-segment transverse incision and requests that the nurse perform surgical skin preparation.

55. Which method of cleansing the abdomen is most appropriate?
[ ] **1.** The nurse cleanses the entire abdomen beginning at the level of the nipple line.
[ ] **2.** The nurse cleanses the entire abdomen beginning at the top of the uterine fundus.
[ ] **3.** The nurse cleanses the entire abdomen beginning at the level of the umbilicus.
[ ] **4.** The nurse cleanses the entire abdomen beginning 6″ (15 cm) above the mons pubis.

The cesarean birth is performed without complications. About 1½ hours after surgery, the client is transferred in stable condition to the postpartum unit. The abdominal dressing is dry and intact, the indwelling catheter is patent and draining clear yellow urine, and I.V. fluids are infusing at the prescribed rate. The client also has a continuous infusion of epidural morphine sulfate.

56. While the client is receiving epidural morphine sulfate, the nurse closely monitors the client for which adverse reaction?
[ ] **1.** Urinary incontinence
[ ] **2.** Pupil dilation
[ ] **3.** Respiratory depression
[ ] **4.** Elevated blood pressure

57. Which medication should the nurse plan to have readily available while the client is receiving epidural morphine sulfate?
[ ] **1.** Buprenorphine hydrochloride (Buprenex)
[ ] **2.** Calcium gluconate (Calsan)
[ ] **3.** Atropine sulfate (Atropair)
[ ] **4.** Naloxone hydrochloride (Narcan)

Twenty-four hours after surgery, the physician writes orders to discontinue the morphine epidural, I.V. therapy, and indwelling catheter and to administer meperidine hydrochloride (Demerol) 50 mg P.O. every 3 to 4 hours p.r.n. for pain. The physician also removes the abdominal dressing and tells the client that she may shower and get out of bed.

58. Which assessment finding best indicates the presence of infection of the abdominal incision line?
[ ] **1.** The client states that the incision line feels numb.
[ ] **2.** The client's oral temperature is 99° F (37.2° C).
[ ] **3.** The incision line is approximated.
[ ] **4.** The incision line is red and swollen.

The day after surgery, the client complains of abdominal pain and bloating. The nurse notes that the client's abdomen is distended.

59. Which intervention is most appropriate to relieve the client's discomfort?
[ ] **1.** Assist the client to ambulate in the hall.
[ ] **2.** Insert a rectal tube to monitor bowel function.
[ ] **3.** Administer the prescribed pain medication.
[ ] **4.** Instruct the client to use a straw when drinking fluids.

The client tells the nurse that she is disappointed that she had to deliver by cesarean section. She asks the nurse, "If I have another baby, will I have to have another cesarean?"

60. Which response by the nurse is most accurate regarding a vaginal birth after a cesarean birth (VBAC)?
[ ] **1.** "It may be possible to have a vaginal birth after a cesarean birth if the previous cesarean incision was a classical incision."
[ ] **2.** "A vaginal birth is not recommended after a cesarean birth because of the danger of uterine rupture."
[ ] **3.** "A vaginal birth is just as painful as a cesarean birth because an episiotomy has to be performed."
[ ] **4.** "A vaginal birth after a cesarean birth may be possible if there is no history of medical conditions that prohibit it."

Nursing Care of Clients Having an Emergency Delivery

A 25-year-old primigravid client is in the active phase of the first stage of labor when her membranes rupture. The nurse notes a decrease in the fetal heart tones on the electronic monitor. Upon inspection of the perineum, the nurse observes that the umbilical cord is protruding through the vagina.

61. Which action is most appropriate for the nurse to take initially?
[ ] **1.** Turn the client on her left side and administer oxygen.
[ ] **2.** Notify the physician of the findings.
[ ] **3.** Place the client in Trendelenburg's position.
[ ] **4.** Prepare a sterile field for delivery of the baby.

A 32-year-old client with a history of precipitous labor is admitted to the hospital. She states that her contractions are occurring every 2 to 3 minutes. When the nurse observes the client's perineum, she notes that the baby's head is crowning. The nurse is alone with the client and unable to obtain assistance.

62. At this point, what is most appropriate for the nurse to do after putting on sterile gloves?
[ ] **1.** Gently place one hand on the crowning head, and allow the head to emerge slowly between contractions.
[ ] **2.** Push back firmly on the head, and place pressure on the vaginal meatus until the physician arrives.

[ ] **3.** Place a sterile towel over the perineal area, and have the client bring her legs close together.
[ ] **4.** Slide a finger into the vagina, and enlarge its exit while delivering the head during a contraction.

Nursing Care of Clients Having a Stillborn Baby

A 26-year-old primigravid client at 40 weeks' gestation is admitted to the hospital with a possible fetal demise. The nurse is unable to detect a fetal heartbeat using the external fetal monitor. The physician examines the client and determines that the fetus is dead. An infusion of oxytocin (Pitocin) is ordered for induction of labor. The client is crying and tells the nurse, "This can't be true. You must have made a mistake."

63. Which nursing intervention is most appropriate at this time?
[ ] **1.** Recheck the fetal heart tones with the electronic external fetal monitor so that the client can listen.
[ ] **2.** Express sorrow about the client's loss and encourage the client to express her feelings.
[ ] **3.** Redirect the client's attention to the laboring process and the correct use of breathing techniques.
[ ] **4.** Explain that the baby probably would have been born with severe long-term health problems.

The baby is delivered stillborn. The client's condition is stabilized, and she is transferred to a private room on a wing adjacent to the LDRP unit. The client's husband is present. The client asks the nurse if she can see her baby.

64. Which action is most appropriate for the nurse to take at this time?
[ ] **1.** Prepare a memory packet, including such items as a picture of the baby and footprints, and give it to the client.
[ ] **2.** Bring the infant to the client and her husband, and allow them to visit with the baby privately.
[ ] **3.** Encourage the client to postpone viewing the baby until she and her husband have had an opportunity to receive counseling.
[ ] **4.** Bring the infant to the client and her husband, but do not allow the parents to hold or touch the infant.

Nursing Care of Clients During the Postpartum Period

65. Which finding would the nurse consider abnormal for the postpartum client who delivered within the past 24 hours?
[ ] 1. The client states that she passed a couple of nickel-sized clots.
[ ] 2. The client complains of calf pain when her foot is dorsiflexed.
[ ] 3. The client complains of abdominal cramping while breast-feeding.
[ ] 4. The client states that her vaginal discharge is dark red.

66. In order to prevent hemorrhage, when should the nurse massage the fundus during the postpartal period?
[ ] 1. When the fundus is firm and hard
[ ] 2. When the fundus is at the level of the umbilicus
[ ] 3. When the amount of lochia flow decreases
[ ] 4. When the fundus is soft and boggy

67. The nurse correctly massages the fundus by placing one hand on the fundus and the other hand where?
[ ] 1. Just above the symphysis pubis
[ ] 2. To the right side of the abdomen
[ ] 3. Just below the xiphoid process
[ ] 4. To the left side of the abdomen

A 33-year-old client delivered a healthy baby girl vaginally 6 hours ago. During the delivery, the physician performed a mediolateral episiotomy. The client's condition is stable; however, she is complaining of incisional discomfort.

68. How should the nurse position the client when assessing the perineum after an episiotomy?
[ ] 1. Prone
[ ] 2. Supine
[ ] 3. Sims' position
[ ] 4. Lithotomy position

69. Which nursing intervention is most appropriate for relieving discomfort associated with episiotomy repair?
[ ] 1. Sitz bath
[ ] 2. Ice pack
[ ] 3. Heat lamp
[ ] 4. Topical cortisone

70. Which assessment finding by the nurse best indicates the presence of a perineal hematoma?
[ ] 1. The client complains of a feeling of fullness in the vagina.
[ ] 2. Lochia rubra is heavy and foul-smelling.
[ ] 3. There are separation and purulent drainage from the episiotomy.
[ ] 4. The client complains of severe pain in the perineal area.

During the initial assessment, the nurse notes that the client's fundus is one fingerbreadth above the umbilicus and displaced to the right of the abdominal midline.

71. Which action is most appropriate for the nurse to take in response to this finding?
[ ] 1. Assist with repositioning the client onto her left side.
[ ] 2. Have the client void, and recheck the uterus afterward.
[ ] 3. Massage the fundus until it becomes firm and returns to its normal position.
[ ] 4. Document the findings and continue to check the fundus at least every 8 hours.

The patient care technician assists the client with perineal hygiene.

72. Which observation by the nurse indicates that the technician needs additional instruction?
[ ] 1. The technician applies the peripad from back to front.
[ ] 2. The technician wears gloves while providing perineal care.
[ ] 3. The technician fills the peri bottle with warm tap water.
[ ] 4. The technician washes her hands before giving perineal care.

The client tells the nurse that she feels the urge to urinate but has been unsuccessful.

73. Which nursing action is most appropriate to implement initially?
[ ] 1. Catheterize the client with a straight catheter.
[ ] 2. Assist the client with ambulation.
[ ] 3. Have the client drink more fluids.
[ ] 4. Assist the client with a warm sitz bath.

When reviewing the client's medical records, the nurse notes that the client's rubella titer is low (less than 1:10) and that she is scheduled to receive the rubella vaccine prior to discharge.

74. Before giving the vaccine, the nurse should determine if the client is allergic to which medication?
[ ] **1.** Neomycin sulfate (Mycifradin)
[ ] **2.** Erythromycin estolate (Ilosone)
[ ] **3.** Tetracycline (Panmycin)
[ ] **4.** Doxycycline (Vibramycin)

75. When administering Rho(D) immune globulin (RhoGAM) to an Rh-negative mother who has delivered an Rh-positive infant, which is the maximum length of time the nurse has to give the medication?
[ ] **1.** 48 hours after delivery
[ ] **2.** 72 hours after delivery
[ ] **3.** At the 6-week postpartum checkup
[ ] **4.** Within the first 24 hours after delivery

76. Which finding by the nurse is most suggestive of cystitis in the postpartum client?
[ ] **1.** Boggy uterus displaced to the right of the abdominal midline
[ ] **2.** Complaint of increased thirst and voiding large amounts of urine
[ ] **3.** Urine retention and swelling of the lower extremities
[ ] **4.** Complaint of painful urination and presence of blood in the urine

Twenty-four hours after delivery, the obstetrician writes discharge orders. The nurse reviews home care instructions with the client in anticipation of her discharge.

77. After the nurse instructs the client about ways to avoid constipation, which statement made by the client indicates a need for additional teaching?
[ ] **1.** "I should drink at least 2 to 3 quarts of fluid daily."
[ ] **2.** "I will need to take a stool softener every other day."
[ ] **3.** "I should include raw fruits and vegetables in my diet."
[ ] **4.** "I will need to continue my daily walks."

78. The nurse correctly instructs the client to notify her health care provider if what occurs?
[ ] **1.** She experiences difficulty urinating.
[ ] **2.** Her lochia becomes creamy yellow after the first postpartum week.
[ ] **3.** She experiences unexplained feelings of tearfulness and sadness.
[ ] **4.** Her breasts become slightly firm after 48 hours.

The client informs the nurse that she plans to continue breast-feeding after she is discharged. She asks the nurse what she should do if her breasts become engorged after she gets home.

79. Which nursing instruction is most appropriate regarding breast engorgement?
[ ] **1.** "Pump your breasts between breast-feedings."
[ ] **2.** "Limit your fluid intake for 24 hours."
[ ] **3.** "Feed your baby every 2 to 3 hours."
[ ] **4.** "Apply ice packs to your breasts four times per day."

80. Which instruction should the nurse plan to include in the discharge teaching plan for the client who is at risk for developing mastitis?
[ ] **1.** Wear a breast binder between breast-feedings.
[ ] **2.** Apply petroleum jelly to the nipples before breast-feeding.
[ ] **3.** Clean the nipples with soap and water after breast-feeding.
[ ] **4.** Wash both hands before handling the breast.

The client asks the nurse how long she should wait after discharge before having sexual intercourse.

81. The nurse best explains that sexual intercourse may be resumed at which time?
[ ] **1.** As soon as the lochia has ceased and the perineum is healed
[ ] **2.** As soon as an acceptable birth control method is selected
[ ] **3.** After the postpartum checkup in 4 to 6 weeks
[ ] **4.** After the uterus has returned to its normal position

82. When the client tells the nurse that she is nervous about going home with her new baby, which nursing action is most appropriate?
[ ] **1.** Suggest that the client ask the physician to postpone her discharge.
[ ] **2.** Tell the client that this is a normal feeling that will go away in time.
[ ] **3.** Make sure the client has written instructions on infant care before discharge.
[ ] **4.** Give the client the facility's telephone number, encouraging her to call as needed.

The client is readmitted to the hospital on her fifth postpartum day with a tentative diagnosis of puerperal infection.

83. Which assessment finding is most characteristic of a puerperal infection?
[ ] **1.** Slower than normal pulse rate
[ ] **2.** Complaint of abdominal tenderness
[ ] **3.** A decrease in the size of the uterus
[ ] **4.** Presence of lochia serosa

Nursing Care of the Newborn Client

Two hours after a female newborn is delivered at 39 weeks' gestation, the newborn is admitted to the well-baby nursery. The nurse performs a newborn physical assessment and observes normal variations to the skin.

84. Which variations are considered normal and require no further intervention? Select all that apply.
[ ] **1.** Mongolian spot
[ ] **2.** Milia
[ ] **3.** Epstein's pearls
[ ] **4.** Erythema toxicum
[ ] **5.** Molding
[ ] **6.** Cephalohematoma

85. When the nurse documents the following newborn profile information on the flow sheet, which data require notifying the pediatrician immediately? Select all that apply.
[ ] **1.** Head circumference of 20″ (50 cm)
[ ] **2.** Chest circumference of 13″ (33 cm)
[ ] **3.** Length of 19½″ (50 cm)
[ ] **4.** Heart rate of 100 beats/minute
[ ] **5.** Weight of 11 lb (5 kg)
[ ] **6.** Abdominal circumference of 11½″ (30 cm)

The nurse proceeds with the assessment, observing the newborn's reflexes.

86. Which reflexes would the nurse expect to find in a newborn of this gestational age? Select all that apply.
[ ] **1.** Rooting reflex
[ ] **2.** Moro reflex
[ ] **3.** Tonic neck reflex
[ ] **4.** Extrusion reflex
[ ] **5.** Barlow reflex
[ ] **6.** Ortolani reflex

The length and weight are recorded on the newborn's name card. The weight has been documented in kilograms, and the nurse must convert the weight into pounds.

87. If the newborn weighs 3.5 kg, what is the weight in pounds?

_____

After the newborn's temperature has stabilized, the nurse gives her a bath.

88. Which finding noted by the nurse bathing the newborn should be reported immediately?

[ ] **1.** The hands and feet are bluish in color.
[ ] **2.** The pulse rate is 140 beats/minute.
[ ] **3.** The skin has a yellowish discoloration.
[ ] **4.** The labia are slightly swollen.

After the bath is completed, the nurse rechecks the newborn's axillary temperature and records it as 97° F (36.1° C).

89. Which nursing intervention is most appropriate at this time?
[ ] **1.** Dress and wrap the newborn in a blanket, place her in an open crib, and recheck her temperature every 4 to 8 hours.
[ ] **2.** Place the newborn on a preheated radiant warmer, and gradually rewarm her over a period of 2 or more hours.
[ ] **3.** Dress the newborn, wrap her in double blankets, place her in an open crib, and recheck her temperature in 30 to 60 minutes.
[ ] **4.** Place the newborn on a preheated radiant warmer, and rewarm her over a period of 15 to 30 minutes.

Four hours after admission to the nursery, the newborn's condition is stable and she has no signs of distress. The newborn is taken to the mother's room for a visit.

90. When the nurse begins gathering data for a discussion about methods to keep the baby safe while in the hospital, which information should she include in the teaching plan? Select all that apply.
[ ] **1.** Identification bands must be kept on the newborn at all times.
[ ] **2.** When the client is showering, the crib should be placed outside the bathroom door.
[ ] **3.** Staff should check the baby's name bands when entering the room.
[ ] **4.** Staff must wear a visible, valid hospital ID.
[ ] **5.** The newborn can sleep in bed with the mother.

91. Which of the following observations by the nurse indicate that an appropriate mother-infant bond is occurring? Select all that apply.
[ ] **1.** The mother holds her baby away from her body.
[ ] **2.** The mother makes eye contact with her baby.
[ ] **3.** The mother talks or sings to her baby.
[ ] **4.** The mother discusses the baby's physical attributes.
[ ] **5.** The mother becomes upset because the baby has spit up.
[ ] **6.** The mother repeatedly asks the nurse if the baby is going to live.

The nurse instructs the mother about initial breast-feeding. The client tells the nurse that her breasts are small and asks if she will be able to breast-feed her baby.

92. Which response by the nurse is most appropriate?
[ ] **1.** "The size of your breasts does not affect your ability to breast-feed."
[ ] **2.** "You should attempt to breast-feed and give supplemental formula."
[ ] **3.** "Bottle-feeding is just as nutritious as breast-feeding."
[ ] **4.** "You can do exercises to increase the size of your breasts."

The client informs the nurse that she thinks it is best to give her baby formula until her milk comes in. She tells the nurse that she started to breast-feed her first child but changed to bottle-feeding because the baby "lost lots of weight" before being discharged from the hospital.

93. Which response by the nurse is most appropriate regarding neonatal weight loss?
[ ] **1.** "It's normal for both bottle-fed and breast-fed infants to lose up to 10% of their birth weight during the first few days after birth."
[ ] **2.** "If your baby begins bottle-feeding, she won't be successful with breast-feeding because she will prefer the bottle nipple."
[ ] **3.** "A baby is more prone to lose weight with bottle-feeding than breast-feeding because formula is more difficult to digest."
[ ] **4.** "Until the baby is ready to begin breast-feeding, you should pump your breasts to promote the letdown reflex."

94. The nurse also explains that during the first few days after the newborn's birth, the client's breasts will secrete colostrum, which is beneficial to the baby because it contains which substance?
[ ] **1.** Estrogen, which will prevent the newborn from developing breakthrough bleeding
[ ] **2.** Antibodies, which provide protection against certain types of infections
[ ] **3.** Predigested fats, which increase the newborn's ability to absorb fat-soluble vitamins
[ ] **4.** Digestive enzymes, which increase the newborn's ability to absorb nutrients

The nurse gives the mother verbal instructions about how to breast-feed her baby correctly. She then remains in the room to assist the mother.

95. Which action by the client indicates a need for additional teaching regarding proper breast-feeding technique?

[ ] **1.** The mother uses the thumb of her free hand to gently press the breast away from her baby's nose.
[ ] **2.** The mother gently strokes her baby's lips with her nipple when she is ready to breast-feed.
[ ] **3.** The mother places a breast shield over her nipple before placing the nipple in her baby's mouth.
[ ] **4.** The mother gently pulls down on her baby's chin before removing the nipple from the baby's mouth.

Before leaving the newborn with the parents, the nurse hands the mother a bulb syringe and instructs her on its proper use.

96. Which statement made by the client indicates a need for additional teaching regarding proper use of the bulb syringe?
[ ] **1.** The mother states that her baby's mouth should be suctioned before the nose is suctioned.
[ ] **2.** The mother states that the bulb syringe should be compressed before it is placed in her baby's mouth or nose.
[ ] **3.** The mother states that, when suctioning the mouth, the bulb syringe should not touch the back of her baby's throat.
[ ] **4.** The mother states that the bulb syringe should remain compressed until it is removed from her baby's nose or mouth.

The newborn's father asks the nurse how he should position the baby when placing her in the crib after his wife finishes breast-feeding.

97. The nurse correctly explains that it is best to place the newborn in which position in the crib after feeding?
[ ] **1.** Right side-lying
[ ] **2.** Left side-lying
[ ] **3.** Prone
[ ] **4.** Supine

The client asks the nurse, "How will I know that my baby is getting enough to eat?"

98. The nurse explains that which action would most likely occur in a newborn whose nutritional needs are not being adequately met?
[ ] **1.** Awakening during the night for a feeding
[ ] **2.** Having fewer than six wet diapers per day
[ ] **3.** Having loose, pale-yellow stools
[ ] **4.** Breast-feeding every 2 to 3 hours

The client tells the nurse that she plans to continue breast-feeding after she returns to work and to pump her breasts when she cannot breast-feed. She asks the nurse how long she can store the breast milk that she pumps.

99. The nurse correctly responds that breast milk can be safely stored in the refrigerator for how long after pumping?
[ ] **1.** Up to 4 hours
[ ] **2.** Up to 2 days
[ ] **3.** Up to 1 week
[ ] **4.** Up to 1 month

A postterm male newborn in no apparent distress is admitted to the nursery after an uneventful planned cesarean birth.

100. During an initial assessment, the nurse would expect to note which finding that is characteristic of a postterm newborn?
[ ] **1.** Few sole creases
[ ] **2.** Flat, shapeless ears
[ ] **3.** Legs in a frog-like position
[ ] **4.** Dry, cracked, leatherlike skin

101. Which assessment finding would the nurse consider abnormal for this newborn?
[ ] **1.** A scrotal sac that has numerous rugae
[ ] **2.** An umbilical cord that has one vein and one artery
[ ] **3.** Vernix caseosa in the creases of the groin area
[ ] **4.** Bluish discoloration of the hands and feet

102. Which assessment finding would the nurse consider most indicative of congenital hip dysplasia in a newborn?
[ ] **1.** Asymmetry of the gluteal skin folds
[ ] **2.** Limited adduction of the affected hip
[ ] **3.** No spontaneous movement of the affected leg
[ ] **4.** Exaggerated curvature of the lumbar spine

Six hours after admission to the nursery, the newborn is taken to the mother for his first feeding. The mother states that she wants to bottle-feed her newborn. The nurse reviews basic principles of bottle-feeding with the mother.

103. Which observation by the nurse indicates that the client has an incorrect understanding of the basic principles of bottle-feeding?
[ ] **1.** The mother places the nipple of the bottle on top of her baby's tongue.
[ ] **2.** During feeding, the mother places her baby in the supine position.
[ ] **3.** The mother burps her baby after each ounce of formula taken.
[ ] **4.** The mother places her baby in the right side-lying position after the feeding.

The mother asks the nurse why it is important to keep the bottle nipple full of formula.

104. Holding the bottle so that the nipple is always full of formula helps prevent which complication in the newborn?
[ ] **1.** Damaging his gums
[ ] **2.** Getting tired while feeding
[ ] **3.** Regurgitating the formula
[ ] **4.** Swallowing air when sucking

The mother tells the nurse that she plans to use concentrated liquid infant formula at home. The nurse gathers information about formula preparations and reviews this with the mother.

105. Which statement made by the mother indicates a need for additional teaching?
[ ] **1.** "I can wash the formula bottles in a dishwasher."
[ ] **2.** "I should use warm tap water to dilute the concentrate."
[ ] **3.** "The formula should be used immediately after it is prepared."
[ ] **4.** "The lid of the can of formula must be wiped before it is opened."

When the newborn is 3 days old, the nurse observes that the skin is slightly yellow.

106. The nurse correctly documents the infant's skin color using which term?
[ ] **1.** Mottled
[ ] **2.** Jaundiced
[ ] **3.** Acrocyanotic
[ ] **4.** Erythematous

The infant's total bilirubin level is 11 mg/dL. The physician orders phototherapy.

107. When providing care for a newborn receiving phototherapy, which nursing intervention is most appropriate?
[ ] **1.** The nurse removes all of the newborn's clothing when providing treatment.
[ ] **2.** The nurse feeds the newborn through the nasogastric route.
[ ] **3.** The nurse maintains the newborn in the supine position.
[ ] **4.** The nurse monitors the I.V. infusion site at least every 2 hours.

After 2 days of therapy, the newborn's total bilirubin level decreases to 9 mg/dL and phototherapy is discontinued. The pediatrician prepares for a circumcision using the Plastibell technique.

108. Following the circumcision, which nursing action is most appropriate?
[ ] **1.** Maintain a petroleum gauze dressing over the penis.
[ ] **2.** Monitor the vital signs every 15 minutes for the first hour.
[ ] **3.** Frequently monitor the penis for swelling and bleeding.
[ ] **4.** Place the newborn on his abdomen.

The pediatrician writes orders for the newborn to be discharged if no complications occur within 4 hours of the circumcision. Prior to discharge, the nurse reviews home care of the circumcision.

109. Which statement by the parents indicates that teaching has been effective?
[ ] **1.** "We'll notify the pediatrician if we see any drainage from the baby's penis."
[ ] **2.** "We'll clean the baby's penis three times a day with alcohol."
[ ] **3.** "We'll remove the Plastibell ring in 1 week if it has not fallen off by then."
[ ] **4.** "We'll apply petroleum jelly to the baby's penis with each diaper change."

Prior to discharge, the nurse prepares to perform a phenylketonuria (PKU) test.

110. Which information is most important for the nurse to assess prior to performing the PKU test?
[ ] **1.** Whether the newborn has been feeding for at least 2 to 3 days
[ ] **2.** Whether the newborn was large for his gestational age at birth
[ ] **3.** Whether the mother had gestational diabetes during her pregnancy
[ ] **4.** Whether there is a family history of mental retardation

111. When obtaining the blood specimen for the PKU test, which action by the nurse is incorrect?
[ ] **1.** Warm the newborn's heel for 5 to 10 minutes prior to obtaining the specimen.
[ ] **2.** Puncture the lateral aspect of the newborn's heel.
[ ] **3.** Discard the first drop of blood obtained.
[ ] **4.** Apply pressure with an alcohol wipe after the specimen is obtained.

Nursing Care of Newborns with Complications

A 38-year-old multiparous client gave birth a day ago to a full-term newborn with a myelomeningocele.

112. Which assessment finding best indicates that the client is grieving over the loss of her "perfect" baby?
[ ] **1.** The client states that she has not selected a name for her baby.
[ ] **2.** The client visits the nursery frequently but only stays for a few minutes.
[ ] **3.** The client asks her physician to postpone her discharge from the hospital.
[ ] **4.** The client leaves the nursery when her baby receives treatments.

113. Which action by the nurse best facilitates the client's acceptance and care of the newborn with a myelomeningocele?
[ ] **1.** Show the client "before" and "after" pictures of other infants born with myelomeningocele.
[ ] **2.** Serve as a role model for the client by feeding, holding, and changing the newborn in the client's presence.
[ ] **3.** Explain to the client that surgery will most probably eliminate the defect and its consequences.
[ ] **4.** Assure the client that social agencies will most likely assume full care of the newborn.

A male newborn is born at 27 weeks' gestation and is taken to the neonatal intensive care unit at a nearby hospital in respiratory distress.

114. Which nursing intervention is essential for preventing retinopathy of prematurity (ROP) in the preterm newborn?
[ ] **1.** Monitor the oxygen concentration level.
[ ] **2.** Monitor the bilirubin level.
[ ] **3.** Check the hemoglobin level.
[ ] **4.** Check the pupil response.

After the newborn's respiratory condition stabilizes and he is weaned from the ventilator, the neonatologist writes an order to begin feedings.

115. When feeding the preterm newborn, which method is most appropriate?
[ ] **1.** Feed him every hour.
[ ] **2.** Give him no more than 3 to 4 ounces per feeding.
[ ] **3.** Feed him by the nasogastric route.
[ ] **4.** Give him glucose feedings for the first month.

The parents of a preterm newborn ask the nurse why their baby is being monitored for signs of infection.

116. The nurse correctly explains that preterm newborns are at risk for developing infections primarily for which reason?
[ ] **1.** Their fragile skin may tear.
[ ] **2.** They lack antibody protection from their mothers.
[ ] **3.** They are exposed to numerous sources of bacterial organisms.
[ ] **4.** They need to undergo many invasive procedures.

117. Which nursing action best ensures that the thermoregulation needs of the preterm newborn are being met?
[ ] **1.** The newborn is wrapped in a blanket.
[ ] **2.** The nursery temperature is maintained between 75° and 79° F (23.9° and 26.1° C)
[ ] **3.** The newborn is placed in an Isolette or a radiant warmer.
[ ] **4.** The crib is positioned away from sources of drafts.

A gravida II, para I client in her 38th week of pregnancy comes to the emergency department in active labor. She delivers an Rh-positive newborn with congenital hemolytic disease caused by Rh incompatibility.

118. Which assessment finding is most indicative of the presence of Rh incompatibility?
[ ] **1.** A slow and irregular respiratory rate
[ ] **2.** Absence of newborn reflexes
[ ] **3.** Limited movement in the lower extremities
[ ] **4.** Jaundice within 24 to 36 hours after birth

A direct Coombs' test is ordered to confirm the diagnosis of hemolytic disease.

119. The nurse should be prepared to assist with the collection of a blood specimen from which source?
[ ] **1.** The newborn's father
[ ] **2.** The newborn's mother
[ ] **3.** The newborn's sibling
[ ] **4.** The umbilical cord

The nurse documents that the direct Coombs' test is positive and the newborn's bilirubin level is elevated. The physician writes orders to begin phototherapy.

120. When initiating phototherapy, what should the nurse do first?
[ ] **1.** Place protective eye shields over the newborn's eyes.
[ ] **2.** Monitor the newborn's vital signs every 15 minutes for the first hour.

[ ] **3.** Catheterize the newborn, and place him on strict intake and output.
[ ] **4.** Place the newborn on NPO status until therapy is completed.

A newborn is delivered at 32 weeks' gestation to a gravida I, para I human immunodeficiency virus (HIV)-positive mother.

121. When providing care for this newborn, the nurse should follow which precautions?
[ ] **1.** Standard precautions
[ ] **2.** Airborne precautions
[ ] **3.** Droplet precautions
[ ] **4.** Contact precautions

The mother asks the nurse when her baby will be tested for HIV, and how long it usually takes before HIV-positive babies develop acquired immunodeficiency syndrome (AIDS).

122. Which statement by the nurse about HIV testing is most appropriate?
[ ] **1.** "Your baby won't be tested because babies of HIV-positive mothers are already HIV-positive."
[ ] **2.** "Your baby will be tested immediately for anti-HIV antibodies to facilitate early treatment."
[ ] **3.** "Your baby won't be tested for anti-HIV antibodies until he is 3 months old."
[ ] **4.** "Your baby will be tested for anti-HIV antibodies for 4 years or until test results are positive."

123. It would be correct for the nurse to explain that most children who contract HIV in utero typically develop AIDS symptoms at which age?
[ ] **1.** At birth
[ ] **2.** By age 6 months
[ ] **3.** By age 12 months
[ ] **4.** By age 2 years

The client asks the nurse if she can breast-feed her baby.

124. Which explanation by the nurse is most appropriate regarding breast-feeding this newborn?
[ ] **1.** "It's OK to breast-feed your baby if the anti-HIV test results are positive."
[ ] **2.** "It's OK to breast-feed your baby as long as he is symptom-free."
[ ] **3.** "You can't breast-feed your baby because you are HIV-positive."
[ ] **4.** "You can't breast-feed your baby if you have developed symptoms of AIDS."

Correct Answers and Rationales

Admission of the Client to a Labor and Delivery Facility

1. **3.** A sudden gush of fluid from the vagina indicates that the bag of water has ruptured. The client should report to the hospital or designated health care facility because once the membranes rupture, she is at increased risk for intrauterine infection and umbilical cord prolapse if the fetal head has not engaged. A sudden burst of energy, also known as the *nesting instinct,* is a preliminary sign of approaching labor and may occur a few days prior to the beginning of labor; it does not require reporting to the health care facility. Urinary frequency may occur as the fetus settles into the pelvic brim. The primigravid client may experience urinary frequency as early as 2 to 3 weeks prior to the beginning of labor. The client is generally told to report to the hospital or health care facility when contractions are 5 minutes apart.
   Client Needs Category—Health promotion and maintenance
   Client Needs Subcategory—None

2. **2.** Upon admittance to the hospital, the least pertinent question to ask a woman who is experiencing uterine contractions is whether she has ever had an enema. Not every client requires an enema, so the best time to ask about this is shortly before administering one. It is more pertinent to ask upon admission whether the client's membranes have ruptured, when her contractions started, and when she last ate. The timing of the last meal is especially important in case the client requires anesthesia for delivery.
   Client Needs Category—Health promotion and maintenance
   Client Needs Subcategory—None

3. **1.** Braxton Hicks contractions are irregular, painless contractions that occur intermittently (in some cases, every 10 to 20 minutes). They tend to disappear with walking and sleeping and become more uncomfortable closer to delivery. Primiparous clients often have difficulty determining the difference between false labor, as evidenced by Braxton Hicks contractions, and true labor. However, there are differences that the nurse can explain to the client. Because of their irregularity, Braxton Hicks contractions cannot be timed, and they do not increase in frequency or intensity. These contractions begin and remain in the abdomen, whereas true labor contractions begin in the lower back and progress to the abdomen. The main difference between true labor and false labor contractions, however, is that Braxton Hicks contractions do not dilate the cervix.
   Client Needs Category—Health promotion and maintenance
   Client Needs Subcategory—None

4. **4.** To obtain the most accurate blood pressure reading, the blood pressure should be assessed between contractions, with the client in the left side-lying position. This method minimizes the possibility of obtaining an inaccurate reading that can occur when the blood pressure is measured during a contraction (when circulating blood volume decreases) or when the client is in any other position (the enlarged uterus may compress the inferior vena cava and affect blood flow).
   Client Needs Category—Health promotion and maintenance
   Client Needs Subcategory—None

Nursing Care of Clients During the First Stage of Labor

5. **1.** When performing a vaginal examination, the examiner wears a pair of sterile gloves to avoid the introduction of bacteria and the risk of infection. The client should be assisted to the supine (not side-lying) position and assisted to use breathing techniques (breathing slowly through an open mouth) to help her relax. An enema is not usually part of client preparation for a vaginal examination.
   Client Needs Category—Safe, effective care environment
   Client Needs Subcategory—Safety and infection control

6. **4.** Dilation and effacement of the cervix are the only definite, reliable indicators of true labor. Regular, progressing contractions and the presence of bloody show are also signs of labor, but they are not considered as reliable.
   Client Needs Category—Health promotion and maintenance
   Client Needs Subcategory—None

7. **2.** The normal fetal heart rate ranges from 120 to 160 beats/minute. During the latent phase of the first stage of labor, the contractions occur every 5 to 30 minutes. The perineum does not begin to bulge until the transition phase of the first stage of labor, and early decelerations usually occur late in labor as a result of head compression.
   Client Needs Category—Health promotion and maintenance
   Client Needs Subcategory—None

8. 2. During the latent phase of the first stage of labor, the client is encouraged to drink clear liquids to prevent dehydration. If the client's membranes are intact and her contractions are not very frequent or intense, she may be allowed to ambulate and take a warm shower or Jacuzzi bath. The client usually uses a panting breathing pattern during the transition phase of the first stage of labor.

Client Needs Category—*Health promotion and maintenance*
Client Needs Subcategory—*None*

9. 3. The fetal heart rate should be assessed every 30 minutes during the latent phase of the first stage of labor, every 15 minutes during the active phase of the first stage of labor, and every 5 minutes during the second stage of labor.

Client Needs Category—*Health promotion and maintenance*
Client Needs Subcategory—*None*

10. 2. Epidural anesthesia can be administered at any time, but it is usually administered to a primigravid client when she is 5 to 6 centimeters dilated. If the client is multigravid, an epidural is generally given when she is 3 to 4 centimeters dilated.

Client Needs Category—*Health promotion and maintenance*
Client Needs Subcategory—*None*

11. 3. Contractions during the active phase of labor usually occur every 3 to 5 minutes and last between 45 and 60 seconds. Contractions last up to 30 seconds during the latent phase of the first stage of labor. They can last up to 90 seconds during the transition phase of the first stage of labor as well as during the second stage of labor.

Client Needs Category—*Health promotion and maintenance*
Client Needs Subcategory—*None*

12. 3. During the transition phase of the first stage of labor, the client usually has an increase in bloody show and the contractions last up to 90 seconds. Crowning of the presenting part does not occur until the cervix is completely dilated, during the second stage of labor.

Client Needs Category—*Health promotion and maintenance*
Client Needs Subcategory—*None*

13. 2. During the transition phase of the first stage of labor, the client is at risk for losing control because of intense discomfort, fatigue, and frequency and length of the contractions. Praising the client's efforts frequently at this time can help her to maintain control of the situation. During the transition phase of labor, the

membranes usually rupture if they have not already done so, and the client may receive an opioid analgesic or regional anesthetic; therefore, ambulation is not usually recommended. The client should not push until the cervix is completely dilated, which occurs during the second stage of labor. Application of sacral pressure can relieve back discomfort. Some women have a low tolerance to touch during this phase of labor; therefore, every client should be assessed individually to determine her preference.

Client Needs Category—*Psychosocial integrity*
Client Needs Subcategory—*None*

14. 1. When the fetus presents in the posterior instead of the anterior position, the client experiences back discomfort and there is a danger of maternal laceration if the fetus does not rotate before delivery. Also, the posterior position usually prolongs labor, so preparing for a precipitous delivery is not necessary. The client should be assisted to a more comfortable position. The knee-chest position is commonly recommended because it relieves discomfort associated with the posterior presentation of the head and facilitates rotation of the head. Trendelenburg's position does not assist with rotation of the head to the anterior position. During this phase, the client should avoid lying on her back to avoid vena cava compression by the uterus. The uterus usually is not displaced with a posterior presentation, so having the client void is inappropriate.

Client Needs Category—*Safe, effective care environment*
Client Needs Subcategory—*Safety and infection control*

15. 4. The client should be encouraged to void every 2 hours to minimize bladder distention, which may prolong labor. The client should be encouraged to drink clear liquids at frequent intervals to prevent dehydration. The I.V. infusion rate is not decreased unless ordered by the physician. Maintaining the prescribed I.V. infusion rate also prevents dehydration. No solid foods are given during labor because peristalsis is slowed during this time, and nausea and vomiting can occur.

Client Needs Category—*Health promotion and maintenance*
Client Needs Subcategory—*None*

16. 1. The contraction duration is defined as the time interval between the beginning of a contraction and the end of the same contraction. The time interval between the end of one contraction and the beginning of the next contraction is called the relaxation period. The time interval between the beginning of one contraction and the end of the next contraction is insignificant when assessing the client's labor pattern and is not generally measured. The time interval between the beginning of one contraction and the beginning of the next contraction is defined as the frequency of the contractions.

> ***Client Needs Category**—Health promotion and maintenance*
> ***Client Needs Subcategory**—None*

17. 1. The nurse should palpate the fundus of the uterus, which is usually located just above the umbilicus in the full-term client. The fundus is palpated because muscular contractions are strongest and easiest to assess at this location.

> ***Client Needs Category**—Health promotion and maintenance*
> ***Client Needs Subcategory**—None*

18. 3. The fetal heart rate is assessed every 15 minutes during the active phase of the first stage of labor, every 30 minutes during the latent phase of the first stage of labor, and every 5 minutes during the second stage of labor.

> ***Client Needs Category**—Health promotion and maintenance*
> ***Client Needs Subcategory**—None*

19. 1. When there is a question about whether or not the membranes have ruptured, a nitrazine test may be performed. Amniotic fluid turns the nitrazine test strip blue because amniotic fluid is alkaline. The nitrazine test remains yellow when exposed to vaginal secretions and urine, which are usually acidic. Red and green are not colors associated with nitrazine testing.

> ***Client Needs Category**—Health promotion and maintenance*
> ***Client Needs Subcategory**—None*

20. 4. The fetal heart rate should be checked immediately after the membranes rupture. A drop in the fetal heart rate may indicate umbilical cord prolapse. Prolapse of the umbilical cord may occur because of the sudden gush of fluid from the vagina, especially if the presenting part is not engaged. The client's pulse is not affected by the rupturing of the membranes. The registered nurse usually performs vaginal examinations, and an indwelling catheter is not usually indicated when the membranes rupture.

> ***Client Needs Category**—Safe, effective care environment*
> ***Client Needs Subcategory**—Safety and infection control*

21. 1. The client's temperature should be assessed every hour after the membranes rupture because of the increased risk of infection. The temperature is assessed every 4 hours if the membranes are intact.

> ***Client Needs Category**—Safe, effective care environment*
> ***Client Needs Subcategory**—Safety and infection control*

22. 1. Internal electronic fetal monitoring requires the application of an electrode to the fetal scalp. Infection and soft-tissue injury can occur with the use of internal electronic fetal monitoring, but both are rare. A soft, water-filled catheter is inserted into the uterus for internal electronic monitoring of uterine contractions. A transducer is applied to the mother's abdomen when external electronic monitoring is used. A suction cup is applied to the fetal scalp when a vacuum extraction is being performed to assist with delivery of the fetal head.

> ***Client Needs Category**—Health promotion and maintenance*
> ***Client Needs Subcategory**—None*

23. 3. The presence of green amniotic fluid indicates that the fetus has passed a meconium stool in utero. Passage of meconium in utero when the fetus is presenting in the vertex position is an indication of fetal distress and should be reported immediately. To avoid meconium aspiration, the mouth, nose, and throat should be suctioned prior to the delivery of the body. The normal range for the fetal heart rate is 120 to 140 beats/minute. It is normal for the fetal heart rate to accelerate. An increase in bloody show usually indicates that the second stage of labor is imminent.

> ***Client Needs Category**—Safe, effective care environment*
> ***Client Needs Subcategory**—Safety and infection control*

24. 4. Solid foods are not usually given when the client is in labor because they may cause nausea and vomiting due to the fact that peristalsis is slowed during labor. Solid foods are not known to alter the absorption of regional anesthetics or to alter the duration and frequency of contraction; they also do not cause fetal distress.

> ***Client Needs Category**—Health promotion and maintenance*
> ***Client Needs Subcategory**—None*

25. 1. When the fetus presents in the vertex position, the head descends into the birth canal first. If the feet or buttocks enter the birth canal first, the presentation is considered a breech. Both breech and shoulder presentations are considered malpresentations and make delivery more difficult.

> ***Client Needs Category**—Health promotion and maintenance*
> ***Client Needs Subcategory**—None*

26. 4. A drop in the fetal heart rate after the contraction acme is defined as a late deceleration. Late decelerations are usually a sign of fetal distress and should be reported immediately. The other options describe processes that normally occur during the active phase of the first stage of labor.

> *Client Needs Category—Physiological integrity*
> *Client Needs Subcategory—Reduction of risk*
> *potential*

27. 2. Tocolytic agents such as terbutaline sulfate (Brethine) should be withheld if the client's cervix is dilated 4 centimeters or more or effaced 50% or more. Tocolytic agents should also be withheld when the client is hemorrhaging or has severe pregnancy-induced hypertension, or when fetal distress is evident. The presence of mild contractions indicates that the client continues to be in premature labor, so it would be appropriate to give the client the tocolytic medication. Fetal heart variability is a normal finding and indicates fetal well-being. The client's perception that contractions are occurring less frequently is not substantial enough to withhold the medication; more objective data are necessary.

> *Client Needs Category—Physiological integrity*
> *Client Needs Subcategory—Pharmacological*
> *therapies*

Nursing Care of Clients During the Second Stage of Labor

28. 1. The perineum usually begins to bulge and the presenting part begins to crown during the second stage of labor. The contractions usually last for 60 to 90 seconds, and the cervix is completely dilated (10 cm). The level of the uterus is not an indicator of the stage of labor.

> *Client Needs Category—Health promotion and*
> *maintenance*
> *Client Needs Subcategory—None*

29. 1. Preparation for delivery for a multiparous client should begin when she is 6 to 7 centimeters dilated. Preparation for a primiparous client is usually delayed until the client is completely dilated (10 cm) because it generally takes longer to achieve full dilation with a woman's first delivery. The arrival time of the physician or midwife varies and usually is not used as an indicator for when to begin preparing for delivery.

> *Client Needs Category—Health promotion and*
> *maintenance*
> *Client Needs Subcategory—None*

30. 3. A vaginal examination is performed to determine whether or not the cervix is 10 centimeters dilated and 100% effaced. The client's cervix should be completely dilated and effaced before she begins to push; this precaution prevents edema or lacerations to the cervix that would prolong labor and possibly require delivery by cesarean birth. The other options are appropriate if the client is fully dilated.

> *Client Needs Category—Health promotion and*
> *maintenance*
> *Client Needs Subcategory—None*

31. 3. If an opioid analgesic such as nalbuphine (Nubain) is given too late during labor, the medication can cross the placental barrier and may be present after the newborn is delivered, resulting in respiratory depression. Conversely, giving an opioid analgesic too early in labor may interfere with labor progression and decrease the contractions' effectiveness. Administration of an opioid analgesic is not associated with uterine rupture or increased fetal activity.

> *Client Needs Category—Physiological integrity*
> *Client Needs Subcategory—Pharmacological*
> *therapies*

32. 1. A saddle block, also called a subarachnoid block, is a form of epidural anesthesia. Epidural blocks provide pain relief during labor and delivery by blocking the pain sensations transmitted to the brain. Blocks are also useful for clients who have preexisting conditions, such as heart disease, pulmonary disease, or diabetes. A saddle block usually takes effect immediately and reaches its maximum potency within 3 to 5 minutes of administration.

> *Client Needs Category—Physiological integrity*
> *Client Needs Subcategory—Pharmacological*
> *therapies*

33. 1. During the immediate postprocedural period, the client's blood pressure should be assessed and evaluated for the presence of hypotension; a drop in blood pressure occasionally occurs secondary to sympathetic blockade and may decrease the oxygen supply to the fetus, which is manifested by fetal bradycardia (not tachycardia). Paralysis of the lower extremities is an expected result of a saddle block. The client may experience a spinal headache within 24 to 72 hours after the procedure, but not immediately. Ensuring that the client is well hydrated (usually via I.V. infusion) before, during, and after the procedure minimizes both maternal hypotension and spinal headache.

> *Client Needs Category—Physiological integrity*
> *Client Needs Subcategory—Pharmacological*
> *therapies*

34. 2. The client who has had saddle block (subarachnoid block) anesthesia is instructed when to push because she is unable to feel contractions. Oxygen is not routinely required unless complications arise. The client is not usually catheterized following this type of anesthesia, and the saddle block anesthesia is usually given late in labor (second stage) or for cesarean birth; thus, it usually does not slow the progress of labor, which would require the use of oxytocin (Pitocin).

Client Needs Category—Physiological integrity
Client Needs Subcategory—Pharmacological therapies

35. 1. When cleaning the perineum in preparation for delivery, the nurse should use the technique that poses the least possibility of infection and increases visibility of the area. The usual procedure of cleaning the area is as follows: pubic bone to lower abdomen, the inner thighs (both), the right and left labia, and the vagina to the anus. The vagina is always the last area cleaned.

Client Needs Category—Safe, effective care environment
Client Needs Subcategory—Safety and infection control

36. 3. An episiotomy is an incision made into the perineum tissue to enlarge the vaginal opening. It is usually performed to prevent lacerations of or damage to the perineum. An episiotomy also diminishes the possibility of prolonged pressure on the fetal head and speeds the delivery process. Episiotomies are not associated with uterine rupture, postpartum infection, or bowel trauma.

Client Needs Category—Health promotion and maintenance
Client Needs Subcategory—None

Nursing Care of Clients During the Third Stage of Labor

37. 3. The priority need of the newborn immediately after delivery is establishment of a patent airway. This is best accomplished by bulb-suctioning the newborn's nose and mouth after the head is delivered but before complete delivery of the body. Oxygen is not given before the airway is cleared; it is only administered if needed. Applying the cord clamp and warming the newborn do not take priority over establishment and maintenance of respirations.

Client Needs Category—Health promotion and maintenance
Client Needs Subcategory—None

38. 4. An Apgar score of 7 to 10 is considered good and does not require any intervention. A score between 4 and 6 indicates moderate distress, in which case the newborn requires close monitoring and possible intervention. A score between 0 and 3 is considered poor and indicates a definite need for resuscitation efforts and medical intervention.

Client Needs Category—Health promotion and maintenance
Client Needs Subcategory—None

39. 2. The newborn should be dried first to prevent heat loss secondary to evaporation, placed on the mother's abdomen in skin-to-skin contact, and then covered with a warmed blanket. The mother's abdomen is usually warm, so direct newborn-mother contact does not pose a danger of heat loss. The other options either interfere with maintaining the newborn's warmth or do not promote mother-infant attachment.

Client Needs Category—Health promotion and maintenance
Client Needs Subcategory—None

40. 3. The preferred site for I.M. injections in a newborn is the vastus lateralis, located on the outside aspect of the thigh. The rectus femoris may also be used. The ventrogluteal muscle and the gluteus maximus muscles are not used in newborns because of the risk of sciatic nerve damage. The deltoid muscle should not be used until a child is 3 years old.

Client Needs Category—Safe, effective care environment
Client Needs Subcategory—Safety and infection control

41. 3. Bacteria normally found in the intestines synthesize vitamin K. The newborn is given vitamin K (AquaMEPHYTON) at birth because his intestines are sterile and he cannot synthesize his own vitamin K. Vitamin K is needed for formation of prothrombin and other clotting factors that help prevent bleeding. Vitamin K does not stimulate respirations, start peristalsis, or increase calcium absorption.

Client Needs Category—Physiological integrity
Client Needs Subcategory—Pharmacological therapies

42. 1. Neonatal blindness can occur as a result of eye infections caused by gonococcal and chlamydial organisms. Erythromycin (Ilotycin) ophthalmic ointment is used prophylactically in the newborn to prevent blindness that may result from exposure to these organisms during passage through the mother's birth canal. *Candida albicans* causes yeast infections and *Pneumocystis carinii* is associated with acquired immunodeficiency syndrome.

Client Needs Category—Physiological integrity
Client Needs Subcategory—Pharmacological therapies

43. 2. The infant may experience temporary blurred vision following administration of erythromycin (Ilotycin) ophthalmic ointment. The infant's eyes may

swell, but this is more likely the result of pressure exerted on the soft tissue of the lids during passage through the birth canal. Purulent eye drainage and conjunctival hemorrhage are not associated with the use of this drug.
Client Needs Category—Health promotion and maintenance
Client Needs Subcategory—None

44. 3. The technician or nurse should keep one hand over the newborn while weighing it. Keeping a hand on the newborn will affect the weight's accuracy. Undressing the newborn before the weight is obtained, placing a diaper or paper barrier on the scale before balancing it, and cleaning the scale with an antiseptic before and after use are all correct techniques to implement when weighing a newborn.
Client Needs Category—Safe, effective care environment
Client Needs Subcategory—Safety and infection control

45. 1. To prevent the risk of the mother receiving the wrong baby, matching identification bracelets should be placed on both the newborn and mother prior to the newborn's leaving the delivery area. Eye prophylaxis and administration of vitamin K (AquaMEPHYTON) are usually delayed to facilitate early bonding between the mother and baby but are completed in the delivery room or in the nursery. PKU testing should be performed when the baby has begun to eat.
Client Needs Category—Safe, effective care environment
Client Needs Subcategory—Safety and infection control

46. 4. The placenta is delivered after it has separated from the wall of the uterus. This is usually accomplished by having the client bear down. In some cases, the attending health care provider may manually express the placenta. Breathing slowly and deeply, assuming a side-lying position, and tightening and relaxing the perineum do not facilitate delivery of the placenta.
Client Needs Category—Health promotion and maintenance
Client Needs Subcategory—None

47. 3. A rise of the fundus in the abdomen, lengthening of the umbilical cord, and a sudden gush of blood from the vagina are signs of impending delivery of the placenta. The perineum does not bulge with delivery of the placenta.
Client Needs Category—Health promotion and maintenance
Client Needs Subcategory—None

Nursing Care of Clients During the Fourth Stage of Labor

48. 2. The client's needs are best met by applying a warmed blanket over her. The nurse can also explain that the shaking is a normal response due to sudden physiological changes and fluid shifts; however, this will not relieve her shaking and coldness. Suggesting that the client try not to think about the shaking will not resolve the underlying cause; therefore, this does not adequately address the client's complaint. Notifying the physician is unnecessary because this is a normal physiological process.
Client Needs Category—Physiological integrity
Client Needs Subcategory—Basic care and comfort

49. 1. Following delivery of the placenta, the fundus of the uterus should be firmly contracted and located at, or just below, the level of the umbilicus.
Client Needs Category—Health promotion and maintenance
Client Needs Subcategory—None

50. 4. A systolic blood pressure of 100 mm Hg or less should be reported because it could indicate that the client is hemorrhaging. Signs of hypovolemic shock occur when about 400 to 500 ml of blood have been lost. Besides a drop in blood pressure, other signs of shock related to hemorrhage include increased pulse rate, increased respiratory rate, cold and clammy skin, decreased urine output, and dizziness. The normal pulse rate is slightly lower during the fourth stage of labor than during previous stages because of decreased cardiac strain. The pulse rate can range between 40 and 80 beats/minute and still be considered normal. During the fourth stage of labor, the lochia is usually dark red with a fleshy, not foul, odor. The client may saturate one perineal pad within 1 hour.
Client Needs Category—Physiological integrity
Client Needs Subcategory—Reduction of risk potential

51. 3. Oxytocin (Pitocin) decreases the risk of hemorrhage after delivery because the medication causes uterine contractions. The client's blood pressure should be monitored closely because hypertension is a side effect of this medication. Also, uterine rupture may occur with the administration of oxytocin (Pitocin) if hyperstimulation of the uterus secondary to a toxic dose of the medication occurs. Administering oxytocin (Pitocin) will not prevent the uterus from inverting. When palpating the uterus, the nurse commonly supports it just above the symphysis pubis to prevent the uterus from inverting.
Client Needs Category—Physiological integrity
Client Needs Subcategory—Pharmacological therapies

Nursing Care of Clients Having a Cesarean Birth

52. 2. The client is catheterized prior to abdominal surgery to prevent bladder trauma that may occur if the bladder becomes distended during surgery. Such catheterization is not performed to reduce postpartum hemorrhage, provide a landmark for the physician, or provide a safe way of collecting urine specimens.
> *Client Needs Category—Safe, effective care environment*
> *Client Needs Subcategory—Safety and infection control*

53. 1. When a cesarean birth is performed using epidural anesthesia, the client may feel pressure but does not experience pain or stinging because the nerve roots (source of pain) are blocked. Clients are not asleep when this type of anesthesia is used.
> *Client Needs Category—Physiological integrity*
> *Client Needs Subcategory—Physiological adaptation*

54. 3. The client's husband (or partner or coach) is usually allowed in the operating room during the cesarean birth. However, because of the sterile environment, he must first scrub and change into the appropriate attire before being brought into the surgical area when the procedure is ready to begin. Then he is usually seated near the client's head.
> *Client Needs Category—Psychosocial integrity*
> *Client Needs Subcategory—None*

55. 1. Prior to a cesarean birth, the nurse performs an abdominal-perineal preparation. The area prepared begins at the nipple line and extends vertically to the perineal area visible when the legs are parallel and then horizontally from one side of the abdomen to the other side of the abdomen.
> *Client Needs Category—Safe, effective care environment*
> *Client Needs Subcategory—Safety and infection control*

56. 3. The client should be monitored for respiratory depression when receiving morphine by the epidural route. Respiratory depression is the most serious adverse reaction associated with administration of opioids by this route. The client may also experience urine retention, pinpoint pupils, and circulatory collapse.
> *Client Needs Category—Physiological integrity*
> *Client Needs Subcategory—Pharmacological therapies*

57. 4. An opioid antagonist such as naloxone hydrochloride (Narcan) should be readily available in case respiratory depression occurs. If Narcan is used, the nurse should monitor the client for extreme pain. The medications identified in the other options are not required when the client is receiving epidural morphine sulfate.
> *Client Needs Category—Physiological integrity*
> *Client Needs Subcategory—Pharmacological therapies*

58. 4. Redness and swelling around the incision usually indicate the presence of an infection. Other signs of infection include an elevated temperature (100.4° F [38° C] or greater orally) 2 to 3 days after delivery, severe pain, and incisional drainage. It is normal for the incision line to feel numb for several months following a cesarean birth.
> *Client Needs Category—Safe, effective care environment*
> *Client Needs Subcategory—Safety and infection control*

59. 1. Ambulation, a diet low in gas-forming foods, small enemas, and antiflatulence medications are some methods used to reduce abdominal discomfort that may be experienced by the client who has had a cesarean birth. Pain medications, such as meperidine hydrochloride (Demerol) and morphine sulfate, can contribute to the abdominal discomfort instead of relieving it because they slow peristalsis. Rectal tubes are not usually used postpartally. Drinking from a straw is discouraged because it causes the client to swallow more air, which further aggravates the problem.
> *Client Needs Category—Physiological integrity*
> *Client Needs Subcategory—Basic care and comfort*

60. 1. VBAC is possible if the client has had a classical (low transverse) incision and wishes to attempt to have a vaginal birth. The client must also have no history of medical conditions that prohibit a vaginal birth.
> *Client Needs Category—Health promotion and maintenance*
> *Client Needs Subcategory—None*

Nursing Care of Clients Having an Emergency Delivery

61. 3. If the nurse observes prolapse of the umbilical cord, the client should be placed in the Trendelenburg's or knee-chest position. Both positions help to relieve the pressure of the presenting part on the umbilical cord. The nurse may also attempt to lift the presenting part off the cord with a gloved finger or hand until the physician or midwife arrives. Oxygen is usually administered, but the client is not positioned on the left side. The newborn is usually delivered by cesarean birth; however, preparation of the delivery area and notification of the physician do not take priority over relieving the cord compression.

Client Needs Category—Physiological integrity
Client Needs Subcategory—Reduction of risk potential

62. 1. When birth is imminent and no help is available, the nurse should gently control the delivery of the head, allow it to emerge, and deliver the newborn between contractions. The nurse should not hold back the baby's head to prevent birth or attempt to enter or enlarge the vaginal opening.
Client Needs Category—Safe, effective care environment
Client Needs Subcategory—Safety and infection control

Nursing Care of Clients Having a Stillborn Baby

63. 2. The nurse should encourage the client to express her feelings, including sorrow over her baby's loss. These actions allow the client to sort through her feelings and facilitate the establishment of a trusting relationship between the client and nurse. The fetal heart rate should be checked only once by an experienced nurse; any rechecking may give the client false hope, which is inappropriate. Redirecting the client's attention to the laboring process does not allow the client the opportunity to sort through her feelings. Explaining that the baby probably would have been born with severe long-term health problems is not necessarily an accurate statement and also does nothing to ease the client's sorrow.
Client Needs Category—Psychosocial integrity
Client Needs Subcategory—None

64. 2. Allowing the parents to visit with their baby affords them an opportunity to say their last goodbyes and helps them accept the infant's death. The infant is bathed and diapered, and the parents are allowed to hold and touch the infant. Although a memory packet may also be presented, it does not substitute for an actual visit if the parents desire one. Postponing the visit may interfere with the grieving process.
Client Needs Category—Psychosocial integrity
Client Needs Subcategory—None

Nursing Care of Clients During the Postpartum Period

65. 2. Calf pain when the foot is dorsiflexed is a manifestation of thrombophlebitis. This response is also called a positive Homans' sign. Thrombophlebitis, the inflammation of the lining of a blood vessel with clot formation, can involve superficial or deep veins. Clients at risk for developing thrombophlebitis include obese

women, those with varicose veins, multiparas, and those over age 30. It is normal for the client to pass a couple of nickel-sized clots during the first 24 hours after delivery. The client may experience abdominal cramping similar to contraction pain during labor; these contractions are caused by the release of oxytocin when the client is breast-feeding and are more common in multiparous clients. The vaginal discharge is normally dark red during this time.
Client Needs Category—Physiological integrity
Client Needs Subcategory—Physiological adaptation

66. 4. A soft and boggy fundus can lead to uterine bleeding. Normally, the fundus is firm, hard, and located at, or just below, the level of the umbilicus. The uterus should be massaged if there is any increase in the lochia flow.
Client Needs Category—Physiological integrity
Client Needs Subcategory—Reduction of risk potential

67. 1. Placing one hand on the fundus of the uterus and the other hand just above the symphysis pubis prevents the uterus from becoming inverted. The hand placement in the other options will not prevent the uterus from inverting.
Client Needs Category—Health promotion and maintenance
Client Needs Subcategory—None

68. 3. An episiotomy is the surgical incision made by the physician to avoid perineal tears during delivery. When assessing the perineum of the client who received an episiotomy, the nurse should assist the client to the left side-lying position with the right leg flexed at the knee (Sims' position). The upper buttock is lifted to expose the anus and perineum. This technique allows the best visualization of the perineal area. The positions identified in the other options do not allow for maximal visualization of this area.
Client Needs Category—Health promotion and maintenance
Client Needs Subcategory—None

69. 2. An episiotomy is a surgical cut into the perineum to widen the vaginal opening. If the client has an episiotomy, ice is applied to the perineum to reduce the swelling and subsequently decrease the discomfort that may occur from swelling. Sitz baths, heat lamp treatments, and topical cortisone are usually ordered for use after the fourth stage of labor.
Client Needs Category—Physiological integrity
Client Needs Subcategory—Basic care and comfort

70. 4. A hematoma is the collection of blood in tissue that occurs when a vessel ruptures. A client who develops a perineal hematoma usually complains of a great deal of pain in the perineal area, especially when sutures were needed to repair the episiotomy. The condition should be reported promptly. A hematoma is not associated with a feeling of fullness in the vagina, the presence of heavy and foul-smelling lochia rubra, or separation and purulent drainage from an episiotomy.

> *Client Needs Category—Physiological integrity*
> *Client Needs Subcategory—Physiological adaptation*

71. 2. A high fundus that is displaced from the midline is consistent with urine retention. Therefore, the nurse should encourage the client to void and then recheck the fundus afterward. The client may need to be catheterized if she cannot void voluntarily. Repositioning the client and massaging the uterus will not resolve the urine retention.

> *Client Needs Category—Health promotion and maintenance*
> *Client Needs Subcategory—None*

72. 1. The peripad is always applied and removed from front to back to avoid contamination of the perineum. Peripads are changed frequently during the first few days because blood harbors microorganisms that can lead to infection. The technician should wash her hands before and after assisting with pericare. She should also wear gloves for the procedure. A peri bottle, if used, should be filled with warm water.

> *Client Needs Category—Safe, effective care environment*
> *Client Needs Subcategory—Safety and infection control*

73. 4. Clients typically have an increase in urine output within the first 24 hours following delivery and void frequently during that time. If an ambulatory client cannot void, the nurse may try giving a warm sitz bath or having the client shower to help her void. If these techniques are unsuccessful, the client would be catheterized with a straight catheter to avoid bladder complications. If the client has to be catheterized more than once, the health care provider may order the insertion of an indwelling catheter. Having the client drink more fluid usually makes the situation worse because it increases the bladder distention.

> *Client Needs Category—Physiological integrity*
> *Client Needs Subcategory—Basic care and comfort*

74. 1. The client should be asked if she is allergic to neomycin sulfate (Mycifradin) because the rubella vaccine contains neomycin. It is unnecessary to ask the client if she is allergic to any of the medications listed in the other options because the rubella vaccine does not contain those drugs.

> *Client Needs Category—Physiological integrity*
> *Client Needs Subcategory—Pharmacological therapies*

75. 2. During the postpartum period, Rho(D) immune globulin (RhoGAM) should be administered within 72 hours after delivery of the newborn. If RhoGAM is not administered within this time frame, the mother is at increased risk for developing antibodies that can cause hemolytic disease if she has an Rh-positive infant in the future.

> *Client Needs Category—Physiological integrity*
> *Client Needs Subcategory—Pharmacological therapies*

76. 4. Dysuria and hematuria are clinical manifestations of a urinary tract infection (cystitis). A boggy, displaced uterus is usually associated with bladder distention. Urinary retention and swelling of the lower extremities are associated with kidney or circulatory problems. Increased thirst (polydipsia) and voiding large amounts of urine (polyuria) are common symptoms of diabetes mellitus.

> *Client Needs Category—Physiological integrity*
> *Client Needs Subcategory—Physiological adaptation*

77. 2. Stool softeners should be used only when the client has difficulty passing stools. Drinking at least 2 to 3 quarts of fluids daily, including raw fruits and vegetables in the diet, and taking daily walks are effective ways of preventing constipation.

> *Client Needs Category—Health promotion and maintenance*
> *Client Needs Subcategory—None*

78. 1. Normal bladder function usually returns within a few days after delivery. Therefore, the client should notify the health care provider of any difficulty with urination, including burning on urination and the inability to void. These are considered danger signs and may indicate infection or some other complication. Changes in lochia color, tearfulness, and breast engorgement are all considered normal findings during the postpartum period.

> *Client Needs Category—Health promotion and maintenance*
> *Client Needs Subcategory—None*

79. 3. The best method for alleviating breast engorgement is to breast-feed the newborn frequently. Pumping the breast usually increases the milk supply and further aggravates engorgement. Limiting fluid intake and applying cold compresses or ice packs will suppress lactation and interfere with the production of an adequate amount of milk for feeding. The client can try applying warmth to the breast area instead or wearing a support bra.

> *Client Needs Category—Physiological integrity*
> *Client Needs Subcategory—Basic care and comfort*

80. **4.** To prevent contamination and inflammation of the breast (mastitis), it is important for the client to wash her hands thoroughly before handling her breasts. A client who is breast-feeding should not wear a breast binder, which may suppress milk production. The nipples should not be cleaned with soap because soap contributes to drying and cracking of the nipples. Petroleum jelly also should not be applied to the nipples.

> *Client Needs Category—Safe, effective care environment*
> *Client Needs Subcategory—Safety and infection control*

81. **1.** The client may resume sexual intercourse when the perineum is healed and the lochia has ceased. This generally occurs by the third postpartum week, which may be before the postpartum checkup. It is unnecessary to wait for complete involution of the uterus before having sexual intercourse. Also, the client should decide about whether or not to use birth control before resuming intercourse, especially if she wants to avoid becoming pregnant so soon. However, the choice of an appropriate method of birth control is not necessarily the most significant factor to consider when deciding when to resume sexual relations.

> *Client Needs Category—Health promotion and maintenance*
> *Client Needs Subcategory—None*

82. **4.** The client who feels nervous about going home with a new baby will benefit most from knowing that she can contact the health care facility after her discharge if she has questions. Some facilities also make follow-up phone calls to check on the new mother. The client will probably have the same nervous feeling at the time of the rescheduled discharge if the discharge is postponed, so this action will only relieve the nervousness temporarily. Nervousness is not usually an acceptable reason for postponing the client's discharge. The nurse should acknowledge that the client's feelings are normal and provide her with written instructions on infant care, but these actions alone probably will not alleviate her nervousness.

> *Client Needs Category—Psychosocial integrity*
> *Client Needs Subcategory—None*

83. **2.** An elevated temperature, abdominal tenderness, foul-smelling lochia, an abnormally large uterus, and chills are all manifestations of a puerperal infection. When infection is present, the pulse usually in-

creases. The presence of lochia serosa on the fifth postpartum day is considered within normal limits.

> *Client Needs Category—Physiological integrity*
> *Client Needs Subcategory—Physiological adaptation*

Nursing Care of the Newborn Client

84. **1, 2, 3, 4.** A Mongolian spot is bluish gray pigmentation found on the sacrum, buttocks, or scrotum of children of Asian, southern European, and African American descent. This pigmentation fades by school age and is considered a normal variation of the skin. Milia are pinpoint papules that are unopened sebaceous glands found on the nose and cheek. They disappear after a couple of weeks and are also considered a normal variation of the skin. Epstein's pearls are small, hard, shiny white specks on the gums and hard palate. They disappear a few days after birth and are of no significance. Erythema toxicum, commonly called newborn rash, is found on the cheeks. It disappears by the third day and is a normal variation of the skin.

Molding refers to the shape the newborn's head assumes and retains as it molds to the cervix during delivery. Although a normal finding (especially in primiparous women), it is not associated with the skin. A cephalohematoma is a collection of blood between the periosteum and skull bones that occurs about 1 day after delivery. Although a fairly common finding in newborns, cephalohematoma is not a normal variation of the skin.

> *Client Needs Category—Health promotion and maintenance*
> *Client Needs Subcategory—None*

85. **1, 4, 5.** The normal head circumference of a term newborn is 13″ to 14½″ (34 to 35 cm). Therefore, a head circumference of 20″ (50 cm) is quite large and should be reported immediately because it may be an indication of hydrocephalus resulting from a neural tube disorder. The heart rate of a normal newborn is between 140 and 160 beats/minute; consequently, a heart rate of 100 beats/minute indicates bradycardia and requires immediate attention. A weight of 11 lb (5 kg) is also considered abnormal and requires immediate notification. A newborn's weight is generally between 5½ and 10 lb (2.5 and 4.7 kg); any weight above this range may be caused by gestational diabetes. Because newborns of diabetic mothers are generally larger, these newborns are prone to low blood glucose levels and require frequent glucose level monitoring.

A chest circumference of 13″ (33 cm) is within the normal range of 12½″ to 14″ (31.8 to 35.6 cm) for a newborn. Also, a length of 19½″ (50 cm) is within the normal range of 19 to 21 (48 to 53 cm). Generally, the chest and abdominal circumferences should be similar

in measurement. An abdominal circumference of 11½″ (30 cm) is within normal range for a term newborn.
Client Needs Category—Health promotion and maintenance
Client Needs Subcategory—None

86. **1, 2, 3, 4.** The nurse should expect to find the rooting, Moro, tonic neck, and extrusion reflexes in a normal newborn. The rooting reflex serves to help the newborn find food. It is manifested when stroking the newborn's cheek or mouth causes him to turn his head toward the same direction. The rooting reflex disappears at about 2 months, when the infant's eyesight improves. The Moro reflex, also called the startle reflex, is a protective mechanism that fades by the 4th to 5th month, when the infant can roll away from danger.

The tonic neck reflex is described as a fencing position: When the newborn lies on his back, his head is usually turned to the side, and the arm and leg on the same side are extended while the arm and leg on the opposite side are contracted. The tonic neck reflex does not appear to have a particular function, as the other reflexes do. The extrusion reflex is a protective mechanism that prevents the infant from swallowing inedible substances. It is manifested by protrusion of the tongue when any substance is placed on its tip (the infant looks as if he is spitting out the substance). This reflex usually fades at about 4 months, at which time solid foods are usually introduced. Barlow and Ortolani are not reflexes. The terms are associated with the assessment of congenital hip dislocation.
Client Needs Category—Health promotion and maintenance
Client Needs Subcategory—None

87. **7.** Remember that 1 kg = 2.2 lb. To convert, multiply 3.5 kg by 2.2 lb = 7 lb.
Client Needs Category—Health promotion and maintenance
Client Needs Subcategory—None

88. **3.** Yellow skin discoloration within 24 hours of the newborn's birth indicates pathologic jaundice. This finding should be reported immediately so that the health care provider can order the appropriate treatment. Bluish discoloration of the hands and feet, a pulse rate of 140 beats/minute, and slightly swollen labia are all normal findings in a female newborn.
Client Needs Category—Physiological integrity
Client Needs Subcategory—Physiological adaptation

89. **2.** The axillary temperature of a normal newborn ranges from 97.7° to 98.6° F (36.5° and 37°C). Any lower temperature is associated with hypothermia. The hypothermic newborn should be placed on a prewarmed radiant warmer and rewarmed gradually over a period

of approximately 2 hours. Warming the newborn too rapidly can result in apnea and acidosis. When the temperature is within the acceptable range, the newborn can be dressed, wrapped in a blanket, and placed in an open crib; the temperature should be rechecked again in 4 to 8 hours.
Client Needs Category—Physiological integrity
Client Needs Subcategory—Physiological adaptation

90. **1, 3, 4.** Newborn safety is a major focus in the hospital. Therefore, addressing this issue with the parents is the prudent thing to do. The nurse should instruct the parents to look at their baby's ID band during each visit because these bracelets are prone to fall off and become lost when dressing and undressing the newborn. The mother (and, in some cases, the father or significant other) should also wear an ID bracelet throughout her stay. Hospital personnel should check the name bracelets of both the mother and baby upon entering the room. Because only authorized hospital personnel should be allowed in the mother's room, the nurse should instruct the mother to look for a valid hospital ID on anyone entering the room. She should also instruct her to never leave her baby unattended. If she plans to take a shower or must leave the room, she should ask that the baby be taken back to the nursery.

After delivery, most mothers are extremely tired. Having the newborn sleep in bed with the mother is not considered safe practice. Mothers should also be advised not to breast-feed or bottle-feed their babies in bed during the night after returning home.
Client Needs Category—Safe, effective care environment
Client Needs Subcategory—Safety and infection control

91. **2, 3, 4.** Mother-infant bonding is usually a natural occurrence after delivery. To adequately assess bonding, the nurse should observe the mother's interactions with the baby and listen to what she is saying. The nurse should also assess the mother's nonverbal cues, such as how she looks at the baby during the first few hours following birth and while breast-feeding. The mother should be touching the baby and making good eye contact. Talking or singing to the baby and discussing the baby's physical attributes are also good signs of mother-infant bonding. To facilitate bonding, the mother should hold her baby close to her (not far away). Becoming upset because the baby spits up should alert the nurse that further observation is warranted. Repeatedly asking if the baby is going to live indicates an unwillingness to invest in the bonding process.
Client Needs Category—Health promotion and maintenance
Client Needs Subcategory—None

92. **1.** Each breast consists of lobules that house the milk-secreting cells. The size of the breast is determined by the amount of adipose tissue, not the milk-secreting cells. Thus, breast size has nothing to do with a woman's ability to breast-feed.

> ***Client Needs Category***—*Health promotion and maintenance*
> ***Client Needs Subcategory***—*None*

93. **1.** During the first few days after delivery, all newborns normally lose up to 10% of their birth weight. It is not necessarily true that a newborn who bottle-feeds first will not successfully breast-feed because of her preference for a bottle nipple. The nurse should advise the client that it is preferable to breast-feed rather than pump the breast because the infant's sucking stimulates production of an adequate amount of milk to meet the newborn's needs. Also, breast-fed newborns benefit from the colostrum initially present in breast milk.

> ***Client Needs Category***—*Health promotion and maintenance*
> ***Client Needs Subcategory***—*None*

94. **2.** Colostrum is a thin, yellowish fluid that contains maternal antibodies, salt, protein, and fat. The maternal antibodies found in colostrum provide the newborn with limited immunity to certain disorders. Also, colostrum has a laxative effect and helps the newborn expel the thick meconium normally present in the intestinal tract at birth. Colostrum does not contain estrogen, predigested fats, or digestive enzymes.

> ***Client Needs Category***—*Health promotion and maintenance*
> ***Client Needs Subcategory***—*None*

95. **3.** A breast shield is not routinely used for breast-feeding. A breast shield is worn when the nipple is flat or inverted and occasionally when the nipple is sore and cracked. The other options identify correct breast-feeding techniques.

> ***Client Needs Category***—*Health promotion and maintenance*
> ***Client Needs Subcategory***—*None*

96. **4.** When suctioning the newborn with a bulb syringe, the bulb should be compressed before it is placed in the nose or mouth, and then decompressed once it is inserted so that mucus can be aspirated. The mouth should be suctioned before the nose to prevent aspiration during the gasp response. Also, the back of the throat should not be touched when suctioning the mouth because the gag reflex may be stimulated.

> ***Client Needs Category***—*Health promotion and maintenance*
> ***Client Needs Subcategory***—*None*

97. **4.** The newborn should be placed supine (on the back) when positioned in the crib. Placing a newborn or infant in the prone position (on the stomach) is associated with sudden infant death syndrome. The left-side lying position may prevent aspiration, but does not facilitate gastric emptying.

> ***Client Needs Category***—*Health promotion and maintenance*
> ***Client Needs Subcategory***—*None*

98. **2.** A newborn whose nutritional needs are not being met is at risk for developing dehydration. One indication of dehydration in a newborn is having fewer than six wet diapers per day. It is normal for a breast-fed newborn to have loose, pale-yellow stools, to awaken during the night for a feeding, and to feed every 2 to 3 hours.

> ***Client Needs Category***—*Health promotion and maintenance*
> ***Client Needs Subcategory***—*None*

99. **2.** Breast milk can be stored in the refrigerator for up to 2 days (48 hours). It can be stored in a freezer (one with separate refrigerator and freezer doors) for up to 3 months or in a deep-freezer for up to 12 months. Breast milk should be refrigerated immediately after being pumped; it should not be allowed to sit at room temperature.

> ***Client Needs Category***—*Health promotion and maintenance*
> ***Client Needs Subcategory***—*None*

100. **4.** Postterm newborns (delivered at 41 weeks' gestation or more) are at risk for such complications as meconium aspiration if the pregnancy is allowed to progress longer than 42 weeks. Usually, labor needs to be induced. Postterm newborns are usually lighter in weight because of placental insufficiency and have dry, cracked, leathery skin. They also lack vernix and have longer than normal fingernails. Premature babies tend to have flat, shapeless ears; legs in a froglike position; and few sole creases.

> ***Client Needs Category***—*Health promotion and maintenance*
> ***Client Needs Subcategory***—*None*

101. **2.** The umbilical cord has two arteries and one vein. Variations in this configuration are associated with congenital anomalies, particularly kidney defects. Normal findings include a pendulous scrotum with numerous rugae; vernix caseosa, especially in body creases; and bluish discoloration of the hands and feet (acrocyanosis).

> ***Client Needs Category***—*Health promotion and maintenance*
> ***Client Needs Subcategory***—*None*

102. **1.** Asymmetry of the gluteal skin folds, limited abduction of the affected hip, and apparent shortening of the femur are signs of congenital hip dysplasia. Absence of spontaneous leg movement may be associated with other musculoskeletal disorders and usually is not seen in a newborn with congenital hip dysplasia. An exaggerated curvature of the lumbar spine (lordosis) is unrelated to congenital hip dysplasia.

Client Needs Category—Physiological integrity
Client Needs Subcategory—Physiological adaptation

103. **2.** The newborn should not be placed in the supine position during feeding because of the danger of aspiration. Infants seem to bottle-feed best when held close and at a 45-degree angle. The techniques stated in the other options are correct for bottle-feeding the newborn.

Client Needs Category—Health promotion and maintenance
Client Needs Subcategory—None

104. **4.** Positioning the bottle so that the nipple remains full of formula throughout the feeding prevents the baby from swallowing air. Keeping the nipple full of formula does not affect the infant's gums, nor will it prevent regurgitation. Also, this technique does not appear to prevent the infant from getting tired while feeding.

Client Needs Category—Health promotion and maintenance
Client Needs Subcategory—None

105. **3.** Prepared formula can be refrigerated for up to 48 hours. However, any formula remaining in the bottle when the newborn has finished feeding should be discarded. Bottles can be washed in a dishwasher or with hot, soapy water or warm tap water. If the water source is questionable, tap water should be boiled first. Also, the lid of the can of formula concentrate should be wiped before being opened.

Client Needs Category—Health promotion and maintenance
Client Needs Subcategory—None

106. **2.** A yellowish skin discoloration is known as jaundice. Acrocyanosis indicates a bluish discoloration of the hands and feet. Erythematous means that the skin is red. Mottling is an irregular skin discoloration that is associated with hypothermia or oxygen depravation.

Client Needs Category—Physiological integrity
Client Needs Subcategory—Physiological adaptation

107. **1.** The nurse should remove the newborn's clothes when preparing him for phototherapy and ap-

ply protective eye shields to protect his retinas from damage caused by the ultraviolet lights used in the treatment. The nurse should monitor the newborn's temperature frequently, assessing for hypothermia (from being unclothed) and hyperthermia (because of exposure to the light source). I.V. infusions and nasogastric tube feedings are not required for phototherapy. The infant's position should be changed frequently to ensure exposure of all body surface areas to the ultraviolet light.

Client Needs Category—Physiological integrity
Client Needs Subcategory—Physiological adaptation

108. **3.** Following circumcision, the newborn's penis should be frequently assessed for signs of swelling and bleeding, the most common complications associated with the circumcision procedure. If penile swelling occurs, the urinary meatus may be occluded, affecting urine output. Therefore, monitoring intake and output is an appropriate nursing intervention. Petroleum gauze dressings are not required when a Plastibell is in place. In most cases, it is unnecessary to check the vital signs more frequently unless there are complications such as hemorrhage. Bacteriostatic ointments may be applied if a Gomco circumcision has been performed; otherwise, the health care provider should be consulted for further instructions when an infection is suspected. Placing the newborn on his abdomen is inappropriate because the nurse cannot assess the amount of bleeding if it occurs; also, newborns should not be positioned this way because of the risk of sudden infant death syndrome.

Client Needs Category—Physiological integrity
Client Needs Subcategory—Physiological adaptation

109. **1.** The physician should be notified if there is any drainage from the penis, if there are any blood spots larger than the size of a quarter, if the infant is not voiding, and if the Plastibell ring has not fallen off in 7 days. The Plastibell ring should not be removed manually. The penis should be gently cleaned with soap and water. It is unnecessary to apply petroleum jelly to the penis if a Plastibell ring is in place.

Client Needs Category—Health promotion and maintenance
Client Needs Subcategory—None

110. **1.** The newborn should be drinking breast milk or formula for at least 2 to 3 days before a PKU test is performed. If the newborn has not been receiving formula for the prescribed time, the result may be inaccurate. Newborns discharged prior to this time should have the test performed within the prescribed amount of time in an outpatient setting, such as the pediatrician's office or a clinic. The data identified in the remaining options are not needed when performing the PKU test.

> *Client Needs Category*—*Health promotion and maintenance*
> *Client Needs Subcategory*—*None*

111. 4. After the heel stick, the nurse should apply pressure to the newborn's heel with dry gauze to prevent further bleeding. The nurse is correct to warm the heel, puncture the lateral aspect of the heel, and discard the first drop of blood when performing the PKU test.

> *Client Needs Category*—*Safe, effective care environment*
> *Client Needs Subcategory*—*Safety and infection control*

Nursing Care of Newborns with Complications

112. 1. A client who is experiencing grief may delay naming her newborn, may be reluctant to visit the baby in the nursery, or may focus on equipment and treatments rather than the baby when visiting. Asking the physician to postpone her discharge from the hospital is not a sign of anticipatory grieving; instead, this request is often made because the client does not want to leave the newborn.

> *Client Needs Category*—*Psychosocial integrity*
> *Client Needs Subcategory*—*None*

113. 2. A myelomeningocele is a neural tube defect that occurs during the embryonic development of the nervous system, when the spinal column fails to cover the spinal cord. This defect is evident by the presence of the meninges and spinal cord protruding outside the vertebral column. Because of the exposure of the meninges, meningitis is a realistic complication. Motor and sensory functions are affected beyond the point of the defect, resulting in paralysis of the lower extremities and loss of bowel and bladder function. Hydrocephalus and clubfoot are common findings in conjunction with this defect.

To facilitate acceptance and care of the newborn with this defect, the nurse should act as a role model by demonstrating the proper way to feed, hold, and change the newborn. This will encourage the parents to interact with their baby and promote early bonding. Although surgery will result in closure of the defect, it may not correct the neurologic deficit that accompanies this condition. Showing the parents "before" and "after" surgery pictures is usually more effective when the surgical intervention results in correction of the deformity or disorder; however, this is not the case with myelomeningocele. Social agencies usually do not take custody or assume care of a child unless there is due cause, such as neglect or abuse.

> *Client Needs Category*—*Psychosocial integrity*
> *Client Needs Subcategory*—*None*

114. 1. When oxygen is given in high concentrations to a premature newborn in respiratory distress, he becomes especially vulnerable to developing blindness due to hemorrhage of blood vessels in the eyes followed by retinal detachment. Therefore, frequent monitoring of the oxygen concentration is necessary to ensure that excessive amounts are not given. Assessment of the bilirubin level, hemoglobin level, and pupillary response will not assist the nurse in preventing ROP.

> *Client Needs Category*—*Safe, effective care environment*
> *Client Needs Subcategory*—*Safety and infection control*

115. 3. Preterm newborns may have weak or absent sucking and swallowing reflexes. These infants may require nasogastric formula or breast milk feeding, or feedings of parenteral fluids (TPN and lipids) by an umbilical catheter or peripheral vein. The normal interval between formula or breast milk feedings is 2 to 3 hours. The amount fed depends on the infant's weight, but it may be as little as 1 to 5 ml for each feeding. If glucose is tolerated, the physician may order a formula similar to that fed to normal-sized newborns.

> *Client Needs Category*—*Physiological integrity*
> *Client Needs Subcategory*—*Physiological adaptation*

116. 2. The primary reason that a preterm newborn is at risk for developing infections is the lack of maternal antibodies that are normally supplied during the third trimester of pregnancy and the newborn's inability to produce antibodies independently. Care is taken to prevent exposure to bacterial and viral infections; procedures are done using strict asepsis. The preterm newborn does have fragile skin, but appropriate measures are taken to prevent skin breakdown.

> *Client Needs Category*—*Physiological integrity*
> *Client Needs Subcategory*—*Physiological adaptation*

117. 3. The preterm newborn is kept in an Isolette or radiant warmer because of the increased risk of cold stress secondary to the immaturity of the brain's temperature-regulating centers, the absence of subcutaneous fat, and the large surface area of the newborn's head. The other actions are appropriate to maintain thermoregulation in a full-term newborn but are inadequate for the preterm newborn's special needs.

> *Client Needs Category*—*Physiological integrity*
> *Client Needs Subcategory*—*Physiological adaptation*

118. **4.** Jaundice within 24 to 36 hours after birth indicates congenital hemolytic disease (erythroblastosis fetalis). Physiological jaundice, which occurs in some newborns, is seen 3 to 4 days after birth. Alterations in the respiratory rate, newborn reflexes, and movement of extremities are not usual manifestations associated with Rh incompatibility.

> *Client Needs Category—Physiological integrity*
> *Client Needs Subcategory—Physiological adaptation*

119. **4.** The direct Coombs' test requires a sample of the newborn's blood. The usual procedure is to obtain a specimen from the umbilical cord after the newborn is delivered and the cord is cut. An indirect Coombs' test is performed using a specimen of maternal blood. Paternal blood and sibling blood are not used for a direct or indirect Coombs' test.

> *Client Needs Category—Safe, effective care environment*
> *Client Needs Subcategory—Safety and infection control*

120. **1.** Infants with congenital hemolytic disease are treated with phototherapy to reduce the amount of circulating bilirubin. This requires covering the newborn's eyes with eye shields to protect the retinas from damage. Vital signs are monitored every 4 hours. Fluids are given by mouth to maintain hydration and promote excretion of bilirubin via urine and feces. A small covering is commonly placed over the genitalia to serve the same purpose as a diaper.

> *Client Needs Category—Physiological integrity*
> *Client Needs Subcategory—Physiological adaptation*

121. **1.** Nursing care of an HIV-positive client should include standard precautions. Standard precautions were developed by the U.S. Centers for Disease Control and Prevention in an effort to reduce the risk of transmission of blood-borne and other pathogens in hospitals. All clients are cared for using standard precautions guidelines. The other forms of isolation are not necessary unless additional protection is needed for a specific disorder.

> *Client Needs Category—Safe, effective care environment*
> *Client Needs Subcategory—Safety and infection control*

122. **3.** Between 30% and 50% of children who are HIV-positive contract the virus via perinatal transmission. Infants of HIV-positive mothers are not tested for anti-HIV antibodies before they are 3 months old because the mother's antibodies may be present in the baby's blood for at least that long and may cause a false-positive reading of HIV antibody test. Infants of HIV-positive mothers are usually tested periodically for at least 2 years.

> *Client Needs Category—Physiological integrity*
> *Client Needs Subcategory—Physiological adaptation*

123. **4.** Infants who are HIV-positive are typically asymptomatic at birth but usually develop symptoms of AIDS by age 2 years.

> *Client Needs Category—Physiological integrity*
> *Client Needs Subcategory—Physiological adaptation*

124. **3.** HIV can be transmitted via breast milk; therefore, HIV-positive mothers are instructed not to breast-feed their newborns because of the possibility of transmitting the disease. HIV transmission can occur even if the mother does not exhibit signs and symptoms of AIDS. An infant whose test result is positive for the anti-HIV antibodies may have maternal anti-HIV antibodies; thus, the infant may not actually have the virus even though his test result is positive. Because of this, the infant should not be breast-fed regardless of whether or not an anti-HIV antibody test is positive. Absence of symptoms in the newborn would be more indicative of the absence of HIV rather than the presence of the disease; therefore, breast-feeding this uninfected infant could expose him to the virus.

> *Client Needs Category—Physiological integrity*
> *Client Needs Subcategory—Reduction of risk potential*

[UNIT III]

The Nursing Care of Children

The Nursing Care of Infants, Toddlers, and Preschool Children

⇨ *Normal Growth and Development of Infants, Toddlers, and Preschool Children*
⇨ *Nursing Care of an Infant with Myelomeningocele*
⇨ *Nursing Care of an Infant with Hydrocephalus*
⇨ *Nursing Care of an Infant with Cleft Lip*
⇨ *Nursing Care of an Infant with Pyloric Stenosis*
⇨ *Nursing Care of an Infant with Bilateral Clubfoot*
⇨ *Nursing Care of a Child with Otitis Media*
⇨ *Nursing Care of a Child with a Congenital Heart Defect*
⇨ *Nursing Care of a Child with an Infectious Disease*
⇨ *Nursing Care of a Child with HIV Infection*
⇨ *Nursing Care of a Child with Atopic Dermatitis*
⇨ *Nursing Care of a Toddler with Sickle Cell Crisis*
⇨ *Nursing Care of a Toddler with Cystic Fibrosis*
⇨ *Nursing Care of a Toddler with Asthma*
⇨ *Nursing Care of a Toddler Who Has Swallowed a Toxic Substance*
⇨ *Nursing Care of a Toddler with Croup*
⇨ *Nursing Care of a Toddler with Pneumonia*
⇨ *Nursing Care of a Preschooler with Seizure Disorder*
⇨ *Nursing Care of a Preschooler with Leukemia*
⇨ *Nursing Care of a Preschooler with Strabismus*
⇨ *Nursing Care of a Preschooler Having a Tonsillectomy and Adenoidectomy*
⇨ *Correct Answers and Rationales*

Directions: *With a pencil, blacken the space in front of the option you have chosen for your correct answer.*

Normal Growth and Development of Infants, Toddlers, and Preschool Children

The nurse in a well-baby clinic assesses the growth and development of healthy infants and toddlers and uses that information as a basis for teaching.

1. Which assessment finding would the nurse consider normal for a 3-month-old infant?
[ ] **1.** Able to hold a bottle
[ ] **2.** Able to lift head and shoulders
[ ] **3.** Able to roll from back to abdomen
[ ] **4.** Able to sit with support

2. Following routine immunizations, which of the following symptoms should the nurse instruct the parents of a 15-month-old child to report?
[ ] **1.** Fever that occurs within 7 to 10 days of the immunization
[ ] **2.** Rash that appears 2 to 4 days following the immunization
[ ] **3.** Crying for more than 3 hours, even after comfort measures are taken
[ ] **4.** Soreness, redness, and swelling at the injection site

3. During a home health visit to a family with a 20-month-old child, the nurse would expect to discuss childhood safety issues with the parent when noticing which finding?

[ ] **1.** Electrical outlets are covered.
[ ] **2.** The child is eating raw carrots.
[ ] **3.** Furniture has rounded edges.
[ ] **4.** The child is building a tower with large blocks.

4. Which artery is the best site to assess the pulse of a 2-year-old child who is brought to the clinic for a well-child checkup?

[ ] **1.** Apical
[ ] **2.** Brachial
[ ] **3.** Carotid
[ ] **4.** Radial

The nurse provides instructions about the proper administration of oral medications in liquid form to the parents of an infant.

5. The nurse can assume the parents understood the medication instructions when they make which statement?

[ ] **1.** "We'll add the medication to the bottle of formula."
[ ] **2.** "We should pinch the baby's nose when we're giving him the medicine."
[ ] **3.** "We need to use a rubber-tipped medicine dropper to give the medicine."
[ ] **4.** "We should give the baby the medicine while he's lying on his back."

6. Which assessment technique is most accurate for counting the respirations of an infant during a well-child checkup?

[ ] **1.** Count the respirations for 10 seconds and multiply by 6.
[ ] **2.** Count the respirations for 15 seconds and multiply by 4.
[ ] **3.** Count the respirations for 30 seconds and multiply by 2.
[ ] **4.** Count the respirations for 60 seconds or one full minute.

7. Which statement by a toddler's mother suggests the need for further teaching about signs of readiness for toilet-training?

[ ] **1.** "I won't start toilet training my daughter until she's at least 18 months old because sphincter control isn't usually accomplished before then."
[ ] **2.** "I should begin bladder training before bowel training."
[ ] **3.** "I'll wait until my daughter can communicate when she needs to go to the bathroom."
[ ] **4.** "I should wait to begin toilet training until my daughter can remove her underwear by herself."

8. Which is the best advice a nurse can give parents who are helping a 3-year-old child overcome the rivalry created by the birth of a sibling?

[ ] **1.** Enroll the child immediately in a day-long preschool program.
[ ] **2.** Arrange for the child to have extended visits with grandparents.
[ ] **3.** Find ways that the child can assist with the infant's care.
[ ] **4.** Invite other similarly aged children to play with the child.

9. Which teaching aid is developmentally appropriate for a preschooler who is about to have a bone marrow puncture?

[ ] **1.** Dolls or puppets
[ ] **2.** Pamphlets or booklets
[ ] **3.** Colored diagrams
[ ] **4.** Commercial videotapes

10. Which action by parents of a 16-month-old toddler indicates that they understand how to best minimize separation anxiety during their child's hospitalization?

[ ] **1.** The parents bring the child's favorite toy to the hospital.
[ ] **2.** The parents explain all procedures to the child.
[ ] **3.** The parents remain with the child during the hospital stay.
[ ] **4.** The parents bring the siblings to visit the child.

11. Which instruction would the nurse include when teaching the parents about introducing solid foods to a 4-month-old infant?

[ ] **1.** Begin with plain strained fruits and vegetables.
[ ] **2.** Do not breast- or bottle-feed until after solid food has been given.
[ ] **3.** Introduce one food at a time at an interval of every 4 to 5 days.
[ ] **4.** Postpone introduction if the infant pushes food out of his mouth with his tongue.

12. Which assessment finding would the nurse consider abnormal for an 18-month-old child?

[ ] **1.** Vocabulary of about 6 words
[ ] **2.** Uses a spoon when eating
[ ] **3.** Walks with support
[ ] **4.** Shows readiness for toilet training

13. Which observation by the nurse indicates that the parents of a toddler need additional teaching regarding household safety?

[ ] **1.** Household cleaners are in their original containers.

[ ] **2.** Medicines are stored on a high shelf out of the child's reach.

[ ] **3.** The hot water heater thermostat is set at 120° F (48.8° C).

[ ] **4.** The number for the poison control center is posted by the telephone.

14. If the father of a 4-year-old child tells the nurse that he is concerned because his child frequently talks about a make-believe playmate, which response by the nurse is best?

[ ] **1.** "This type of behavior is normal for a preschooler."

[ ] **2.** "Can you identify any stressors that may be causing this regression?"

[ ] **3.** "You may need a referral to see a child psychologist."

[ ] **4.** "Give a time out when this behavior occurs."

A young, first time mother expresses concern that she does not understand normal physical growth and development. The mother states, "I'm unsure when I need to childproof my home."

15. Prioritize the mother's actions in the home with the child's physical development progression. List in ascending chronological order the actions the mother will need to do now through the first year of life. Use all the options.

1. **Cover the electrical outlets.**
2. **Have straps on the changing table.**
3. **Turn pot handles inward when cooking.**
4. **Remove stuffed animals with small pieces from the child's grasp.**
5. **Lower crib mattress.**
6. **Maintain water temperature under 120° F (48.8° C).**

Nursing Care of an Infant with Myelomeningocele

An infant is born with a myelomeningocele high in the spinal column.

16. Which nursing action is most important for the nurse to include during the preoperative period?

[ ] **1.** Keep the diaper area clean to prevent contamination of the myelomeningocele.

[ ] **2.** Position the infant so that there is no pressure on the myelomeningocele.

[ ] **3.** Keep the infant's myelomeningocele clean by washing it with antiseptic soap.

[ ] **4.** Encourage the parents to cuddle and hold the infant to promote bonding.

A surgical repair of the myelomeningocele is successfully completed.

17. Unless the physician orders otherwise, in which position should the infant be placed during the postoperative period?

[ ] **1.** Supine

[ ] **2.** Prone

[ ] **3.** Right- or left side-lying

[ ] **4.** Whichever position is most comfortable for the infant

18. In planning the infant's home care, which expectation about walking should the nurse keep in mind?

[ ] **1.** The infant will be unable to walk without crutches.

[ ] **2.** The infant will have a 50% chance of eventually walking alone.

[ ] **3.** The infant will have a 95% chance of eventually walking alone.

[ ] **4.** The infant will someday be able to walk without crutches.

19. What should the nurse teach the parents to prepare them for managing their child's urinary incontinence at home?
[ ] **1.** How to care for a retention catheter
[ ] **2.** How to insert a straight catheter
[ ] **3.** How to reapply a ureterostomy appliance
[ ] **4.** How to attach an external catheter

The infant also has talipes equinovarus (clubfoot) and congenital hip dysplasia (dislocation of the hips).

20. What is the priority nursing intervention to prevent contractures of the infant's lower extremities?
[ ] **1.** Massage the lower extremities.
[ ] **2.** Reposition the infant frequently.
[ ] **3.** Place sheepskin under the bony prominences.
[ ] **4.** Conduct range-of-motion exercises.

Nursing Care of an Infant with Hydrocephalus

A 1-week-old infant who was born with hydrocephalus is scheduled for surgery.

21. Which assessment finding for an infant with hydrocephalus is most characteristic of the disorder?
[ ] **1.** Increased head size
[ ] **2.** Paralysis of the lower extremities
[ ] **3.** Absence of the sucking reflex
[ ] **4.** Marked depression of the anterior fontanel

The parents ask the nurse to explain why their baby has hydrocephalus.

22. The nurse correctly explains which as the common cause of hydrocephalus?
[ ] **1.** Absence of the dura mater
[ ] **2.** Blockage of cerebrospinal fluid circulation
[ ] **3.** Increased cerebrospinal fluid in the subarachnoid space
[ ] **4.** Occlusion in the cerebral arteries

23. After feeding the infant, the nurse correctly places him in which position?
[ ] **1.** Sitting
[ ] **2.** Supine
[ ] **3.** Prone
[ ] **4.** Side-lying

24. Which measure is most appropriate to reduce the potential for a pressure ulcer developing on the infant's head?
[ ] **1.** Place a sheepskin under the infant's head.
[ ] **2.** Massage the circumference of the infant's skull.
[ ] **3.** Support the infant's head on two pillows.
[ ] **4.** Apply a padded helmet to the infant's head.

25. If a shunting device is placed on the right side of the infant's head, which postoperative position is most appropriate?
[ ] **1.** The right side, to increase absorption of cerebrospinal fluid
[ ] **2.** The abdomen, to prevent obstruction in the shunt catheter
[ ] **3.** The left side, to avoid pressure on the operative site
[ ] **4.** The back, to promote ventricular drainage

26. Postoperatively, which sign provides the best indication that the infant is developing increased intracranial pressure?
[ ] **1.** Depression of the fontanel
[ ] **2.** Decreased pulse and respiratory rates
[ ] **3.** Change in frequency of bowel movements
[ ] **4.** Sudden increase in weight

27. Postoperatively, which nursing action is most appropriate if the nurse observes that the infant's anterior fontanel is sunken?
[ ] **1.** Document the finding and take no further action.
[ ] **2.** Place the infant in the supine position.
[ ] **3.** Elevate the infant's head.
[ ] **4.** Notify the charge nurse or physician immediately.

Nursing Care of an Infant with Cleft Lip

The nurse is caring for a newborn infant with a cleft lip.

28. During the initial data collection process in the nursery, the nurse palpates the roof of the newborn's mouth to assess for which finding?
[ ] **1.** The infant's ability to suck
[ ] **2.** The presence of a gag reflex
[ ] **3.** An opening in the palate
[ ] **4.** Position of the uvula

29. When taking the newborn to the parents for the first visit, which action is the nurse's priority?
[ ] **1.** Teaching the parents how to feed the infant
[ ] **2.** Demonstrating open acceptance of the infant
[ ] **3.** Discussing the plans for surgical repair of the defect
[ ] **4.** Showing the parents how to use a bulb syringe

30. Which observation by the nurse indicates that the parents understand how to minimize the risk of aspiration?

[ ] **1.** They burp the newborn frequently during feedings.
[ ] **2.** They position the newborn prone for feedings.
[ ] **3.** They feed the newborn formula thickened with rice cereal.
[ ] **4.** They feed the newborn only glucose water until after surgical repair of the defect.

31. Prior to surgery, which utensil is best for the nurse to use when feeding the infant with a cleft lip?

[ ] **1.** Gavage tube
[ ] **2.** Plastic spoon
[ ] **3.** Rubber-tipped syringe
[ ] **4.** Firm rubber nipple

32. Which restraint is best for the nurse to use for a child who has had a cleft lip repair?

[ ] **1.** Papoose board
[ ] **2.** Leg restraints
[ ] **3.** Elbow restraints
[ ] **4.** Posey belt or jacket

33. When developing a care plan for a child who underwent surgery to correct a cleft lip, how frequently should the nurse plan to remove and reapply the restraints?

[ ] **1.** Daily
[ ] **2.** Every 8 hours
[ ] **3.** Every 4 hours
[ ] **4.** Every 2 hours

Nursing Care of an Infant with Pyloric Stenosis

The nurse is caring for a 3-week-old infant who has been admitted to the hospital for surgical correction of pyloric stenosis.

34. Which assessment finding is most significant during the data collection process?

[ ] **1.** The infant is eager to suck.
[ ] **2.** The anterior fontanel is flat.
[ ] **3.** The gastric peristaltic waves are visible.
[ ] **4.** The mucous membranes are dry.

The physician orders an I.V. infusion of dextrose 2.5% normal saline solution.

35. Which information regarding infant I.V. therapy is correct?

[ ] **1.** The infant's head may be shaved at the I.V. site.
[ ] **2.** The infant will be maintained on nothing-by-mouth (NPO) status during I.V. therapy.
[ ] **3.** The infant may be restless during I.V. therapy.
[ ] **4.** The area around the I.V. site will swell slightly.

36. After surgical correction of the defect, the nurse demonstrates to the parents the correct way to feed the infant by placing him in which position?

[ ] **1.** On his abdomen
[ ] **2.** On his side
[ ] **3.** On his back
[ ] **4.** In a comfortable position

Nursing Care of an Infant with Bilateral Clubfoot

A 1-week-old infant with bilateral talipes equinovarus (bilateral clubfoot) is being seen at the pediatrician's office.

37. Which of the following information found in the infant's birth history is most indicative of a true clubfoot condition?

[ ] **1.** The infant was born in the breech position.
[ ] **2.** The heels were drawn in and the feet turned inward.
[ ] **3.** The feet could not be corrected to a neutral position.
[ ] **4.** Both feet were affected at birth.

After nonsurgical treatment failed to correct the infant's defect, bilateral leg casts are applied.

38. When the mother asks why the ends of the cast have adhesive "petals," how should the nurse respond?

[ ] **1.** "The adhesive petals ensure that nothing is placed between the cast and the skin."
[ ] **2.** "The adhesive petals allow air circulation between the cast and the skin."
[ ] **3.** "The adhesive petals prevent the plaster of the cast from irritating the skin."
[ ] **4.** "The adhesive petals allow for stronger bonding of the plaster cast materials."

39. Which finding noted by the nurse best indicates that the infant is experiencing a neurovascular complication?

[ ] **1.** The infant cries 4 hours after the last feeding.
[ ] **2.** The infant's toes are wiggling.
[ ] **3.** The infant's toes are pale and cold.
[ ] **4.** The pedal pulse is 110 beats/minute and regular.

40. Which nursing action will minimize swelling of the infant's feet?
[ ] **1.** Elevate the legs and feet on a pillow.
[ ] **2.** Place the infant in the prone position.
[ ] **3.** Petal the edges of the cast.
[ ] **4.** Apply ice packs over the cast.

41. The nurse correctly informs the infant's parents that initially the casts will be changed how frequently?
[ ] **1.** Every 3 to 7 days
[ ] **2.** Every 1 to 2 weeks
[ ] **3.** On a monthly basis
[ ] **4.** Every other month

When the infant is 8 weeks old, he is seen in the pediatrician's office for a routine cast change. The nurse uses this opportunity to teach the parents ways to promote normal growth and development.

42. Which age-appropriate developmental instruction can the nurse recommend to the parents during this visit?
[ ] **1.** Encouraging the infant to crawl about in the crib
[ ] **2.** Playing peek-a-boo with the infant's favorite blanket
[ ] **3.** Encouraging the infant to reach for cuddly toys
[ ] **4.** Placing a brightly colored mobile over the crib

The parents tell the nurse that they can barely feel the soft spot in the back of the infant's head and ask whether this is normal.

43. Which statement by the nurse is most correct?
[ ] **1.** "Barely feeling the soft spot is normal because the posterior fontanel usually closes between 2 and 3 months."
[ ] **2.** "Barely feeling the soft spot is abnormal because the posterior fontanel usually closes between 9 and 18 months."
[ ] **3.** "Barely feeling the soft spot is abnormal because the posterior fontanel usually remains open longer in children."
[ ] **4.** "Barely feeling the soft spot is normal because the posterior fontanel usually closes earlier in children with congenital skeletal defects."

Nursing Care of a Child with Otitis Media

A 6-month-old infant is examined by the physician and found to have otitis media.

44. Which nursing observation best indicates the presence of ear pain in an infant?

[ ] **1.** The infant refuses to suck a bottle.
[ ] **2.** The infant pulls on one ear.
[ ] **3.** The infant's temperature is elevated.
[ ] **4.** There is drainage from the infant's ear.

The pediatrician prescribes an oral antibiotic for 10 days. The office nurse gives the first dose to the infant.

45. When preparing to give medications, which action by the nurse best ensures that the infant receives a safe dose of the prescribed medication?
[ ] **1.** Reading the physician's orders carefully
[ ] **2.** Determining the infant's weight
[ ] **3.** Determining the infant's medication allergies
[ ] **4.** Reading the medication label carefully

46. When explaining the prescribed antibiotic treatment to the parents, the nurse is most likely to emphasize which instruction?
[ ] **1.** "Position your baby on her side after giving the antibiotic."
[ ] **2.** "Give the antibiotic with feedings."
[ ] **3.** "Store the antibiotic at room temperature."
[ ] **4.** "Give the antibiotic for the full 10 days."

47. The physician orders Pediazole 6 mL P.O. every 8 hours for a child with an ear infection. The child weighs 38 lb (17.2 kg). Pediazole contains erythromycin ethylsuccinate 200 mg and sulfisoxazole acetyl 600 mg in a 5-mL suspension. How many milligrams of erythromycin will the child receive in a 24-hour period?

Nursing Care of a Child with a Congenital Heart Defect

A 2-week-old infant with a diagnosis of coarctation of the aorta is being cared for in the high-risk nursery.

48. Which of the following findings obtained on admission best indicates the presence of coarctation of the aorta?
[ ] **1.** Generalized cyanosis, especially when the infant cries
[ ] **2.** Clubbing of the fingers and toes
[ ] **3.** Bounding brachial pulses and weak femoral pulses
[ ] **4.** Rapid and irregular apical heartbeat

49. The nurse correctly advises the parents that the optimal time for surgical correction is when?
[ ] **1.** As soon as the child's condition stabilizes
[ ] **2.** When the child is 6 months old
[ ] **3.** Before the child is 2 years old
[ ] **4.** When the child is between ages 2 and 4

The infant receives digoxin (Lanoxin) while in the nursery.

50. Which nursing intervention is most important to perform before giving digoxin (Lanoxin)?
[ ] **1.** Check the apical pulse for 1 minute.
[ ] **2.** Position the infant with his head slightly elevated.
[ ] **3.** Check the expiration date on the medication label.
[ ] **4.** Monitor the infant's urine output.

51. The nurse can best facilitate reduction of the heart's workload by which method?
[ ] **1.** Limiting the amount of holding and cuddling by the infant's parents
[ ] **2.** Organizing nursing care so that the infant has longer rest periods
[ ] **3.** Feeding only by the nasogastric route
[ ] **4.** Keeping the infant mildly sedated at all times

The nurse provides discharge instructions regarding medication administration.

52. Which statement by the parents indicates a need for additional teaching about administering digoxin (Lanoxin) at home?
[ ] **1.** "If we miss giving a dose, we should give the next dose at the regularly scheduled time."
[ ] **2.** "We need to check the baby's apical pulse before giving each dose of the medication."
[ ] **3.** "We should mix each dose of the medication in a small amount of formula."
[ ] **4.** "We should never increase or decrease the dose except if ordered by the doctor."

Nursing Care of a Child with an Infectious Disease

After a 7-month-old infant with chickenpox is seen in the emergency department, she is admitted to the hospital because of moderate dehydration. An I.V. infusion is begun.

53. Which isolation category is most appropriate for a child with chickenpox in the early stage of infection?
[ ] **1.** Airborne precautions
[ ] **2.** Droplet precautions
[ ] **3.** Contact precautions
[ ] **4.** Standard precautions

54. Which nursing action is correct when implementing the prescribed isolation precautions?

[ ] **1.** A supply of clean masks is placed in the child's room.
[ ] **2.** Specimens are sent to the laboratory in a zip-closure biohazard bag.
[ ] **3.** The child is assigned to a semiprivate room.
[ ] **4.** A glass thermometer is utilized and wiped with alcohol following use.

55. A child weighing 18 lb (8.2 kg) is receiving maintenance I.V. fluids. What would be the daily I.V. fluid volume for this child?

_____

56. After obtaining all of the following data, which is most important to report to the charge nurse?
[ ] **1.** The child sleeps for short intervals during the day.
[ ] **2.** There is an increase in the frequency and amount of urine.
[ ] **3.** The child occasionally cries when disturbed by noise.
[ ] **4.** There is an increase in the I.V. infusion drip rate.

Nursing Care of a Child with Human Immunodeficiency Virus (HIV) Infection

A 2-month-old infant with HIV infection is discharged from the hospital to go home with her mother. At age 4 months, the infant is seen in the physician's office for a routine checkup.

57. Which of the following assessment data documented by the nurse is considered a high-risk factor for developing acquired immunodeficiency syndrome (AIDS)?
[ ] **1.** The child has pinpoint white spots on her nose.
[ ] **2.** The mother states that her daughter has had thrush twice.
[ ] **3.** The child's respirations have an irregular pattern.
[ ] **4.** The mother states that her daughter wets six diapers per day.

58. While developing a care plan for a 2-year-old child with perinatally acquired HIV infection, which assessment findings would indicate that the child has clinical signs of AIDS? Select all that apply.
[ ] **1.** History of bacterial infections
[ ] **2.** Herpes simplex lesions around the mouth
[ ] **3.** White patch in the mouth and larynx
[ ] **4.** Lung consolidation on a chest X-ray
[ ] **5.** Limited muscle tone
[ ] **6.** Increased blood pressure

Nursing Care of a Child with Atopic Dermatitis

A 2-year-old child in the clinic is diagnosed with atopic dermatitis. The mother asks what caused the child's skin condition and why the physician had many questions about the home environment.

59. The nurse is correct in correlating which factor as a probable cause of this child's atopic dermatitis?
[ ] **1.** Poor nutrition
[ ] **2.** Premature birth
[ ] **3.** Allergic reaction
[ ] **4.** Hormonal imbalance

60. Which disease symptom is the nurse most likely to focus on when providing the mother with preventive care measures?
[ ] **1.** Nausea
[ ] **2.** Vomiting
[ ] **3.** Itching
[ ] **4.** Drowsiness

The physician prescribes hydrocortisone ointment (Cortaid) for the child's skin lesions and instructs the mother to give him colloid baths.

61. On a subsequent visit, which outcome demonstrates that the ointment has been effective?
[ ] **1.** The child's skin is no longer weeping.
[ ] **2.** There is no further spread of the skin lesions.
[ ] **3.** The skin inflammation has decreased.
[ ] **4.** The child's white blood cell count is increased.

62. When instructing the mother on how to give a colloid bath, the nurse correctly explains that a typical colloid bath consists of tepid water and which additive?
[ ] **1.** Cornstarch
[ ] **2.** Mineral oil
[ ] **3.** Liquid glycerin soap
[ ] **4.** Iodized salt

Nursing Care of a Toddler with Sickle Cell Crisis

An acutely ill 21-month-old child is admitted to the hospital with vaso-occlusive sickle cell crisis. The child has a 6-year-old sibling who also has sickle cell disease.

63. When admitting the child, which nursing assessment is an initial priority?
[ ] **1.** Assessing for pain
[ ] **2.** Assessing for dehydration
[ ] **3.** Assessing for hemorrhage
[ ] **4.** Assessing for bradycardia

64. The nurse also anticipates which nursing action related to the progression of the child's disease?
[ ] **1.** Administering an I.V. transfusion of plasma
[ ] **2.** Initiating measures to decrease the hemoglobin level
[ ] **3.** Beginning an administration of large doses of iron
[ ] **4.** Promoting measures to rehydrate the child

The mother informs the nurse that she has the sickle cell trait and the child's father has sickle cell disease.

65. Which statement by the mother indicates that she understands how sickle cell disease is transmitted?
[ ] **1.** "All of my children will have sickle cell disease."
[ ] **2.** "With each pregnancy, there is a 50% chance that my baby will be born with sickle cell disease."
[ ] **3.** "If I conceive again, my baby will be born with sickle cell trait."
[ ] **4.** "With each pregnancy, there is a 75% chance that my baby will be born with sickle cell disease."

66. In order to prevent further sickle cell crisis, which instructions provided by the nurse are essential? Select all that apply.
[ ] **1.** Obtain plenty of rest.
[ ] **2.** Drink plenty of fluids.
[ ] **3.** Use routine pain medication.
[ ] **4.** Complete a full course of antibiotics.
[ ] **5.** Utilize proper hand washing.
[ ] **6.** Avoid crowds.

Nursing Care of a Toddler with Cystic Fibrosis

An 18-month-old toddler with a diagnosis of cystic fibrosis is admitted to the hospital because of increasing respiratory difficulty and repeated respiratory infections.

67. Which documented history finding reported by the parents is typical of a child with cystic fibrosis?
[ ] **1.** The child rarely cries.
[ ] **2.** The child has gained a lot of weight.
[ ] **3.** The child tastes salty when kissed.
[ ] **4.** The child has poor head control.

68. Which assessment finding is most likely to be present in the child with cystic fibrosis?
[ ] **1.** Poor appetite
[ ] **2.** Excessive perspiration
[ ] **3.** Low urine output
[ ] **4.** Bulky, foul-smelling stools

69. Which is the priority goal for the child with cystic fibrosis?

[ ] **1.** The child will consume appropriate nutrients to meet body needs.

[ ] **2.** The child will maintain an effective breathing pattern.

[ ] **3.** The child will consume an adequate amount of fluids to meet body needs.

[ ] **4.** The child will demonstrate a decreased level of anxiety.

The physician prescribes a bronchodilator for the child.

70. The nurse determines that this type of therapy is successful if which outcome is noted?

[ ] **1.** There is decreased mucus in the stools.

[ ] **2.** The serum sodium level decreases.

[ ] **3.** The breathing pattern improves.

[ ] **4.** Excess fat is excreted from the body.

After collecting additional data, the nurse determines that the child has not been receiving the recommended diet.

71. The nurse correctly informs the parents that the child should have which type of diet?

[ ] **1.** High-fat

[ ] **2.** Low-protein

[ ] **3.** Low-salt

[ ] **4.** High-calorie

The parents ask the nurse whether the physician can prescribe a larger dosage of pancrelipase (Pancrease) given twice daily instead of the current dosage, which is given with each meal.

72. The nurse correctly explains that Pancrease must be given with meals for which reason?

[ ] **1.** To prevent gastrointestinal upset

[ ] **2.** To increase nutrient absorption

[ ] **3.** To prevent salt depletion

[ ] **4.** To increase the child's desire to eat

73. The nurse further explains that it is necessary to increase the child's fluid intake for which reason?

[ ] **1.** To prevent kidney failure

[ ] **2.** To increase cardiac function

[ ] **3.** To reduce pain and discomfort

[ ] **4.** To liquefy lung secretions

74. The parents demonstrate their understanding of the child's needs by stating it is most important to protect the child from exposure to which hazard?

[ ] **1.** Airborne pollen

[ ] **2.** Infections

[ ] **3.** Pet dander

[ ] **4.** Bright sunlight

Nursing Care of a Toddler with Asthma

The physician sees a 3-year-old toddler with allergic (extrinsic) asthma because of an upper respiratory tract infection.

75. If the nurse collects all the following data, which condition best indicates that the child is having an acute asthma attack?

[ ] **1.** Presence of expiratory wheezing

[ ] **2.** Respiratory rate between 20 and 30 breaths/minute

[ ] **3.** Thoracic breathing pattern

[ ] **4.** Clear, watery nasal drainage

76. Which nursing action is most appropriate for relieving the child's acute episode of respiratory distress?

[ ] **1.** Distract the child with age-appropriate toys.

[ ] **2.** Position a steam vaporizer at the bedside.

[ ] **3.** Give antibiotics as ordered.

[ ] **4.** Place the child in semi-Fowler's position.

The child responds to treatment and is scheduled to be discharged. The physician has prescribed breathing exercises for the child.

77. Which nursing intervention best facilitates the child's performance of breathing exercises?

[ ] **1.** Promise to give the child a treat after the exercises.

[ ] **2.** Have the parents assist the child with the exercises.

[ ] **3.** Demonstrate the exercise, and then have the child do the exercise.

[ ] **4.** Instruct the parents to have the child blow bubbles.

78. Which nursing instruction is most appropriate to include during discharge teaching?

[ ] **1.** Instruct the parents to give breathing treatments every 2 hours.

[ ] **2.** Instruct the parents to eliminate vegetables from the child's diet.

[ ] **3.** Instruct the parents to limit the child's fluid intake.

[ ] **4.** Instruct the parents to remove area rugs from the home.

Nursing Care of a Toddler Who Has Swallowed a Toxic Substance

The mother of a 15-month-old toddler calls the physician's office and reports that her child swallowed a lye-based cleaner.

79. Which instruction is most appropriate initially?
[ ] **1.** Begin cardiopulmonary resuscitation on the child immediately.
[ ] **2.** Induce vomiting with syrup of ipecac immediately.
[ ] **3.** Give the child water to drink to dilute the substance.
[ ] **4.** Take the child and substance to the nearest emergency department.

The child is taken to the emergency department. After examination, the physician decides to admit the child for further observation.

80. If the nurse documents all the following data on admission, which finding best indicates that the child needs to be monitored with a pulse oximeter?
[ ] **1.** Substernal and intercostal retractions
[ ] **2.** Red, swollen lips
[ ] **3.** Thin, clear mucus drooling from lips
[ ] **4.** Pulse rate of 105 beats/minute

81. In addition to monitoring the child with a pulse oximeter, which intervention would the nurse expect to perform?
[ ] **1.** Administering gastric lavage
[ ] **2.** Implementing pain-relief measures
[ ] **3.** Maintaining the child on nothing-by-mouth status
[ ] **4.** Performing neurovascular checks

After 2 days, the child is discharged from the hospital.

82. Which statement by the mother best indicates that she understands how to prevent the child from ingesting poisonous substances in the future?
[ ] **1.** "I'll remove all toxic substances from my home."
[ ] **2.** "I won't ever let my son out of my sight again."
[ ] **3.** "I'll place all toxic substances out of my son's reach."
[ ] **4.** "I'll keep all toxic substances in a locked cabinet."

Nursing Care of a Toddler with Croup

A 2½-year-old toddler is seen in the pediatrician's office because of coughing and difficulty breathing during the previous night. The physician makes a diagnosis of laryngotracheobronchitis (croup).

83. When the parents ask how croup occurs, the nurse correctly informs them about which pathophysiologic mechanism of the disorder?

[ ] **1.** Croup is most often caused by a virus.
[ ] **2.** Croup occurs in children with chronic asthma.
[ ] **3.** Croup occurs in children who have whooping cough.
[ ] **4.** Croup is often a complication of underdeveloped lungs.

84. Which common characteristic of croup would the nurse expect to document in the child's chart?
[ ] **1.** Moist cough
[ ] **2.** Barky cough
[ ] **3.** Muffled cough
[ ] **4.** Wheezy cough

85. Which recommendation by the nurse commonly relieves the primary symptom associated with laryngeal spasms?
[ ] **1.** Providing central heating
[ ] **2.** Maintaining an air-conditioned room
[ ] **3.** Placing a humidifier in the child's room
[ ] **4.** Ensuring that the child's room is dust-free

86. The nurse appropriately instructs the parents to contact the physician immediately if the child develops which symptom?
[ ] **1.** Mild fever
[ ] **2.** Extreme anxiety
[ ] **3.** Coughing at night
[ ] **4.** Sleeping during the day

87. Which statement by the parents indicates a need for further teaching?
[ ] **1.** "Our son may have recurrent episodes of croup for one or two more nights."
[ ] **2.** "We'll give our son aspirin if his temperature is greater than 101° F (38.3° C)."
[ ] **3.** "We'll place a cool mist humidifier at the head of our son's bed."
[ ] **4.** "We'll offer our son small sips of clear liquids at frequent intervals."

The child develops acute respiratory distress during the night and is taken to the hospital's emergency department. The physician admits the child for further treatment.

88. To prevent aggravation of the child's respiratory distress, which nursing action is most beneficial?
[ ] **1.** Medicate the child with a sedative.
[ ] **2.** Encourage the parents to remain at the child's bedside.
[ ] **3.** Give the child an age-appropriate toy to play with.
[ ] **4.** Postpone unpleasant procedures until the child's condition stabilizes.

89. Which medications should the nurse expect a child with croup to receive?
[ ] **1.** Ampicillin
[ ] **2.** Ferrous sulfate (Feosol)
[ ] **3.** Metoclopramide (Reglan)
[ ] **4.** Racemic epinephrine (Vaponefrin)

90. Which beverage should be avoided when offering liquids to a child with croup?
[ ] **1.** Ginger ale
[ ] **2.** Apple juice
[ ] **3.** Whole milk
[ ] **4.** Cold water

Nursing Care of a Toddler with Pneumonia

A 2½-year-old toddler is admitted to the hospital with a diagnosis of pneumococcal pneumonia. On admission, the child has an intermittent, productive cough. The parents report that the child has been lethargic and anorexic for several days.

91. In addition to the above manifestations, the nurse would expect to find which manifestation of the disease process?
[ ] **1.** Clubbing of the fingers
[ ] **2.** Synchronized chest movement
[ ] **3.** Slow pulse rate
[ ] **4.** Rapid and shallow respirations

92. Which assessment technique is most appropriate for determining the child's hydration status?
[ ] **1.** Urine output
[ ] **2.** Urine pH
[ ] **3.** Blood pressure
[ ] **4.** Respiratory rate

93. If pulse oximetry is ordered, the nurse is correct to report values that consistently remain at which percentage?
[ ] **1.** Below 95%
[ ] **2.** Above 95%
[ ] **3.** Below 100%
[ ] **4.** Above 100%

94. Which medication can the nurse expect to give to the child with pneumonia who has a productive, moist cough?
[ ] **1.** Antibiotic
[ ] **2.** Bronchodilator
[ ] **3.** Expectorant
[ ] **4.** Cough suppressant

The physician leaves orders to give the child a sponge bath for a temperature of 103° F (39.4° C) or more rectally. When the child's temperature remains consistently above that level, the parents ask the nurse if it is all right for them to give the bath.

95. Which instruction regarding the sponge bath is essential for the parents to know?
[ ] **1.** The sponge bath should be given for at least 1 hour.
[ ] **2.** The water temperature of the bath should be cool.
[ ] **3.** The bath should be discontinued if the child begins to shiver.
[ ] **4.** The bath should be given until the temperature is below 101° F (38.3° C).

96. A child with pneumonia is ordered cephalexin monohydrate (Keflex) 0.5 g P.O. every 8 hours. The pharmacy dispenses 500 mg per teaspoon. How many mL would the nurse administer?

_____

After 3 days of treatment, the child's condition improves significantly. The physician writes discharge orders that include instructions for home care. The parents speak some English, but their primary language is Spanish.

97. Which action is best to ensure that the parents understand the discharge instructions?
[ ] **1.** Give the parents a copy of the instructions written in Spanish.
[ ] **2.** Have an interpreter present when instructions are given.
[ ] **3.** Have the physician give the instructions.
[ ] **4.** Instruct the parents to call if questions arise when they get home.

Nursing Care of a Preschooler with Seizure Disorder

A 4½-year-old preschooler is admitted to the hospital with a tentative diagnosis of tonic-clonic seizures.

98. Of the following history findings reported by the parents, which information best indicates that the child had a tonic-clonic seizure?
[ ] **1.** The child had a high fever.
[ ] **2.** The child has begun wetting the bed.
[ ] **3.** The child suddenly dropped to the floor.
[ ] **4.** The child's whole body was jerking.

99. Which nursing action is most appropriate when preparing the hospital room for the child's admission?
[ ] **1.** Padding the side rails on the bed
[ ] **2.** Keeping phenobarbital at the bedside
[ ] **3.** Placing the bed in the Trendelenburg's position
[ ] **4.** Following standard precautions

100. Which equipment is least important to have at the bedside?
[ ] **1.** Suction equipment
[ ] **2.** Oral airway
[ ] **3.** Oxygen sources
[ ] **4.** Cool mist humidifier

The child has a tonic-clonic seizure while the nurse is at the bedside.

101. Which action should the nurse take first?
[ ] **1.** Calling for assistance
[ ] **2.** Placing the child in a side-lying position
[ ] **3.** Inserting a padded tongue blade in the child's mouth
[ ] **4.** Administering oxygen

The child is placed on phenytoin (Dilantin). After several days on the medication, the child has no further seizure activity. The physician writes discharge orders, which include administering Dilantin at home.

102. During the discharge process, which long-term adverse effect of phenytoin (Dilantin) should the nurse include in her instructions to the parents?
[ ] **1.** Poor appetite
[ ] **2.** Urinary incontinence
[ ] **3.** Painful joints
[ ] **4.** Gum overgrowth

103. Which statement by the parents indicates that teaching has been effective?
[ ] **1.** "We'll give Dilantin only on an empty stomach."
[ ] **2.** "We won't restrain our child while he's having a seizure."
[ ] **3.** "We know that our son will develop mental retardation because of his condition."
[ ] **4.** "We're aware that our son should no longer attend preschool."

104. Which statement is most appropriate when communicating with the child about the disorder?
[ ] **1.** Tell the child that the pain will stop eventually.
[ ] **2.** Tell the child that the seizures are not a punishment.
[ ] **3.** Tell the child that he must take the medication.
[ ] **4.** Tell the child that other children also have seizures.

Nursing Care of a Preschooler with Leukemia

A 5-year-old child suspected of having leukemia is admitted to the hospital for diagnosis and treatment.

105. The nurse correctly explains to the parents that the most accurate way to confirm a diagnosis of leukemia is which test?
[ ] **1.** Complete blood count (CBC)
[ ] **2.** Spinal fluid examination
[ ] **3.** Bone marrow aspiration
[ ] **4.** X-ray of long bones

Tests confirm that the child has acute lymphoblastic leukemia (ALL). Induction therapy is begun. The child is started on vincristine sulfate, prednisone, and asparaginase (Elspar). The physician also places the child under protective isolation precautions.

106. Which instruction should the nurse give to those visiting a child on protective isolation?
[ ] **1.** Only washable toys are allowed into the child's room.
[ ] **2.** Children under age 12 are restricted from the room.
[ ] **3.** Fresh fruit that cannot be peeled is prohibited in the room.
[ ] **4.** Only immediate family members may visit in the room.

107. Which route of temperature assessment is contraindicated for a child with leukemia?
[ ] **1.** Axillary
[ ] **2.** Oral
[ ] **3.** Rectal
[ ] **4.** Tympanic

108. Which medication should the nurse have on hand when asparaginase (Elspar) is given?
[ ] **1.** Epinephrine (Adrenalin)
[ ] **2.** Calcium gluconate
[ ] **3.** Sodium bicarbonate
[ ] **4.** Furosemide (Lasix)

The child receives a transfusion of packed red blood cells.

109. Which statement best indicates that the child is having a transfusion reaction?
[ ] **1.** The child complains of being thirsty.
[ ] **2.** The child complains of feeling chilly.
[ ] **3.** The child complains of feeling tired.
[ ] **4.** The child complains of being hungry.

110. Which is the most appropriate initial nursing action if the child experiences a transfusion reaction?
[ ] **1.** Administering oxygen, and being prepared to start cardiopulmonary resuscitation
[ ] **2.** Checking the temperature, and giving acetaminophen (Tylenol)
[ ] **3.** Stopping the transfusion, but keeping the I.V. line open with normal saline solution
[ ] **4.** Notifying the charge nurse, and returning the blood to the blood bank for testing

The child asks the nurse, "Am I going to die?"

111. What is the most appropriate response by the nurse?
[ ] **1.** "Are you feeling especially bad today? Tell me more about how you feel."
[ ] **2.** "You shouldn't worry about things like that. You are only a little girl."
[ ] **3.** "We are all going to die someday. Usually we die when we get old."
[ ] **4.** "Let's talk about something else. What is your favorite television program?"

112. Which statement by the child's father indicates a need for additional teaching about the child's condition?
[ ] **1.** "My daughter should receive only active forms of immunity."
[ ] **2.** "My daughter should avoid high-contact play activities."
[ ] **3.** "My daughter should receive small but frequent high-protein meals."
[ ] **4.** "My daughter shouldn't be around individuals with infections."

Nursing Care of a Preschooler with Strabismus

A 4-year-old child is to be admitted to an ambulatory surgical center for the correction of strabismus (crossed eyes). The day before the surgery, the child and parents go to the surgical center for preoperative teaching.

113. Which preoperative instruction is most important to give the parents in preparation for the surgical procedure?
[ ] **1.** Clean the child's eyelid with povidone-iodine (Betadine) at bedtime.
[ ] **2.** Give the child a Fleet's enema at bedtime.
[ ] **3.** Do not give the child anything by mouth after midnight.
[ ] **4.** Give the child a dose of acetaminophen (Tylenol) at bedtime.

The child asks if the surgery will "hurt."

114. Which response by the nurse is most appropriate?
[ ] **1.** "Don't think about that now."
[ ] **2.** "No, you won't feel any pain."
[ ] **3.** "I don't know. Ask the physician."
[ ] **4.** "Your eye may be sore after surgery."

115. Which type of game best prepares the child for the postoperative period?
[ ] **1.** Tic-Tac-Toe on a large piece of paper
[ ] **2.** Pretending the child is a pirate with a patch
[ ] **3.** Hide-and-seek within the hospital room
[ ] **4.** Peek-a-boo with a member of the hospital staff

The child is admitted the following morning and undergoes surgery.

116. Which statement by the parents indicates a need for additional teaching?
[ ] **1.** "Our child can be up and about after the anesthesia wears off."
[ ] **2.** "Our child can have a regular diet after nausea has ceased."
[ ] **3.** "Our child cannot play with toys for at least 4 weeks."
[ ] **4.** "The restraints can be removed when we are holding our child."

Nursing Care of a Preschooler Having a Tonsillectomy and Adenoidectomy

A 5-year-old child who is scheduled for a tonsillectomy and adenoidectomy arrives in the outpatient department the morning of surgery. The nurse admitting the child assesses the vital signs.

117. Which result should be reported immediately to the charge nurse or physician?
[ ] **1.** Blood pressure of 96/60 mm Hg
[ ] **2.** Temperature of 101° F (38.3° C)
[ ] **3.** Respiratory rate of 20 breaths/minute
[ ] **4.** Pulse rate of 110 beats/minute

Following surgery, the child is admitted to a room in the pediatric unit. The physician leaves orders for pain medication and a clear liquid diet.

118. Which food is most appropriate for the nurse to offer the child following surgery?
[ ] **1.** Orange juice
[ ] **2.** Apple juice
[ ] **3.** Ice cream
[ ] **4.** Cream of chicken soup

119. If the nurse observes all the following behaviors, which one is contraindicated?

[ ] **1.** The ice collar is removed from the child's neck.
[ ] **2.** The child is sucking liquids through a straw.
[ ] **3.** The parents are holding the child.
[ ] **4.** The child is using the bedpan.

120. If the nurse collects all the following data, which observation indicates that the child may have postoperative complications?

[ ] **1.** Small amount of dark red emesis
[ ] **2.** Respiratory rate of 30 breaths/minute
[ ] **3.** Complaint of throat pain
[ ] **4.** Frequent swallowing

121. Which instruction is most appropriate to give to the parents during discharge teaching?

[ ] **1.** The child should be kept quiet for a few days after discharge.
[ ] **2.** The child's fluid intake should be limited for the next 48 hours.
[ ] **3.** The child should be given aspirin for discomfort and fever.
[ ] **4.** The child should resume a regular diet after nausea subsides.

Correct Answers and Rationales

Normal Growth and Development of Infants, Toddlers, and Preschool Children

1. 2. When in the prone position, a 3-month-old infant should be able to raise his head and shoulders 45 to 90 degrees. The other developmental skills are accomplished later in infancy. Sitting with support and rolling from the abdomen to the back occur at approximately 5 months old. Holding a bottle occurs when the infant is about 4½ months old.
  ***Client Needs Category**—Health promotion and maintenance*
  ***Client Needs Subcategory**—None*

2. 3. Crying for long periods of time, even after comfort measures have been used, is unusual and should be reported to the health care provider. The other signs and symptoms mentioned are usual side effects of the measles-mumps-rubella (MMR) inoculation, which is given at 15 months old, and do not require notifying the health care provider.
  ***Client Needs Category**—Health promotion and maintenance*
  ***Client Needs Subcategory**—None*

3. 2. Raw carrots should not be given to the toddler unless they are shredded because they may be a choking hazard. All the other findings observed by the nurse demonstrate that the parents understand the toddler's safety needs.
  ***Client Needs Category**—Health promotion and maintenance*
  ***Client Needs Subcategory**—None*

4. 1. The apical site is preferred when assessing the pulse of a child under age 5. A satisfactory radial pulse cannot be obtained until the child is 2 years old. The carotid site is not routinely used when assessing children; however, it is the preferred site when performing child cardiopulmonary resuscitation (CPR). The brachial site is not routinely used when assessing children, but it is the preferred site when performing infant CPR.
  ***Client Needs Category**—Health promotion and maintenance*
  ***Client Needs Subcategory**—None*

5. 3. The correct way to give the liquid medication is to position the infant upright and slowly administer the medication using a rubber-tipped medicine dropper or a small medicine cup. The medication may also be given through the nipple from a bottle. However, oral medications should not be added to the infant's formula; there is no guarantee that all of the medication will be administered if the infant does not drink all of the formula. Pinching the infant's nose is inappropriate; when the infant inhales through the mouth, it may cause the infant to aspirate the medication. Utilizing the supine position may also cause the child to aspirate the medication or the medication to leak from the side of the mouth.

> ***Client Needs Category***—*Health promotion and maintenance*
> ***Client Needs Subcategory***—*None*

6. 4. An infant's respiratory rate is generally counted for 1 full minute because of normal irregularities. When assessing an older child, respirations may be counted for 30 seconds and then multiplied by 2.

> ***Client Needs Category***—*Health promotion and maintenance*
> ***Client Needs Subcategory***—*None*

7. 2. Bowel control is usually easier to accomplish than bladder control and is usually achieved first. All the other statements indicate the child's readiness to toilet-train.

> ***Client Needs Category***—*Health promotion and maintenance*
> ***Client Needs Subcategory***—*None*

8. 3. Finding age-related tasks that involve nurturing and responsibility tends to promote a feeling that the child's contributions are valued and appreciated. Sending the child to a preschool program or for long visits away from home further reinforces the feeling of abandonment. Although playing with same-age children promotes socialization skills, it does not relieve sibling rivalry.

> ***Client Needs Category***—*Health promotion and maintenance*
> ***Client Needs Subcategory***—*None*

9. 1. Using dolls or puppets as a teaching aid is the most appropriate strategy for a preschooler's cognitive ability. Pamphlets and diagrams are too abstract for the cognitive level of children who are 3, 4, or 5 years of age. The use of a videotape might be confused as a form of entertainment rather than personal instruction.

> ***Client Needs Category***—*Psychosocial integrity*
> ***Client Needs Subcategory***—*None*

10. 3. The most effective means for minimizing separation anxiety is having a parent remain with the child during hospitalization. A familiar toy may help the child deal with the separation, but it is not as effective as a parent actually being there. Likewise, a sibling visit is not a substitute for the parents' presence; it may or may not assist with minimizing separation anxiety, depending on the child's relationship with the siblings. Explaining the procedure to the child will not decrease separation anxiety.

> ***Client Needs Category***—*Psychosocial integrity*
> ***Client Needs Subcategory***—*None*

11. 3. Introducing one food at a time makes it easier to identify food tolerances and allergies. Infants normally push food out of their mouths because of the extrusion reflex. Cereals should be the first solid food introduced. It may be necessary to breast- or bottle-feed a hungry infant prior to giving solid food.

> ***Client Needs Category***—*Health promotion and maintenance*
> ***Client Needs Subcategory***—*None*

12. 3. An 18-month-old child should be able to walk without support and climb stairs while holding onto a railing. The other findings are normal and should have been accomplished by a toddler of this age.

> ***Client Needs Category***—*Health promotion and maintenance*
> ***Client Needs Subcategory***—*None*

13. 2. Medicine and other toxic substances should be kept in a locked cabinet. Merely keeping such substances out of reach is inadequate; the child might be able to climb higher than anticipated, giving him access to unsafe substances. The other observations are correct safety measures.

> ***Client Needs Category***—*Health promotion and maintenance*
> ***Client Needs Subcategory***—*None*

14. 1. It is developmentally normal for a 4-year-old child to talk to an imaginary playmate. Preschoolers usually abandon imaginary playmates when they begin to interact more with children their own age. Because the behavior is not pathologic, it would be inappropriate to look for unusual stressors, recommend the services of a child psychologist, or invoke a disciplinary time-out period.

> ***Client Needs Category***—*Health promotion and maintenance*
> ***Client Needs Subcategory***—*None*

15.

6.	Maintain water temperature under 120° F (48.8° C).
2.	Have straps on the changing table.
4.	Remove stuffed animals with small pieces from the child's grasp.
1.	Cover the electrical outlets.
3.	Turn pot handles inward when cooking.
5.	Lower crib mattress.

Water temperatures should be set under 120° F to assure the fragile skin of the newborn is maintained. Due to the child's placement on top of tables, straps should be placed on the changing table. Parents should not leave the child unattended. Stuffed animals with small pieces should be removed from the child's environment so that he does not place the pieces in his mouth. When the child begins to crawl, electrical outlet plugs should be included in childproofing the home. As the child begins to pull himself up from the floor, pot handles should be turned inward so as not to have hot objects spilled. As the child becomes tall enough to extend over crib rails, the crib mattress should be lowered.

> ***Client Needs Category***—*Health promotion and maintenance*
> ***Client Needs Subcategory***—*None*

Nursing Care of an Infant with Myelomeningocele

16. **2.** The most important nursing measure would be to avoid pressure on and prevent injury to the sac. This is important because a break in the sac could lead to serious infection. Washing the area would not be appropriate because of the danger of injury to the sac. Preventing skin breakdown is important but not as important as preventing injury to the sac. The normal care of the diaper area is maintained because the sac is high in the spinal column. Parents are encouraged to bond with the infant utilizing touch and eye contact. Cuddling and holding the infant could potentially cause trauma to the sac.

> ***Client Needs Category***—*Physiological integrity*
> ***Client Needs Subcategory***—*Reduction of risk potential*

17. **2.** The prone position (lying on the abdomen) is used after surgical repair of a myelomeningocele. This position is maintained until the operative site heals. To prevent infection, it is important to keep the operative site clean and free of pressure. Infants undergoing this procedure should not be placed supine (on the back) or on their side, as this may put stress on the operative site. The most comfortable position may not be the most appropriate position for care of the surgical site.

> ***Client Needs Category***—*Physiological integrity*
> ***Client Needs Subcategory***— *Reduction of risk potential*

18. **1.** A child born with spina bifida with a myelomeningocele located high in the spinal column has a poor prognosis for being able to walk alone. The child may be able to use a wheelchair or possibly braces and crutches. When the myelomeningocele is low in the spine (in or near the sacral area, for example), only minimal weakness of the lower extremities may be evident.

> ***Client Needs Category***—*Physiological integrity*
> ***Client Needs Subcategory***— *Physiological adaptation*

19. **2.** Urinary and bowel control problems are usually seen in children with spina bifida and myelomeningocele. Because intermittent catheterization is required in most cases, the parents should be instructed in how to insert a straight catheter using a clean technique. During the early school years, the child will also be taught how to perform this procedure. The infant with myelomeningocele usually does not require a retention catheter or ureterostomy.

> ***Client Needs Category***—*Health promotion and maintenance*
> ***Client Needs Subcategory***—*None*

20. **4.** Infants with spina bifida and a myelomeningocele commonly have clubfoot and congenital hip dysplasia. Because the defect typically causes a loss of motion in the lower extremities, range-of-motion exercises are most effective in preventing contractures. Although massaging the lower extremities, repositioning the infant, and placing sheepskin under the bony prominences are good nursing interventions, they will not prevent contractures.

> ***Client Needs Category***—*Health promotion and maintenance*
> ***Client Needs Subcategory***—*None*

Nursing Care of an Infant with Hydrocephalus

21. 1. An increase in head size is the most prominent characteristic of hydrocephalus. Some hydrocephalic infants also have spina bifida with a myelomeningocele and may have lower extremity paralysis, but this neurologic deficit is not a prominent symptom of hydrocephalus. The presence or absence of the sucking reflex also is not considered a prominent sign. Usually, hydrocephalus causes a bulging of the fontanel and separation of the skull sutures.
> *Client Needs Category—Physiological integrity*
> *Client Needs Subcategory—Physiological adaptation*

22. 2. The cause of hydrocephalus in most infants is a blockage (obstruction) that prevents proper circulation of cerebrospinal fluid. This is known as the noncommunicating type of congenital hydrocephalus. Absence of the dura mater, increased cerebrospinal fluid in the subarachnoid space, and blockage of the cerebral arteries are not known to cause hydrocephalus.
> *Client Needs Category—Physiological integrity*
> *Client Needs Subcategory—None*

23. 4. The side-lying position is the preferred way to place an infant with hydrocephalus after feeding. Because such infants are at risk for vomiting as a result of increased intracranial pressure, placing them on their side allows vomitus to easily escape, decreasing the chance of aspiration. The positions identified in the remaining options may result in aspiration.
> *Client Needs Category—Safe, effective care environment*
> *Client Needs Subcategory—Safety and infection control*

24. 1. The head and ears of an infant with hydrocephalus are especially prone to the development of pressure ulcers. The primary reason for using a sheepskin in this situation is to help relieve pressure on the head and ears. The infant's position should also be changed frequently to prevent complications due to inactivity. The other options are incorrect because they will not relieve pressure on the infant's head.
> *Client Needs Category—Safe, effective care environment*
> *Client Needs Subcategory—Reduction of risk potential*

25. 3. The position of choice after installing a shunting device in an infant with hydrocephalus is on the side opposite the site of the surgical incision. This position prevents damage to the shunt valve and suture line. The infant described in this question should be placed on the left side postoperatively because the surgical site of entry was on the right side of the head.
> *Client Needs Category—Physiological integrity*
> *Client Needs Subcategory—Physiological adaptation*

26. 2. Signs of increased intracranial pressure in an infant include bulging or tense fontanels, decreased pulse and respiratory rates, irritability, and vomiting. Changes in weight and bowel elimination are not common indicators of increased intracranial pressure.
> *Client Needs Category—Physiological integrity*
> *Client Needs Subcategory—Physiological adaptation*

27. 2. When an infant's anterior fontanel is sunken, the most appropriate action is to keep him flat in a supine position. This position will prevent a rapid decrease in intracranial pressure. If the fontanel is bulging, the head would be elevated. It would be appropriate to notify the charge nurse or physician after positioning the infant.
> *Client Needs Category—Physiological integrity*
> *Client Needs Subcategory—Physiological adaptation*

Nursing Care of an Infant with Cleft Lip

28. 3. Upon admission to the nursery, the nurse checks for any defects, such as cleft lip and cleft palate. A cleft lip is easily identified during inspection due to the obvious appearance of the lip. However, a cleft palate is a fissure in the midline of the palate and therefore requires palpating the roof of the mouth. A congenital defect, cleft palate occurs in about 50% of those born with a cleft lip, especially bilateral cleft lip. The nurse does not palpate the roof of the mouth to elicit the gag reflex or to assess the infant's sucking ability or position of the uvula.
> *Client Needs Category—Physiological integrity*
> *Client Needs Subcategory—Physiological adaptation*

29. 2. One of the nurse's primary considerations when caring for an infant with a cleft lip is dealing with the parents' reaction to the child's appearance. The nurse can facilitate parental adjustment by demonstrating acceptance of the child, encouraging the parents to express their feelings, and acknowledging the appropriateness of their feelings. Discussions about the infant's special needs, including feeding, surgical repair, and use of the bulb syringe, are important; however, the parents must first begin to adjust to their child's appearance before they can deal with other issues.
> *Client Needs Category—Psychosocial integrity*
> *Client Needs Subcategory—None*

30. **1.** Infants with cleft lip swallow more air than usual; therefore, they should be burped frequently to decrease the chance of vomiting and subsequent aspiration. Lying horizontal with the face down in the prone position should be avoided because this position makes feeding difficult and the risk for aspiration is high. An infant schedules for cleft lip repair is fed regular formula before surgery.

> ***Client Needs Category***—*Health promotion and maintenance*
> ***Client Needs Subcategory***—*None*

31. **3.** Of the four options, a rubber-tipped syringe is the best method of feeding the infant with cleft lip. A small medicine dropper and a specially designed nipple are other methods sometimes used. Feeding the infant with a plastic spoon or firm rubber nipple may still result in aspiration through the opening in the palate. Gavage feeding is not usually necessary because the remainder of the gastrointestinal tract is intact.

> ***Client Needs Category***—*Physiological integrity*
> ***Client Needs Subcategory***—*Reduction of risk potential*

32. **3.** Elbow restraints allow the infant to move the arms but prevent him from touching his face. A papoose board or a mummy restraint prevents movement of the entire body; these forms of restraint are not usually necessary for this type of surgery. A Posey belt or jacket will not prevent a child from touching his face; such devices are used to keep a client in bed or in a wheelchair. Leg restraints are not utilized because the infant cannot use the leg to injure the surgical site.

> ***Client Needs Category***—*Safe, effective care environment*
> ***Client Needs Subcategory***—*Safety and infection control*

33. **4.** Unless the physician orders otherwise, most restraints are removed and reapplied at least every 2 hours.

> ***Client Needs Category***—*Safe, effective care environment*
> ***Client Needs Subcategory***—*Safety and infection control*

Nursing Care of an Infant with Pyloric Stenosis

34. **4.** Dry mucous membranes are an indication of dehydration. The infant must be rehydrated and electrolytes must be within normal limits prior to undergoing surgery. The anterior fontanel is normally flat. Hunger and visible gastric peristaltic waves are present with pyloric stenosis, but they do not indicate the same health risk as dehydration.

> ***Client Needs Category***—*Physiological integrity*
> ***Client Needs Subcategory***—*Physiological adaptation*

35. **1.** The site of choice for I.V. therapy in infants is the scalp vein because of the supply of superficial veins. Use of scalp veins may require shaving the infant's hair. Restlessness and swelling are not usual findings, so they should be reported immediately because they may indicate I.V. infiltration. I.V. therapy does not require that the infant be kept NPO; the infant with pyloric stenosis may be given feedings of thickened formula prior to going to surgery.

> ***Client Needs Category***—*Physiological integrity*
> ***Client Needs Subcategory***—*Physiological adaptation*

36. **2.** After feeding, the infant should be placed on the right side or in an infant seat. These positions aid in emptying the stomach and preventing aspiration. The left side does not facilitate gastric emptying. The prone position is not recommended because of its association with the occurrence of sudden infant death syndrome. Placing the infant on his or her back creates a greater risk for aspiration of stomach contents. The most comfortable position may not necessarily be the best choice for this infant, given the nature of the infant's condition.

> ***Client Needs Category***—*Health promotion and maintenance*
> ***Client Needs Subcategory***—*None*

Nursing Care of an Infant with Bilateral Clubfoot

37. **3.** The infant should be evaluated carefully because the feet may appear to be clubbed but actually be the result of *in utero* positioning. True clubfoot is fixed and cannot be corrected to the neutral or natural position. One or both feet may be involved. In both the infant with true clubfoot and the infant with false clubfoot, the heels may be drawn in and the feet turned inward. Not all infants who are born breech develop clubfoot.

> ***Client Needs Category***—*Physiological integrity*
> ***Client Needs Subcategory***—*Physiological adaptation*

38. **3.** Adhesive petals are placed around the cast edges to prevent the plaster from irritating the skin. The material is smooth and placed on the opening at the top of the cast and around the toes. Such petaling is not used to keep materials from getting between the cast and the skin or to keep air circulating between the skin and the cast. It is also not intended or needed to make the cast stronger.

> ***Client Needs Category***—*Physiological integrity*
> ***Client Needs Subcategory***—*Reduction of risk potential*

39. 3. Pale, cold extremities are signs of impaired circulation caused by the pressure of the cast. This problem must be reported immediately. Crying 4 hours after the last feeding is normal because the infant is likely to be hungry, but unexplained crying may indicate pain or discomfort. Wiggling the toes is a sign that the nervous system has not been compromised by application of a cast. A pulse rate of 110 beats/minute is normal.

Client Needs Category—*Physiological integrity*
Client Needs Subcategory—*Reduction of risk potential*

40. 1. After a cast is applied to the lower extremities, the extremities are elevated on pillows to improve circulation and prevent swelling. The infant's position is usually changed every 2 hours to promote even drying. Petaling the edges is performed to prevent skin breakdown. Ice packs are not used to decrease swelling associated with casting.

Client Needs Category—*Physiological integrity*
Client Needs Subcategory—*Physiological adaptation*

41. 1. The purpose of casting is to gradually correct the defect without causing trauma; therefore, the casts are changed every few days initially, then every 1 to 2 weeks. Correction is usually achieved in approximately 6 to 8 weeks.

Client Needs Category—*Health promotion and maintenance*
Client Needs Subcategory—*None*

42. 4. An infant develops the ability to look at surroundings during the first month of life. By 2 months old, the infant can follow an object with both eyes; therefore, a mobile is an appropriate amusement for a child of this age. By 4 months old, the infant typically can reach for objects. By 7 to 9 months old, he usually can crawl and play peek-a-boo. It would be inappropriate, however, to encourage an infant in a cast to crawl.

Client Needs Category—*Health promotion and maintenance*
Client Needs Subcategory—*None*

43. 1. A fontanel is a space covered by tough membranes between the bones of an infant's cranium. The posterior fontanel normally closes between 2 and 3 months of age. All the other options provide inaccurate information.

Client Needs Category—*Health promotion and maintenance*
Client Needs Subcategory—*None*

Nursing Care of a Child with Otitis Media

44. 2. A young child with otitis media typically pulls at or rubs the affected ear in response to the pain occurring secondary to fluid pressure on the tympanic membrane. Although the other options may be present with otitis media, they are not caused by or related to the pain.

Client Needs Category—*Physiological integrity*
Client Needs Subcategory—*Physiological adaptation*

45. 2. Even though the physician prescribes the amount of medication to be given, the nurse is responsible for determining whether the prescribed dose is within the recommended safe dosage range. The most reliable method of determining the recommended safe dosage range requires use of the child's weight. The other options are important steps in medication administration but do not relate specifically to determining the safe dose.

Client Needs Category—*Physiological integrity*
Client Needs Subcategory—*Pharmacological therapies*

46. 4. The nurse should instruct the parents to complete the full course of antibiotics even though the infant's condition may improve after 2 to 3 days of treatment. Failure to complete the full course of antibiotics may lead to recurrent infection and other associated complications. Whether the antibiotic is given with food and how the antibiotic is stored varies, depending on the specific antibiotic. Placing the infant on his side after giving an antibiotic is not usually required unless the medication was instilled by eardrop. In this case, the infant is receiving an oral antibiotic.

Client Needs Category—*Health promotion and maintenance*
Client Needs Subcategory—*None*

47. 720. Erythromycin is supplied as 200 mg/5 mL or 40 mg/mL. When the child is receiving 6 mL, the child is receiving 240 mg every 8 hours. Multiplied by three 8-hour periods in 24 hours, the child receives 720 mg/day.

Client Needs Category—*Physiological integrity*
Client Needs Subcategory—*Pharmacological therapies*

Nursing Care of a Child with a Congenital Heart Defect

48. 3. In the child with coarctation of the aorta, the pulses are typically bounding in the upper extremities and weak in the lower extremities. Also, the blood pressure is higher in the upper extremities than in the lower extremities. This happens because of the narrowing of the aorta that occurs with coarctation. The other choices may develop at some point, but they may also be associated with other defects.

> **Client Needs Category**—*Physiological integrity*
> **Client Needs Subcategory**—*Physiological adaptation*

49. **3.** Initially, the infant with coarctation of the aorta may be given prostaglandin E to dilate the narrowed aorta. However, the corrective treatment is surgical repair, which is usually performed before the child is 2 years old. If correction is not performed, life-threatening complications may develop.

> **Client Needs Category**—*Physiological integrity*
> **Client Needs Subcategory**—*Physiological adaptation*

50. **1.** The nurse should check the infant's apical pulse for 1 full minute before giving digoxin (Lanoxin). If the pulse is less than the normal lower limit, the nurse should withhold the medication and notify the physician. When giving any medication, not just digoxin, an infant's head should be slightly elevated. The nurse should always check the expiration date before giving any medication to a client. The infant's kidney function should be adequate because medications are primarily excreted by the kidneys; however, these factors are not unique to digoxin (Lanoxin).

> **Client Needs Category**—*Physiological integrity*
> **Client Needs Subcategory**—*Pharmacological therapies*

51. **2.** Organizing nursing care to allow for longer rest periods decreases the infant's energy demands, thereby decreasing the workload of the heart. The nurse should encourage the parents to hold and cuddle their infant. A nasogastric route is used only if the infant has a poor suck reflex or the feedings take too long, which increases the energy expenditure. The infant would not be routinely sedated.

> **Client Needs Category**—*Physiological integrity*
> **Client Needs Subcategory**—*Physiological adaptation*

52. **3.** Digoxin (Lanoxin) should not be mixed in the infant's formula or food. Administering medication this way does not ensure that the child will receive the full dose, especially if all of the formula or food is not ingested. All the other statements are correct and indicate that the parents understood the nurse's instructions.

> **Client Needs Category**—*Health promotion and maintenance*
> **Client Needs Subcategory**—*None*

Nursing Care of a Child with an Infectious Disease

53. **1.** Although standard precautions are used in the care of all clients, airborne precautions are added for clients who have illnesses that are transmitted by airborne droplet nuclei, such as chickenpox during the early stage of infection. Droplet precautions are initiated when a client is known or suspected to have illnesses transmitted by large-particle droplets. Contact precautions are initiated for clients when direct patient contact or contact with client items may spread the disease.

> **Client Needs Category**—*Safe, effective care environment*
> **Client Needs Subcategory**—*Safety and infection control*

54. **2.** Specimens are placed in a zip-closure biohazard bag before being sent to the laboratory. The zip-closure prevents contamination of the environment during transportation. The infant is in airborne precautions; therefore, masks and personal protective equipment are placed outside the room because the room environment is considered contaminated. The infant is placed in a private room to prevent the potential spread of chickenpox to other clients. A disposable thermometer, which can be sterilized, is placed in the room and then disposed of or sent for proper cleaning upon discharge.

> **Client Needs Category**—*Safe, effective care environment*
> **Client Needs Subcategory**—*Safety and infection control*

55. **820.** The formula to calculate the daily rate of pediatric maintenance I.V. fluids is:

> 100 mL/kg/day for the first 10 kg of body weight
>
> 50 mL/kg/day for the next 10 kg of body weight
>
> 20 mL/kg/day for each kg above 20 kg of body weight

Convert lb into kg: $\dfrac{18\ lb}{2.2\ kg} = 8.1\ kg$

> 100 mL/kg/day $\times$ 8.1 = 820 mL

> **Client Needs Category**—*Physiological integrity*
> **Client Needs Subcategory**—*Physiological adaptation*

56. **4.** It is important to monitor the infusion rate carefully to prevent circulatory overload. Therefore, any increase in the rate should be reported immediately to the charge nurse. Normal behaviors for a child include voiding frequently, sleeping, and crying when disturbed by noise.

> **Client Needs Category**—*Physiological integrity*
> **Client Needs Subcategory**—*Reduction of risk potential*

Nursing Care of a Child with Human Immunodeficiency Virus (HIV)

57. 2. Infants who are HIV-positive and develop AIDS often present with thrush, mouth sores, and severe diaper rashes. In some cases, such children also develop bacterial infections and *Pneumocystis carinii* pneumonia. The other options are examples of normal infant behaviors or characteristics.

    Client Needs Category—*Physiological integrity*
    Client Needs Subcategory—*Physiological adaptation*

58. 1, 2, 3, 4, 5. The Centers for Disease Control and Prevention developed a classification system to describe the spectrum of HIV disease in children (AIDS Defining Conditions). The system indicates the severity of clinical signs or symptoms and the degree of immunosuppression. A history of bacterial infections, herpes simplex disease, oral and pulmonary candidiasis (white patches in the mouth and larynx), *Pneumocystis carinii* or lymphoid interstitial pneumonia (consolidation areas of a chest X-ray), and wasting syndrome (limited muscle tone) all indicate a moderate status for AIDS Defining Conditions. An increase in blood pressure may be associated with a disease process but is not closely linked to an AIDS Defining Condition.

    Client Needs Category—*Physiological integrity*
    Client Needs Subcategory—*Physiological adaptation*

Nursing Care of a Child with Atopic Dermatitis

59. 3. It is thought that atopic dermatitis (infantile eczema) is caused, at least in part, by an allergic reaction to an irritant, which is why the physician asked about the home environment. Hereditary factors may also play a role. Poor nutrition, premature birth, and hormonal imbalances are not associated with the development of atopic dermatitis.

    Client Needs Category—*Health promotion and maintenance*
    Client Needs Subcategory—*None*

60. 3. An infant with atopic dermatitis experiences severe itching of the skin lesions. The nurse must provide the parents with itch-relief measures to prevent the child from scratching and introducing microorganisms into the lesions, which will cause a secondary infection to develop. Nausea, vomiting, and drowsiness are not usual symptoms of atopic dermatitis.

    Client Needs Category—*Health promotion and maintenance*
    Client Needs Subcategory—*None*

61. 3. Hydrocortisone (Cortaid) is an anti-inflammatory drug. It helps reduce inflammation and its symptoms, such as swelling, redness, heat, and discomfort. This medication does not influence the weeping of lesions, spread of the disease, or white blood cell count.

    Client Needs Category—*Physiological integrity*
    Client Needs Subcategory—*Reduction of risk potential*

62. 1. Colloid baths have been found effective for their soothing effects on the irritated and itching skin of a child with atopic dermatitis. The most commonly used type of colloid bath preparation is cornstarch added to tepid water. Other colloid bath preparations include cooked oatmeal and commercial bath preparations. Mineral oil, liquid glycerin soap, and salt are not components of a colloid bath.

    Client Needs Category—*Health promotion and maintenance*
    Client Needs Subcategory—*None*

Nursing Care of a Toddler with Sickle Cell Crisis

63. 1. The sickle-shaped cells tend to clump together in vessels and obstruct normal blood flow. A thrombus may form and cause death of tissue because of poor blood circulation. Severe pain in the affected body parts is the characteristic symptom when tissue is denied normal blood circulation. Bradycardia and hemorrhage are not usually associated with sickle cell crisis. Although dehydration may lead to a potential sickle cell crisis, this is not the initial nursing priority.

    Client Needs Category—*Physiological integrity*
    Client Needs Subcategory—*Physiological adaptation*

64. 4. The child with sickle cell crisis is prone to dehydration. The child is encouraged to drink fluids. It is helpful to offer the child appealing fluids, such as juices, popsicles, and gelatins. It may be necessary during the acute stage to rehydrate the child with I.V. fluids. Whole-blood transfusions may be given to increase hemoglobin levels. Iron is of no value in the treatment of this blood disorder.

    Client Needs Category—*Physiological integrity*
    Client Needs Subcategory—*Physiological adaptation*

65. 2. Sickle cell disease occurs when the child inherits the trait from both parents. If one parent has the disease and one parent has the trait, then all offspring will have at least the trait. Furthermore, there is a 50% chance that the offspring will have sickle cell disease. Information about the probability of offspring having sickle cell disease or trait can be given only in terms of each conception. The only instance in which it is possible to predict that all offspring will definitely have the disease is when both parents are known to have sickle cell disease.

> *Client Needs Category*—*Health promotion and maintenance*
> *Client Needs Subcategory*—*None*

66. **1, 2, 4, 5, 6.** Because infection is the major cause of sickle cell crisis and death, the nurse needs to stress the importance of measures to reduce infection. Obtaining plenty of rest, utilizing proper hand-washing techniques, and avoiding crowds, especially during cold and flu season, are all important measures. Some individuals are placed on antibiotic therapy prophylactically. It is important to finish the full course of the antibiotic therapy. Maintaining good hydration is an important step in preventing cell sickling. Utilizing pain medication is not typical in preventing a sickle cell crisis.

> *Client Needs Category*—*Health promotion and maintenance*
> *Client Needs Subcategory*—*None*

Nursing Care of a Toddler with Cystic Fibrosis

67. **3.** In many cases, the parents of a child with cystic fibrosis report that their child tastes salty when kissed. This is because the child's perspiration, tears, and saliva contain abnormally high concentrations of salt. Consequently, sweat analysis is an important diagnostic tool when children are examined for cystic fibrosis. These children are typically underweight. Infrequent crying, weight gain, and poor head control are findings that may be associated with the presence of other disorders.

> *Client Needs Category*—*Physiological integrity*
> *Client Needs Subcategory*—*Physiological adaptation*

68. **4.** Typically, the stools of a child with cystic fibrosis are large, sticky, and foul smelling. The condition is due to diminished or absent flow of pancreatic enzymes, which leads to faulty absorption of nutrients, especially fat-soluble vitamins. Other signs and symptoms of cystic fibrosis include malnutrition despite a hearty appetite, chronic coughing, and a distended abdomen. Children with cystic fibrosis usually eat very well but fail to gain weight. Typically, they also do not perspire excessively or have a low urine output.

> *Client Needs Category*—*Physiological integrity*
> *Client Needs Subcategory*—*Physiological adaptation*

69. **2.** The cause of death in children with cystic fibrosis is most often related to respiratory or cardiac failure; thus, the priority goal would be maintenance of an effective breathing pattern. All the other goals are appropriate for the child with cystic fibrosis, but maintaining respiratory function is the priority.

> *Client Needs Category*—*Physiological integrity*
> *Client Needs Subcategory*—*Reduction of risk potential*

70. **3.** The air passages of the lungs of persons with cystic fibrosis become clogged with mucus, thus decreasing the amount of oxygen reaching the lungs. A bronchodilator increases the diameter of the bronchi, thereby allowing more air to enter the lungs so breathing is improved. Characteristics of the stool, serum sodium levels, and fat excretion by the body are not affected by bronchodilators.

> *Client Needs Category*—*Physiological integrity*
> *Client Needs Subcategory*—*Pharmacological therapies*

71. **4.** A child with cystic fibrosis may need 1½ to 2 times the normal caloric intake to meet caloric needs. The diet should be high in protein and carbohydrates. No restrictions on fat intake are necessary if the child is taking pancrelipase (Pancrease) as prescribed. However, the child should not consume excessive amounts of fat. The child may require an increase in the intake of salt, especially during summer months, when excessive sweating may occur.

> *Client Needs Category*—*Physiological integrity*
> *Client Needs Subcategory*—*Physiological adaptation*

72. **2.** Commercially prepared pancreatic enzymes should be given with meals and snacks to facilitate nutrient absorption. Pancreatic enzyme preparations have no relationship to the child's appetite, prevention of salt depletion, or prevention of gastric upset.

> *Client Needs Category*—*Physiological integrity*
> *Client Needs Subcategory*—*Physiological adaptation*

73. **4.** In children with cystic fibrosis, sodium and chloride become trapped in the cells of the lungs' lining. The salt draws liquids from the airways and causes the mucus in the airways to become thick and sticky. Maintaining adequate fluid intake will help liquefy secretions in the airways, which ultimately helps improve breathing. The goal of increased fluid intake for the child with cystic fibrosis is not to prevent kidney failure, improve cardiac function, or reduce pain and discomfort.

> *Client Needs Category*—*Physiological integrity*
> *Client Needs Subcategory*—*Reduction of risk potential*

74. 2. Children with cystic fibrosis are very susceptible to infections, especially infections of the respiratory tract. The parents should be taught to guard against exposing the child to infections to the greatest extent possible. Immunization against childhood diseases is highly recommended, especially against diseases that may place the respiratory tract at risk. Airborne pollen and pet dander are usually avoided when the child has a history of respiratory symptoms secondary to environmental allergies. Avoiding exposure to bright sunlight is not necessarily important unless this poses the risk of excessive sweating, which would result in excessive sodium loss. However, protecting the child against infection takes priority over preventing exposure to bright sunlight.

    Client Needs Category—Physiological integrity
    Client Needs Subcategory—Physiological adaptation

Nursing Care of a Toddler with Asthma

75. 1. Wheezing and a dry, hacking cough are major manifestations of an acute asthma attack. The normal respiratory rate for a 3-year-old child is 20 to 30 breaths/minute. Children also begin to assume a thoracic breathing pattern around this age. Clear, watery nasal drainage is usually seen in upper respiratory tract disorders, not acute asthma attacks.

    Client Needs Category—Physiological integrity
    Client Needs Subcategory—Physiological adaptation

76. 4. The most effective method of relieving acute respiratory distress in a young child is to place him in semi-Fowler's position. An older child may be more comfortable leaning forward on a pillow on an overbed table. Cool mist humidifiers, not steam vaporizers, may be used as well. Antibiotics will not relieve the acute respiratory distress. Distracting the child with age-appropriate toys is not an effective strategy when the child is experiencing acute distress.

    Client Needs Category—Physiological integrity
    Client Needs Subcategory—Physiological adaptation

77. 4. If breathing exercises are incorporated into play activities such as blowing bubbles, the child is more likely to enjoy them and may practice the exercises more. This is a creative teaching strategy. Promises of treats, parental assistance with the exercise, demonstrations, and return demonstrations are not likely to be as effective as incorporating exercises into play activities.

    Client Needs Category—Health promotion and maintenance
    Client Needs Subcategory—None

78. 4. When a client has asthma due to an allergy to one or more environmental factors, general control of the environment is necessary to reduce chances of future asthma attacks. Removing area rugs helps to eliminate a potential allergen and control the environment. The physician orders breathing treatments every 2 hours in the acute stage of the disease process. A generous fluid intake is recommended because fluid is lost through sweating and an increased respiratory rate. A well-balanced diet is necessary, especially for a growing child. Asthma cannot be cured, but it can often be controlled.

    Client Needs Category—Health promotion and maintenance
    Client Needs Subcategory—None

Nursing Care of a Toddler Who Has Swallowed a Toxic Substance

79. 3. When a caustic substance is ingested, water or milk should be given to dilute the substance. Vomiting should not be induced because the substance may cause additional injury when regurgitated. There is also a danger of respiratory complications secondary to aspiration of vomitus. It is important to address life-threatening concerns immediately before taking the child to the emergency department. Cardiopulmonary resuscitation may or may not be necessary, depending on the specific injury incurred.

    Client Needs Category—Physiological integrity
    Client Needs Subcategory—Physiological adaptation

80. 1. Substernal and intercostal retractions indicate that the child is experiencing respiratory distress. This child's oxygen saturation level should be monitored to assist in determining the need for additional therapy to relieve or minimize respiratory distress. The child may manifest all the other symptoms, but they do not indicate respiratory distress.

    Client Needs Category—Physiological integrity
    Client Needs Subcategory—Physiological adaptation

81. 2. The child may experience pain related to burns on the lips and in the mouth from the lye-based substance. Gastric lavage is not performed when caustic substances have been ingested; however, a gastrostomy may be necessary with severe damage. The child is given liquids by mouth as tolerated. Neurovascular checks are not usually required.

    Client Needs Category—Physiological integrity
    Client Needs Subcategory—Physiological adaptation

82. **4.** All poisonous substances should be placed in locked compartments or cabinets. Children are often capable of climbing and reaching areas higher than anticipated. It would be unrealistic to remove all poisonous substances from the home or to keep a constant eye on the child.
> *Client Needs Category—Health promotion and maintenance*
> *Client Needs Subcategory—None*

Nursing Care of a Toddler with Croup

83. **1.** A virus is the usual cause of croup. Croup affects the upper and lower respiratory tracts and occurs primarily in infants and young children. It is unrelated to whooping cough or inadequate lung development. Croup may occur in toddlers with or without a history of asthma.
> *Client Needs Category—Physiological integrity*
> *Client Needs Subcategory—Physiological adaptation*

84. **2.** The child with croup has a cough that sounds hoarse, much like a loud, barking, metallic sound. The cough is usually dry rather than moist, loud, and muffled. Wheezing is a term used to describe breath sounds, not cough characteristics.
> *Client Needs Category—Physiological integrity*
> *Client Needs Subcategory—Physiological adaptation*

85. **3.** To help liquefy secretions and reduce laryngeal spasms, the child with croup should breathe air that is high in humidity. A mist tent or a cool mist vaporizer may be used for this purpose. A dust-free environment is required for children who are allergic to dust. Dry or hot air does not provide relief for children with croup.
> *Client Needs Category—Physiological integrity*
> *Client Needs Subcategory—Physiological adaptation*

86. **2.** Extreme anxiety is a sign of respiratory difficulty and may indicate more serious involvement of the trachea and bronchial tree. The physician should be contacted immediately in this case. Mild fever, coughing during the night, and sleeping during the day are not considered signs of a worsening condition or more serious complications.
> *Client Needs Category—Physiological integrity*
> *Client Needs Subcategory—Physiological adaptation*

87. **2.** Aspirin, a salicylate, is contraindicated in young children with a fever, flulike symptoms, or chickenpox. Its use has been associated with Reye's syndrome. All the other options reflect a correct understanding of croup and appropriate measures to treat it.
> *Client Needs Category—Health promotion and maintenance*
> *Client Needs Subcategory—None*

88. **2.** The parents are encouraged to remain close to the child because emotional upset can cause an increase in respiratory distress. The child with croup is not usually sedated. Typically, age-appropriate toys do not interest a child during acute respiratory distress. Sometimes to stabilize or improve the child's condition, it is necessary to perform procedures that may be unpleasant to the child; postponing them may not be an option.
> *Client Needs Category—Psychosocial integrity*
> *Client Needs Subcategory—None*

89. **4.** The physician may order racemic epinephrine (Vaponefrin) via nebulizer to reduce edema and airway obstruction. Because a virus is the usual cause of croup, antibiotics such as ampicillin are not typically used. The other two medications also are not routinely given to children with croup.
> *Client Needs Category—Physiological integrity*
> *Client Needs Subcategory—Pharmacological therapies*

90. **3.** Milk and milk products should be avoided because they increase mucus production. Croup is accompanied by a severe cough and often requires expectorants to loosen secretions. Clear liquids, such as ginger ale, Popsicles, apple juice, and gelatin, are permitted because they help to liquefy secretions and allow easier expectoration.
> *Client Needs Category—Physiological integrity*
> *Client Needs Subcategory—Reduction of risk potential*

Nursing Care of a Toddler with Pneumonia

91. **4.** The respiratory pattern in children with pneumonia is usually rapid and shallow. The rapid respiratory rate is the body's way of compensating for decreased ventilation in the lungs. The pulse is usually elevated in the child with pneumonia. Clubbing of the fingers is seen in chronic illnesses associated with a chronic lack of oxygen. Synchronized breathing is characteristic of a normal breathing pattern.
> *Client Needs Category—Physiological integrity*
> *Client Needs Subcategory—Physiological adaptation*

92. **1.** Recording the child's urine output will assist in determining fluid needs. Fluid loss commonly occurs because of the high fever, vomiting, and increased respiratory rate associated with pneumonia. Such loss results in a decreased amount of urine, which is usually dark in color with a high specific gravity. To ensure that fluid needs are met, the nurse should monitor the child's fluid intake as well. The pH of the urine will indicate whether the urine is acidic or alkalotic; it will not indicate hydration status. A child may have a normal blood pressure yet still be dehydrated. A drop in blood pressure occurs with circulatory collapse, which is a late sign dehydration. An increased respiratory rate may result in an increased insensible fluid loss, which indicates a risk of dehydration, but this does not indicate the child's hydration status.

> *Client Needs Category—Physiological integrity*
> *Client Needs Subcategory—Physiological adaptation*

93. **1.** Pulse oximetry is used to determine oxygen saturation in the blood. A value less than 95% indicates that the saturation level may be insufficient to meet the client's oxygen demand. In this case, the charge nurse or physician should be notified.

> *Client Needs Category—Physiological integrity*
> *Client Needs Subcategory—Reduction of risk potential*

94. **3.** Expectorants help to loosen secretions so that the client can cough up and get rid of mucus that has accumulated in the airways. Suppressants prevent the child from coughing. A moist cough indicates secretions in the airway that need to be removed. Antibiotics and bronchodilators have no effect on the cough.

> *Client Needs Category—Physiological integrity*
> *Client Needs Subcategory—Pharmacological therapies*

95. **3.** If the child is observed shivering, the bath should be stopped immediately because shivering will further increase the core body temperature. The bath should not be given for more than 30 minutes. Tepid water is used for the bath. The child's temperature should drop, but not below 101° F.

> *Client Needs Category—Safe, effective care environment*
> *Client Needs Subcategory—Safety and infection control*

96. **5.** Equivalents:

> 1 g = 1,000 mg
>
> 1 tsp = 5 mL
>
> 0.5 g = 0.5 × 1,000 = 500 mg

5 mL would fulfill the physician's order.

> *Client Needs Category—Physiological integrity*
> *Client Needs Subcategory—Pharmacological therapies*

97. **2.** Having an interpreter present when instructions are given allows the nurse to give clear instructions as well as validate the parents' understanding of the instructions. Providing a copy of the instructions in Spanish should be used as reinforcement; it does not guarantee that the parents understand the instructions. Having the physician give the instructions is unnecessary unless the physician speaks Spanish. The parents should be encouraged to call if questions arise after discharge, but the nurse must ensure that they have a basic understanding of the instructions before they leave.

> *Client Needs Category—Health promotion and maintenance*
> *Client Needs Subcategory—None*

Nursing Care of a Preschooler with Seizure Disorder

98. **4.** Generalized involuntary body movement is characteristic of tonic-clonic seizures. A child may have seizures associated with fever, but not all children who have a fever have seizures. The child could also drop to the floor with other disorders, such as muscle weakness and unconsciousness. The child may wet the bed after a seizure has ceased, but bedwetting could occur for other reasons.

> *Client Needs Category—Physiological integrity*
> *Client Needs Subcategory—Physiological adaptation*

99. **1.** The priority nursing action for a child experiencing a generalized seizure is protection from injury. Padding the side rails is one means of protecting the child. Phenobarbital may be given to a child who has tonic-clonic seizures, but the medication is not usually kept in the child's room. The other options are not routinely used in caring for the child with tonic-clonic seizures.

> *Client Needs Category—Safe, effective care environment*
> *Client Needs Subcategory—Safety and infection control*

100. **4.** It is unnecessary to have a cool mist humidifier at the bedside of a child subject to seizure activity. Suction equipment may be required to remove mucus from the child's mouth. An oral airway and oxygen may be needed in the case of respiratory arrest, which can occur with generalized seizures.

> *Client Needs Category—Safe, effective care environment*
> *Client Needs Subcategory—Safety and infection control*

101. **2.** Placing the child in the side-lying position establishes a patent airway and prevents aspiration of

saliva. Inserting a padded tongue blade is no longer recommended because injury to the mouth and teeth may occur. The nurse should be prepared to administer oxygen after the seizure, if required. The nurse should implement necessary measures to minimize injury to the child before calling for assistance.
Client Needs Category—Physiological integrity
Client Needs Subcategory—Physiological adaptation

102. 4. Prolonged use of phenytoin (Dilantin) tends to cause an overgrowth of gum tissues. Poor appetite, urinary incontinence, and painful joints are not associated with the use of this medication.
Client Needs Category—Physiological integrity
Client Needs Subcategory—Pharmacological therapies

103. 2. The child should not be restrained during seizure activity because this may injure the child rather than protect him. The parents should be encouraged to maintain as normal a lifestyle as possible for the child. Mental retardation does not always occur with seizure disorder. To reduce stomach irritation, phenytoin (Dilantin) should be given with food or immediately after meals.
Client Needs Category—Health promotion and maintenance
Client Needs Subcategory—None

104. 2. The preschool child often thinks that illness or painful treatments are a punishment for having done something bad. It is important to explain to the child that the seizure activity is not a punishment. The nurse must always be honest with the child. Pain should be addressed and rated by the child using a pain scale appropriate for the age because it is the child's perception of pain that is important. It is not comforting to tell the child that the pain will eventually stop. The nurse may explain that the medication must be taken and that other children have seizures, but it should be done in terms that are developmentally appropriate.
Client Needs Category—Health promotion and maintenance
Client Needs Subcategory—None

Nursing Care of a Preschooler with Leukemia

105. 3. Bone marrow aspiration is commonly used to confirm a diagnosis of leukemia. The bone marrow of the child with leukemia is characterized as being hypercellular, lacking fat globules, and containing blast cells (immature white cells). The CBC and spinal fluid examinations are part of the battery of tests a client may undergo when leukemia is suspected, but they do not confirm the diagnosis. An X-ray of the long bones also does not confirm the diagnosis.
Client Needs Category—Physiological integrity
Client Needs Subcategory—Physiological adaptation

106. 3. Fresh fruits that cannot be peeled should not be taken into the child's room because they may harbor organisms that can cause life-threatening illnesses in someone with leukemia. The risk of contracting a life-threatening illness is increased because of the child's compromised immune system. Allowing only washable toys is appropriate for a child with a contagious disease who is in isolation to prevent the spread of infection to other individuals. However, in this case, the child's disease is not contagious; also, he is more likely to contract an infection than spread one to someone else. Visitation requirements vary by facility. Generally, family members, including children under age 12, are permitted to visit as long as they do not have any type of active infectious disease.
Client Needs Category—Safe, effective care environment
Client Needs Subcategory—Safety and infection control

107. 3. Because of the child's immunosuppressed state, the nurse should avoid taking rectal temperatures. This route increases the child's risk of developing a perirectal abscess, which can lead to a life-threatening complication. Temperatures taken by the axillary, oral, or tympanic routes are appropriate for the child with leukemia.
Client Needs Category—Physiological integrity
Client Needs Subcategory—Reduction of risk potential

108. 1. Epinephrine (Adrenalin) and oxygen should be on hand when giving asparaginase (Elspar) because of the increased risk of an anaphylactic reaction. The other medications are not required.
Client Needs Category—Physiological integrity
Client Needs Subcategory—Reduction of risk potential

109. 2. Signs of a transfusion reaction include feeling cold and having chills, fever, and a rapid pulse rate. The child may also complain of itching and low back pain. If the child experiences chilliness very early in a blood transfusion, it may be the result of the cold transfused blood entering the body. Nevertheless, the nurse should suspect a transfusion reaction until proven otherwise. Complaints of hunger, thirst, and tiredness are not common indicators of a blood transfusion reaction.
Client Needs Category—Physiological integrity
Client Needs Subcategory—Reduction of risk potential

110. **3.** If a client is having a reaction to blood, the nurse should first clamp the tubing to stop the blood flow. Then the clamp on the second bottle (normal saline solution) should be immediately opened to maintain I.V. access. The temperature is taken, and acetaminophen (Tylenol) may be given if ordered and necessary. The charge nurse should be notified, but not before the infusion is stopped.

Client Needs Category—Physiological integrity
Client Needs Subcategory—Physiological adaptation

111. **1.** Preschoolers have a limited ability to grasp complex concepts such as death and dying. "Am I going to die?" is a question that can be answered in different ways. However, the nurse's response should encourage the child to ventilate feelings about dying. The nurse should avoid responses that would either make the child feel guilty or discourage him from talking about anxieties experienced. Also, the nurse's response should not reinforce feelings of denial and unrealistic perceptions of the child's prognosis. When dealing with children, it is important to answer questions honestly based on the child's level of understanding and development.

Client Needs Category—Psychosocial integrity
Client Needs Subcategory—None

112. **1.** Children with leukemia should postpone live-virus vaccines for 6 to 12 months after chemotherapy has been discontinued and after blood count levels are within normal ranges. All the other statements by the parents are consistent with the recommended treatment plan.

Client Needs Category—Health promotion and maintenance
Client Needs Subcategory—None

Nursing Care of a Preschooler with Strabismus

113. **3.** Foods and fluids are generally withheld for 6 to 12 hours before surgery to reduce the risk of aspirating vomitus when the client is under anesthesia or recovering from anesthesia. Preparation of the eyelids is usually carried out in the clinical setting. A Fleet's enema is not routinely needed for eye surgery. Acetaminophen (Tylenol) is not usually given as a preparation for eye surgery.

Client Needs Category—Safe, effective care environment
Client Needs Subcategory—Safety and infection control

114. **4.** Some soreness may occur after this type of eye surgery. The child's question should not be ignored or minimized and deserves an honest response. Any re-

sponses or explanations should be developmentally appropriate.

Client Needs Category—Psychosocial integrity
Client Needs Subcategory—None

115. **2.** Pretending the child is a pirate affords an opportunity to wear an eye patch, thereby restricting the child's vision and giving him a perception of the postoperative experience. Done in a nonthreatening manner, this game will decrease the child's anxiety during the postoperative period. The other games do not relate to preparation of the child's postoperative needs.

Client Needs Category—Psychosocial integrity
Client Needs Subcategory—None

116. **3.** Unless both of the child's eyes are bandaged, there is no reason why he cannot play with toys while under an adult's supervision. In most cases, the child can resume a regular diet and activity as soon as nausea has ceased and the anesthesia has worn off. Restraints are removed while the child is under adult supervision.

Client Needs Category—Health promotion and maintenance
Client Needs Subcategory—None

Nursing Care of a Preschooler Having a Tonsillectomy and Adenoidectomy

117. **2.** It is important to promptly report an elevated temperature of a preoperative client along with any other signs of infection, such as a sore throat, cough, or excessive nasal discharge. Surgery will be canceled if the child has an infection. The other vital signs listed are normal for a child of this age.

Client Needs Category—Safe, effective care environment
Client Needs Subcategory—Coordinated care

118. **2.** Clear liquids include clear broth, gelatin, synthetic juices, water, and ice chips. Natural juices, such as orange juice, are irritating to the throat and are not clear. When a full liquid diet can be tolerated, such foods as ice cream, puddings, creamed soups, and custards can be added to the menu.

Client Needs Category—Physiological integrity
Client Needs Subcategory—Physiological adaptation

119. **2.** The child should not be allowed to drink from a straw because sucking can dislodge clots and sutures and lead to hemorrhage. An ice collar is typically applied to promote comfort; however, it may be removed if the child is more comfortable without one. The child may prefer to use the bedpan or urinal during the immediate postoperative period; it also may be safer for the child, particularly if he is receiving pain medication. It is appropriate for the parents to hold the child following surgery.

Client Needs Category—*Physiological integrity*
Client Needs Subcategory—*Physiological adaptation*

120. **4.** Signs of excessive bleeding following a tonsillectomy include frequent swallowing (which may be due to blood trickling down the back of the throat), a rapid pulse rate, restlessness, and vomiting bright red blood. Vomiting dark (old) blood is expected and should not cause concern unless there is a large amount of emesis. Throat pain is a common postoperative finding. A respiratory rate of 30 breaths/minute is within the normal range for a 5-year-old child.

Client Needs Category—*Physiological integrity*
Client Needs Subcategory—*Physiological adaptation*

121. **1.** It is recommended to keep a child quiet for a few days following a tonsillectomy to discourage bleeding at the operative site. Fluids and soft foods can be taken as desired, but a regular diet is not usually recommended for several days because certain food may cause irritation and bleeding of the operative site. Aspirin is contraindicated for a child of this age because its use has been associated with Reye's syndrome. Aspirin may also affect the blood's ability to clot and therefore increases bleeding tendencies.

Client Needs Category—*Health promotion and maintenance*
Client Needs Subcategory—*None*

The Nursing Care of School-Age Children and Adolescents

⇨ Nursing Care of a Child with Rheumatic Fever
⇨ Nursing Care of a Child with Diabetes Mellitus
⇨ Nursing Care of a Child with Partial- and Full-Thickness Burns
⇨ Nursing Care of a Child with Juvenile Rheumatoid Arthritis
⇨ Nursing Care of a Child with an Injury
⇨ Nursing Care of a Child with a Head Injury
⇨ Nursing Care of a Child with a Brain Tumor
⇨ Nursing Care of a Child in Traction
⇨ Nursing Care of a Child with a Kidney Disorder
⇨ Nursing Care of a Child with a Blood Disorder
⇨ Nursing Care of a Child with a Communicable Disease
⇨ Nursing Care of a Child with a Nutritional Deficiency
⇨ Nursing Care of a Child with Musculoskeletal Disability
⇨ Nursing Care of an Adolescent with Appendicitis
⇨ Nursing Care of an Adolescent with Dysmenorrhea
⇨ Nursing Care of an Adolescent Who Is Abusing Drugs
⇨ Nursing Care of an Adolescent with a Sexually Transmitted Disease
⇨ Nursing Care of an Adolescent with Scoliosis
⇨ Dosage Calculations for Children and Adolescents
⇨ Correct Answers and Rationales

Directions: With a pencil, blacken the space in front of the option you have chosen for your correct answer.

Nursing Care of a Child with Rheumatic Fever

A 7-year-old child is admitted to the hospital with possible rheumatic fever.

1. If the parents report all the following history findings, which one is most closely correlated with an increased risk of rheumatic fever?
[ ] **1.** The child was exposed to measles within the last 4 weeks.
[ ] **2.** The child had a severe sore throat within the last 2 weeks.
[ ] **3.** The child is no longer interested in schoolwork.
[ ] **4.** The child received a bump on the head while playing.

2. Which finding documented by the nurse is most indicative of rheumatic fever?
[ ] **1.** Slow, irregular heartbeat
[ ] **2.** Blotchy, diffuse erythema
[ ] **3.** Decreased antistreptolysin O titer (ASO titer)
[ ] **4.** Generalized migrating joint tenderness

The child is placed on bed rest and started on penicillin V (Pen-Vee-K) and acetylsalicylic acid (aspirin).

3. Which diversional activity is most appropriate for the child during the acute phase of rheumatic fever?
[ ] **1.** Playing with action figures
[ ] **2.** Playing video games
[ ] **3.** Reading an adventure story
[ ] **4.** Pounding wooden pegs with a mallet

4. The nurse would expect to withhold penicillin V (Pen-Vee-K) and notify the physician if the child had a previous allergic reaction to a medication from which drug group?
[ ] **1.** Aminoglycosides
[ ] **2.** Cephalosporins
[ ] **3.** Macrolides
[ ] **4.** Sulfonamides

The parents ask why the child is receiving aspirin instead of acetaminophen (Tylenol).

5. Which response by the nurse best explains why aspirin is preferred to acetaminophen (Tylenol) in the treatment of rheumatic fever?
[ ] **1.** Aspirin controls fever better.
[ ] **2.** Aspirin prevents infections.
[ ] **3.** Aspirin relieves joint inflammation.
[ ] **4.** Aspirin prevents cardiac enlargement.

6. Which statement by the parents indicates that the nurse's teaching has been effective?
[ ] **1.** "We'll give the penicillin for 10 days."
[ ] **2.** "Our child isn't allowed to play in bright, direct sunlight."
[ ] **3.** "Our child must take seizure medication every day."
[ ] **4.** "We'll notify the physician if our child has a sore throat."

7. If the child develops shortness of breath when ambulating to the bathroom, which intervention should the nurse add to the care plan?
[ ] **1.** Have the child use a bedside commode for elimination.
[ ] **2.** Administer oxygen after the child uses the bathroom.
[ ] **3.** Instruct the child to call for assistance when ambulating to the bathroom.
[ ] **4.** Provide a walker for the child to use when ambulating to the bathroom.

Nursing Care of a Child with Diabetes Mellitus

A 9-year-old child is admitted to the hospital with a tentative diagnosis of type 1 (insulin-dependent) diabetes mellitus. The parents state that the child has been complaining of feeling bad for several days. The physician states that the child has signs and symptoms of diabetic ketoacidosis. The physician writes orders for an I.V. infusion of insulin, hourly blood glucose checks, and urine checks every 8 hours.

8. Which finding by the nurse best indicates that the child is experiencing diabetic ketoacidosis?
[ ] **1.** Blood glucose level of 120 mg/dL
[ ] **2.** Fruity-smelling breath
[ ] **3.** Pale-colored face
[ ] **4.** Excessive perspiration

9. What should the nurse be assessing when testing this child's urine?
[ ] **1.** Blood in the urine
[ ] **2.** Bilirubin in the urine
[ ] **3.** Ketones in the urine
[ ] **4.** White blood cells in the urine

10. Which type of insulin is most appropriate when giving the child's insulin intravenously?
[ ] **1.** Regular insulin (Humulin R)
[ ] **2.** Isophane insulin suspension (Humulin N)
[ ] **3.** Insulin zinc suspension (Humulin L)
[ ] **4.** Insulin zinc suspension, extended (Humulin U)

After further tests, the diagnosis of type 1 diabetes mellitus is confirmed. The child's condition improves. The physician writes orders to discontinue the I.V. infusion and to begin subcutaneous Humulin R insulin. The physician also orders a dietary consultation.

11. When is the correct time for the nurse to administer the child's morning dose of regular insulin?
[ ] **1.** 30 minutes before breakfast is served
[ ] **2.** 15 minutes before breakfast is served
[ ] **3.** 30 minutes after breakfast is served
[ ] **4.** 15 minutes after breakfast is served

12. Which finding best indicates that the child is having a hypoglycemic reaction?
[ ] **1.** The child complains of being thirsty.
[ ] **2.** The child's breathing is labored and prolonged.
[ ] **3.** The child's urine tests positive for glucose.
[ ] **4.** The child complains of feeling shaky.

13. What is the priority nursing action if the child develops hypoglycemia?
[ ] **1.** Give the child orange juice to drink.
[ ] **2.** Give the child 10% glucose I.V.
[ ] **3.** Notify the physician immediately.
[ ] **4.** Administer a second dose of insulin.

The child's parents ask the nurse why the child cannot receive the insulin in the form of a pill.

14. Which response by the nurse best explains why insulin must be given subcutaneously?

[ ] **1.** "The oral form of insulin can lead to the development of birth defects."

[ ] **2.** "Insulin is destroyed by digestive enzymes when given by mouth."

[ ] **3.** "Insulin causes vomiting and dehydration when given by mouth."

[ ] **4.** "The oral form of insulin isn't effective in treating children with diabetes."

The child has completely recovered from ketoacidosis and is receiving regular insulin (Humulin R) and isophane insulin suspension (Humulin N) subcutaneously. The blood glucose levels have stabilized, and the physician requests that diabetic home care teaching be started.

15. The nurse correctly explains to the child and parents that insulin injection sites should be rotated for which reason?

[ ] **1.** To slow the absorption of insulin from the subcutaneous tissue

[ ] **2.** To prevent accumulation of insulin in the subcutaneous tissue

[ ] **3.** To decrease the duration of the action of insulin

[ ] **4.** To prevent lipodystrophy of subcutaneous tissue

16. Which statement by the child indicates to the nurse that diabetic teaching has been effective?

[ ] **1.** "If I eat more food, I won't need as much insulin."

[ ] **2.** "If I'm more active, I won't need as much insulin."

[ ] **3.** "If I get an infection, I won't need as much insulin."

[ ] **4.** "If I get real upset, I won't need as much insulin."

The parents state that their child is very active in sports and likes to swim, play basketball, and soccer. The parents ask the nurse if the child will be able to continue these activities.

17. Which is the best response by the nurse?

[ ] **1.** "You should redirect you child to participate in activities that require less energy."

[ ] **2.** "You should encourage swimming because it lowers the metabolism, but discourage him from playing basketball or soccer."

[ ] **3.** "You should allow your child to continue these activities but accompany him when he goes swimming."

[ ] **4.** "You should permit your child to play basketball and soccer, but keep in mind that swimming will increase his insulin needs."

18. If the child is athletic and very competitive, the nurse should recommend checking the child's blood glucose level how often?

[ ] **1.** Twice daily, 30 minutes before eating

[ ] **2.** Before participating in athletics

[ ] **3.** Every 4 hours throughout the day

[ ] **4.** When a hypoglycemic reaction occurs

19. The nurse is caring for a diabetic child whose 11 a.m. blood glucose monitoring check is 269 mg/dL. The physician orders the following coverage schedule:

150 to 200 mg/dL—2 units of Humulin R

201 to 250 mg/dL—4 units of Humulin R

251 to 300 mg/dL—6 units of Humulin R

301 to 350 mg/dL—8 units of Humulin R

351 to 399 mg/dL—10 units of Humulin R

Over 400 mg/dL—Call the physician

Indicate the correct area on the syringe representing the amount of insulin that should be drawn into the syringe.

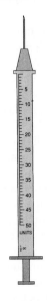

The diabetic child begins using an insulin pump. A diabetic nurse educator has been consulted to assist with insulin pump education and regulation.

20. Which statement by a diabetic child indicates a need for additional instructions on how to use an insulin pump?

[ ] **1.** "I like the insulin pump because I can wear it under my clothes without anyone noticing I have it on."

[ ] **2.** "I like the insulin pump because I only have to change the needle site every 24 to 48 hours."

[ ] **3.** "I like the insulin pump because when I need extra insulin, all I have to do is push a button on the pump."

[ ] **4.** "I like the insulin pump because I don't have to check my blood glucose level; the pump checks the level for me."

Nursing Care of a Child with Partial- and Full-Thickness Burns

An 8-year-old child is hospitalized for treatment of extensive partial- and full-thickness burns on his face, neck, anterior chest, and left arm.

21. Which manifestation of the full-thickness burns would the nurse anticipate on the face, neck, anterior chest, and left arm?
[ ] **1.** Pain due to exposed nerve endings
[ ] **2.** Edema formation throughout the area
[ ] **3.** The appearance of blister formation
[ ] **4.** Noted destruction of the epidermis

22. The nurse should plan to keep which equipment or supplies in the child's room in case an emergency arises?
[ ] **1.** An extra supply of sterile dressing
[ ] **2.** An endotracheal tube and oxygen supply
[ ] **3.** Equipment to administer pain medication
[ ] **4.** A bag of I.V. fluid

23. Which nursing interventions are essential to restore the child's fluid and electrolyte balance during the emergent phase of burn care and treatment? Select all that apply.
[ ] **1.** Initiate the administration of I.V. fluids.
[ ] **2.** Track the child's vital signs.
[ ] **3.** Give the child sips of water.
[ ] **4.** Encourage the child to consume protein-rich feedings.
[ ] **5.** Monitor the child's urine output.
[ ] **6.** Insert a small-bore catheter.

24. During early postburn care, it is especially important for the nurse to closely monitor which of the following?
[ ] **1.** Unburned skin
[ ] **2.** Bowel elimination
[ ] **3.** I.V. fluid therapy
[ ] **4.** Pupillary response to light

The physician orders hourly measurement of the child's urine output.

25. The nurse is correct to immediately notify the physician or charge nurse if the urine output is greater than which amount?
[ ] **1.** 1 mL/kg/hour
[ ] **2.** 1.5 mL/kg/hour
[ ] **3.** 2 mL/kg/hour
[ ] **4.** 2.5 mL/kg/hour

26. Which finding by the nurse would best indicate that the I.V. opioid analgesic is effective?

[ ] **1.** The respiratory rate is within normal limits.
[ ] **2.** The child no longer complains of nausea.
[ ] **3.** The child no longer complains of pain.
[ ] **4.** The urine output is 30 mL/hour.

27. Which nursing action best prevents the development of footdrop in a child confined to bed?
[ ] **1.** Apply braces to the feet and ankles.
[ ] **2.** Keep the child in the side-lying position.
[ ] **3.** Keep sheets tucked in at the foot of the bed.
[ ] **4.** Rest the child's feet against a footboard.

28. Which finding documented by the nurse is most indicative of the presence of a Curling's ulcer?
[ ] **1.** Absence of bowel sounds
[ ] **2.** A positive hemoccult test
[ ] **3.** An elevated hematocrit
[ ] **4.** A distended abdomen

After the child's condition stabilizes, he is placed on a high-protein diet.

29. If the following snacks are available, which one is best to meet the child's need for protein?
[ ] **1.** Strawberry milk shake
[ ] **2.** Apple sprinkled with cinnamon
[ ] **3.** Cubes of flavored gelatin
[ ] **4.** Chocolate candy bar

30. Which diversional activity is best for meeting the child's developmental needs?
[ ] **1.** Reading the newspaper
[ ] **2.** Coloring simple designs
[ ] **3.** Playing with a coin collection
[ ] **4.** Playing a solitary card game

Nursing Care of a Child with Juvenile Rheumatoid Arthritis

A 10-year-old child who has juvenile rheumatoid arthritis is seen in the joint disorders specialty clinic 2 weeks after an acute episode of the disorder. The nurse discusses home care with the child and parents.

31. Which statement by the child indicates teaching about ibuprofen (Motrin) use has been effective?
[ ] **1.** "I should take Motrin every day to control my joint inflammation."
[ ] **2.** "I should take Motrin when my temperature is 101° F (38.3° C) or higher."
[ ] **3.** "I should take Motrin only when I'm having muscle spasms."
[ ] **4.** "I should take Motrin every day to thin my blood."

32. The nurse correctly explains that the toxic effects of acetylsalicylic acid (aspirin) include which manifestations?

[ ] **1.** Constipation, weight gain, and fluid retention
[ ] **2.** Ringing in the ears, nausea, and diarrhea
[ ] **3.** Anorexia, weight loss, and double vision
[ ] **4.** Headache, dry mouth, and dental cavities

33. Which activity is most appropriate for the child with juvenile rheumatoid arthritis?

[ ] **1.** Skipping rope
[ ] **2.** Softball
[ ] **3.** Gymnastics
[ ] **4.** Swimming

34. Which statement by the parents indicates they understand the home care instructions given by the nurse?

[ ] **1.** "We've made arrangements for a homebound teacher."
[ ] **2.** "We'll put ice packs on our child's joints during episodes of inflammation."
[ ] **3.** "We'll serve meals that prevent excess weight gain."
[ ] **4.** "We'll keep our child in bed most of the time."

35. The nurse advises the parents that, to detect possible complications of juvenile rheumatoid arthritis, the child will require which periodic evaluation?

[ ] **1.** Chest X-rays
[ ] **2.** Dental examinations
[ ] **3.** Hearing examinations
[ ] **4.** Eye examinations

Nursing Care of a Child with an Injury

A nurse in a rural community clinic provides nursing care and age-appropriate instruction for pediatric clients with minor injuries. Throughout the day, children with a variety of injuries come for medical care.

36. Which nursing instruction concerning ice applications is appropriate to give the parents of a 12-year-old child with a sprained ankle?

[ ] **1.** Ice can be applied and left on until the swelling is gone.
[ ] **2.** Ice can be applied but must be removed every 30 minutes to 1 hour.
[ ] **3.** Ice should not be used for treating sprains; heat should be used instead.
[ ] **4.** There is no danger associated with the application of ice.

37. Which nursing action is most appropriate when caring for a school-age child who is experiencing a nosebleed?

[ ] **1.** Tilt the child's head backward, and apply an ice pack to the nose.
[ ] **2.** Position the child's head forward while gently pinching the nostrils.
[ ] **3.** Pack the affected nostril with a small amount of clean cotton.
[ ] **4.** Clean the affected nostril, and instill saline nose drops.

38. When a 10-year-old child falls from a bicycle and loses a permanent incisor tooth, which advice can the nurse provide the parents before they take him to see a dentist?

[ ] **1.** Submerge the tooth in water.
[ ] **2.** Have the child hold the tooth under the tongue.
[ ] **3.** Wrap the tooth in a clean cloth.
[ ] **4.** Clean the tooth with alcohol.

39. Which intervention is most appropriate initially for an 8-year-old child who has a score of 4 on the Wong-Baker FACES Pain Rating Scale?

[ ] **1.** Take no action; the child is pain-free.
[ ] **2.** Provide diversional activities to relieve the child's pain.
[ ] **3.** Document findings, and recheck the child later.
[ ] **4.** Give the prescribed analgesic to relieve the pain.

Nursing Care of a Child with a Head Injury

A 9-year-old child is admitted to the hospital for observation after falling off a bicycle. The parents state that the child's head hit the pavement during the fall.

40. If the nurse collects the following data, which finding best indicates the presence of increased intracranial pressure?

[ ] **1.** Rapid bilateral pupillary response to light
[ ] **2.** Tympanic temperature of 97.9° F (36.6° C)
[ ] **3.** Blood pressure of 150/90 mm Hg
[ ] **4.** Deep tendon reflexes +2

41. Which assessment finding should the nurse report immediately to the charge nurse or physician?

[ ] **1.** Clear, watery nasal drainage
[ ] **2.** Glasgow Coma Scale score of 15
[ ] **3.** Child does not know the time of day
[ ] **4.** Apical pulse of 80 beats/minute

The child is monitored overnight and no complications are observed. The physician discharges him. Prior to leaving the clinic, the nurse reviews safety needs with the child and parents.

42. Which statement by the child indicates a need for further teaching about bicycle safety?
[ ] **1.** "I'll wear my helmet whenever I ride my bicycle."
[ ] **2.** "I'll ride my bicycle in the opposite direction of traffic flow."
[ ] **3.** "I'll stop at all intersections and look both ways before proceeding."
[ ] **4.** "I won't ride my bicycle after dark on the street."

Another child is being assessed in the emergency department following a blow to the head. The physician determines that the child may be discharged to home. The nurse provides discharge instructions to the client and parents.

43. Which instruction is essential to give the parents prior to discharge?
[ ] **1.** Return the child for a follow-up visit in 3 to 5 days.
[ ] **2.** Give the child nothing by mouth for the next 12 hours.
[ ] **3.** Check the child's pupillary response every 4 hours.
[ ] **4.** Awaken the child every 4 hours during the first night.

Nursing Care of a Child with a Brain Tumor

An 11-year-old child is admitted to the hospital with complaints of headaches, dizziness, and vomiting. The physician orders X-rays of the head and a magnetic resonance imaging (MRI) scan.

44. Which of the following information reported by the parents indicates a high risk for the presence of a brain tumor?
[ ] **1.** The child vomits when first getting out of bed.
[ ] **2.** The child frequently complains of nausea.
[ ] **3.** The child does not like going to school anymore.
[ ] **4.** The child's head tilts toward the side when sleeping.

45. Which statement by the nurse would best prepare the child for the MRI?
[ ] **1.** "You'll be placed in a tunnel-like scanner with a special call button."
[ ] **2.** "You'll experience a slight headache when the dye is injected."
[ ] **3.** "You'll be given medicine that will make you sleep during the test."
[ ] **4.** "You'll have little electrodes placed on your head with a special gel."

The results of the MRI show that the child has a brain tumor, and the child is taken immediately to surgery. A craniotomy is performed, and the tumor is partially removed. When the child returns from surgery, the nurse observes a moderate amount of clear drainage on the head dressing.

46. Which action by the nurse is most appropriate at this time?
[ ] **1.** Change the dressing; then notify the physician or charge nurse.
[ ] **2.** Remove the dressing and monitor the child for active drainage.
[ ] **3.** Reinforce the dressing until the physician can change it.
[ ] **4.** Leave the dressing intact and document findings.

The child's parents express their feelings of helplessness and anxiety to the nurse after learning about their child's diagnosis.

47. Which statement by the nurse would best help the parents cope with their feelings?
[ ] **1.** "Perhaps you'd feel better if you visited your child for shorter periods of time."
[ ] **2.** "Don't worry. You're doing a great job, and everything will work out for the best."
[ ] **3.** "This is painful for you. Let's identify things you can do to help make your child feel good."
[ ] **4.** "It's sad that you feel helpless. What do you usually do to take your mind off your worries?"

The oncologist visits and writes orders for the child to begin chemotherapy.

48. Which nursing action would best help the child to cope with the effects of the chemotherapy?
[ ] **1.** Serve the child a well-balanced meal before beginning the chemotherapy.
[ ] **2.** Give the child an antiemetic before beginning the chemotherapy.
[ ] **3.** Encourage the child to get plenty of rest before beginning the chemotherapy.
[ ] **4.** Give the child an enema before beginning the chemotherapy.

The physician orders an I.V. line to maintain fluid replacement for this child.

49. If the child weighs 30 kg, what is the hourly flow rate in milliliters?

_____

After losing hair from the chemotherapy treatments, the child cries and says, "Everybody is going to laugh at me. I never want to go to school again!"

50. Which nursing action best facilitates the child's reestablishment of friendships with peers?
[ ]   **1.** Encourage the child to make friends with children who have a similar problem.
[ ]   **2.** Tell the child that real friends do not care how you look on the outside.
[ ]   **3.** Encourage the child's friends to visit while the child is still in the hospital.
[ ]   **4.** Tell the child that the appearance changes are temporary and not that bad.

The physician orders a lumbar puncture for a child suspected of having a brain tumor.

51. How should the nurse position a child who is about to undergo a lumbar puncture?
[ ]   **1.** Prone position
[ ]   **2.** Trendelenburg's position
[ ]   **3.** Supine position
[ ]   **4.** Side-lying position

Nursing Care of a Child in Traction

A 9-year-old girl is admitted to the pediatric unit with a fractured right femur. The child is in skeletal traction.

52. Which nursing intervention should be included in the care plan of a child in skeletal traction?
[ ]   **1.** Maintain the child in the prone position.
[ ]   **2.** Clean the pin site every 8 hours.
[ ]   **3.** Perform range-of-motion exercises on the child's legs.
[ ]   **4.** Release weights on the traction every 2 hours.

53. The nurse correctly assesses for evidence of skin breakdown in which area?
[ ]   **1.** Over the child's calves
[ ]   **2.** Over the child's scapulae
[ ]   **3.** On the child's knees
[ ]   **4.** On the child's buttocks

54. Which assessment finding should the nurse report immediately to the physician or charge nurse?
[ ]   **1.** The pin protrudes through the skin on both sides.
[ ]   **2.** The foot of the bed is elevated on blocks.
[ ]   **3.** The weights of the traction are hanging freely.
[ ]   **4.** A traction rope is out of the pulley groove.

55. Which intervention is best to prevent complications associated with traction and immobility?

[ ]   **1.** Offer the child fluids on a frequent basis.
[ ]   **2.** Assist the child to select low-fiber foods.
[ ]   **3.** Assist the child with right leg exercises daily.
[ ]   **4.** Reposition the child onto her side every 2 hours.

56. Which assessment finding may indicate a serious neurovascular problem that should be reported immediately to the charge nurse or physician?
[ ]   **1.** The pulse is palpable in the right foot.
[ ]   **2.** The toes of both feet are cool to the touch.
[ ]   **3.** The child is unable to wiggle the toes of the right foot.
[ ]   **4.** The capillary refill in the toes of the right foot is 2 seconds.

Nursing Care of a Child With a Kidney Disorder

A 7-year-old child is brought to the pediatrician's office when the mother notes that the child is voiding dark-colored urine. The child is being evaluated for acute glomerular nephritis.

57. Which finding best indicates that a school-age child has acute glomerular nephritis?
[ ]   **1.** Periorbital edema
[ ]   **2.** Excessive urination
[ ]   **3.** Increased appetite
[ ]   **4.** Low blood pressure

A toddler is examined by the pediatrician and diagnosed with nephrotic syndrome. The parents are concerned due to the generalized edema throughout the toddler's body.

58. Which nursing action is most appropriate to include in the care plan of a child with nephrotic syndrome?
[ ]   **1.** Restricting the intake of protein
[ ]   **2.** Weighing the child daily
[ ]   **3.** Completing range-of-motion exercises
[ ]   **4.** Measuring head circumference

A 12-year-old child is diagnosed with renal tubular dysfunction. Blood chemistry results reveal a potassium level of 2.5 mEq/L.

59. Which finding by the nurse strongly indicates that a child is experiencing hypokalemia?
[ ]   **1.** Full, bounding pulses
[ ]   **2.** Muscle weakness
[ ]   **3.** Elevated blood pressure
[ ]   **4.** Hyperactive bowel sounds

The mother of a 4-year-old child notes that the child's clothes do not fit around the waist due to a lump in the abdomen. Following evaluation, the child is diagnosed with Wilms' tumor.

60. Which nursing action should be avoided when giving care to a child diagnosed with Wilms' tumor?
[ ] **1.** Palpating the child's abdomen
[ ] **2.** Giving the child a ball
[ ] **3.** Feeding the child
[ ] **4.** Combing the child's hair

Nursing Care of a Child with a Blood Disorder

A 2-year-old child is brought to the public health office for a routine checkup.

61. Which of the following findings during a routine wellness checkup best indicates that a child has iron deficiency anemia?
[ ] **1.** Weight gain and hypertension
[ ] **2.** Nervousness and diarrhea
[ ] **3.** Nausea and vomiting
[ ] **4.** Pallor and listlessness

The nurse is providing discharge instructions to the parents of a client recently diagnosed with hemophilia.

62. The nurse correctly advises the parents of a child who has hemophilia to avoid medications containing which ingredient?
[ ] **1.** Aspirin
[ ] **2.** Caffeine
[ ] **3.** Barbiturate
[ ] **4.** Antacid

Nursing Care of a Child with a Communicable Disease

A public health nurse is presenting information on communicable diseases at the local health fair. Following the presentation, as the individuals are picking up brochures with specific information of interest, many ask questions of the nurse.

63. Which statement by the mother of a school-age child with tinea capitis indicates that the nurse's teaching was effective?

[ ] **1.** "I'll comb my child's hair with a fine-tooth comb dipped in vinegar to remove the nits."
[ ] **2.** "I'll give the griseofulvin (Grisactin) with whole milk to increase absorption of the medication."
[ ] **3.** "I'll give the medication for the full 2 weeks to prevent spreading of the lesions."
[ ] **4.** "I'll apply the medication to my child's scalp three times a day until the lesions are gone."

One family asks if there is any literature on pinworms. They state that their nephew had them and they are wondering if their son does as well.

64. Which finding would the nurse most expect the parents to report if their child is suspected of having pinworms?
[ ] **1.** Teeth grinding
[ ] **2.** Abdominal pain
[ ] **3.** Anal itching
[ ] **4.** Bulky, greasy stools

A father expresses frustration because his daughter has frequent outbreaks of impetigo. The nurse assesses his knowledge of the disease process.

65. Which statement by the father indicates that he requires additional teaching?
[ ] **1.** "I can give oral antihistamines to decrease the inflammation and itching."
[ ] **2.** "Antibiotic treatment isn't necessary because the infection is self-limiting."
[ ] **3.** "I'll be sure to trim my child's nails to prevent scratching of the lesions."
[ ] **4.** "I'll take the necessary precautions to prevent my child from spreading the infection to others."

Nursing Care of a Child with a Nutritional Deficiency

Orphans from another country are brought to the United States for adoption. Following a complete physical examination, the children are found to be in generally good health but thin, and several of the children are diagnosed with rickets.

66. When developing a care plan for a child with rickets, the nurse appropriately includes providing nutritional sources of which vitamin?
[ ] **1.** Vitamin A
[ ] **2.** Vitamin B_{12}
[ ] **3.** Vitamin C
[ ] **4.** Vitamin D

The school nurse identifies a 7-year-old child who does not like to drink milk as possibly being deficient in calcium.

67. Which of the following foods provide an excellent source of calcium for this school-age child? Select all that apply.

[ ] **1.** A serving of broccoli
[ ] **2.** Blueberry yogurt
[ ] **3.** Chocolate ice cream
[ ] **4.** A serving of chicken
[ ] **5.** Cheese and crackers
[ ] **6.** A medium-sized apple

Nursing Care of a Child with a Musculoskeletal Disability

A pediatric nurse is providing guidance to parents whose child was recently diagnosed with cerebal palsy.

68. When discussing cerebral palsy with the parents of a newly diagnosed child, which information is correct?

[ ] **1.** Cerebral palsy is a nonprogressive disease caused by damage to the brain.
[ ] **2.** Brain surgery commonly helps or even cures children with cerebral palsy.
[ ] **3.** Physical therapy is of little value to a child with cerebral palsy.
[ ] **4.** Cerebral palsy is the result of injury to the sensory areas of the brain.

A 3-year-old boy is brought to the pediatrician's office for a follow up visit because the child has fallen behind in developmental milestones. The parents state, "His muscles don't seem to be as strong as they once were, and he has to rest after limited activity." Following a genetic testing, an electromyelogram, and muscle biopsy, the child has been diagnosed with Duchenne's muscular dystrophy.

69. If the parents of a child with Duchenne's muscular dystrophy are having a difficult time accepting the diagnosis, which nursing action is most beneficial to the family?

[ ] **1.** Recommend that the parents place the child in a long-term health care facility.
[ ] **2.** Recommend that the parents contact the local social welfare agency.
[ ] **3.** Recommend that the parents talk with other parents who have children with muscular dystrophy.
[ ] **4.** Recommend that the parents read as much literature as possible about treatment of muscular dystrophy.

Nursing Care of an Adolescent with Appendicitis

A 15-year-old boy is seen in the emergency department with an elevated temperature and complaint of generalized abdominal pain. The physician suspects appendicitis, and the boy is admitted for observation and possible appendectomy.

70. If the nurse documents all the following data, which finding should be reported immediately?

[ ] **1.** Refusal to eat
[ ] **2.** Complaint of nausea
[ ] **3.** Absent bowel sounds
[ ] **4.** Temperature of 101° F (38.3° C) orally

71. During preoperative preparation, which nursing action is most appropriate?

[ ] **1.** Give analgesics.
[ ] **2.** Give nothing by mouth (NPO).
[ ] **3.** Give an enema.
[ ] **4.** Apply heat to the abdomen.

Surgery is performed, and the appendix is removed intact. The boy is returned to the pediatric unit with an I.V. infusion in progress and an abdominal dressing in place. The physician has written orders to continue the I.V. infusion at a rate of 1,000 mL over 8 hours.

72. The nurse would be correct to set the infusion pump for which hourly rate?

[ ] **1.** 50 mL
[ ] **2.** 75 mL
[ ] **3.** 100 mL
[ ] **4.** 125 mL

73. Which nursing measure is most appropriate to prevent respiratory complications during the postoperative period?

[ ] **1.** Give a bronchodilator by inhalation.
[ ] **2.** Administer oxygen by nasal cannula.
[ ] **3.** Give the child a corticosteroid.
[ ] **4.** Have the child use an incentive spirometer.

The physician visits on the second postoperative day and writes an order to ambulate the boy t.i.d. The nurse enters the boy's room and begins to assist with ambulation. The boy begins to cry and states, "I'm scared."

74. Which statement by the nurse is most therapeutic in addressing the boy's behavior?

[ ] **1.** "There's nothing to be scared of. This won't hurt."
[ ] **2.** "The stitches are strong. They won't come out."
[ ] **3.** "I know you're scared, but you must be brave."
[ ] **4.** "Let's do this later, when you're better prepared."

The parents ask when the boy will be able to return to school.

75. The nurse advises the parents that, in most cases, children who have had an appendectomy usually return to school within what time frame?

[ ] **1.** 5 days
[ ] **2.** 2 weeks
[ ] **3.** 4 weeks
[ ] **4.** 6 weeks

Nursing Care of an Adolescent with Dysmenorrhea

A mother brings her 16-year-old daughter to the pediatric clinic because of recurrent complaints of pain and discomfort during the teenager's menstrual cycle. The physician diagnoses primary dysmenorrhea and recommends the use of acetylsalicylic acid (aspirin) or ibuprofen (Advil) for the pain and discomfort. The physician also asks the nurse to discuss other measures that can be taken to reduce the pain and discomfort.

76. Which suggestion by the nurse would be most helpful in relieving the teenager's menstrual pain and discomfort?

[ ] **1.** "Stay in bed until cramping is relieved, increase your fluid intake, and eat a low-fat diet."
[ ] **2.** "Drink plenty of cold liquids, add extra salt to your diet, and take a nap in the afternoon."
[ ] **3.** "Apply ice packs to the abdomen, eat a high-calorie diet, and have your largest meal at noon."
[ ] **4.** "Get at least 8 hours of sleep, eat a well-balanced diet, and apply heat to your abdomen."

77. Which information regarding the use of acetylsalicylic acid (aspirin) is best for the nurse to discuss with the client?

[ ] **1.** Aspirin should be discarded if not used within 2 years of first being opened.
[ ] **2.** Ringing in the ears is a common side effect of aspirin that will go away eventually.
[ ] **3.** If aspirin alone does not help, take one or two ibuprofen (Advil) along with the aspirin.
[ ] **4.** It is best to take aspirin with food to prevent gastrointestinal upset.

The adolescent tells the nurse, "One of my friends says she is scared because the physician told her she has amenorrhea. What does that word mean?"

78. What does the nurse correctly explain that amenorrhea means?

[ ] **1.** Absence of menstruation
[ ] **2.** Excessive vaginal bleeding
[ ] **3.** Discomfort before menstruation
[ ] **4.** The first menstrual period

The adolescent is also upset that she has outbreaks of acne vulgaris on her face, back, and shoulders prior to her menstrual cycle. The adolescent is started on systemic and topical medications to treat the acne.

79. Which statement by an adolescent with acne vulgaris indicates that additional teaching about taking tetracycline hydrochloride (Panmycin) is needed?

[ ] **1.** "I'll take the medication with a full glass of water."
[ ] **2.** "I won't take any antacids with this medication."
[ ] **3.** "I'll take this medication with food."
[ ] **4.** "I'll avoid sun exposure while taking this medication."

Nursing Care of an Adolescent Who Is Abusing Drugs

The parents of a 14-year-old adolescent call the pediatrician because they have discovered amphetamine capsules in the child's room and suspect that he is abusing the substance.

80. Which information about amphetamine use is most accurate and important for the parents to know?

[ ] **1.** Amphetamines are tried by most adolescents and cause no harm.
[ ] **2.** Amphetamines are known to lead to psychological dependence.
[ ] **3.** Amphetamines are a central nervous system depressant.
[ ] **4.** Amphetamines are harmful only if taken intravenously.

81. Which symptom reported by the parents is the best indicator of amphetamine abuse by the adolescent?

[ ] **1.** Watery eyes
[ ] **2.** Drowsiness
[ ] **3.** Excessive nasal drainage
[ ] **4.** Marked nervousness

The parents ask the nurse, "What's wrong with our child? Why has this happened?" The parents tell the nurse that the child associates with a gang that is known to get in trouble and abuse drugs.

82. The nurse correctly explains that, during adolescence, being with a peer group and trying out peer group values is part of the process of achieving which developmental task?
[ ] **1.** Identity
[ ] **2.** Intimacy
[ ] **3.** Integrity
[ ] **4.** Idealism

The parents ask the nurse whether they should force their child to enter a drug treatment program.

83. Which response by the nurse would be most helpful in this situation?
[ ] **1.** "You should attempt to discuss the dangers of drug abuse with your child before deciding that treatment is necessary."
[ ] **2.** "It will be necessary to get a court order before you can force your child to enter a drug treatment program."
[ ] **3.** "The success of the drug treatment program will depend on your child's desire to become drug-free."
[ ] **4.** "It's best that you force your child into the treatment program because he won't participate in the program otherwise."

While the boy is talking with the physician, the nurse reviews the child's immunization records and discovers that the last immunization received was when he was 6 years old.

84. The nurse advises the parents that the child is due to receive which of the following immunization boosters?
[ ] **1.** *Haemophilus influenzae* type b (Hib)
[ ] **2.** Polio (IPV)
[ ] **3.** Smallpox
[ ] **4.** Tetanus

Nursing Care of an Adolescent with a Sexually Transmitted Disease

A 16-year-old girl has learned that she has been exposed to gonorrhea. She visits the clinic for diagnosis and treatment.

85. When preparing the adolescent for the examination, the nurse correctly explains that she needs to collect which specimen to send to the laboratory?

[ ] **1.** Blood sample
[ ] **2.** Urine sample
[ ] **3.** Vaginal smear
[ ] **4.** Biopsy of the cervix

The physician confirms the diagnosis of gonorrhea and informs the client that she also has Chlamydia trachomatis *infection, another sexually transmitted disease. The physician orders an I.M. injection of ceftriaxone (Rocephin) to treat the gonorrhea and a prescription for oral doxycycline (Vibramycin) to treat the chlamydia.*

86. Which instruction is most appropriate to give to the client regarding doxycycline (Vibramycin)?
[ ] **1.** "The medication normally causes a dark orange discoloration of urine."
[ ] **2.** "Take the medication 1 hour before or 2 hours after a meal."
[ ] **3.** "Don't drink water for at least 30 minutes after taking the medication."
[ ] **4.** "Report any symptoms of gastrointestinal upset to the health care provider."

Before leaving the clinic, the client asks the nurse, "When can I be certain that I'm no longer infectious?"

87. The nurse correctly advises the client that she is still considered infectious until which time?
[ ] **1.** She no longer has foul-smelling vaginal discharge.
[ ] **2.** She no longer experiences discomfort during her menstrual periods.
[ ] **3.** She has a negative culture after being off antibiotics for at least 7 days.
[ ] **4.** She has received the prescribed doses of ceftriaxone (Rocephrin) for 1 day.

A 17-year-old adolescent is seen in the sexually transmitted diseases specialty clinic and is diagnosed with genital herpes (herpes simplex type 2).

88. Which term best describes the type of lesions manifested in genital herpes?
[ ] **1.** Macules
[ ] **2.** Vesicles
[ ] **3.** Papules
[ ] **4.** Fistulas

89. Which statement by the client indicates a need for additional teaching about genital herpes?

[ ] **1.** "Males who have genital herpes need a yearly prostate-specific antigen (PSA) test."

[ ] **2.** "Females who have genital herpes need a Papanicolaou (Pap) test every 6 months."

[ ] **3.** "Genital herpes is closely associated with the occurrence of sterility."

[ ] **4.** "Genital herpes is closely associated with Hodgkin's disease."

Oral and topical forms of acyclovir (Zovirax) are prescribed for the client.

90. Which medication instruction provided by the nurse is most accurate?

[ ] **1.** "Taking your acyclovir as prescribed will prevent the recurrence of lesions."

[ ] **2.** "Your sex partners also need to be treated for 10 days with oral acyclovir."

[ ] **3.** "Use a glove to apply topical acyclovir."

[ ] **4.** "Take the oral acyclovir even when the disease is in remission."

The nurse discusses the sexual transmission of herpes with the client.

91. Which statement by the client indicates that teaching has been effective?

[ ] **1.** "Males must use a condom when lesions are present to prevent transmission."

[ ] **2.** "Douching after intercourse prevents females from becoming infected."

[ ] **3.** "Applying acyclovir to lesions before intercourse prevents transmission."

[ ] **4.** "One way to prevent spreading the disease is to avoid sexual contact, especially when lesions or symptoms are present."

The client asks the nurse, "What are the symptoms of AIDS?"

92. The nurse informs the client that acquired immunodeficiency syndrome (AIDS) is commonly associated with which symptoms?

[ ] **1.** Increased appetite and night sweats

[ ] **2.** Tachycardia, dyspnea, and constipation

[ ] **3.** Fatigue, fever, and persistent yeast infections

[ ] **4.** Weight gain, peripheral edema, and jaundice

The client also asks the nurse if human immunodeficiency virus (HIV) infection can be contracted from a sex partner who has no symptoms of AIDS.

93. Which response by the nurse provides the best clarification about the disease process?

[ ] **1.** "If you're afraid of getting HIV, you'll be safer if you avoid having sex with past sex partners."

[ ] **2.** "An HIV-positive individual may not develop symptoms of AIDS for years."

[ ] **3.** "HIV can only be transmitted when symptoms of AIDS are present."

[ ] **4.** "The medication prescribed for AIDS also protects against HIV infection."

The client is diagnosed with AIDS and is experiencing oral complications.

94. Which diet is most appropriate for an adolescent with thrush and herpes simplex infections of the oral cavity secondary to AIDS?

[ ] **1.** High-calorie, bland diet

[ ] **2.** Soft, low-protein diet

[ ] **3.** Low-residue, low-fat diet

[ ] **4.** High-residue, low-cholesterol diet

After being diagnosed with a sexually transmitted disease, a 16-year-old boy asks the nurse about safe sex practices.

95. If the client asks the nurse for instructions on safe condom use, which information needs to be stressed?

[ ] **1.** Condoms should be stored in a warm, dry place to prevent damage.

[ ] **2.** Condoms are generally lubricated with mineral oil or petroleum jelly.

[ ] **3.** A condom should be applied before the penis becomes erect.

[ ] **4.** During application, a ½-inch space should be left at the end of the condom.

The client also tells the nurse that he is concerned about developing testicular cancer because he recently lost his father to it.

96. When teaching an adolescent male client about testicular self-examination, which instruction should the nurse include?

[ ] **1.** "Do the examination after a warm bath or shower."

[ ] **2.** "Report any difference in the size of your testicles to the physician."

[ ] **3.** "Malignant lumps are usually located on the front side of the testicles."

[ ] **4.** "Both testicles should be examined simultaneously to detect differences."

Nursing Care of an Adolescent with Scoliosis

A 14-year-old girl is referred for further evaluation after the school nurse discovers lateral spinal curvature during routine scoliosis screening.

97. Which of the following statements made by the adolescent best supports the nurse's suspicion that she has scoliosis?
[ ] 1. "My friends are getting taller faster than I am."
[ ] 2. "One of my sleeves is always shorter than the other."
[ ] 3. "I have a difficult time sleeping on my side at night."
[ ] 4. "I always roll crooked when I am doing a somersault."

98. Which question is most important for the nurse to ask the adolescent in preparation for her X-rays?
[ ] 1. "Is there any possibility that you're pregnant?"
[ ] 2. "Have you eaten anything in the past 24 hours?"
[ ] 3. "Have you taken any medications in the past 24 hours?"
[ ] 4. "Are you allergic to iodine or shellfish?"

A diagnosis of structural scoliosis is confirmed, and the physician determines that the adolescent has a 35-degree curvature. The parents ask the nurse if treatment is really necessary.

99. Which explanation by the nurse is most accurate?
[ ] 1. "Curvatures of this degree may improve without treatment."
[ ] 2. "Without treatment, your daughter may develop problems with bladder control."
[ ] 3. "Without treatment, your daughter may develop problems with bowel control."
[ ] 4. "Without treatment, your daughter may develop breathing problems."

The child is to be fitted for a Milwaukee brace. The adolescent asks if the brace has to be worn when she is at school.

100. The nurse correctly advises the adolescent that the brace has to be worn during which time period?
[ ] 1. At all times, except when bathing
[ ] 2. At least 8 hours each day
[ ] 3. At night while sleeping
[ ] 4. At all times, without exception

101. Which nursing action would best promote the adolescent's compliance with the treatment plan?

[ ] 1. Advising the parents to keep a constant watch on their daughter to make sure she wears her brace
[ ] 2. Suggesting that the parents help their daughter find stylish clothing that will hide the brace
[ ] 3. Telling the parents that it might be best to arrange for a homebound teacher during treatment
[ ] 4. Telling the adolescent that the problem will only get worse if she does not wear her brace

Dosage Calculations for Children and Adolescents

102. The physician orders cefaclor (Ceclor) 125 mg P.O. If the Ceclor suspension is available in 250 mg/5 mL, how many milliliters should the nurse give the pediatric client?

_____

103. The nurse is caring for a 52-lb child with an elevated temperature. If the recommended dosage of acetaminophen (Tylenol) for children is 10 to 15 mg/kg P.O. every 4 to 6 hours, what is the highest single dose of acetaminophen that would be safe for this child?

_____

Correct Answers and Rationales

Nursing Care of a Child with Rheumatic Fever

1. 2. The exact cause of rheumatic fever is not clearly understood. However, evidence suggests that rheumatic fever may be associated with a recent bacterial infection caused by group A beta-hemolytic streptococci. These microorganisms cause some, but not all, sore throats; therefore, of the symptoms reported, a sore throat is most closely correlated with rheumatic fever and should be brought to the physician's attention. Measles is caused by a viral infection, not streptococci. A bump on the head and a disinterest in schoolwork probably are not related to rheumatic fever but should be recorded in the health history.
> *Client Needs Category—Physiological integrity*
> *Client Needs Subcategory—Reduction of risk potential*

2. 4. Migrating joint pain is a major manifestation of rheumatic fever. The ASO titer and the pulse rate are usually elevated with this disease. The child may also have erythema marginatum, which is a distinctive rash found on the trunk and extremities.
> *Client Needs Category—Physiological integrity*
> *Client Needs Subcategory—Physiological adaptation*

3. 3. Reading an adventure story would be the most appropriate activity for the child during the acute phase of the illness. The child will need both physical and emotional rest; therefore, quiet, age-appropriate activities are recommended to prevent overexertion as well as boredom and emotional upset that may occur if the child is not permitted any activity. Preschoolers usually enjoy playing with action figures; also, this activity may cause excitement, which will increase energy consumption. Video games may also cause too much excitement. Toy mallets and wooden pegs are more appropriate for a toddler.
> *Client Needs Category—Health promotion and maintenance*
> *Client Needs Subcategory—None*

4. 2. There is a slight cross-sensitivity between medications in the penicillin group and those in the cephalosporin group. Therefore, the nurse should exercise caution and notify the charge nurse or physician before giving the medication. There is no cross-sensitivity between penicillin and the other medication categories listed.
> *Client Needs Category—Physiological integrity*
> *Client Needs Subcategory—Pharmacological therapies*

5. 3. Despite the risk of Reye's syndrome, acetylsalicylic acid (aspirin) is given instead of acetaminophen because it not only controls fever but also relieves joint inflammation, which is a major manifestation of rheumatic fever. Aspirin is not necessarily more effective in reducing fever than acetaminophen, and it does not prevent infection or cardiac enlargement.
> *Client Needs Category—Physiological integrity*
> *Client Needs Subcategory—Pharmacological therapies*

6. 4. A child who has had rheumatic fever may develop the disease again. Although streptococci do not cause all sore throats, the child would be at risk for a recurrence of the disease if he develops a sore throat. Therefore, any sign of a sore throat should be reported promptly to facilitate immediate diagnosis and treatment. Antibiotics should be taken for the prescribed course unless otherwise indicated by the physician. Sunlight has no effect on rheumatic heart disease. Seizure medication is not prescribed for this disease.
> *Client Needs Category—Health promotion and maintenance*
> *Client Needs Subcategory—None*

7. 1. The use of a bedside commode is an appropriate alternative to reduce the heart's workload. Shortness of breath indicates that the heart is unable to adapt to the demands required during ambulation. Giving oxygen after elimination or having the child continue to ambulate, even with the assistance of the nurse or a walker, is not likely to prevent or reduce the heart's effort in response to activity.
> *Client Needs Category—Physiological integrity*
> *Client Needs Subcategory—Physiological adaptation*

Nursing Care of a Child with Diabetes Mellitus

8. 2. Fruity-smelling breath is a manifestation of diabetic ketoacidosis. Excessive perspiration and pallor are signs of hypoglycemia. A blood glucose reading of 120 mg/dL is within the normal range.
> *Client Needs Category—Physiological integrity*
> *Client Needs Subcategory—Physiological adaptation*

9. 3. A client experiencing diabetic ketoacidosis will have glucose and ketones in the urine. Blood, white blood cells, and bilirubin are not usually present in ketoacidosis.
> *Client Needs Category—Physiological integrity*
> *Client Needs Subcategory—Physiological adaptation*

10. **1.** Regular insulin (Humulin R) is the only type of insulin given intravenously. Regular insulin can also be given subcutaneously along with insulin zinc suspension (Humulin L), insulin zinc suspension, extended (Humulin U), and isophane insulin suspension (Humulin N).

> *Client Needs Category—Physiological integrity*
> *Client Needs Subcategory—Pharmacological therapies*

11. **1.** Regular insulin (Humulin R) is given 30 minutes before a meal because the onset of action is 30 minutes to 1 hour. Giving the insulin within a shorter period might result in inadequate coverage because the insulin will not have had a chance to take effect. Giving the insulin after eating will not provide coverage for the food already consumed.

> *Client Needs Category—Physiological integrity*
> *Client Needs Subcateogry—Pharmacological therapies*

12. **4.** Shakiness is a common sign of hypoglycemia. Other symptoms of hypoglycemia include sweating, tremors, weakness, and hunger. The remaining options are signs and symptoms of hyperglycemia.

> *Client Needs Category—Physiological integrity*
> *Client Needs Subcategory—Pharmacological therapies*

13. **1.** Hypoglycemia must be corrected immediately. If the child is awake and able to swallow, the nurse should offer a concentrated source of sugar such as orange juice. I.V. administration of glucose is reserved for those who have a change in level of consciousness and are unable to swallow. Insulin would not be given because the child already has too much insulin. The physician should be notified after the problem is corrected or if the child's condition worsens.

> *Client Needs Category—Physiological integrity*
> *Client Needs Subcategory—Physiological adaptation*

14. **2.** Persons with type 1 diabetes mellitus require insulin to control the disease. The hormone insulin cannot be given by mouth because digestive enzymes would destroy the insulin before it reaches the site of action. Also, the child is not a candidate for oral hypoglycemic agents because the pancreas has to be capable of producing some insulin for the child to benefit from the oral hypoglycemics; this is not the case with a child with type 1 diabetes mellitus.

> *Client Needs Category—Physiological integrity*
> *Client Needs Subcategory—Pharmacological therapies*

15. **4.** If insulin sites are not rotated following a planned rotation schedule, atrophy (lipodystrophy) of subcutaneous fat may occur. Lipodystrophy can interfere with insulin absorption if insulin is given in areas affected by this problem. Rotating the injection sites does not slow the absorption of, prevent accumulation of, or decrease the duration of insulin.

> *Client Needs Category—Health promotion and maintenance*
> *Client Needs Subcategory—None*

16. **2.** Activity requires glucose for energy. Therefore, increasing activity uses up glucose and, consequently, the body requires less-than-usual amounts of insulin. Eating too much, having an infection, and experiencing emotional stress are situations in which a diabetic tends to require more, not less, insulin.

> *Client Needs Category—Health promotion and maintenance*
> *Client Needs Subcategory—None*

17. **3.** The diabetic child can participate in normal activities. However, certain precautions are necessary to promote safety. For example, the parents should ensure that the child goes swimming with an adult or responsible person who knows that the child is diabetic. The child can participate in activities requiring increased energy expenditure, such as basketball and soccer, as long as the activity is taken into consideration when planning the child's meals and insulin requirements. Generally, the child should consume a snack before engaging in the activity or have a simple form of glucose on hand in case a hypoglycemic reaction should occur.

> *Client Needs Category—Health promotion and maintenance*
> *Client Needs Subcategory—None*

18. **2.** It is important for the newly diagnosed diabetic athlete to check his blood glucose level before participating in exercises or athletics. If the blood glucose level is high, additional glucagon, growth hormone, and catecholamines may be released. This causes the liver to release more glucose, resulting in a higher blood glucose level. If the child's blood glucose level is within the normal range or lower, exercise may help to lower it. Some individuals are instructed to eat a carbohydrate snack before engaging in exercise to prevent unexpected hypoglycemia.

> *Client Needs Category—Physiological integrity*
> *Client Needs Subcategory—Physiological adaptation*

19. The child's blood glucose level is 269 mg/dL, thus falling within the 6-unit range (251 to 300 mg/dL) specified by the physician. Therefore, the nurse would administer 6 units of Humulin R insulin.
   Client Needs Category—*Physiological integrity*
   Client Needs Subcategory—*Pharmacological therapies*

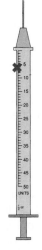

20. **4.** The child will need to continue to monitor blood glucose levels because the insulin pump only delivers the insulin; it does not monitor the blood glucose level. The other options indicate the child correctly understands how to use an insulin pump.
   Client Needs Category—*Health promotion and maintenance*
   Client Needs Subcategory—*None*

Nursing Care of a Child with Partial- and Full-Thickness Burns

21. **4.** A burn is classified according to the depth of tissue destruction. Burns may be superficial partial-thickness injuries, deep partial-thickness injuries, or full-thickness injuries. A full-thickness burn involves total destruction of the epidermis and usually the dermis and underlying tissues. The wound color ranges widely from white to red, brown, or black and may contain blister formation. The burned area is painless because nerve fibers are destroyed. Edema may be present.
   Client Needs Category—*Physiological integrity*
   Client Needs Subcategory—*Physiological adaptation*

22. **2.** It is important for the nurse to remain alert for the possibility of respiratory distress from a blocked airway following burns to the head, face, neck, and chest. Therefore, it is imperative to keep an endotracheal tube and oxygen supply on hand in the burned client's room. An oral airway should also be readily available. The other devices and equipment mentioned in the remaining options are not appropriate for treating an emergency arising from respiratory distress.
   Client Needs Category—*Physiological integrity*
   Client Needs Subcategory—*Physiological adaptation*

23. **1, 2, 5, 6.** The emergent phase marks the first 24 to 48 hours following a burn injury. During this time, the primary emphasis is on the treatment of burn shock, specifically restoring the child's fluid and electrolyte balance. Careful tracking of vital signs, urine output, and I.V. infusion is essential. Large-bore I.V. catheters are used whenever possible because of the potential need for rapid infusions or blood products. The child would receive nothing by mouth during the emergent phase because of the risk of a paralytic ileus.
   Client Needs Category—*Physiological integrity*
   Client Needs Subcategory—*Physiological adaptation*

24. **3.** A burn victim is placed on I.V. fluid therapy during the first 24 hours to restore fluid and electrolyte balance and to maintain perfusion of vital organs. During I.V. fluid therapy, the child is at risk for fluid overload; therefore, the nurse must closely monitor the I.V. infusion. Monitoring skin integrity and bowel elimination is a regular, ongoing assessment consideration. Checking pupillary response to light is part of a neurologic assessment; this would typically be done only if the child's neurologic status was compromised.
   Client Needs Category—*Physiological integrity*
   Client Needs Subcategory—*Physiological adaptation*

25. **4.** A urine output of 1 to 2 mL/kg/hour is considered within the normal range. Excessive output requires reducing the rate of the I.V. infusion.
   Client Needs Category—*Physiological integrity*
   Client Needs Subcategory—*Physiological adaptation*

26. **3.** Because severe burns produce considerable pain, an opioid analgesic is commonly used as part of treatment. If the child no longer complains of pain or rates the pain as 0 to 2 on a pain scale (in which 0 represents no pain and 10, the worst pain imaginable), the pain medication is considered effective. Opioid analgesics do not prevent nausea or maintain the respiratory rate within the normal range. Rather, nausea, respiratory depression, and urine retention are adverse effects of these drugs.
   Client Needs Category—*Physiological integrity*
   Client Needs Subcategory—*Physiological adaptation*

27. **4.** A footboard is an effective device that the nurse can use to help prevent footdrop by keeping the child's feet from dangling forward or to the side. Braces cannot be used without a physician's order. Keeping the child in a side-lying position will not prevent footdrop; this problem can only be prevented when the feet are supported in a normal position. The top sheet should fit loosely over the feet to assist with preventing footdrop.
   Client Needs Category—*Physiological integrity*
   Client Needs Subcategory—*Reduction of risk potential*

28. 2. Stress ulcers, also called *Curling's ulcers,* commonly occur in the stomach or duodenum as a complication of burns. If the ulcer bleeds, the client will have blood in the stool, which is detected by a positive hemoccult test and black, tarry stools. The other findings are not usual manifestations of Curling's ulcers.

Client Needs Category—Physiological integrity
Client Needs Subcategory—Physiological adaptation

29. 1. The child requires a diet rich in protein to help rebuild body tissues destroyed by the burns. A milk shake is a good source of protein. Apples, candy, and gelatin contain little or no protein.

Client Needs Category—Physiological integrity
Client Needs Subcategory—Physiological adaptation

30. 3. Of the diversional activities described in this item, an 8-year-old is likely to enjoy playing with a coin collection. Television may also provide diversion. Playing a solitary game of cards, reading the newspaper, or coloring a simple design probably would not appeal to a child of this age.

Client Needs Category—Health promotion and maintenance
Client Needs Subcategory—None

Nursing Care of a Child with Juvenile Rheumatoid Arthritis

31. 1. The primary reason for using ibuprofen (Motrin) in the treatment of juvenile rheumatoid arthritis is the drug's ability to reduce inflammation. Although ibuprofen (Motrin) also lowers the body temperature, this is not the foremost reason for using this drug. Muscle spasms are not prevented by the administration of ibuprofen (Motrin). Ibuprofen (Motrin) does not increase the prothrombin time; however, this is not part of the treatment for rheumatoid arthritis.

Client Needs Category—Physiological integrity
Client Needs Subcategory—Pharmacological therapies

32. 2. Side effects of aspirin are the same as symptoms of aspirin toxicity, which include tinnitus (ringing in the ears), nausea, vomiting, difficulty hearing, lassitude, dizziness, diarrhea, and mental confusion. The signs and symptoms identified in the other options are not usual manifestations of aspirin toxicity.

Client Needs Category—Physiological integrity
Client Needs Subcategory—Pharmacological therapies

33. 4. Of the four activities listed, swimming would most likely be the safest form of exercise for a child with rheumatoid arthritis because it causes the least trauma to the affected joints.

Client Needs Category—Health promotion and maintenance
Client Needs Subcategory—None

34. 3. This child needs to avoid gaining excessive weight because extra weight places additional stress on the joints. Serving well-balanced meals is an effective way to ensure that the child receives enough of the right nutrients to promote growth while keeping the weight in check. After the acute phase, the child should be encouraged to lead as normal a life as possible, which includes going to school and participating in age-appropriate activities. Heat, not cold, should be applied to joints to treat inflammation.

Client Needs Category—Health promotion and maintenance
Client Needs Subcategory—None

35. 4. Uveitis, an inflammatory disorder of the eye, is a complication of juvenile rheumatoid arthritis that can occur without any noticeable symptoms. Therefore, children with juvenile rheumatoid arthritis should have regular eye examinations. Chest X-rays, dental checkups, and routine hearing examinations are not recommended any more frequently than for a child without juvenile rheumatoid arthritis.

Client Needs Category—Health promotion and maintenance
Client Needs Subcategory—None

Nursing Care of a Child with an Injury

36. 2. An ice bag can be used safely as long as it is removed every 30 minutes to 1 hour to check the skin and allow the area to return to normal. Continuous application of cold results in vasoconstriction, which, if allowed to continue, could result in a loss of blood supply to the affected part and possible gangrene.

Client Needs Category—Physiological integrity
Client Needs Subcategory—Reduction of risk potential

37. 2. A child experiencing a nosebleed should be placed in a sitting position with the head tilted forward while the nostrils are gently compressed between the thumb and forefinger. Tilting the head backward may lead to nausea, vomiting, and aspiration. Applying ice may or may not help stop the bleeding. If bleeding does not stop, the nose should be packed with a small piece of gauze that is preferably impregnated with petroleum jelly or a solution such as aqueous epinephrine (1:1000).

Client Needs Category—Physiological integrity
Client Needs Subcategory—Physiological adaptation

38. 2. Temporarily holding the root of a tooth under the tongue or placing the tooth in milk preserves the tooth. Water, alcohol, and exposure to air can damage the root and reduce the potential success of implantation.

> ***Client Needs Category***—*Physiological integrity*
> ***Client Needs Subcategory***—*Physiological adaptation*

39. 4. A score of 4 indicates that the child is experiencing a lot of pain; therefore, the child should be medicated with the prescribed analgesic. Diversional activities can be used with analgesics to increase their effectiveness, or alone when the child has mild pain. Documenting the child's pain and rechecking later do not relieve or change the pain that the child is currently experiencing.

> ***Client Needs Category***—*Physiological integrity*
> ***Client Needs Subcategory***—*Physiological adaptation*

Nursing Care of a Child with a Head Injury

40. 3. The classic signs of increased intracranial pressure are a change in the level of consciousness, a rise in blood pressure, an increase in body temperature, a decrease in the pulse rate, and a widening pulse pressure. Brisk pupillary response to light, tympanic temperature of 97.9° F, and +2 deep tendon reflexes are indicative of normal central nervous system function.

> ***Client Needs Category***—*Physiological integrity*
> ***Client Needs Subcategory***—*Physiological adaptation*

41. 1. Cerebrospinal fluid is commonly seen leaking from the nose of the child who has sustained a basilar skull fracture. The presence of this finding should be reported immediately because this is the most serious type of skull fracture. A child who has had a head injury may have lost consciousness and may not remember the time of day. A Glasgow Coma Scale score of 15 and an apical pulse of 80 beats/minute are within the normal ranges.

> ***Client Needs Category***—*Physiological integrity*
> ***Client Needs Subcategory***—*Physiological adaptation*

42. 2. When riding a bicycle, the child should travel in the same direction as the flow of traffic. The other options are correct safety measures that should be followed when riding a bicycle.

> ***Client Needs Category***—*Health promotion and maintenance*
> ***Client Needs Subcategory***—*None*

43. 4. The person sustaining a head injury should be observed for signs of intracranial bleeding, which can occur even after a mild or slight head injury. Because signs of bleeding are most likely to occur in the first 24 hours, the parents are instructed to awaken the child every 4 hours during the first night to check for altered level of consciousness or other neurologic changes. Examples of changes requiring prompt notification of the health care provider include slurred speech, headache, visual problems, or difficulty arousing the child from sleep.

> ***Client Needs Category***—*Health promotion and maintenance*
> ***Client Needs Subcategory***—*None*

Nursing Care of a Child with a Brain Tumor

44. 1. The signs and symptoms of a brain tumor usually occur as a result of increased intracranial pressure. Vomiting, especially early in the morning, is one sign seen in the child with a brain tumor. Nausea is not a common symptom. The child may not want to go to school and that should be documented, but this is not considered a risk factor for the presence of a brain tumor. Tilting the head to one side while sleeping does not correspond with a diagnosis of a brain tumor.

> ***Client Needs Category***—*Physiological integrity*
> ***Client Needs Subcategory***—*Physiological adaptation*

45. 1. The child will be placed in a tunnel-like scanner with a special call button. Sedation is used only if the client is restless or claustrophobic. Electrodes are not placed on the child's head, and headaches do not usually occur during this procedure.

> ***Client Needs Category***—*Physiological integrity*
> ***Client Needs Subcategory***—*Physiological adaptation*

46. 3. The head dressing of a child who has undergone a craniotomy may become damp from cerebrospinal fluid drainage. The nurse should reinforce the dressing until the physician can change it. The child will require further intervention to prevent the possibility of an infection at the operative site; however, complications may occur if the dressing is changed or removed.

> ***Client Needs Category***—*Physiological integrity*
> ***Client Needs Subcategory***—*Reduction of risk potential*

47. 3. The nurse should encourage the parents to express their feelings without concern about being judged by the nurse. The parents need to know that the feelings they are experiencing are normal. Besides listening, the nurse can suggest ways in which the parents can cope with their feelings. Suggesting that the parents identify things they can do to make the child feel good will assist them in coping with their feelings of helplessness.

> **Client Needs Category**—*Psychosocial integrity*
> **Client Needs Subcategory**—*None*

48. 2. Most chemotherapeutic agents cause some degree of nausea and vomiting. To lessen or prevent this side effect, the nurse should give a prescribed antiemetic prior to administering the chemotherapeutic agent. The child should always consume well-balanced meals. Serving the child a meal prior to chemotherapy may cause increased nausea and vomiting. The child should get plenty of rest whether receiving chemotherapy or not. Administration of an enema is not usually indicated prior to beginning chemotherapy.

> **Client Needs Category**—*Physiological integrity*
> **Client Needs Subcategory**—*Reduction of risk potential*

49. 71. To find the answer, use this formula as a guide:

> 100 mL/kg/day for the first 10 kg of body weight
>
> 50 mL/kg/day for the next 10 kg of body weight
>
> 20 mL/kg/day for each kilogram above 20 kg of body weight

Calculate:

> 100 mL/kg/day × 10 kg = 1,000 mL/day (for the first 10 kg)
>
> 50 mL/kg/day × 10 kg = 500 mL/day (for the next 10 kg)
>
> 20 mL/kg/day × 10 kg = 200 mL/day (for the remaining 10 kg)

Total the amounts:

> 1,000 mL/day + 500 mL/day + 200 mL/day = 1,700 mL/day

To find the hourly rate, divide by 24:

> 1,700 ÷ 24 = 70.9 or 71

> **Client Needs Category**—*Physiological integrity*
> **Client Needs Subcategory**—*Pharmacological therapies*

50. 3. The nurse should encourage early and consistent visits from the child's friends to promote support and acceptance of his condition and enable him to deal with the reactions of friends. Although any changes in appearance resulting from treatment are usually temporary, such changes can be very distressing to a child and the nurse should not minimize the child's feelings. None of the remaining options adequately addresses the child's concerns.

> **Client Needs Category**—*Psychosocial integrity*
> **Client Needs Subcategory**—*None*

51. 4. The side-lying position with knees drawn up is the position of choice when a lumbar puncture is performed. This position widens the space between the vertebrae, thereby aiding with insertion of the needle. The supine and Trendelenburg's positions are not suitable for this procedure because they do not allow exposure of the lumbar region. The prone position does not facilitate widening of intervertebral spaces; thus, it also is not used.

> **Client Needs Category**—*Physiological integrity*
> **Client Needs Subcategory**—*Physiological adaptation*

Nursing Care of a Child in Traction

52. 2. Because of the added risk of infection with skeletal traction, the pin site should be monitored for signs of infection and cleaned as prescribed by the physician. The child should be placed in the supine position. Range-of-motion exercises cannot be performed on the right leg because of the traction, and the weights should not be released.

> **Client Needs Category**—*Physiological integrity*
> **Client Needs Subcategory**—*Reduction of risk potential*

53. 2. Pressure areas and skin breakdown are most likely to develop first over bony prominences, such as the heels, elbows, sacrum, ankles, and scapulae.

> **Client Needs Category**—*Physiological integrity*
> **Client Needs Subcategory**—*Reduction of risk potential*

54. 4. A traction rope that has slipped out of a pulley should be replaced in the pulley groove. The physician or the registered nurse skilled in orthopedic care should perform this. The other findings are appropriate for the child in traction.

> **Client Needs Category**—*Physiological integrity*
> **Client Needs Subcategory**—*Physiological adaptation*

55. 1. A high fluid intake and a diet high in fiber are recommended to prevent constipation and other complications of immobilization such as kidney stones. The right leg, which is in traction, is kept immobile. Turning the client is not routinely performed.

> **Client Needs Category**—*Physiological integrity*
> **Client Needs Subcategory**—*Physiological adaptation*

56. **3.** The child should be able to move the toes freely; an inability to do so may indicate an alteration in neurovascular status. If the toes on both feet are cool, it is probably due to the environmental temperature rather than neurovascular impairment. The other parameters indicate intact neurovascular function.

> **Client Needs Category**—*Physiological integrity*
> **Client Needs Subcategory**—*Physiological adaptation*

Nursing Care of a Child with a Kidney Disorder

57. **1.** Periorbital edema that is worse in the morning, decreased urination, anorexia, and hypertension are all signs of acute glomeruli nephritis.

> **Client Needs Category**—*Physiological integrity*
> **Client Needs Subcategory**—*Physiological adaptation*

58. **2.** Nephrotic syndrome results in a large amount of protein excreted in the urine, which in turn results in hypoalbuminemia and edema. The child with nephrotic syndrome should be weighed daily to monitor the amount of edema present. The abdominal circumference, not head circumference, is also measured. The child is able to maintain range of motion and perform activities of daily living on his own. A high-protein, low-sodium diet is commonly required as part of the treatment plan.

> **Client Needs Category**—*Physiological integrity*
> **Client Needs Subcategory**—*Physiological adaptation*

59. **2.** Weak pulse, hypotension, muscular weakness, diminished reflexes, loss of peristalsis, and cardiac arrest are signs and symptoms of hypokalemia.

> **Client Needs Category**—*Physiological integrity*
> **Client Needs Subcategory**—*Physiological adaptation*

60. **1.** A Wilms' tumor is a congenital, cancerous tumor of the kidney. Feeling, touching, or handling the client's abdomen may result in rupture of the renal capsule and the spread of cancerous tumor cells. Feeding the client, combing the client's hair, or giving the client a ball will not exert pressure on the renal capsule.

> **Client Needs Category**—*Physiological integrity*
> **Client Needs Subcategory**—*Reduction of risk potential*

Nursing Care of a Child with a Blood Disorder

61. **4.** Pallor, listlessness, and irritability are observable signs of iron deficiency anemia. The child's history may also reveal anorexia, weight loss, and a decrease in normal activity. The signs and symptoms mentioned in the remaining options are unrelated to iron deficiency anemia.

> **Client Needs Category**—*Health promotion and maintenance*
> **Client Needs Subcategory**—*None*

62. **1.** Salicylates prolong bleeding time by interfering with the blood's ability to clot. Acetylsalicylic acid (aspirin), a salicylate, is contraindicated for anyone with a bleeding disorder because it is usually extremely difficult to stop the bleeding. A child who receives aspirin could bleed to death from even a relatively small lesion. Although caffeine, barbiturates, and antacids are not contraindicated for those with hemophilia, they are not routinely given.

> **Client Needs Category**—*Health promotion and maintenance*
> **Client Needs Subcategory**—*None*

Nursing Care of a Child with a Communicable Disease

63. **2.** The preferred treatment for tinea capitis is oral griseofulvin (Grisactin) for a minimum of 6 weeks. It is recommended that the medication be taken with milk or ice cream to increase its absorption. Nits are found in pediculosis capitis, not tinea capitis. Topical medications alone are ineffective in the treatment of tinea capitis.

> **Client Needs Category**—*Health promotion and maintenance*
> **Client Needs Subcategory**—*None*

64. **3.** The most common manifestation of pinworms is anal itching. Teeth grinding, abdominal pain, and bulky, greasy stools are not usual findings.

> **Client Needs Category**—*Physiological integrity*
> **Client Needs Subcategory**—*Physiological adaptation*

65. **2.** Impetigo is a contagious disorder caused by a streptococcal or staphylococcal skin infection. Both systemic and topical antibiotics are usually prescribed. The lesions are itchy, and oral antihistamines are sometimes ordered to decrease the inflammation and itching.

> **Client Needs Category**—*Psychosocial integrity*
> **Client Needs Subcategory**—*Physiological adaptation*

Nursing Care of a Child with a Nutritional Deficiency

66. 4. Rickets is caused by a lack of sufficient vitamin D in the diet. The vitamin is essential for proper calcium and phosphorus use in the normal development of bone and teeth. Signs of rickets include delayed closure of the fontanels, delayed tooth growth, dental caries, and deformities of the long bones.
> **Client Needs Category**—*Physiological integrity*
> **Client Needs Subcategory**—*Physiological adaptation*

67. 2, 3, 5. The best dietary sources of calcium are dairy products (including milk, yogurt, and cheese products), soybeans, fortified orange juice, dark green leafy vegetables, sardines, clams, and oysters. Chicken is a good source of protein, and apples have vitamins and antioxidant properties. Broccoli is not a dark green leafy vegetable, and it only has 62 mg of calcium per 1 cup serving.
> **Client Needs Category**—*Health promotion and maintenance*
> **Client Needs Subcategory**—*None*

Nursing Care of a Child with a Musculoskeletal Disability

68. 1. Cerebral palsy is a nonprogressive neuromuscular disorder caused by an injury to the motor-coordinating areas of the brain. Brain surgery cannot help or cure those with this disorder. Physical therapy and other disciplines, such as occupational, speech, and recreational therapy, are often of great benefit to those with cerebral palsy.
> **Client Needs Category**—*Physiological integrity*
> **Client Needs Subcategory**—*Physiological adaptation*

69. 3. Parents with children who have the same disability are often able to provide emotional support. When these parents meet, they share a common bond and a common burden, and they learn from one another about how to overcome obstacles. Recommending that the child be placed in a long-term care facility, referring the parents to a social welfare agency, or giving them literature to read probably will not help them cope with their problems as effectively as would talking with someone with a similar experience.
> **Client Needs Category**—*Psychosocial integrity*
> **Client Needs Subcategory**—*None*

Nursing Care of an Adolescent with Appendicitis

70. 3. Absent bowel sounds may be a sign of inflammation and possible obstruction and should be reported immediately. The other findings do not pose as great a threat to the adolescent's health at this time.
> **Client Needs Category**—*Physiological integrity*
> **Client Needs Subcategory**—*Physiological adaptation*

71. 2. Before surgery, the teenager should be kept NPO to reduce the risk of aspiration during surgery. Analgesics can mask clinical signs and symptoms needed for a diagnosis; therefore, they should not be given before surgery. Enemas and laxatives should be avoided because they increase peristalsis, which may rupture the appendix. Applying heat to the abdomen is contraindicated because it also may rupture the appendix.
> **Client Needs Category**—*Physiological integrity*
> **Client Needs Subcategory**—*Physiological adaptation*

72. 4. If a total of 1,000 mL is to be given over 8 hours, the nurse needs to divide the amount to be given (1,000 mL) by the total number of hours (8).

$$1{,}000 \text{ mL} \div 8 \text{ hours} = 125 \text{ mL/hour.}$$

> **Client Needs Category**—*Safe, effective care environment*
> **Client Needs Subcategory**—*Safety and infection control*

73. 4. Incentive spirometry and deep breathing help to prevent respiratory complications that may be experienced by persons having abdominal surgery. Bronchodilators, oxygen, and corticosteroids are used to treat respiratory complications; they are not preventative measures.
> **Client Needs Category**—*Physiological integrity*
> **Client Needs Subcategory**—*Reduction of risk potential*

74. 2. Many clients, children and adults alike, are afraid their sutures will pull out if they walk or move too much. The nurse should reassure such clients that the sutures are designed to endure movement and walking. Telling the teenager that walking will not cause discomfort is not true. Although acknowledging the boy's fear is appropriate, the nurse should attempt to respond in a way that helps to resolve the fear. Putting off ambulation is not therapeutic and will not help him to face and resolve his fear.
> **Client Needs Category**—*Psychosocial integrity*
> **Client Needs Subcategory**—*None*

75. **2.** A child with no complications may return to school within 1 to 2 weeks following an appendectomy; this generally allows sufficient time for healing and recovery. Limited activities are generally recommended throughout the recovery period.

> *Client Needs Category—Health promotion and maintenance*
> *Client Needs Subcategory—None*

Nursing Care of an Adolescent with Dysmenorrhea

76. **4.** Proper sleep, a well-balanced diet, warm tub baths, application of heat to the abdomen, drinking warm liquids, and moderate exercise are some recommendations the nurse can make to relieve dysmenorrhea (painful menstruation). The other options are not known to relieve menstrual cramps or pain.

> *Client Needs Category—Health promotion and maintenance*
> *Client Needs Subcategory—None*

77. **4.** If gastrointestinal distress occurs, aspirin may be taken with food or milk. If gastrointestinal distress persists, the physician should be contacted. An open bottle of aspirin has a short shelf life, usually within a year of purchase. Ringing in the ears is not a common adverse effect of aspirin when taken in normal doses. If ringing in the ears occurs, the physician should be notified because this condition may indicate toxicity. Aspirin should not be taken with a nonsteroidal anti-inflammatory agent such as ibuprofen (Advil).

> *Client Needs Category—Health promotion and maintenance*
> *Client Needs Subcategory—None*

78. **1.** *Amenorrhea* means the absence of menstruation. Excessive vaginal bleeding is called *menorrhagia*. Discomfort prior to menstruation is related to premenstrual tension, and the first menstrual period is called *menarche*.

> *Client Needs Category—Physiological integrity*
> *Client Needs Subcategory—Physiological adaptation*

79. **3.** The client should take tetracycline hydrochloride (Panmycin) when the stomach is empty and wait 1 hour before eating after taking the drug. The other options are appropriate when taking this medication.

> *Client Needs Category—Health promotion and maintenance*
> *Client Needs Subcategory—None*

Nursing Care of an Adolescent Who Is Abusing Drugs

80. **2.** Amphetamines, which are central nervous system stimulants, do not cause physical dependence but are associated with psychological dependence. Those who abuse amphetamines may also be involved with the abuse of other substances. It is untrue to state that amphetamines are tried by "most" adolescents and cause no harm. Amphetamines are most commonly administered orally.

> *Client Needs Category—Health promotion and maintenance*
> *Client Needs Subcategory—None*

81. **4.** Symptoms of amphetamine abuse include marked nervousness, restlessness, excitability, talkativeness, and excessive perspiration. The remaining symptoms are not characteristic of amphetamine abuse.

> *Client Needs Category—Physiological integrity*
> *Client Needs Subcategory—Pharmacological therapies*

82. **1.** Adolescents normally try to develop self-identity. One way of achieving this is through identifying with peers and their values. The search for intimate relationships usually occurs between ages 18 and 40. Generally, adults demonstrate integrity, not adolescents. Idealism refers to the pursuit of ideas; it is most likely unrelated to amphetamine abuse.

> *Client Needs Category—Health promotion and maintenance*
> *Client Needs Subcategory—None*

83. **3.** The successful treatment of substance abuse largely depends on the person's desire to become drug-free. Someone who is forced to enter a drug rehabilitation program probably has less of a chance of remaining drug-free than someone who enters a program willingly. Usually a court order is not necessary for participation in a drug abuse program. Merely discussing the dangers of drug abuse is not likely to change the teenager's pattern of substance abuse.

> *Client Needs Category—Psychosocial integrity*
> *Client Needs Subcategory—None*

84. **4.** Booster doses of tetanus toxoid are recommended during adolescence and once every 10 years thereafter. Smallpox vaccination is no longer advised because it is believed that the disease has been essentially eradicated. The last polio vaccine is given between ages 4 and 6. The Hib vaccine is completed at 15 months.

> *Client Needs Category—Health promotion and maintenance*
> *Client Needs Subcategory—None*

Nursing Care of an Adolescent with a Sexually Transmitted Disease

85. **3.** A diagnosis of gonorrhea is confirmed when the microorganism is found in the client's vaginal discharge. This is usually accomplished by viewing a smear sample under a microscope, although cultures of the discharge may also be taken. Cervical biopsy and blood and urine specimen examinations are not used to confirm a diagnosis of gonorrhea.

> *Client Needs Category—Physiological integrity*
> *Client Needs Subcategory—Physiological adaptation*

86. **4.** Gastrointestinal upset is one of the adverse reactions to doxycycline (Vibramycin). Potentially serious adverse reactions should be immediately reported to the physician. This medication does not usually discolor the urine. The medication should be taken with a full glass of water; it can also be taken with food or dairy products.

> *Client Needs Category—Health promotion and maintenance*
> *Client Needs Subcategory—None*

87. **3.** One or preferably two follow-up smears or cultures should be taken after therapy is completed for clients who have gonorrhea. If the cultures and smears are negative, the client is considered noninfectious. It is unsafe to assume that a client is no longer infectious based on cessation of vaginal discharge, pain-free menstrual periods, or taking prescribed medication; follow-up studies are essential.

> *Client Needs Category—Physiological integrity*
> *Client Needs Subcategory—Physiological adaptation*

88. **2.** The initial lesions of genital herpes can be described as fluid-filled vesicles. The lesions may become pustules, which in time may become crusted. The other terms do not accurately describe genital herpes lesions.

> *Client Needs Category—Physiological integrity*
> *Client Needs Subcategory—Physiological adaptation*

89. **3.** Genital herpes is not associated with sterility; however, current studies have identified a close link with prostate cancer in men and cervical cancer in women. It has also been closely associated with the occurrence of Hodgkin's disease. Female clients with genital herpes are advised to have Pap tests every 6 months, and male clients are advised to have rectal examinations and PSA tests yearly.

> *Client Needs Category—Physiological integrity*
> *Client Needs Subcategory—Physiological adaptation*

90. **3.** Topical acyclovir (Zovirax) should be applied with a glove or finger cot to prevent spreading the infection. Acyclovir (Zovirax) does not provide protection against or prevent recurrence of the disease; however, it does prolong remission and decrease the pain associated with the presence of lesions. Sex partners do not need to be treated with topical acyclovir (Zovirax) because it is used to decrease pain and prevent recurrence.

> *Client Needs Category—Physiological integrity*
> *Client Needs Subcategory—Pharmacological therapies*

91. **4.** Sexual contact should be avoided, especially during active disease. The herpes virus can cross the condom membrane; therefore, wearing a condom will not ensure protection. Also, douching and taking acyclovir (Zovirax) will not protect against virus transmission.

> *Client Needs Category—Health promotion and maintenance*
> *Client Needs Subcategory—None*

92. **3.** Malaise, fever, and opportunistic infections are some common symptoms of AIDS. Female clients with AIDS also tend to experience recurrent yeast infections. Other symptoms may include anorexia, weight loss, sore throat, diarrhea, lymph node enlargement, and abdominal cramps. Some people have few or no early symptoms.

> *Client Needs Category—Health promotion and maintenance*
> *Client Needs Subcategory—None*

93. **2.** Symptoms of AIDS may appear months or years after the original infection; therefore, the absence of symptoms is no assurance that a sexual partner does not have AIDS. AIDS cannot be cured and the spread of AIDS cannot be controlled with antiviral drugs. The drugs currently in use may slow disease progression in some people. Telling the adolescent to cease sexual activity is rarely effective.

> *Client Needs Category—Physiological integrity*
> *Client Needs Subcategory—Physiological adaptation*

94. **1.** A high-calorie, bland diet served in small amounts at frequent intervals is best for the adolescent for two reasons. The bland foods will not irritate the lesions in the adolescent's mouth, and the additional calories are needed to prevent weight loss, which is a common finding in adolescents with AIDS. The other diets mentioned may not provide the nutrients needed or may aggravate other problems found in adolescents with AIDS.

> *Client Needs Category—Physiological integrity*
> *Client Needs Subcategory—Physiological adaptation*

95. 4. A ½-inch space should be left at the tip of the condom to allow for collection of the ejaculate and to prevent tearing of the condom. Condoms can be damaged by heat and, therefore, should be stored in a cool place. A condom should be applied after the penis is erect. Condoms are not prelubricated; therefore, if lubrication is desired, a water-based lubricant should be used.

>*Client Needs Category*—*Health promotion and maintenance*
>*Client Needs Subcategory*—*None*

96. 1. The client should examine his testicles individually, one at a time, after a warm bath or shower. One testicle is usually slightly larger than the other. Lumps, if detected, are usually found on the sides of the testicles.

>*Client Needs Category*—*Health promotion and maintenance*
>*Client Needs Subcategory*—*None*

Nursing Care of an Adolescent with Scoliosis

97. 2. Children with scoliosis often complain of having difficulty with their clothes fitting properly. Common complaints include an uneven hemline and uneven sleeve length. The other findings are not usually reported with scoliosis.

>*Client Needs Category*—*Health promotion and maintenance*
>*Client Needs Subcategory*—*None*

98. 1. X-rays are used to confirm a diagnosis of scoliosis. Because the radiation emitted by X-rays carries a risk of causing genetic mutation that may lead to birth defects in offspring, the nurse should first determine whether there is a possibility that the client is pregnant. The client's allergy status, medication use, and consumption of food are not pertinent to this type of radiologic test.

>*Client Needs Category*—*Health promotion and maintenance*
>*Client Needs Subcategory*—*None*

99. 4. Any curvature greater than 20 degrees requires treatment. If treatment is not implemented, the curvature will continue to increase and the child will be at risk for developing cardiopulmonary problems.

>*Client Needs Category*—*Physiological integrity*
>*Client Needs Subcategory*—*Physiological adaptation*

100. 1. Curvatures between 20 and 40 degrees usually respond to nonsurgical treatment such as a Milwaukee brace. The brace is worn an average of 22 to 23 hours per day and should be removed only when the child is taking a bath or swimming.

>*Client Needs Category*—*Physiological integrity*
>*Client Needs Subcategory*—*Physiological adaptation*

101. 2. Adolescents are very concerned about appearances and fitting in with their peer group. Because the Milwaukee brace must be worn almost continually, the nurse should discuss ways to help the child find appropriate, stylish attire that hides the brace. This should help the child feel more acceptable to peers and ensure better compliance with the treatment plan. The other options are inappropriate.

>*Client Needs Category*—*Health promotion and maintenance*
>*Client Needs Subcategory*—*None*

Dosage Calculations for Children and Adolescents

102. 2.5.

$$\frac{\text{Desired dose}}{\text{Dose on hand}} \times \text{Total quantity} = \text{Dose to administer}$$

$$\frac{125 \text{ mg}}{250 \text{ mg}} = \frac{X \text{ ml}}{5 \text{ ml}}$$

$$250X = 625$$

$$X = 2.5$$

>*Client Needs Category*—*Safe, effective care environment*
>*Client Needs Subcategory*—*Safety and infection control*

103. 354. Begin by converting pounds to kilograms:

$$\frac{52}{2.2} = 23.6 \text{ kg}$$

Next, use the recommended dose range:

$$15 \text{ mg/kg} \times 23.6 \text{ kg} = 354 \text{ mg}$$

Highest single dose that would be safe:

$$354 \text{ mg/kg}$$

>*Client Needs Category*—*Physiological integrity*
>*Client Needs Subcategory*—*Pharmacological therapies*

The Nursing Care of Clients with Mental Health Needs

The Nursing Care of Infants, Children, and Adolescents with Mental Health Needs

⇨ *Mental Health Needs During Infancy*
⇨ *Mental Health Needs During Childhood*
⇨ *Mental Health Needs During Adolescence*
⇨ *Correct Answers and Rationales*

Directions: *With a pencil, blacken the space in front of the option you have chosen for your correct answer. .*

Mental Health Needs During Infancy

A couple who has been childless for 10 years become parents of a newborn boy with Down syndrome.

1. To help the parents cope with their disappointment and loss of their "perfect" baby, which nursing action is most appropriate initially?
[ ] **1.** Encourage the parents to verbalize their feelings.
[ ] **2.** Treat the child as though he is a normal newborn.
[ ] **3.** Refer the couple to community resources for assistance.
[ ] **4.** Encourage the parents to consider long-term institutional placement.

When the nurse brings the baby to the mother's room, the father says, "These doctors don't know anything. We're going to consult specialists."

2. Which response by the nurse is most appropriate at this time?
[ ] **1.** "The physicians here are very well qualified."
[ ] **2.** "This diagnosis is difficult for you to accept."
[ ] **3.** "Why do you feel you need a second opinion?"
[ ] **4.** "It's not as bad as it may seem right now."

The nurse recognizes that the parents are working through the stages of grieving as a result of having a newborn with Down syndrome.

3. Place the following stages of the grieving process in ascending chronological order according to the most likely order in which they will occur. Use all the options.

1. Depression	
2. Anger	
3. Denial	
4. Bargaining	
5. Acceptance	

4. Which of the following information documented by the nurse provides the best evidence that the mother is bonding with her newborn with Down syndrome?
[ ] **1.** The mother smiles and talks to her baby.
[ ] **2.** The mother asks questions about infant care.
[ ] **3.** The mother wants to see visitors who come.
[ ] **4.** The mother feeds and burps her baby.

The nurse also documents that the mother appears nervous when the newborn cries during his bath.

5. Which nursing action is most appropriate at this time?
[ ] **1.** Briefly take over bathing the newborn for the mother.
[ ] **2.** Advise the mother to discontinue the bath.
[ ] **3.** Give all future baths in the nursery.
[ ] **4.** Point out what a good job she is doing.

6. The nurse describes to the parents which physical characteristics they can expect their child with Down syndrome to develop as he grows?
[ ] **1.** Large head and curved index fingers
[ ] **2.** Long fingers and protruding tongue
[ ] **3.** Small head and upward-slanting eyes
[ ] **4.** Simian creases on the soles of the feet

A nurse is assigned to care for several infants in the newborn nursery.

7. Which withdrawal symptom is the nurse most likely to note while observing the newborn of a mother who used heroin during her pregnancy?
[ ] **1.** Unresponsiveness
[ ] **2.** Dilated pupils
[ ] **3.** Persistent crying
[ ] **4.** Impaired sucking

8. When caring for a newborn experiencing opioid withdrawal, which nursing intervention should be included in the care plan initially?
[ ] **1.** Reduce the newborn's exposure to environmental stimuli.
[ ] **2.** Touch the newborn frequently.
[ ] **3.** Stroke the newborn's skin gently.
[ ] **4.** Leave the newborn unwrapped.

9. To ensure optimum mental health of an infant born with a congenital defect such as myelomeningocele, the nurse explains that it is essential for the parents to meet which of the following needs?
[ ] **1.** Autonomy
[ ] **2.** Love
[ ] **3.** Respect
[ ] **4.** Identity

A teenage mother brings her 6-month-old female infant to the clinic. She tells the nurse that her baby cries a lot, and she is concerned that the baby is ill.

10. Which information is most appropriate for the nurse to collect at this time?
[ ] **1.** The infant's weight and length
[ ] **2.** The infant's breath and heart sounds
[ ] **3.** The infant's head and chest circumference
[ ] **4.** The infant's sucking and grasp reflex

On examination of the teenager's infant, no signs of illness are identified.

11. What information is most helpful for the nurse to obtain next?
[ ] **1.** The mother's expectations of an infant's behavior
[ ] **2.** How many more children the mother wants to have
[ ] **3.** If the mother plans to finish high school
[ ] **4.** The kinds of toys the mother has for the baby

The mother tells the nurse that she is afraid of spoiling her baby, so she frequently puts her in the crib when she cries.

12. Which information given to the teenage mother is most appropriate?
[ ] **1.** Holding her baby will not result in spoiling her.
[ ] **2.** Grandparents usually spoil babies.
[ ] **3.** Babies need to be spoiled.
[ ] **4.** Toddlers are more likely to be spoiled.

13. Which instruction is most important for the nurse to recommend to the teenage mother regarding parenting her infant?
[ ] **1.** Give the baby a pacifier whenever she cries.
[ ] **2.** Turn on a radio in the room with the baby.
[ ] **3.** Cuddle and talk to the baby frequently.
[ ] **4.** Place a brightly colored mobile above the crib.

14. If the teenage mother expresses that she feels inexperienced and inadequate in caring for her baby, which referral is best?
[ ] **1.** Project Head Start
[ ] **2.** Planned Parenthood
[ ] **3.** Parent-Teacher Association
[ ] **4.** Parenting classes

15. The nurse is correct in assuming that without adequate nurturing during infancy, the child of the teenage mother is at risk for developing which psychosocial characteristic?
[ ] **1.** Inferiority
[ ] **2.** Mistrust
[ ] **3.** Doubt
[ ] **4.** Isolation

The teenage mother returns to the clinic 4 months later, stating that she thinks her baby is sick. The nurse assesses the infant and notifies the pediatrician. After further investigation, the pediatrician makes a diagnosis of failure to thrive.

16. Which assessment findings are most characteristic of a 10-month-old infant with the diagnosis of failure to thrive? Select all that apply.
[ ] 1. The infant cries vigorously when handled.
[ ] 2. The infant has a delay in developmental milestones.
[ ] 3. The infant appears pale and lethargic.
[ ] 4. The infant eats vigorously when fed.
[ ] 5. The infant has delayed understanding of speech.

The nurse reviews the mother's history to identify factors that may have led to the diagnosis of the infant's failure to thrive.

17. Which of the following risk factors would the nurse expect to note when assessing for failure to thrive? Select all that apply.
[ ] 1. The pregnancy was unplanned and unwanted.
[ ] 2. The baby's father left the mother during the pregnancy or shortly after delivery.
[ ] 3. The mother is an adolescent.
[ ] 4. The mother's socioeconomic status is low.
[ ] 5. The mother has a history of alcohol and drug abuse.
[ ] 6. The infant has several other siblings.

Mental Health Needs During Childhood

A public health nurse assesses a 2-year-old girl at the immunization clinic.

18. Which assessment finding is most indicative that the child is developmentally delayed?
[ ] 1. The child is being bottle-fed.
[ ] 2. The child is not toilet-trained.
[ ] 3. The child has no language skills.
[ ] 4. The child cannot draw a picture.

19. Which test should the nurse use to more objectively assess the toddler's overall development?
[ ] 1. Denver II Developmental Screening Test
[ ] 2. Scholastic Aptitude Test (SAT)
[ ] 3. Stanford-Binet test
[ ] 4. Weber's test

20. If the mother asks the nurse how to appropriately discipline a child of this age, which response by the nurse is most appropriate?
[ ] 1. By pre-identifying the consequences of unacceptable behavior
[ ] 2. By showing disapproval immediately after an unacceptable act
[ ] 3. By administering some form of moderate physical punishment
[ ] 4. By explaining to the toddler why certain behavior is undesirable

A nursing assistant becomes frustrated by the 2-year-old child's persistent response of "No" whenever she asks her to do something. The nursing assistant asks the nurse for help.

21. The nurse correctly explains that this is normal behavior for toddlers who are developing which psychosocial characteristic?
[ ] 1. Integrity
[ ] 2. Identity
[ ] 3. Autonomy
[ ] 4. Generativity

22. What is the best suggestion the nurse can give the nursing assistant caring for the 2-year-old child at this time?
[ ] 1. Let the child choose from two acceptable alternatives.
[ ] 2. Withhold something the child desires until she complies.
[ ] 3. Identify what is expected of the child, rather than ask.
[ ] 4. Tell the child that her mother will be told if she refuses to cooperate.

A 3-year-old-child is brought to the emergency department for a sudden, acute episode of an illness with vague symptoms. The child has a history of multiple hospital admissions. The health care team is beginning to suspect Munchausen syndrome by proxy.

23. If this diagnosis is accurate, it is most important for the nurse to assess for which characteristic finding?
[ ] 1. The mother is obsessed with the fear that her child will die.
[ ] 2. The mother is ignorant of normal health patterns among children.
[ ] 3. The mother is responsible for creating the child's symptoms.
[ ] 4. The mother is overreacting to minor variations in her child's health.

A 3½-year-old child is scheduled for cardiac surgery. The parents are informed that hospitalization will be prolonged.

24. Which nursing strategy is best to help the child overcome the fear of being in the unfamiliar hospital environment?
[ ] 1. Bringing a favorite blanket from home
[ ] 2. Providing age-specific toys such as a stuffed animal
[ ] 3. Having one or both parents nearby at all times
[ ] 4. Placing the child in a room with a same-aged child

The parents notice that their child has begun to suck his thumb. They explain to the nurse that he has not sucked his thumb for over a year.

25. Which response by the nurse provides the best explanation of the child's behavior?
[ ] **1.** Thumb sucking is a primitive form of self-stimulation and security.
[ ] **2.** Thumb sucking is a regressive behavior with a comforting effect.
[ ] **3.** Thumb sucking substitutes for the postoperative restriction of fluids.
[ ] **4.** Thumb sucking satisfies the child's increased need for a familiar touch.

The nurse uses simple, age-appropriate language to explain to the child the purpose and procedure for starting an I.V. line.

26. Which additional nursing action is most beneficial for reducing the child's anxiety?
[ ] **1.** Tell the child that the pain will be minimal.
[ ] **2.** Offer the child a reward for good behavior.
[ ] **3.** Let the child handle some of the equipment.
[ ] **4.** Show the child others who have I.V. infusions in place.

27. Which of the following behaviors exhibited by the child demonstrates the most severe reaction to prolonged hospitalization?
[ ] **1.** Clinging to the parents
[ ] **2.** Shaking the crib frantically
[ ] **3.** Throwing himself about
[ ] **4.** Ignoring the parents

A mother brings her 2-year-old girl to the emergency department for treatment of a fractured femur.

28. Which assessment finding would lead the nurse to suspect physical abuse?
[ ] **1.** The child protests when approached by the nurse.
[ ] **2.** The child has varying lengths of hair on her head.
[ ] **3.** The child has a fresh bruise on her forehead.
[ ] **4.** The child has an abrasion on her right knee.

29. What information strongly suggests that the child's fractured femur is the result of physical abuse?
[ ] **1.** The nurse notes evidence of other healed fractures.
[ ] **2.** Only the mother witnessed the injury.
[ ] **3.** The child is not fully immunized yet.
[ ] **4.** The child is underweight for her height.

After assessing for physical abuse, the nurse suspects that the toddler has also been sexually abused.

30. If the nurse's suspicions are true, which assessment findings require further investigation? Select all that apply.
[ ] **1.** The child demonstrates sexual activity with a doll.
[ ] **2.** The child has a gonorrheal infection.
[ ] **3.** The child is underweight for her height.
[ ] **4.** The child complains of burning during urination.
[ ] **5.** The child is afraid to be left alone with the suspected parent.
[ ] **6.** The child has trouble sleeping through the night.

31. Which strategy is most appropriate for developing a positive, therapeutic relationship with the injured child at the time of assessment?
[ ] **1.** The nurse should make an effort to have prolonged eye contact with the child.
[ ] **2.** The nurse should maintain her body position at the same level as the child.
[ ] **3.** The nurse should separate the child from the mother during the interview.
[ ] **4.** The nurse should ask the child direct questions about her mother's parenting.

32. If the following facts are present in the social history of a person suspected of child abuse, which one is most similar to the profile of other child abusers?
[ ] **1.** The person grew up in a divorced household.
[ ] **2.** The person's income is at or below poverty level.
[ ] **3.** The person was the victim of child abuse.
[ ] **4.** The person became a parent after the age of 25.

33. If the nurse suspects that a child is the victim of physical abuse, which nursing action is most appropriate to take initially?
[ ] **1.** Refer the parents to Parents Anonymous.
[ ] **2.** Recommend that the child be made a ward of the court.
[ ] **3.** Contact a relative to care for the child.
[ ] **4.** Report the facts to child protective services.

34. When interacting with a person suspected of committing child abuse, which attitude is most conducive for facilitating a referral to a support group?
[ ] **1.** An impersonal attitude
[ ] **2.** An indifferent attitude
[ ] **3.** A sympathetic attitude
[ ] **4.** A nonjudgmental attitude

A mother who is distressed by the fact that her 3-year-old male child has been publicly masturbating asks a nurse for advice.

35. Which nursing suggestion is most helpful for preventing the child from feeling guilty about masturbating?
[ ] **1.** Interrupt the child casually when masturbation is observed.
[ ] **2.** Explain to the child that this is an unacceptable practice.
[ ] **3.** Tell the child that the genitals can be touched only when urinating.
[ ] **4.** Relate that touching the genitals is something that is done privately.

A nurse observes a 4-year-old girl with her mother and infant sibling.

36. Which is the best example that the 4-year-old child is going through the developmental process called identification?
[ ] **1.** The child recognizes and names animals correctly.
[ ] **2.** The child calls her sibling by name.
[ ] **3.** The child pretends to feed her doll.
[ ] **4.** The child accurately points to colors.

A pediatric office nurse prepares a 4-year-old child for his preschool physical examination. The child's mother has also brought her newborn for his first immunization.

37. Which statement is most indicative that the preschooler is experiencing anxiety in relation to his new sibling?
[ ] **1.** The child wants to use his father's tools.
[ ] **2.** The child is taking shorter naps in the afternoon.
[ ] **3.** The child cries when his toys become broken.
[ ] **4.** The child has been wetting and soiling himself.

38. The nurse correctly explains that the behavior the preschooler is demonstrating is based on a need to feel what?
[ ] **1.** Powerful
[ ] **2.** Secure
[ ] **3.** Confident
[ ] **4.** Dependent

39. Which advice given to the preschooler's mother is most appropriate for relieving the 4-year-old child's anxiety?
[ ] **1.** Give him some new toys to play with.
[ ] **2.** Let him stay up later at night.
[ ] **3.** Invite the grandparents to visit.
[ ] **4.** Spend more time alone with him.

The mother of the 4-year-old child asks the nurse what is most helpful in preparing her preschooler for kindergarten.

40. Which suggestion is likely to be most beneficial to the mother?
[ ] **1.** Give him simple responsibilities to perform.
[ ] **2.** Teach him to print his first and last names.
[ ] **3.** Buy a set of mathematic flash cards that teach addition.
[ ] **4.** Have him watch children's daytime television programs.

The mother states that when her 2-year-old child asks her to buy candy at the grocery store and she refuses, he throws a temper tantrum. She resorts to buying the candy so he stops kicking and screaming.

41. What is the most appropriate recommendation for eliminating tantrums when the 2-year-old child does not get his way?
[ ] **1.** Give him candy before entering the store.
[ ] **2.** Ignore the unacceptable behavior.
[ ] **3.** Explain to him that his behavior is childish.
[ ] **4.** Remind him that he is a big boy now.

The parents of a 3-year-old child with infantile autism bring their child to a mental health clinic on a regular basis. Today, a care conference is planned with the mental health team and the family.

42. When the social worker, who has not had experience with autistic children, asks the nurse to identify signs and symptoms of the disorder, the nurse correctly identifies which finding as most characteristic?
[ ] **1.** Repetitive body movements
[ ] **2.** Intense attachment to one parent
[ ] **3.** Early sexual development
[ ] **4.** Profound mental retardation

43. When providing care for the 3-year-old autistic child, which behavior is the nurse most likely to note?
[ ] **1.** Constant use of the words "I" and "me"
[ ] **2.** Insensitivity to pain
[ ] **3.** Flexibility in normal routine
[ ] **4.** Increased interest in others' actions

44. When planning care for an autistic child, which nursing intervention is most appropriate?
[ ] **1.** Providing interactive play activities
[ ] **2.** Using soft restraints while in bed
[ ] **3.** Using a consistent caregiver
[ ] **4.** Providing a rocking chair for calming the child

45. If the 3-year-old child is typical of other autistic children, what would the nurse expect the child's response to his parents to be?
[ ] **1.** Indifference
[ ] **2.** Friendliness
[ ] **3.** Submissiveness
[ ] **4.** Impatience

46. Based on the nurse's knowledge of autistic behavior, which nursing diagnosis is most likely to be a priority at the team conference?
[ ] **1.** *Ineffective health maintenance*
[ ] **2.** *Chronic low self-esteem*
[ ] **3.** *Risk for activity intolerance*
[ ] **4.** *Risk for self-directed violence*

During the care conference, the mother of the autistic child says that he helps dress himself but he will not eat unless he is fed.

47. Which suggestion by the nurse would be most beneficial for the child's nutrition at this time?
[ ] **1.** Continue to feed the child until he tries to pick up food.
[ ] **2.** Try giving the child finger foods while he is dressing.
[ ] **3.** Leave the food until he becomes hungry enough to eat it.
[ ] **4.** Demonstrate how to use a spoon at every meal.

48. If and when the autistic child actually makes an effort to self-feed, which of the following suggestions is most appropriate for the nurse to make?
[ ] **1.** Note if the self-feeding effort is repeated.
[ ] **2.** Stop feeding the child thereafter.
[ ] **3.** Demonstrate approval in some way.
[ ] **4.** Offer food more frequently during the day.

49. When discussing the home environment with the parents, the nurse should explain that which is the most appropriate environment for an autistic child?
[ ] **1.** Stimulating, with a variety of sensory experiences
[ ] **2.** Consistent, with a minimum amount of physical change
[ ] **3.** Flexible, with the freedom to do as desired
[ ] **4.** Strict, with narrow limits for acceptable behavior

The parents express a desire to leave their autistic child with a responsible person for a few hours occasionally so that they can have relief from the constant care and supervision required.

50. Which is the most appropriate community resource for the nurse to recommend for respite services?
[ ] **1.** Aid to Dependent Children
[ ] **2.** Association on Mental Deficiency
[ ] **3.** A local children's day-care facility
[ ] **4.** A home health care agency

The school nurse is conducting a class for parents whose children are about to enter first grade.

51. When describing the characteristic developmental stage of school-age children, which statement by the nurse is most accurate?
[ ] **1.** "School-age children begin developing long-lasting friendships."
[ ] **2.** "School-age children are learning to work beside and with others."
[ ] **3.** "School-age children are preoccupied with finding a sense of purpose in life."
[ ] **4.** "School-age children are striving for independence from others."

The school nurse meets a 7-year-old child and his parents to follow up on the child's progress since being diagnosed with attention deficit hyperactivity disorder (ADHD). The child is being treated with methylphenidate hydrochloride (Ritalin).

52. The nurse recognizes that methylphenidate hydrochloride (Ritalin) is classified as which type of drug?
[ ] **1.** Central nervous system depressant
[ ] **2.** Central nervous system stimulant
[ ] **3.** Antidepressant
[ ] **4.** Tranquilizer

53. The nurse advises the parents to look for which change as evidence that methylphenidate hydrochloride (Ritalin) is achieving its desired effect?
[ ] **1.** The child is more alert and active.
[ ] **2.** The child is less easily distracted.
[ ] **3.** The child does not seem fatigued.
[ ] **4.** The child's moods are more stable.

54. When the parents ask about the side effects of taking methylphenidate hydrochloride (Ritalin), the nurse correctly explains that the child may have which common cluster of signs and symptoms?
[ ] **1.** Nausea, vomiting, and diarrhea
[ ] **2.** Fatigue, drowsiness, and dry mouth
[ ] **3.** Insomnia, tachycardia, and anorexia
[ ] **4.** Hypotension, bradycardia, and constipation

55. Which assessment finding best indicates that a child taking methylphenidate hydrochloride (Ritalin) is experiencing undesirable side effects?
[ ] **1.** The child has altered elimination patterns.
[ ] **2.** The child develops intolerance to certain foods.
[ ] **3.** The child has an elevated blood pressure.
[ ] **4.** The child has evidence of skin breakdown.

56. The nurse should advise the parents of a child taking methylphenidate hydrochloride (Ritalin) that, to avoid potentiating the drug's effects, it is best if their child refrains from consuming which food?
[ ] **1.** Dairy products
[ ] **2.** Cola beverages
[ ] **3.** Processed meats
[ ] **4.** Saturated fats

An 8-year-old girl is tentatively diagnosed with leukemia. A bone marrow puncture is part of the diagnostic workup.

57. If this child is typical of others her age with a serious illness, which concept is the most commonly held belief about being ill?
[ ] **1.** Illness is not life-threatening; recovery is assured.
[ ] **2.** Significant others can prevent serious consequences.
[ ] **3.** Discomfort is a punishment for some wrongdoing.
[ ] **4.** Failure to comply with treatment results in parental rejection.

58. To minimize this child's apprehension about the bone marrow puncture, which nursing strategy is most appropriate?
[ ] **1.** Explain the procedure to her shortly before it is done.
[ ] **2.** Give her information as soon as the test is scheduled.
[ ] **3.** Postpone teaching about the procedure until she asks specific questions.
[ ] **4.** Wait for the physician to explain the procedure to her.

59. The nurse is aware that whenever a school-age child is prepared for a procedure, test, or medical treatment, which is the most important information to convey?
[ ] **1.** When the procedure will take place
[ ] **2.** Who will perform the procedure
[ ] **3.** Where the procedure will be performed
[ ] **4.** What will happen to the child during the procedure

The child fails to respond to drug therapy for leukemia, and her condition eventually becomes terminal. The parents are unsure of how, or if, they should tell their daughter about her prognosis.

60. Which rationale is the best justification for openly discussing the child's prognosis with her?

[ ] **1.** The child will eventually guess that she is dying.
[ ] **2.** Sharing prevents the child from dealing with fears alone.
[ ] **3.** Concealing the truth will be very difficult.
[ ] **4.** Being less than honest is immoral and unethical.

61. Which outcome would the nurse expect a seriously ill school-age child to demonstrate by providing honest explanations, including discussion about unpleasant experiences?
[ ] **1.** Confidence in caregivers
[ ] **2.** Perseverance in hardship
[ ] **3.** Courage in crises
[ ] **4.** Hope in suffering

A single parent consults the school nurse for help in dealing with her 8-year-old daughter, who has been diagnosed with a learning disability.

62. Which nursing suggestion is most important for preserving the child's self-esteem?
[ ] **1.** Set realistic, achievable goals.
[ ] **2.** Obtain professional tutoring.
[ ] **3.** Help the child with homework.
[ ] **4.** Offer rewards for good grades.

A 9-year-old student is frequently absent from school. When he attends school, he talks out of turn, fights with classmates, moves about in the classroom during a lesson, and does not complete his assignments or homework. His current grades are inconsistent with his past performance. The school nurse plans to speak with the student to determine if he has a health problem that is causing these changes.

63. Which approach is most appropriate when the school nurse speaks with the child about his health status?
[ ] **1.** Sit down at the lunch table with him.
[ ] **2.** Arrange to see him in the nursing office before school.
[ ] **3.** Call him aside in the hallway on the way to his classroom.
[ ] **4.** Meet with him on the playground during recess.

64. If the student reveals all the following information to the nurse, which situation is most likely affecting his recent acting-out behavior?
[ ] **1.** His parents are involved in divorce proceedings.
[ ] **2.** His pet turtle just died.
[ ] **3.** He just acquired a neighborhood paper route.
[ ] **4.** He is confused because he has a crush on a girl.

The school nurse meets with the teacher to discuss the child's disruptive behavior.

65. Which approach would the nurse recommend for helping the child maintain acceptable behavior in school?
[ ] **1.** Send him to the principal's office when he misbehaves.
[ ] **2.** Suspend him until a family conference has been conducted.
[ ] **3.** Have the school counselor see him on a daily basis.
[ ] **4.** Consistently enforce reasonable limits for behavior.

A school nurse observes four students who are all approximately 10 years old.

66. If the school nurse observes a group of 10-year-old children socializing, which child is most likely demonstrating behavior commonly associated with firstborn children?
[ ] **1.** The child who has a low tolerance for frustration
[ ] **2.** The child who tends to compromise willingly
[ ] **3.** The child who conforms to adult expectations
[ ] **4.** The child who is flexible when given choices

A 9-year-old girl is brought to the emergency department with ketoacidosis, which is found to be related to undiagnosed type 1 diabetes mellitus.

67. If the following actions are observed as the child improves, which one best indicates that she is having difficulty accepting her diagnosis?
[ ] **1.** She stays up later than usual watching television.
[ ] **2.** She makes angry remarks to the nurse and her mother.
[ ] **3.** She avoids completing her homework assignments.
[ ] **4.** She talks on the phone for long periods of time.

68. If the nursing care plan includes the following activities, which one provides the newly diagnosed diabetic child with the most sense of control over her disease?
[ ] **1.** Informing her of laboratory test results
[ ] **2.** Providing her with calorie-controlled dietary instructions
[ ] **3.** Supervising her self-testing of capillary blood glucose levels
[ ] **4.** Teaching her the parts of an insulin syringe

The nurse is caring for a 12-year-old boy who is being seen for Tourette syndrome.

69. Besides helping the client and family cope with the child's repetitive, purposeless movements, which other problem associated with Tourette syndrome is essential for the nurse to address?
[ ] **1.** Verbal obscenities
[ ] **2.** Social withdrawal
[ ] **3.** Pathological lying
[ ] **4.** Mood swings

The physician prescribes haloperidol (Haldol) to treat the Tourette syndrome. The nurse provides the child and his parents with information about significant side effects.

70. Besides involuntary tremors, which other side effect should the nurse advise the family to anticipate?
[ ] **1.** Muscle spasms
[ ] **2.** Muscle weakness
[ ] **3.** Muscle atrophy
[ ] **4.** Muscle contractures

The parents tell the nurse that they are concerned their son's self-esteem may be jeopardized because of peer ridicule.

71. Which suggestion is most appropriate for the nurse to offer the parents in this situation?
[ ] **1.** Try home-schooling the child.
[ ] **2.** Praise the child's deserved accomplishments.
[ ] **3.** Avoid discussing peer comments.
[ ] **4.** Show disapproval of negative labels.

Mental Health Needs During Adolescence

A 13-year-old student takes a gun to school and murders a teacher.

72. Based on the principles of crisis intervention, when is the best time to provide assistance to those most affected by this incident?
[ ] **1.** After the funeral
[ ] **2.** Within 6 months
[ ] **3.** Immediately
[ ] **4.** Six weeks later

73. If the adolescents who witnessed the violence at school are typical of others who experience crises, how are they most likely feeling?
[ ] **1.** Helpless
[ ] **2.** Depressed
[ ] **3.** Angry
[ ] **4.** Fortunate

74. When crisis intervention is provided, which nursing action takes priority?
[ ] **1.** Explaining the benefits of professional counseling
[ ] **2.** Encouraging the survivors to talk about the event
[ ] **3.** Reassuring the survivors that they will adapt
[ ] **4.** Advising consulting a physician for drug therapy

A 15-year-old girl is being treated in an eating disorders unit for bulimia.

75. When reviewing the assessment data, the nurse would expect to note which characteristic physical finding?
[ ] **1.** Extremely low body weight
[ ] **2.** Erosion of dental enamel
[ ] **3.** Cessation of menstruation
[ ] **4.** Patchy loss of hair

A 17-year-old female client is assessed in the emergency department and admitted to the hospital after she fainted at school. She is more than 25% below the normal weight for her height. She is believed to be suffering from anorexia nervosa.

76. During the initial physical examination, the nurse is most likely to assess which finding related to anorexia?
[ ] **1.** Growth of fine body hair
[ ] **2.** Bruises over her upper torso
[ ] **3.** Hyperactive bowel sounds
[ ] **4.** Club-shaped fingertips

77. Which assessment finding differentiates anorexia nervosa from bulimia in an adolescent with a suspected eating disorder?
[ ] **1.** Body image distortion
[ ] **2.** Purging following meals
[ ] **3.** Decreased self-esteem
[ ] **4.** Binge eating

The nurse reviews the client's history obtained during admission.

78. Which of the following data best correlates with the profile of a person with anorexia nervosa?
[ ] **1.** The client is the middle child of three siblings.
[ ] **2.** The client is a high achiever in school and activities.
[ ] **3.** The client thinks her classmates don't like her.
[ ] **4.** The client experienced many illnesses during childhood.

The nursing team meets to plan the anorectic client's care.

79. Which nursing goal is the highest priority at this time?
[ ] **1.** To improve the client's distorted body image
[ ] **2.** To help the client use healthier coping techniques
[ ] **3.** To restore normal nutrition
[ ] **4.** To help the client develop assertiveness

The client's mother visits at dinnertime. She is overheard to say, "Look at you; you're so thin. Please eat something."

80. Which is most therapeutic for the nurse to say privately to the mother in this situation?
[ ] **1.** "All children know how to frustrate parents."
[ ] **2.** "You need to stop pleading with her to eat."
[ ] **3.** "You're concerned that she's starving herself."
[ ] **4.** "I know how you're feeling; I'm a parent, too."

The mental health technician is frustrated and angry when she sees the anorectic client rearranging the food on her tray but not eating any of it.

81. What is the best guidance the nurse can give the mental health technician caring for the anorectic client?
[ ] **1.** Blend the food and administer it by tube feeding.
[ ] **2.** Remind the client that her intake is being recorded.
[ ] **3.** Review the treatment goals with the client again.
[ ] **4.** Remove the food without making any comments.

Just before the anorectic client is to be weighed, the mental health technician tells the nurse that she observed the client drinking a full pitcher of water.

82. Which nursing action is most appropriate at this time?
[ ] **1.** Postpone weighing the client until later.
[ ] **2.** Confront the client about what was observed.
[ ] **3.** Say nothing and weigh the client as usual.
[ ] **4.** Subtract 2 lb (0.9 kg) from the client's weight.

A 16-year-old with moderate retardation is admitted for treatment of a ruptured appendix. His mother reports that her son has an IQ in the range of 35 to 50, which approximates that of a 5- to 7-year-old child.

83. If this developmentally disabled client is typical of others of his mental age, for what should the nurse assess?
[ ] **1.** Distress when separated from his mother
[ ] **2.** An exaggerated response to pain
[ ] **3.** Difficulty making his needs known
[ ] **4.** Concern over his change in body image

84. If the admitting nurse documents all the following maternal behaviors, which behavior is most likely to suppress this child's ability to reach his maximum potential for development?
[ ] **1.** The mother dresses and undresses her son.
[ ] **2.** The mother answers all the medical questions.
[ ] **3.** The mother exaggerates her son's abilities.
[ ] **4.** The mother blames herself for her son's condition.

A nursing assistant assigned to the mentally retarded adolescent reports that he struck her while she was attempting to help him out of bed.

85. Which statement is the best explanation for the adolescent's behavior?
[ ] **1.** Aggression is a common behavior manifested by mentally retarded people.
[ ] **2.** Aggression is a response that occurs when a person feels threatened.
[ ] **3.** Aggression is an indication that the client has a poor opinion of his care.
[ ] **4.** Aggression is a common way for children to communicate they are experiencing pain.

86. When the nurse documents this incident, which wording is most appropriate?
[ ] **1.** "Became angry for no reason and an assault occurred."
[ ] **2.** "Hit caregiver unexpectedly even though not provoked."
[ ] **3.** "Struck nursing assistant when being helped from bed."
[ ] **4.** "Attacked nursing assistant without prior warning."

The retarded adolescent's behavioral outburst is discussed at a team conference.

87. Of the following suggestions, which one would best prevent nursing personnel from becoming injured when providing the adolescent with care?
[ ] **1.** Apply soft wrist restraints before ambulating the client.
[ ] **2.** Ask the mother to care for the client.
[ ] **3.** Explain steps involved in care before touching the client.
[ ] **4.** Medicate the client immediately before ambulating him.

A 16-year-old male client is brought to the emergency department for treatment of a stab wound following a gang-related fight. The client is eventually ordered by the court to receive counseling at the community mental health clinic.

88. Which area of the adolescent's social history is most appropriate for the clinic nurse to assess?
[ ] **1.** Peer relationships
[ ] **2.** School performance
[ ] **3.** Church attendance
[ ] **4.** Employment records

89. If the nurse obtains the following data, which factor has the strongest influence on the teenager's developing antisocial behavior?
[ ] **1.** Parental discipline is inconsistent.
[ ] **2.** There are more than three siblings.
[ ] **3.** The family relies on public welfare.
[ ] **4.** Role models do not value education.

90. Which information is most important to communicate each time the adolescent attends a group meeting?
[ ] **1.** The date and time of the next meeting
[ ] **2.** The qualifications of the participating therapists
[ ] **3.** That everyone should use first names only
[ ] **4.** That client information is kept confidential

91. If the adolescent who is involved in gang activities demonstrates the following behaviors during group meetings, which is most indicative that he is resisting therapy?
[ ] **1.** The adolescent borrows cigarettes from others.
[ ] **2.** The adolescent laughs inappropriately.
[ ] **3.** The adolescent keeps checking his watch.
[ ] **4.** The adolescent fidgets in his chair.

Family therapy is included in the counseling plan for the adolescent gang member. The client's father arrives late and is intoxicated.

92. If the adolescent is typical of others who have grown up in an alcoholic family, the nurse would expect to assess for problems in which area?
[ ] **1.** Low self-esteem
[ ] **2.** Managing stress
[ ] **3.** Long-term learning
[ ] **4.** Fear of authority

93. Of the following community resources, which referral is the nurse most likely to suggest for this client?
[ ] **1.** Alcoholics Anonymous
[ ] **2.** Al-Anon
[ ] **3.** Alateen
[ ] **4.** The Substance Abuse Council

94. If the adolescent benefits from therapy that focuses on growing up in an alcoholic household, the nurse is most likely to observe that he is developing an ability to do what?
[ ] **1.** Keep promises
[ ] **2.** Trust others
[ ] **3.** Solve problems
[ ] **4.** Honor commitments

A 16-year-old has been selected to play on the junior varsity football team. He spends several hours a day in a weight-training facility.

95. When the gym owner asks the teenager if he would like a drug to help him increase his muscle mass, which factor will most likely influence his desire to accept?
[ ] **1.** Several teammates are taking this drug.
[ ] **2.** The team is having a winning season.
[ ] **3.** His parents support his interest in football.
[ ] **4.** He can afford to pay for a substantial supply.

After taking the unidentified drug for some time, the adolescent's weight increases dramatically and his muscles become larger and well defined.

96. If the unprescribed drug is an anabolic steroid, which other physical effect is common?
[ ] **1.** Decreased lung capacity
[ ] **2.** Bronzed skin
[ ] **3.** Occurrence of or worsened acne
[ ] **4.** Brittle nails

97. Which of the following are behavioral effects of anabolic steroids?
[ ] **1.** Aggression and rage
[ ] **2.** Confusion and doubt
[ ] **3.** Anxiety and depression
[ ] **4.** Paranoia and suicidal ideation

After being suspended from the team for taking anabolic steroids, the teenager tells his mother, "I might as well be dead. My football career is over." The mother calls the physician's office asking for help.

98. What advice is most appropriate to give the mother at this time?
[ ] **1.** Tell her to disregard her son's behavior; he is behaving normally.
[ ] **2.** Advise her to tell her son to snap out of it; his life is not over.
[ ] **3.** Suggest transferring her son to another school.
[ ] **4.** Advise her to ask her son if he is having any thoughts of suicide.

The nurse advises the football player's mother about warning signs of suicide.

99. Which warning signs of suicide should the nurse include? Select all that apply.
[ ] **1.** Withdrawal
[ ] **2.** Apathy
[ ] **3.** Angry outbursts
[ ] **4.** Low standardized scores in reading and math
[ ] **5.** Delusions
[ ] **6.** Incoherent speech

100. Which behavior best indicates that the adolescent is at increased risk for suicide?
[ ] **1.** Disregarding family rules sometimes
[ ] **2.** Arguing with siblings
[ ] **3.** Letting his grade average drop from a 92 to 90
[ ] **4.** Depression over a recent breakup with a girlfriend

A 17-year-old girl has been dating a classmate secretly because the relationship is a constant source of parental conflict. She has also stopped attending church and started smoking cigarettes—something her parents strongly dislike—and she has had sexual intercourse. She has not had a menstrual period for 2 months.

101. When the teenager makes an appointment at a birth control clinic, which nursing attribute is most important to communicate during the initial meeting?
[ ] **1.** Efficiency
[ ] **2.** Intelligence
[ ] **3.** Sympathy
[ ] **4.** Acceptance

102. Which nursing action best conveys an interest in this client and her situation?
[ ] **1.** Making frequent eye contact with her
[ ] **2.** Providing her with free clinic literature
[ ] **3.** Writing down information the client provides
[ ] **4.** Avoiding long pauses between questions

As the adolescent talks with the clinic nurse, she reveals that her parents disapprove of her friends, ideas, and actions.

103. It is normal for adolescents to test previously accepted values in order to establish which need?
[ ] **1.** Ingenuity
[ ] **2.** Identity
[ ] **3.** Intuition
[ ] **4.** Insight

The receptionist calls the nurse out of the room and tells her that the teenager's mother is on the phone, demanding to know why her daughter is being seen.

104. After conferring with the nurse, which response by the receptionist to the mother is most appropriate at this time?

[ ] **1.** "The clinic cannot release that information."
[ ] **2.** "Your daughter will return the phone call shortly."
[ ] **3.** "You may talk to your daughter after her examination."
[ ] **4.** "Your daughter came to the clinic for birth control."

A pregnancy test is performed before a method of birth control is prescribed for the adolescent client. The test result is positive.

105. After receiving the news about her pregnancy, which of the following is most beneficial to the pregnant adolescent at this time?
[ ] **1.** A positive mothering instinct
[ ] **2.** Making plans for marriage
[ ] **3.** Financial support from her boyfriend
[ ] **4.** Emotional support from her family

A nursing assistant asks the nurse why the pregnant adolescent asked for contraceptive assistance when she probably suspected she was pregnant already.

106. The nurse correctly explains that this client's behavior is an example of which psychological defense mechanism?
[ ] **1.** Displacement
[ ] **2.** Regression
[ ] **3.** Denial
[ ] **4.** Compensation

The parents of an 18-year-old bring their daughter to a mental health clinic after she reports hearing voices that tell her she is a bad person.

107. When the parents ask if their daughter is psychotic, the nurse who is performing the initial interview is most correct in explaining which as a behavior psychotic people exhibit?
[ ] **1.** They adjust poorly to new situations.
[ ] **2.** They have difficulty in relationships.
[ ] **3.** They cannot differentiate reality from unreality.
[ ] **4.** They feel helpless in resolving problems.

108. When performing a brief check of the client's mental status, which question is most appropriate for assessing her orientation?
[ ] **1.** "What is today's date?"
[ ] **2.** "How did you get here?"
[ ] **3.** "Where were you born?"
[ ] **4.** "Who is the president of the United States?"

As the nurse is documenting in her notes, the hallucinating client asks to read what she is writing.

109. Which nursing action is most appropriate in this situation?
[ ] **1.** Asking the client why she is so suspicious
[ ] **2.** Putting the notes away
[ ] **3.** Handing the client the form to read
[ ] **4.** Telling the client that it is illegal for her to read her client record

The 18-year-old client refuses to be admitted to the psychiatric unit of the local hospital.

110. Which statement regarding hospital admittance is most accurate?
[ ] **1.** The client cannot be committed involuntarily unless she is uncooperative at this time.
[ ] **2.** The client cannot be committed involuntarily unless she poses harm to herself or others.
[ ] **3.** The client cannot be committed involuntarily unless she does not keep office appointments.
[ ] **4.** The client cannot be committed involuntarily unless she refuses to take medications.

The psychiatrist prescribes the antipsychotic drug haloperidol (Haldol) for this client.

111. Which nursing instruction is most appropriate when teaching a client who self-administers haloperidol (Haldol)?
[ ] **1.** Take the pills on an empty stomach.
[ ] **2.** Do not skip meals while taking the drug.
[ ] **3.** Stop taking the drug if sedation occurs.
[ ] **4.** Rise slowly from a sitting position.

112. Which is the best indication that haloperidol (Haldol) is achieving a therapeutic effect?
[ ] **1.** The client no longer hears voices.
[ ] **2.** The client sleeps more than before.
[ ] **3.** The client thinks of herself as a good person.
[ ] **4.** The client feels more energetic and rested.

113. When the client calls the nurse to report the following physical changes, which symptom is considered a serious side effect of haloperidol (Haldol) that needs to be reported immediately to the prescribing physician?
[ ] **1.** Frequent diarrhea
[ ] **2.** Severe sore throat
[ ] **3.** Gradual weight loss
[ ] **4.** Ringing of the ears

Correct Answers and Rationales

Mental Health Needs During Infancy

1. **1.** Verbalizing feelings is an appropriate step toward processing emotional trauma. Emphasizing the newborn's emotional normalcy regardless of his cognitive ability and referring the parents to agencies that provide early intervention would be appropriate eventually, after the parents have had time to react emotionally themselves. It would be inappropriate for the nurse to encourage the parents to seek institutionalization. Any decisions about how to care for their child should be left up to the parents.
   Client Needs Category—Psychosocial integrity
   Client Needs Subcategory—None

2. **2.** Reflecting is an effective communication technique that involves responding to both feelings and content verbalized. Reflecting requires empathic responses that facilitate further therapeutic interaction. Defensiveness (option 1) is a nontherapeutic communication technique that implies to the client that his feelings and actions are unnecessary and foolish. Asking a "why" question (option 3) demands an explanation from the client. This form of communication is nontherapeutic because most clients are not able to verbalize their rationales. Disagreeing (option 4) implies that the client has no right to feel as he does.
   Client Needs Category—Psychosocial integrity
   Client Needs Subcategory—None

3.

3. Denial
2. Anger
4. Bargaining
1. Depression
5. Acceptance

   Grieving is a highly individual experience based on one's coping mechanisms, life experiences, resources, and support system. Although the grieving process encompasses five stages and in many cases follows a progressive course, the parents who are coping with the loss of their "perfect" baby will need to work through the various stages of grief in their own particular order and on their own timeline.

Generally, the first stage of grief involves shock and disbelief, which results in denial. Denial is a coping mechanism that eases the anxiety and pain of the experience. During this stage, the parents ask, "Why me?" and require proof that something is wrong (such as needing to see laboratory values and X-rays). They may request second, third, or fourth opinions; they also may minimize the child's condition, making it seem less serious that it really is.

Anger, the second stage, is commonly directed at others (such as the other spouse, baby, health care provider, or hospital services). The parents may verbalize the unfairness of the situation. They may even express their anger by focusing on inconsequential things such as the light being too bright.

During the bargaining stage (typically the third stage), the parents try to correct their actions and bargain with God or a higher power. They promise to be a better spouse or parent and attempt to fix the problem.

Depression, the fourth stage of grieving, is commonly manifested by crying. The parents feel sad and alone and begin planning how to tell their family or friends. Acceptance, the last stage of the grieving process, is characterized by the parents' ability to make plans for their child's future; they may also return to work or their normal routine during this stage.
   Client Needs Category—Psychosocial integrity
   Client Needs Subcategory—None

4. **1.** Evidence of bonding includes eye contact, skin contact, touching and stroking, smiling and talking to the infant, and cuddling. Other evidence involves providing basic care, such as changing the baby's diaper and feeding him. The other behaviors are normal and appropriate, but they are not the best evidence of bonding.
   Client Needs Category—Health promotion and maintenance
   Client Needs Subcategory—None

5. **4.** Allowing the mother to provide basic care promotes bonding. A mother's self-concept and self-confidence are increased when the nurse offers supportive encouragement. Interfering with parenting skills contributes to the mother's feelings of insecurity and decreases her confidence.
   Client Needs Category—Psychosocial integrity
   Client Needs Subcategory—None

6. **3.** A small head, upward-slanting eyes, protruding tongue, curved little finger, round face, flat nose, and simian crease on the palms are characteristic of the physical features of someone with Down syndrome.
   Client Needs Category—Physiological integrity
   Client Needs Subcategory—Physiological adaptation

7. 3. Withdrawal from heroin and other abused drugs, whether in a newborn or an adult, is characterized by symptoms somewhat opposite of the drug's action. For example, in heroin withdrawal, newborns are typically hyperactive and irritable, they cry constantly, and they are unable to be consoled. These particular symptoms place the infant at high risk for child abuse. They are also poor feeders, putting them at risk for failure to thrive.

Client Needs Category—*Physiological integrity*
Client Needs Subcategory—*Physiological adaptation*

8. 1. Because opioid withdrawal is characterized by central nervous system stimulation, reducing environmental stimuli is a priority when caring for a newborn experiencing its effects. Touching and stroking increase tactile stimuli and are more appropriate when caring for normal newborns. Most infants, including those experiencing withdrawal, are comforted by being wrapped snugly in a blanket.

Client Needs Category—*Physiological integrity*
Client Needs Subcategory—*Physiological adaptation*

9. 2. Meeting an infant's need for love is one of the best foundations for future mental health, regardless of the child's physical or mental status. Love helps the child feel secure and helps him to build self-esteem and trust in others. The needs for autonomy, respect, and identity are also important, but they represent higher-level needs.

Client Needs Category—*Health promotion and maintenance*
Client Needs Subcategory—*None*

10. 1. Excessive crying is a manifestation of infantile anxiety. Severe anxiety leads to weight loss and stunted, slowed growth, commonly referred to as failure to thrive. Failure to thrive can occur from an unsatisfactory relationship with a caregiver. Listening to the heart and breath sounds and measuring the head and chest are appropriate, but they do not readily indicate how this child's growth compares with norms for infants her age. Assessing the sucking and grasp reflex is more appropriate for a newborn infant.

Client Needs Category—*Physiological integrity*
Client Needs Subcategory—*Physiological adaptation*

11. 1. A certain amount of crying is normal for an infant because it is the baby's only means of communicating distress. How the mother reacts to the baby's crying is important. Finding out her expectations helps the nurse determine whether the mother has a realistic perception of her infant's behavior. The other selections do not provide significant additional data needed to analyze the young mother's complaint.

Client Needs Category—*Health promotion and maintenance*
Client Needs Subcategory—*None*

12. 1. "Spoiling a baby" is a commonly used phrase that refers to the notion that frequent holding, cuddling, or immediately responding to an infant's cries ultimately promotes the infant's dependence on the caregiver. Such "spoiling" was previously viewed by many as a negative behavior that increased a baby's desire for attention; thus, infants were often allowed to cry. However, research has found that neglecting and isolating an infant promotes stress and affects normal development. Infants cannot develop negative effects from being held and touched in an affectionate manner, and they are extremely sensitive to the attitudes and actions of those caring for them. All humans, not just babies or toddlers, need physical and social contact with other humans for adequate nurturing.

Client Needs Category—*Health promotion and maintenance*
Client Needs Subcategory—*None*

13. 3. Touching and hearing a parent's voice are essential for optimal emotional growth during infancy. Receiving affectionate sensory stimulation helps the infant develop a feeling of trust, the major developmental task during infancy. Inanimate sensory stimulation is appropriate, but physical human interaction is a priority.

Client Needs Category—*Health promotion and maintenance*
Client Needs Subcategory—*None*

14. 4. People with expertise in successful child-rearing techniques teach parenting classes. Participants learn by imitating and modeling the behavior of others in the group. Group members support one another by sharing common experiences. Project Head Start is for preschool children. Planned Parenthood is concerned with family planning. Parent-teacher associations are for parents of school-age children.

Client Needs Category—*Health promotion and maintenance*
Client Needs Subcategory—*None*

15. 2. Mistrust is the characteristic most likely to develop if infants are not nurtured adequately. Such infants begin to view the world as unsafe and unreliable. The other characteristics—inferiority, doubt, and isolation—are negative attributes acquired at later stages of unfulfilled development.

Client Needs Category—*Health promotion and maintenance*
Client Needs Subcategory—*None*

16. **2, 3, 5.** Failure to thrive is a condition in which the infant falls below the third percentile for weight and length. There are two main reasons why this occurs: organic causes that result from congenital or other physiological problems, and nonorganic causes that result from poor maternal bonding and lack of parenting skills. Nonorganic causes are regarded as a form of child neglect. In some cases, failure to thrive results from a combination of both causes.

Typical characteristics of an infant who is diagnosed with failure to thrive include a delay in developmental milestones after about the third month and delayed understanding of speech related to the lack of interaction. These infants are typically pale and lethargic. They lack subcutaneous fat, making them thin and wrinkled, often with skin breakdown. They do not cry when handled, but instead stare intensely at people who approach. They are often poor feeders because they lack the strength to eat.

> ***Client Needs Category***—*Health promotion and maintenance*
> ***Client Needs Subcategory***—*None*

17. **1, 2, 3, 4, 5.** Several risk factors—all nonorganic causes—are known to lead to failure to thrive. Most are associated with an interruption in the maternal attachment process or inadequacy of parenting skills. These risks include an unplanned or unwanted pregnancy, maternal history of teenage pregnancy, alcohol or drug abuse, low socioeconomic status, and a father that is no longer available to provide support. The fact that the infant has several siblings is not necessarily a risk factor for failure to thrive.

> ***Client Needs Category***—*Health promotion and maintenance*
> ***Client Needs Subcategory***—*None*

Mental Health Needs During Childhood

18. **3.** A 2-year-old child typically uses at least single words like "no" and "me" to make his ideas understood. Therefore, the absence of language skills would suggest a developmental delay. The other behaviors do not necessarily indicate delayed development. Most children begin drinking from a glass and toilet-training at this stage of development. The ability to draw a picture depends on the development of fine motor skills, which typically begins as a toddler with scribbling and is refined as the child grows older and is able to draw simple figures and pictures.

> ***Client Needs Category***—*Health promotion and maintenance*
> ***Client Needs Subcategory***—*None*

19. **1.** The Denver II Developmental Screening Test measures four major areas of development and can identify developmental delays from infancy through preschool ages. The SAT is administered to high school students and estimates academic success. The Stanford-Binet test is an IQ (intelligence) test. Weber's test is used for conducting hearing assessments.

> ***Client Needs Category***—*Health promotion and maintenance*
> ***Client Needs Subcategory***—*None*

20. **2.** Demonstrating disapproval immediately after unacceptable behavior helps the child associate the undesirable behavior with negative consequences. This approach takes time and consistent reinforcement, but it is the most appropriate form of discipline for a toddler. Toddlers are too young to control their impulses just by identifying potential consequences or receiving explanations for behavioral expectations. Physical punishment tends to teach impressionable youngsters that it is appropriate to be physically violent.

> ***Client Needs Category***—*Health promotion and maintenance*
> ***Client Needs Subcategory***—*None*

21. **3.** To exercise autonomy, toddlers often become defiant and refuse to cooperate with requests, routines, and regulations. At this time, the toddler does not understand the need to abide by rules and requests outside of his or her wants. This often frustrates parents who are trying to guide the toddler. The psychosocial characteristics of integrity, identity, and generativity are acquired at later stages of development.

> ***Client Needs Category***—*Health promotion and maintenance*
> ***Client Needs Subcategory***—*None*

22. **1.** To avoid a power struggle, it is best to give the child an opportunity to choose between two acceptable alternatives. Withholding something desirable is not likely to meet with success because a child of this age tends to be quite oppositional when challenged. The child is too young to comprehend abstract explanations. Threatening the child is not a therapeutic approach to gain cooperation.

> ***Client Needs Category***—*Health promotion and maintenance*
> ***Client Needs Subcategory***—*None*

23. **3.** A parent causing physical symptoms in a dependent child is characteristic of Munchausen syndrome by proxy. Consequently, the victim (typically a young child) is subjected to a variety of unnecessary medical procedures. The parent's sole purpose in intentionally producing an illness in a dependent child is to draw attention to herself for the pain or work associated with caring for an ill child. This condition is considered a form of child abuse and must be reported to the authorities.

> *Client Needs Category*—*Psychosocial integrity*
> *Client Needs Subcategory*—*None*

24. 3. Having one or both parents within sight and touch helps to prevent separation anxiety and provides one of the best coping strategies for dealing with the pain and suffering that the child may experience. The other options listed have secondary therapeutic value.

> *Client Needs Category*—*Health promotion and maintenance*
> *Client Needs Subcategory*—*None*

25. 2. Regressive behavior such as thumb sucking is considered a coping mechanism that relieves anxiety. Given the child's circumstances and behavioral observations among others who have experienced stressful situations, this is the most credible explanation among the given options for the phenomenon.

> *Client Needs Category*—*Health promotion and maintenance*
> *Client Needs Subcategory*—*None*

26. 3. Handling equipment whenever possible helps children overcome some of their initial fears. It is important to be honest with children when procedures involve pain. However, the term "minimal" is relative; from the child's perspective, the pain may be more than minimal. Bribing a child by offering a reward is not a therapeutic means of gaining cooperation. Seeing others who have I.V. lines will not necessarily diminish the child's unique feelings and expectations concerning the upcoming procedure.

> *Client Needs Category*—*Psychosocial integrity*
> *Client Needs Subcategory*—*None*

27. 4. The toddler who is ignoring his parents is practicing a form of detachment, the third stage in typical hospital adjustment. This stage represents the most severe reaction that can occur in a toddler who is hospitalized for a prolonged time. All the remaining options characterize the initial (protest) stage of hospital adjustment. The second (despair) stage is characterized by apathy and withdrawal.

> *Client Needs Category*—*Psychosocial integrity*
> *Client Needs Subcategory*—*None*

28. 2. Hair of varying lengths or bald areas may be attributed to pulling on the child's hair during abusive acts. The nurse who finds this during a physical assessment should suspect child abuse. A 2-year-old child is typically very curious and clumsy. It is not unusual to find bruises and abrasions over bony prominences (such as elbows and knees) sustained during falls. However, a bruise over soft tissue such as the abdomen should arouse suspicion. It is also not unusual for a toddler to protest when approached by a health care provider, especially if past experiences with health care providers have been unpleasant.

> *Client Needs Category*—*Psychosocial integrity*
> *Client Needs Subcategory*—*None*

29. 1. One classic sign of physical abuse is evidence of scars, bruises, and fractures in various stages of healing. Being underweight and not fully immunized may raise suspicions of neglect or that the family is financially needy; however, these findings alone do not strongly suggest abuse. Injuries can occur without an adult witness.

> *Client Needs Category*—*Psychosocial integrity*
> *Client Needs Subcategory*—*None*

30. 1, 2, 4, 5, 6. Any sexual activity between a child under 18 years old and an adult is classified as sexual abuse. Signs of sexual abuse include demonstrating sexual acts on a doll or other toy, having a sexually transmitted disease (such as gonorrhea), being afraid to be left alone with the perpetrator, or difficulty sleeping (or napping). Other signs of sexual abuse include discussing sexual acts with heightened awareness and vocabulary for the child's age; pregnancy younger than age 15; vaginal or anal tearing; perineal, anal, or vaginal inflammation; symptoms of increased anxiety, such as tics, stuttering, or nail biting; and poor school performance. Burning upon urination, especially in young girls, may be a sign of a urinary tract infection; this is not uncommon in toddlers and preschoolers due to poor hygiene and wiping techniques during toileting. However, it does require further investigation because it may be related to a sexually transmitted disease or sexual abuse. Being underweight may be a sign of neglect, not sexual abuse.

> *Client Needs Category*—*Psychosocial integrity*
> *Client Needs Subcategory*—*None*

31. 2. The nurse should position herself at a young child's level, regardless of the reason for interaction, to reduce the child's risk of feeling threatened. Prolonged eye contact tends to heighten anxiety. Victims of child abuse often protect their abusers. Therefore, separating the child from her mother and asking direct questions are not appropriate strategies; they also do not promote a positive nurse-client relationship.

> *Client Needs Category*—*Psychosocial integrity*
> *Client Needs Subcategory*—*None*

32. 3. Commonly, child abusers have been victims of child abuse. Although there are significant stressors for persons raised by a single parent or who are not financially secure, these factors are not uniquely contributory to child abuse. Parents who abuse their children are more often young and immature when the violence begins.

Client Needs Category—*Psychosocial integrity*
Client Needs Subcategory—*None*

33. 4. Nurses are among those required by law to report suspected child abuse. Not reporting suspected child abuse is considered a crime. The child protective services agency is responsible for finding a temporary and safe environment such as foster care for the child in future danger. Parents Anonymous is an organization that provides support to those who wish to break the cycle of child abuse. However, the priority at this time is the child's safety.

Client Needs Category—*Safe, effective care environment*
Client Needs Subcategory—*Safety and infection control*

34. 4. Perpetrators of child abuse, as well as those with other social problems, are more likely to be receptive to seeking help if the nurse conveys a nonjudgmental attitude during the interaction. The other options are not necessarily inappropriate, but they are unlikely to motivate clients toward self-help.

Client Needs Category—*Psychosocial integrity*
Client Needs Subcategory—*None*

35. 4. Giving the child permission to masturbate privately sets limits as to where this is done but does not imply that masturbation is a deviant behavior. Interrupting the practice or providing the child with another alternative may temporarily stop the activity; however, the child would not understand the purpose of the diversion. The other choices imply that experiencing pleasure from touching one's body is objectionable.

Client Needs Category—*Health promotion and maintenance*
Client Needs Subcategory—*None*

36. 3. Feeding a doll (or changing the doll's diaper or clothes) is most suggestive of the identification process. Identification is behavior that imitates the same-sex parent or other adult. The other behaviors are examples of the child's cognitive development.

Client Needs Category—*Health promotion and maintenance*
Client Needs Subcategory—*None*

37. 4. A preschooler who is not accustomed to sharing attention may feel that the new child is taking his place. He may behave like an infant to regain attention, or he may resort to behavior manifested during an earlier period of development (such as wetting and soiling himself) to feel more secure. It is normal for a 4-year-

old child to begin identifying with and imitating the same-sex parent (such as trying to use his father's tools). Preschoolers begin to need less daytime sleep. At this age, crying is a natural emotional response to disappointing events.

Client Needs Category—*Health promotion and maintenance*
Client Needs Subcategory—*None*

38. 2. Anxiety occurs when a person perceives he is in a threatening situation. The perceived threat creates a feeling of insecurity. Mental mechanisms such as regression are unconsciously or subconsciously used to eliminate or reduce conflict, protect one's self-image, and resolve an emotional dilemma.

Client Needs Category—*Health promotion and maintenance*
Client Needs Subcategory—*None*

39. 4. Anxiety that results from competing for attention is diminished if the parent spends time alone with the child. The other options are appropriate, but they wll not necessarily relieve the child's anxiety.

Client Needs Category—*Health promotion and maintenance*
Client Needs Subcategory—*None*

40. 1. A school-age child must learn to follow directions and carry out a task. Therefore, providing the preschooler with tasks within his level of accomplishment promotes success and a positive feeling about his own competence. Printing the first name may be beneficial, but printing both first and last names is a skill not usually accomplished by 4-year-olds. A preschooler usually has no immediate use for flash cards that teach addition. This skill is typically reserved for 7- to 8-year-old children in first and second grades. Daytime television programs are not necessarily educational.

Client Needs Category—*Health promotion and maintenance*
Client Needs Subcategory—*None*

41. 2. Children learn how to manipulate others through certain types of behavior. When a child realizes that a tantrum will not obtain the desired result, the child will most likely discontinue that behavior. Therefore, ignoring behavior is the best choice. Giving candy beforehand contradicts the principle that candy is not allowed at this time. A young child is more likely to behave based on his emotions rather than intellectual logic. Therefore, the preschool child is not likely to accept an explanation about the inappropriateness of his behavior or pleas to act differently.

Client Needs Category—*Health promotion and maintenance*
Client Needs Subcategory—*None*

42. 1. Autism is a psychiatric condition with no known cause. More common among boys, this disorder is characterized by unawareness of external reality, limited or no social interaction, abnormal speech patterns and conversational ability, preoccupation with repetitive behaviors, and a low range of interest in self or others. Autistic children tend to display bizarre body movements. For example, they rock their bodies, bang their heads, or touch their hands to their faces in peculiar mannerisms. If these movements are interrupted, violent temper tantrums may result. None of the other items describes characteristics of autism.
    Client Needs Category—*Physiological integrity*
    Client Needs Subcategory—*Physiological adaptation*

43. 2. Autistic children are prone to repetitive body movements such as continuous hand clapping. If the behavior is interrupted, they often act impulsively, becoming aggressive and causing self-injury. Therefore, they commonly demonstrate insensitivity to pain. Mental retardation is common; diagnosis depends on the clinical presentation and the child's inability to reach developmental milestones. Because of their abnormal speech patterns and inability to communicate effectively, autistic children rarely use the words "I" and "me." Autistic children are also inflexible (not flexible) with normal routines, and they show little to no interest in the actions of others.
    Client Needs Category—*Psychosocial integrity*
    Client Needs Subcategory—*None*

44. 3. A consistent caregiver or primary nurse facilitates development of a trusting relationship. Autistic children have a limited ability to interact with others. Restraints are inappropriate to use on a continual basis because they increase the risk of injury; close supervision is preferred. Rocking is inappropriate because autistic children do not easily tolerate physical contact.
    Client Needs Category—*Psychosocial integrity*
    Client Needs Subcategory—*None*

45. 1. The characteristics of autism are divided into three categories: inability to relate to others, inability to communicate with others, and limited activities and interests. Autistic children tend to show little or no ability to relate to other humans, including their parents. All the remaining examples require interaction with and response to one or more people. This is unrealistic for a child with autism.
    Client Needs Category—*Psychosocial integrity*
    Client Needs Subcategory—*None*

46. 4. One common behavior among autistic children is a tendency to cause self-harm by head banging, biting, and pulling out hair and fingernails. An autistic child is incapable of, or not responsible for, maintaining his own health. Self-esteem is established on the basis of receiving approval or disapproval from others. Because an autistic child is indifferent to the physical presence and opinion of others, low self-esteem is not likely to be a problem. An autistic child's general physical health is unaffected by his mental disorder. Therefore, if the child cannot tolerate activity, it is due to another, unrelated condition.
    Client Needs Category—*Safe, effective care environment*
    Client Needs Subcategory—*Safety and infection control*

47. 1. Children with autism have varying levels of impairment and require full assistance with some or all activities of daily living. When the child demonstrates an attempt at self-feeding, it is appropriate to encourage him to participate in this aspect of self-care. Learning takes place when a person is ready. Until an autistic child demonstrates some interest, attempts to gain his cooperation are likely to be frustrating for the child and the parent.
    Client Needs Category—*Physiological integrity*
    Client Needs Subcategory—*Basic care and comfort*

48. 3. Rewards, even in the form of praise, tend to promote repetition of a desired behavior. Noting whether the behavior is repeated is appropriate, but it is not the best technique to use first. It would be unrealistic to expect the child to continue self-feeding after only one attempt. Giving the child more food does not necessarily encourage self-feeding behavior; if it does, obesity is a possible consequence.
    Client Needs Category—*Health promotion and maintenance*
    Client Needs Subcategory—*None*

49. 2. If an autistic child's possessions, routines, or environment are altered, he is likely to become upset and combative toward others or himself. A stimulating environment creates chaos and distress for an autistic child. A flexible environment with no routines causes anxiety; the child cannot appreciate choices within the flexibility. Limit setting is important, but a rigid, inflexible atmosphere can be distressing.
    Client Needs Category—*Psychosocial integrity*
    Client Needs Subcategory—*None*

50. 4. Private home health care agencies employ various levels of health practitioners. An agency of this type selects the surrogate caregiver most appropriate for the type of client and level of care needed. Aid to Dependent Children is a social welfare agency that provides economic assistance to a parent who is unable to financially support the care of one or more children. The Association on Mental Deficiency is concerned with people who are mentally retarded, not mentally ill. Mental

retardation usually begins in childhood and is characterized by a deficit in intellect and motor and adaptive skills. Autism, however, is a psychiatric (mental) illness with no known cause. *Mental illness* is a term that describes a broad range of mental and emotional conditions. Most day-care facilities do not provide evening care and might not accept a child with special needs.
> ***Client Needs Category**—Safe, effective care environment*
> ***Client Needs Subcategory**—Coordinated care*

51. 2. Children between the ages of 6 and 11 are acquiring industry, which is characterized by learning to work beside and cooperatively with others. They learn to accept success and defeat, and how to give support to others. The other characteristics are associated with later stages of development.
> ***Client Needs Category**—Health promotion and maintenance*
> ***Client Needs Subcategory**—None*

52. 2. Methylphenidate hydrochloride (Ritalin) is a central nervous system stimulant that acts primarily on the cerebral cortex. The drug decreases hyperactivity and impulsiveness and appears to act in a manner similar to amphetamines. Methyphenidate hydrochloride (Ritalin) is effective in 70% to 80% of children.
> ***Client Needs Category**—Physiological integrity*
> ***Client Needs Subcategory**—Pharmacological therapies*

53. 2. Some of the chief characteristics of ADHD include distractibility, difficulty following directions, inability to remain focused on a task, and difficulty sustaining attention. Relief of these symptoms indicates a therapeutic response. Although methylphenidate hydrochloride (Ritalin) is a central nervous system stimulant, it should not cause a child to be more alert, active, or less fatigued than he was before treatment with the drug. In fact, overstimulation indicates a nontherapeutic or adverse response to the drug. Methylphenidate hydrochloride (Ritalin) may cause a child to be less irritable and aggressive, but altering mood is not the primary reason for administering this drug.
> ***Client Needs Category**—Physiological integrity*
> ***Client Needs Subcategory**—Pharmacological therapies*

54. 3. Because methylphenidate hydrochloride (Ritalin) is a central nervous system stimulant, side effects reflect overstimulation as evidenced by insomnia, tachycardia, and anorexia. Some people experience an intense degree of these symptoms, even with low dosages. The remaining choices are not associated with this particular drug.
> ***Client Needs Category**—Physiological integrity*
> ***Client Needs Subcategory**—Pharmacological therapies*

55. 3. Common undesirable side effects of methylphenidate hydrochloride (Ritalin) include tachycardia, hypertension, nervousness, sleep disturbances, and decreased growth rate. Food intolerances, altered elimination patterns, and altered skin integrity are not associated with this drug.
> ***Client Needs Category**—Physiological integrity*
> ***Client Needs Subcategory**—Pharmacological therapies*

56. 2. Caffeine is present in 75% of all soft drinks. It is an ingredient in all cola products, except those labeled caffeine-free. Caffeine is a stimulating drug that contributes to overstimulation in a child who is taking methylphenidate hydrochloride (Ritalin).
> ***Client Needs Category**—Health promotion and maintenance*
> ***Client Needs Subcategory**—None*

57. 3. School-age children tend to view disease and its treatment as a form of punishment, even though they cannot identify the transgression. They have anxiety related to the hospitalization and often perceive parental anxiety. Although school-age children consider adults quite powerful, they are aware that serious illnesses have unpredictable outcomes.
> ***Client Needs Category**—Health promotion and maintenance*
> ***Client Needs Subcategory**—None*

58. 1. School-age children tend to fantasize and exaggerate a potentially unpleasant experience. Therefore, it is best to avoid providing information far in advance. However, the child may be totally unprepared if the teaching is postponed until questions are asked or if the nurse assumes that the physician will provide all the information the child needs to know.
> ***Client Needs Category**—Psychosocial integrity*
> ***Client Needs Subcategory**—None*

59. 4. Most children are primarily concerned with how they will be affected by a diagnostic test, procedure, or medical treatment. The nurse must provide honest information and support the child through the procedure. The other information is secondary to this.
> ***Client Needs Category**—Psychosocial integrity*
> ***Client Needs Subcategory**—None*

60. 2. Although all the reasons for discussing the prognosis with the dying child are basically true, the best rationale for encouraging open communication is that it facilitates coping and emotional support for both the child and her family while they prepare for the child's inevitable death. Families who have left something unsaid often feel guilt and remorse.
> ***Client Needs Category**—Psychosocial integrity*
> ***Client Needs Subcategory**—None*

61. 1. Providing an ill child with honest explanations about the nature of her condition and upcoming procedures or treatments promotes confidence and trust in caregivers, especially when the reality of the experience is congruent with the teaching. The other characteristics may be acquired, but not as a consequence of an honest nurse-client relationship.
>**Client Needs Category**—*Psychosocial integrity*
>**Client Needs Subcategory**—*None*

62. 1. Setting achievable goals allows the child the potential for success. Success instills a sense of pride in accomplishment and motivation for improvement. The other suggestions are not inappropriate; however, they are not the best techniques for supporting the child's self-esteem.
>**Client Needs Category**—*Psychosocial integrity*
>**Client Needs Subcategory**—*None*

63. 2. Privacy is an essential component of a therapeutic environment. Selecting a location where the person cannot be observed or overheard by others facilitates open communication and a therapeutic relationship.
>**Client Needs Category**—*Psychosocial integrity*
>**Client Needs Subcategory**—*None*

64. 1. In addition to the death of a parent, divorce is one of the most disruptive events a child can experience. Changes in family structure jeopardize a child's sense of security. Acting out is a behavioral manifestation of conflict. The death of a pet turtle, acquiring a paper route, and confusion about a crush on a girl are situations that do not match the manifested behavior. Although these incidences may be stressful to the child, they would not have as intense an emotional impact as parental divorce.
>**Client Needs Category**—*Health promotion and maintenance*
>**Client Needs Subcategory**—*None*

65. 4. Discipline delivered immediately, fairly, and consistently helps a child understand the limits of acceptable and unacceptable behavior. Anxious people need reassurance that someone will enforce limitations if they are unable to remain in control. Sending the child to the principal indicates that the teacher is evading personal responsibility for controlling classroom behavior. Suspension isolates the child from any helpful resource and is likely to contribute to continued low academic performance. Sending the child to the counselor on a daily basis is premature and too severe for the behavior manifested at this time. However, the counselor should be informed of the student's behavior and his home situation.
>**Client Needs Category**—*Psychosocial integrity*
>**Client Needs Subcategory**—*None*

66. 3. The oldest child in a family tends to be one who conforms to the expectations of adults and who is more affected by criticism, more responsible, and more behaviorally rigid. The youngest child is likely to be less tolerant of frustration and more dependent on others. Middle children are more flexible and independent.
>**Client Needs Category**—*Health promotion and maintenance*
>**Client Needs Subcategory**—*None*

67. 2. Making angry remarks suggests that this child is demonstrating displacement. Displacement is a psychological defense mechanism in which a person releases feelings onto someone or something else other than the true object of the anger, which in this case is the illness. The other behaviors are more indicative of normal behavior for a child this age, especially one whose usual routine is unstructured due to unusual circumstances.
>**Client Needs Category**—*Psychosocial integrity*
>**Client Needs Subcategory**—*None*

68. 3. Taking an active role in one's care is the most effective way to acquire a sense of control over a disease. Thus, actually performing self-testing of blood glucose levels is therapeutic. The other activities are important, but less effective in promoting a sense of control.
>**Client Needs Category**—*Psychosocial integrity*
>**Client Needs Subcategory**—*None*

69. 1. Tourette syndrome is a genetic disorder that begins manifesting at about age 7. More common among boys, the disorder causes the child to suffer from various tics (rapid, repetitive movements), including vocal tics (repeated use of words or phrases, coughing, barking, snorting, or throat clearing) and motor tics (such as eye movements, neck jerking, facial grimacing, jumping, and touching). Those with Tourette syndrome tend to utter verbal obscenities or other socially unacceptable words (coprolalia) and make other vocal sounds embarrassing to all concerned. The bizarre activities, which are difficult to control, tend to make the client an object of ridicule or avoidance by those unfamiliar with the condition. If other symptoms in the remaining options occur, they are secondary to the diagnosis or unique to the client.
>**Client Needs Category**—*Psychosocial integrity*
>**Client Needs Subcategory**—*None*

70. 1. Antipsychotic drugs such as haloperidol (Haldol) cause a cluster of side effects known as extrapyramidal symptoms. Parkinsonianlike tremors and sudden strong muscle spasms, especially relating to the neck, are two types of these symptoms. Muscle weakness, muscle atrophy, and muscle contracture are not common symptoms.

> ***Client Needs Category***—*Physiological integrity*
> ***Client Needs Subcategory***—*Pharmacological therapies*

71. 2. Self-esteem develops as a consequence of experiencing deserved praise from people the child respects. Positive reinforcement is preferable to focusing on negative behavior. Praise is considered a far healthier approach than sheltering and protecting the child physically or emotionally from peers.

> ***Client Needs Category***—*Psychosocial integrity*
> ***Client Needs Subcategory***—*None*

Mental Health Needs During Adolescence

72. 3. The best outcomes are obtained when crisis intervention is initiated immediately after the precipitating event. Although crises tend to become resolved even without professional support, the outcomes are less than optimal as time passes.

> ***Client Needs Category***—*Psychosocial integrity*
> ***Client Needs Subcategory***—*None*

73. 1. Most people who experience a crisis have an overwhelming feeling of helplessness. This feeling is a direct consequence of having inadequate coping strategies. The other emotional responses may occur among some individuals, but they are not characteristic of the majority of individuals experiencing crises.

> ***Client Needs Category***—*Psychosocial integrity*
> ***Client Needs Subcategory***—*None*

74. 2. The first step toward resolving a crisis is to have survivors process the event from their perspective. Some individuals require professional counseling, but most do not if crisis intervention is initiated soon after the event. Reassuring survivors that they will adapt may be appropriate, but it is not the most important action to take initially. Drug therapy in the form of minor tranquilizers is usually unnecessary; also, tranquilizing may be detrimental because it tends to interfere with processing the reality of the crisis.

> ***Client Needs Category***—*Psychosocial integrity*
> ***Client Needs Subcategory***—*None*

75. 2. Bulimia is a mental illness that is characterized by a preoccupation with food and body weight. Bulimics control their weight by a cycle of purging after eating binges. The disorder is more common among female adolescents and young adults (in their twenties). Most bulimic clients experience a period of depression or guilt after binging on large quantities of high-calorie foods. Because consuming such large amounts causes abdominal distention and pain, the bulimic client typically vomits to lessen the discomfort. Deterioration of

dental structures and erosion of tooth enamel results from repeated contact between gastric acid and teeth from self-induced vomiting. Bulimic clients usually maintain a normal weight. Anorectic clients are more likely to cease menstruating when their body fat is depleted. Loss of hair is also correlated more with the malnutrition of anorexia nervosa.

> ***Client Needs Category***—*Psychosocial integrity*
> ***Client Needs Subcategory***—*None*

76. 1. Anorexia nervosa is a mental illness characterized by preoccupation with food, body weight, and extreme weight loss caused by fasting or excessive exercise. Anorexia nervosa usually occurs in young women between ages 13 and 20 and is more common in families who have already had an occurrence of the disorder. Low self-esteem and a distorted body image are major characteristics of the illness. Clients with anorexia nervosa commonly manifest lanugo, a growth of fine downy hair similar to that of newborn infants. It is thought that this occurs to promote or maintain normal body temperature in people who have little or no body fat. Bruises may indicate a vitamin deficiency, but they would not be limited to the upper torso. Generally, bowel sounds are normal in anorectic clients. Clubbing of the fingers is characteristic of conditions causing chronic hypoxia.

> ***Client Needs Category***—*Psychosocial integrity*
> ***Client Needs Subcategory***—*None*

77. 4. The distinguishing clinical difference between anorexia nervosa and bulimia is binge eating. Adolescents with bulimia often binge and then purge what they have eaten. Both anorexia nervosa and bulimia disorders have similar symptoms of body image distortion, purging following meals, and decreased self-esteem.

> ***Client Needs Category***—*Psychosocial integrity*
> ***Client Needs Subcategory***—*None*

78. 2. Generally, anorectic clients are characterized as being "perfect" children with above-average scholastic achievement, perhaps due to a fear of failure. They often adhere to a strict program of exercise and are ritualistic in their behaviors. None of the other characteristics listed are unique to clients with anorexia nervosa.

> ***Client Needs Category***—*Psychosocial integrity*
> ***Client Needs Subcategory***—*None*

79. 3. Initial treatment of a client with anorexia nervosa focuses on meeting physiological needs. When nutrients, fluids, vitamins, and electrolytes are administered, attention shifts to the client's psychosocial problems.

> ***Client Needs Category***—*Physiological integrity*
> ***Client Needs Subcategory***—*Physiological adaptation*

80. 3. Validation is a therapeutic communication technique in which the nurse interprets what is perceived to be the underlying meaning of the words. If the interpretation is correct, it increases rapport and forms a basis for future collaboration. The techniques of generalizing, giving advice, and responding with a stereotypical statement are examples of nontherapeutic ways of communicating.

Client Needs Category—*Psychosocial integrity*
Client Needs Subcategory—*None*

81. 4. Controlling the desire to eat is a nonverbal technique that the anorectic client uses to demonstrate power and control. Getting attention as a result of this behavior reinforces its effectiveness. Consequently, the most appropriate way to handle this situation is to simply remove the food without making any comments. Until a client's malnutrition becomes life-threatening, forced feeding is unethical and inappropriate. Recording intake is not an incentive for eating. The fear of becoming fat is often greater than a prior commitment to collaborated goals.

Client Needs Category—*Psychosocial integrity*
Client Needs Subcategory—*None*

82. 2. Confrontation is an effective therapeutic communication technique that allows the nurse to point out differences between an expected behavior and the actual action. Postponing weighing is likely to result in more accurate assessment data. However, this choice of action—as well as saying nothing or subtracting 2 lb from the client's weight—avoids the greater issue of dealing with the behavior.

Client Needs Category—*Psychosocial integrity*
Client Needs Subcategory—*None*

83. 1. Separation anxiety is a common response when a developmentally disabled client experiences a change in caretakers in an unfamiliar environment. Pain is a subjective experience; it is erroneous to assume that a client who is developmentally disabled will respond any differently to pain than others with normal intelligence. An adolescent with this cognitive capacity should be able to communicate his basic needs despite his disability. An adolescent with normal cognitive ability is typically concerned about changes in body image; however, such concerns are unlikely for someone at this developmental level.

Client Needs Category—*Psychosocial integrity*
Client Needs Subcategory—*None*

84. 1. Assuming responsibility for skills that can be performed independently, such as dressing and undressing, tends to interfere with the ability to achieve maximum levels of self-care. It is normal for a parent to be the medical historian for nonadult children. Self-blame and exaggerating the child's abilities are indica-

tions that the mother is not coping well with the child's condition.

Client Needs Category—*Psychosocial integrity*
Client Needs Subcategory—*None*

85. 2. The client's aggressive response is a defensive reaction not unlike that displayed by younger children who perceive themselves to be in threatening situations. Stating that all mentally retarded people are physically aggressive is an overgeneralization. One incidence of physically lashing out is not sufficient to conclude that the client has a poor opinion of his care. Children commonly demonstrate that they are in pain by crying or moaning, not by being aggressive.

Client Needs Category—*Psychosocial integrity*
Client Needs Subcategory—*None*

86. 3. The nurse should take care to document facts, not opinions. Although stating that the nursing assistant was struck while helping the client out of bed requires more elaboration, it is more appropriate than the other choices. Stating that the aggression was a consequence of feeling angry or that the act was spontaneous is inaccurate. The word "attacked" is an emotionally charged term that suggests more violence than actually occurred.

Client Needs Category—*Safe, effective care environment*
Client Needs Subcategory—*Coordinated care*

87. 3. To avoid any misperceptions, it is best to offer explanations before physically touching the client. Entering the client's personal space without warning may be interpreted as a threatening act. Restraints are unjustified in this situation. The mother should not be asked to assume total responsibility for caring for her son. Medicating the client with an analgesic is justified if the client experiences pain, but it is best to administer it at least 20 to 30 minutes before an activity.

Client Needs Category—*Psychosocial integrity*
Client Needs Subcategory—*None*

88. 1. The adolescent's attitudes and behavior are influenced much more by peers than by school, religion, or employment—although all these affect the dynamics of each individual.

Client Needs Category—*Psychosocial integrity*
Client Needs Subcategory—*None*

89. 1. Inconsistency in setting limits or imposing consequences when limits are violated weaken an adolescent's ability to recognize boundaries for behavior. Discipline provides security even if restrictions are not appreciated at the time. Siblings, social status, and role models influence the teen but are not the strongest influence.

Client Needs Category—Psychosocial integrity
Client Needs Subcategory—None

90. 4. Reassuring clients that the information they divulge will remain confidential is perhaps the most important concept to emphasize. Most therapy meetings are scheduled on a day and time that repeats on a regular basis. It is understood that someone who leads a group is qualified to do so. Using first names is common, but indicating that this is a practice to follow is less important than stressing confidentiality.

Client Needs Category—Psychosocial integrity
Client Needs Subcategory—None

91. 3. Persistently checking a wristwatch is a nonverbal way of saying that one would rather be someplace else or that the therapy session should be over soon. Such nonverbal behaviors suggest that no value is being obtained from the session. Borrowing cigarettes demonstrates irresponsibility. Laughing inappropriately suggests insensitivity. Fidgeting is a sign of anxiety.

Client Needs Category—Psychosocial integrity
Client Needs Subcategory—None

92. 1. Children who have grown up with an alcoholic parent commonly have a problem with low self-esteem. Other dysfunctional attributes include an inability to trust, an extreme need to control, an excessive sense of responsibility, and a denial of feelings, which can be carried into adulthood. The other problems may be present in any person exposed to alcoholism, but they are not commonly shared characteristics.

Client Needs Category—Psychosocial integrity
Client Needs Subcategory—None

93. 3. All the resources listed are helpful in some way to a person growing up in an alcoholic family. However, the one best suited for an adolescent is Alateen. Alateen focuses on providing support for teenagers in alcoholic families and helping them to see how the alcoholism affects their lives. One of the primary goals is to help break the pattern of alcoholism within the family.

Client Needs Category—Psychosocial integrity
Client Needs Subcategory—None

94. 2. Learning to trust others is a major sign of accomplishment for children of alcoholic parents. It is often difficult for such children to understand the concept of "normal" trusting relationships because these children have not yet experienced them. Developing the psychosocial skills in the remaining options would be considered positive accomplishments, but they are not commonly identified needs associated with growing up in an alcoholic household.

Client Needs Category—Psychosocial integrity
Client Needs Subcategory—None

95. 1. The peer group becomes more influential than parents in determining how adolescents behave. Peer behavior is used as a model for establishing what activities are acceptable or unacceptable. The fact that the team is winning is no more a motivation for taking controlled substances than if the team was losing. Affordability is not necessarily a factor in compromising values.

Client Needs Category—Health promotion and maintenance
Client Needs Subcategory—None

96. 3. Anabolic steroids commonly cause acne in both male and female users, regardless of the age-group. The other physical changes are unrelated to the use of anabolic steroids.

Client Needs Category—Physiological integrity
Client Needs Subcategory—Physiological adaptation

97. 1. Anabolic steroids are synthetic drugs chemically related to androgens such as testosterone. Androgens and anabolic steroids are associated with aggressive behavior. Severe mental changes, such as uncontrolled rage and personality changes, are common. The other emotional changes are unrelated to steroid use.

Client Needs Category—Physiological integrity
Client Needs Subcategory—Physiological adaptation

98. 4. The described signs indicate depression. Adolescents are likely to attempt suicide impulsively when they are unable to cope with a significant loss. It is appropriate to ask overtly about suicidal feelings. Talking or asking about suicide does not make a person more likely to act on his feelings; in fact, just the opposite is true. A dramatic change in behavior should never be disregarded. When dealing with crises, adolescents lack the perspective of life experiences to understand that their problems will resolve. Establishing new peer relationships at another school may be equally traumatic for a depressed adolescent.

Client Needs Category—Psychosocial integrity
Client Needs Subcategory—None

99. 1, 2, 3. Suicide is common among school-age children and adolescents. Drugs, alcohol, depression, and behavior problems contribute to the problem. Boys are more likely to succeed at committing suicide, whereas girls make more suicide attempts. The warning signs include withdrawal from family, friends, and school activities; depression; apathy; and angry outbursts or obnoxious behavior that is out of character. Low standardized tests in reading and math may indicate a learning disorder, not a sign of suicide. However, overall poor school performance is a warning sign.

Delusions and incoherent speech are signs commonly associated with schizophrenia.
> ***Client Needs Category***—*Psychosocial integrity*
> ***Client Needs Subcategory***—*None*

100. **4.** Loss of a girlfriend may lead the male adolescent to depression and thoughts of suicide. It is not unusual for adolescents to challenge rules set by their parents and argue with siblings on occasion. These actions would be of concern only if they occur frequently or if the adolescent's behavior becomes violent. A 2-point drop in the adolescent's grades is not significant.
> ***Client Needs Category***—*Psychosocial integrity*
> ***Client Needs Subcategory***—*None*

101. **4.** Acceptance is the basis for developing a therapeutic relationship. An accepting attitude indicates that the client is unique and worthy of respect. Trust develops when a client feels accepted. Empathy, not sympathy, should be demonstrated. The other qualities are desirable but are not as likely to facilitate building trust.
> ***Client Needs Category***—*Psychosocial integrity*
> ***Client Needs Subcategory***—*None*

102. **1.** Eye contact communicates that the nurse is paying attention and considers what the client says as important. Giving away free literature does not communicate a sincere, personal regard for the client. Writing information is a job-related task. Avoiding pauses could be interpreted as disinterest.
> ***Client Needs Category***—*Psychosocial integrity*
> ***Client Needs Subcategory***—*None*

103. **2.** Teenagers normally go through a period when they reject the standards and ideals of their parents and other adults. By experimenting with new behaviors that are often opposite those of the parents, the adolescent emerges with a unique identity and a lasting set of values. Adolescent rebellion is not likely to facilitate ingenuity, intuition, or insight.
> ***Client Needs Category***—*Health promotion and maintenance*
> ***Client Needs Subcategory***—*None*

104. **1.** Client treatment is a confidential matter. Neither the nurse nor other clinic personnel may reveal the client's identity or reason for treatment without the client's consent. All the other actions overtly or covertly divulge a relationship between the clinic and the client; the examples violate the principle of confidentiality.
> ***Client Needs Category***—*Safe, effective care environment*
> ***Client Needs Subcategory***—*Coordinated care*

105. **4.** One important element in resolving a crisis is the emotional support of significant others. The client's mothering instinct, marriage plans, and financial support are not as beneficial as a family's unconditional love and encouragement.
> ***Client Needs Category***—*Psychosocial integrity*
> ***Client Needs Subcategory***—*None*

106. **3.** Denial is a form of behavior that protects one's consciousness from dealing with a catastrophic situation. Denying a situation keeps anxiety at an acceptable level. Displacement involves discharging angry feelings onto an unrelated person or object. Regression occurs when a person resorts to behavior associated with a younger age. Compensation is characterized by pursuing an activity that ensures success to make up for feeling inadequate.
> ***Client Needs Category***—*Psychosocial integrity*
> ***Client Needs Subcategory***—*None*

107. **3.** Clients who are psychotic generally have unrealistic and irrational thoughts. Yet these thoughts seem real and logical to the psychotic person. Many people who are mentally healthy experience difficulty in relationships, have problems adjusting to new situations, and feel helpless in resolving some problems.
> ***Client Needs Category***—*Psychosocial integrity*
> ***Client Needs Subcategory***—*None*

108. **1.** Orientation is the person's ability to identify who and where she is as well as the day, month, and year. Asking how the client arrived is one way to assess her short-term memory. Having the client identify her place of birth assesses her long-term memory. Asking the client to name the current president assesses her knowledge base.
> ***Client Needs Category***—*Psychosocial integrity*
> ***Client Needs Subcategory***—*None*

109. **3.** According to the American Hospital Association, a client has a fundamental right to review his or her own medical records. Also, the Mental Health Systems Act of 1980 contains a model for the mental health client's bill of rights. It states that a client has the right to access his or her mental health care records except for information provided by third parties and information deemed by a mental health professional to be detrimental to the client's health. Therefore, the nurse should hand the client the notes and allow her to read them. Asking a "why" question is a nontherapeutic communication technique because it demands an explanation of the client. Putting the notes away is a nonverbal method of denying the client's request; it may also be misinterpreted by the client as an indication that there is something to hide. It is not illegal for clients to read their own medical records.
> ***Client Needs Category***—*Safe, effective care environment*
> ***Client Needs Subcategory***—*Coordinated care*

110. 2. The most essential criterion for an involuntary commitment is that the client is a clear and present danger to herself or to others. Commitment criteria have been established to protect the client's right to appropriate treatment in the least restrictive setting. There are methods for assessing a client other than involuntary commitment. Neither failure to keep office appointments nor uncooperative behavior is a criterion for involuntary commitment. All competent adults have the right to refuse treatment, which includes not taking medications.

> ***Client Needs Category****—Psychosocial integrity*
> ***Client Needs Subcategory****—None*

111. 4. Orthostatic hypotension is a side effect commonly associated with antipsychotic drugs such as haloperidol (Haldol). Cautioning a client to rise slowly helps moderate the drop in blood pressure, thus minimizing the potential for dizziness, fainting, or falling. Taking the medication on an empty stomach or skipping meals does not affect the drug's therapeutic action. This category of drugs is likely to make the client feel drowsy when treatment is initiated. The client should never omit or discontinue taking an antipsychotic drug without first consulting the physician.

> ***Client Needs Category****—Physiological integrity*
> ***Client Needs Subcategory****—Pharmacological therapies*

112. 1. Antipsychotics are most likely to reduce or eliminate psychotic symptoms, such as delusions and hallucinations. They do so by blocking the receptors of the neurotransmitter dopamine. Increased drowsiness and sleepiness are undesirable side effects of antipsychotics. It is doubtful that the client will feel more energetic and rested because one of the drug's common side effects is sedation. The drug does not alter the client's self-concept.

> ***Client Needs Category****—Physiological integrity*
> ***Client Needs Subcategory****—Pharmacological therapies*

113. 2. Antipsychotic drugs can depress the bone marrow's production of blood cells. A severe sore throat suggests that the client does not have sufficient white blood cells to fight off microorganisms. A complete blood count is needed to assess the possibility of this adverse effect. This drug is likely to cause constipation and weight gain. Ringing of the ears (tinnitus) is not associated with haloperidol (Haldol) use.

> ***Client Needs Category****—Physiological integrity*
> ***Client Needs Subcategory****—Pharmacological therapies*

The Nursing Care of Adult Clients with Mental Health Needs

⇨ *Mental Health Needs During Young Adulthood*
⇨ *Mental Health Needs During Middle Age (35-65)*
⇨ *Mental Health Needs During Late Adulthood (Over 65)*
⇨ *Correct Answers and Rationales*

Directions: *With a pencil, blacken the space in front of the option you have chosen for your correct answer.*

Mental Health Needs During Young Adulthood

A nurse works in a substance abuse clinic where most of the clients are ages 18 to 35.

1. When a 24-year-old with a record of multiple convictions for driving under the influence claims he is not an alcoholic, which is the most pertinent assessment question the nurse can ask?
[ ] 1. "When you drink, do you drink only beer?"
[ ] 2. "Did you begin drinking before or after you were of legal age?"
[ ] 3. "Do you prefer to drink alcohol rather than soft drinks?"
[ ] 4. "Are you unable to recall events that occurred while drinking?"

2. The nurse explains to the client's family the alcoholic's recovery process. What is the first step in recovering from alcohol?
[ ] 1. Admitting an inability to control drinking
[ ] 2. Eliminating nutritional deficiencies
[ ] 3. Resuming some form of religious affiliation
[ ] 4. Developing more willpower to stay sober

3. The nurse refers the alcoholic's family members to a community organization. Which resource is most appropriate in this situation?
[ ] 1. Alcoholics Anonymous
[ ] 2. Recovery Anonymous
[ ] 3. Al-Anon
[ ] 4. Synanon

An anonymous caller phones the clinic and asks the nurse how to tell if someone has been smoking marijuana within the last few hours.

4. The nurse correctly informs the caller that most people have which physical sign after recent marijuana use?
[ ] 1. Shivering
[ ] 2. Inflamed eyes
[ ] 3. Rapid breathing
[ ] 4. Restlessness

5. Which additional symptom is a common effect of marijuana use?
[ ] 1. Drowsiness
[ ] 2. Hyperactivity
[ ] 3. Apprehension
[ ] 4. Suspiciousness

6. Which statement regarding the effects of marijuana smoking is most accurate?
[ ] 1. It suppresses motivation.
[ ] 2. It is physically addicting.
[ ] 3. It can cause lung cancer.
[ ] 4. It can inhibit respiration.

7. The nurse is aware that a client who chronically uses marijuana has which problem?
[ ] 1. The client has difficulty sleeping.
[ ] 2. The client's memory is impaired.
[ ] 3. The client needs to drink large volumes of liquids.
[ ] 4. The client has low tolerance for frustration.

A young couple brings their infant son to the emergency department, where he is pronounced dead on arrival. Sudden infant death syndrome (SIDS) is the tentative cause of death.

8. When resuscitation efforts are unsuccessful, which nursing action is most important next?

[ ] **1.** Ask the parents for permission to perform an autopsy.

[ ] **2.** Ask about the possibility of harvesting the infant's organs for transplantation.

[ ] **3.** Check on the parents' choice for the funeral arrangements.

[ ] **4.** Take the parents to a room where they can be with the baby.

9. Which emotional response are the parents most likely to experience immediately following the sudden death of their infant son?

[ ] **1.** Anger

[ ] **2.** Guilt

[ ] **3.** Fear

[ ] **4.** Depression

10. Which concept is most important for the nurse to convey to the parents after they have been informed of their son's death?

[ ] **1.** The staff did all they could to resuscitate the infant.

[ ] **2.** The infant would have been brain damaged if he had survived.

[ ] **3.** They did not cause nor could they have prevented the death.

[ ] **4.** Grief support groups are available in the community.

During a routine clinic visit, the nurse suspects that a 20-year-old mother is the victim of domestic assault.

11. Which nursing action is most appropriate for determining whether domestic abuse is occurring?

[ ] **1.** Ask directly if domestic abuse is occurring.

[ ] **2.** Arrange a second visit to validate suspicions.

[ ] **3.** Assess the young children for signs of injury.

[ ] **4.** Make inquiries among relatives or neighbors.

12. If the client admits that incidences of domestic abuse are occurring, which nursing intervention is most beneficial?

[ ] **1.** Offering the victim her personal phone number

[ ] **2.** Identifying resources for shelter and safety

[ ] **3.** Recommending that she end the abusive relationship

[ ] **4.** Suggesting joint counseling with a therapist or clergyman

13. If a client is typical of other victims who remain in abusive relationships, what is she most likely to believe?

[ ] **1.** She is not in any serious danger.

[ ] **2.** She can turn to her family for protection.

[ ] **3.** She can prevent the battering behavior.

[ ] **4.** She is free to leave at any time.

A nurse is a volunteer answering telephone calls on a hotline at a crisis center.

14. When the nurse responds to a call from a 22-year-old rape victim, which instruction is most important before referring the woman to the emergency department of the local hospital?

[ ] **1.** "Do not bathe or shower."

[ ] **2.** "Make a sketch of the rapist."

[ ] **3.** "Write down what happened."

[ ] **4.** "Call a 911 operator."

15. When the rape victim arrives at the emergency department, which nursing action is best for relieving the client's anxiety?

[ ] **1.** Determine the victim's last date of menstruation.

[ ] **2.** Collect evidence for criminal prosecution.

[ ] **3.** Assess the extent of the client's injuries.

[ ] **4.** Stay with the client at all times.

16. Which nursing action is the highest priority during the immediate care of a rape victim?

[ ] **1.** Documenting the circumstances of the rape

[ ] **2.** Keeping contact with strangers to a minimum

[ ] **3.** Offering the victim a choice of sedatives

[ ] **4.** Contacting the victim's minister, rabbi, or priest

17. The emergency department nurse describes procedures and their purposes to the rape victim before they are implemented. What is the rationale for the nurse's action?

[ ] **1.** It diminishes feelings of powerlessness.

[ ] **2.** It tends to reduce the client's anxiety.

[ ] **3.** It is a policy of the emergency department.

[ ] **4.** It meets the client's need for teaching.

18. If a rape victim desires medical treatment but objects to having evidence collected for criminal prosecution, which nursing action is most appropriate?

[ ] **1.** Persuading her to change her mind

[ ] **2.** Proceeding because it is required

[ ] **3.** Accepting the rape victim's wishes

[ ] **4.** Advising her to use better judgment

Before being discharged, the rape victim is referred to a rape support counselor who is also a nurse. The counselor recommends that the rape victim attend a group meeting of others who have been raped.

19. Which is the most desired outcome of a self-help group of rape victims?
[ ] **1.** Obtaining mutual assistance with similar problems
[ ] **2.** Receiving authoritative information about rape trauma
[ ] **3.** Establishing new friendships with other victims
[ ] **4.** Developing additional social skills for the future

20. If the rape victim shares all of the following information during a group session, which finding is most indicative of a severe adjustment reaction?
[ ] **1.** The victim reports feeling somewhat anxious.
[ ] **2.** The victim describes having sporadic nightmares.
[ ] **3.** The victim has no appetite but eats out of habit.
[ ] **4.** The victim has occasional doubts about her self-worth.

A public health nurse must inform a 26-year-old male homosexual that he has tested positive for human immunodeficiency virus (HIV)?

21. Which initial reaction would the nurse expect if the client is typical of others who just received news of their diagnosis?
[ ] **1.** Anger
[ ] **2.** Shock
[ ] **3.** Resentment
[ ] **4.** Depression

22. Which action by the client is most suggestive that he is in denial about his illness?
[ ] **1.** He conceals the information from his family.
[ ] **2.** He avoids contact with his homosexual friends.
[ ] **3.** He confronts some of his former sexual partners.
[ ] **4.** He has intercourse without using condoms.

23. If the client has all of the following strengths, which one is most important for coping with his diagnosis?
[ ] **1.** Acceptance by religious leaders
[ ] **2.** A sustained network of support
[ ] **3.** Acquisition of many social acquaintances
[ ] **4.** Sexual tolerance within the community

24. Which statement made by the client would the nurse interpret as the most serious indication of an increased risk for suicide?
[ ] **1.** "I have been having recurring dreams about dying."
[ ] **2.** "How many people have died from HIV?"
[ ] **3.** "Will I be alert when I'm near death?"
[ ] **4.** "Everyone would be better off without me."

The nurse has been working with a bulimic college student to help her control her eating disorder.

25. Which recommendation by the nurse is most likely to be effective in helping the client control her bulimia?
[ ] **1.** Avoid using the bathroom after meals.
[ ] **2.** Take a daily inventory of food offered at the dormitory.
[ ] **3.** Avoid eating in fast-food establishments.
[ ] **4.** Keep a daily calorie count of all foods consumed.

26. If the client has been taking an antidepressant for several weeks, which outcome would be the most desired therapeutic effect?
[ ] **1.** The client is feeling less depressed.
[ ] **2.** The client is eating more nutritiously.
[ ] **3.** The client is having fewer food binges.
[ ] **4.** The client is feeling less suicidal.

The bulimic client attends a group meeting and tells another member who is very emaciated, "You're a real weirdo if you think you've got a weight problem."

27. Which nursing action is most appropriate at this time?
[ ] **1.** Criticize the nature of the client's rude behavior.
[ ] **2.** Support the emaciated client who was targeted by the remark.
[ ] **3.** Invite others in the group to respond to the situation.
[ ] **4.** Embarrass the bulimic client with a similar comment.

An obese 25-year-old man who abuses dextroamphetamine (Dexedrine) also attends the eating disorder group meetings.

28. Which sign is most suggestive that he is taking dextroamphetamine (Dexedrine) at this time?
[ ] **1.** He stares blankly into space.
[ ] **2.** He monopolizes the discussions.
[ ] **3.** He wears sunglasses indoors.
[ ] **4.** He slurs his words as he speaks.

29. Which history finding strongly suggests that the client has not achieved the characteristic developmental level expected at this age in the life cycle?
[ ] **1.** He drifts in and out of relationships.
[ ] **2.** He worries about his financial security.
[ ] **3.** He questions his sexual identity.
[ ] **4.** He hesitates to assert himself.

30. When discussing his obesity, which comment by the client best indicates that he is using the coping mechanism of rationalization to deal with his problems?

[ ] **1.** "I have many health risks from being obese."
[ ] **2.** "I have real difficulty resisting ice cream."
[ ] **3.** "I know you don't like me because I'm fat."
[ ] **4.** "I can't help being overweight; it's in my genes."

A 27-year-old foreign immigrant is admitted to the mental health unit with somatic abdominal pain. The client is apprehensive and speaks very little English. A family member reveals that the client has a history of mental illness.

31. Which translation method is most beneficial for the client when the nurse explains the need to search for contraband?

[ ] **1.** A translation card that includes key words, phrases, and pictures
[ ] **2.** A translator who speaks the client's dialect
[ ] **3.** A hospital housekeeper who speaks the client's language
[ ] **4.** The client's family member who can translate the process

The nurse observes the client's sister placing a knife beneath the client's pillow to "cut" his pain.

32. Which nursing action is most appropriate at this time?

[ ] **1.** Explaining through a translator that analgesic drugs will be administered to control pain
[ ] **2.** Explaining through a translator that sharp objects pose a safety hazard to the client and others
[ ] **3.** Explaining through a translator that a form must be signed relieving the agency of responsibility
[ ] **4.** Explaining through a translator that the staff will leave the knife in place as long as necessary

A 30-year-old man with a history of substance abuse is admitted to the chemical dependency unit at a local hospital.

33. If the client snorts cocaine on a regular basis, which physical assessment will the nurse most likely find?

[ ] **1.** Dry, stuffy nose
[ ] **2.** Perforated nasal septum
[ ] **3.** Congested breath sounds
[ ] **4.** Sinus pain under the eyes

34. If the client's drug screen is positive for cocaine, it is most appropriate for the nurse to advise a staff person to monitor the client closely for which finding?

[ ] **1.** Cardiac arrhythmias
[ ] **2.** Depressed respirations
[ ] **3.** Low blood pressure
[ ] **4.** Elevated blood glucose level

A home health nurse monitors several young adults who have been diagnosed with schizophrenia but who are able to function for extended periods of time in the community.

35. During a home visit, which assessment finding is most suggestive that a client is experiencing auditory hallucinations?

[ ] **1.** The client sings a song as he walks around the room.
[ ] **2.** The client quickly changes the topic of conversation.
[ ] **3.** The client repeats a sentence over and over again.
[ ] **4.** The client cocks his head as if listening to someone.

36. If a schizophrenic client says, "Wing ding, the world is a ring," which response by the nurse is most therapeutic?

[ ] **1.** "How clever. You've made up a poem."
[ ] **2.** "I don't understand what you mean."
[ ] **3.** "Earth does orbit in a circle."
[ ] **4.** "Tell me more about the world."

37. Which assessment finding is most indicative that a community-based client with schizophrenia needs to be rehospitalized?

[ ] **1.** The client neglects eating, hygiene, and sleep.
[ ] **2.** The client has missed some counseling appointments.
[ ] **3.** The client is hesitant about applying for work.
[ ] **4.** The client wants to live with his relatives.

38. When caring for a schizophrenic who is receiving risperidone (Risperdal), the nurse is aware that the medication is likely to have which effect on the client?

[ ] **1.** An increased incidence of extrapyramidal symptoms
[ ] **2.** An increased incidence of insomnia and agitation
[ ] **3.** Urine retention from anticholinergic effects
[ ] **4.** Symptoms of anorexia with profound weight loss

Mental Health Needs
During Middle Age (35-65)

A nurse is assigned to care for a 35-year-old client who sustained a severe head injury and brain damage in a motor vehicle accident.

39. During his initial feeding, the client deliberately spits at the nurse. Which action is most appropriate to take first?
[ ] **1.** Leave the client's room immediately.
[ ] **2.** Indicate that the behavior is unacceptable.
[ ] **3.** Act as if the behavior was accidental.
[ ] **4.** Stand as far from the bed as possible.

40. If the client's spitting becomes habitual, which intervention is best to include in his care plan?
[ ] **1.** Establish a significant consequence, such as no television for 30 minutes.
[ ] **2.** Wear a face shield or other form of barrier protection when feeding the client.
[ ] **3.** Explain how rude it is to spit at other people.
[ ] **4.** Identify the health risks associated with spitting.

41. Which action is most appropriate when performing a mental status assessment on this client?
[ ] **1.** Ask open-ended questions such as "How have you been feeling lately?"
[ ] **2.** Allow extra time for the client to respond to assessment questions.
[ ] **3.** Defer mental status questions to the client's wife.
[ ] **4.** Omit the mental status assessment; the results will be abnormal.

A 42-year-old woman is assessed in the emergency department to determine the etiology of her chest pain.

42. If the client's pain is the result of a panic attack, which finding is the nurse most likely to note during the physical assessment?
[ ] **1.** Tachycardia
[ ] **2.** Hypotension
[ ] **3.** Increased salivation
[ ] **4.** Constricted pupils

43. If a diagnosis of panic disorder is accurate, the nurse would correctly assume that the chest pain is related to which cause?
[ ] **1.** Unknown cause
[ ] **2.** Feigned illness
[ ] **3.** Attention-seeking behavior
[ ] **4.** Intense fear

44. When interacting with a client experiencing a panic attack, which technique by the nurse is most likely to help reduce the client's anxiety level?
[ ] **1.** Stand less than an arm's length from her.
[ ] **2.** Wear a laboratory coat and name tag.
[ ] **3.** Offer her a cup of coffee or tea.
[ ] **4.** Explain all actions and procedures.

45. Which concept is most important for the nurse to convey to a client during a panic attack?
[ ] **1.** The client is safe.
[ ] **2.** The client is believed.
[ ] **3.** The client is trusted.
[ ] **4.** The client is accepted.

46. When the client begins crying and says, "Nurse, I feel like I'm going to die," which response is most therapeutic?
[ ] **1.** "Don't cry. It won't help matters right now."
[ ] **2.** "You don't want the physician to see you this way."
[ ] **3.** "Everyone feels frightened in an emergency."
[ ] **4.** "I'll stay with you until you feel better."

The physician prescribes alprazolam (Xanax) to treat the client's panic disorder.

47. Which information is most appropriate for the nurse to tell the client about taking alprazolam (Xanax)?
[ ] **1.** Avoid consuming alcohol while taking this drug.
[ ] **2.** Long-term use will not cause drug dependency.
[ ] **3.** This drug can cause insomnia in some people.
[ ] **4.** A blood test will be required periodically.

48. The nurse is aware that if the client's panic attacks occur more frequently, she is likely to develop which common reaction?
[ ] **1.** She will seek out referrals for psychiatric treatment.
[ ] **2.** She will fear venturing from home and become reclusive.
[ ] **3.** She will take more than the prescribed amount of medication.
[ ] **4.** She will become psychotic and require psychiatric admission.

The nurse on a mental health unit conducts a group meeting for clients diagnosed with obsessive-compulsive disorder (OCD).

49. Which clients are most likely to be members of an obsessive-compulsive group? Select all that apply.
[ ] **1.** A 30-year-old woman who washes her hands five times per hour
[ ] **2.** A 35-year-old business executive who makes several pots of coffee daily, thinking the coffee is poisoned
[ ] **3.** A 40-year-old woman who is sexually promiscuous
[ ] **4.** A 45-year-old man who drinks a fifth of whiskey daily
[ ] **5.** A 50-year-old man who cannot throw anything away
[ ] **6.** A 60-year-old woman who locks and unlocks her doors

50. The nurse reviews various treatment options with the group members. Which of the following are considered most therapeutic in treating obsessive-compulsive disorder (OCD)? Select all that apply.
[ ] **1.** Selective serotonin reuptake inhibitors (SSRIs) such as fluvoxamine (Luvox)
[ ] **2.** Electroconvulsive therapy (ECT)
[ ] **3.** Cognitive-behavioral therapy
[ ] **4.** Lobotomy
[ ] **5.** Tranquilizers such as diazepam (Valium)

The nurse and a nurse's aide enter the room of a 48-year-old man while he is arguing with his wife on the phone. After hanging up, the client becomes angry and belligerent toward the nurse's aide.

51. The nurse correctly explains to the aide that this is an example of a client using which coping mechanism?
[ ] **1.** Introjection
[ ] **2.** Projection
[ ] **3.** Compensation
[ ] **4.** Displacement

52. Which action is best to use initially when trying to help the angry client maintain self-control?
[ ] **1.** Administer a sedative.
[ ] **2.** Get the client involved in an activity.
[ ] **3.** Remain calm and appear nonthreatening.
[ ] **4.** Offer to talk to the client's wife.

53. If the client's anger continues to escalate to potentially violent behavior, which nursing action is most appropriate?
[ ] **1.** Assemble several staff members.
[ ] **2.** Ask the physician to calm the client.
[ ] **3.** Go alone with the client to his room.
[ ] **4.** Place behavioral restraints within the client's view.

54. If the angry client is out of control and refuses a STAT sedative medication, the nurse has which legal option?
[ ] **1.** The nurse must respect the client's right to refuse the ordered medication.
[ ] **2.** The nurse can administer the medication to protect the safety of self and others.
[ ] **3.** The nurse must get permission from a probate court judge to administer the medication.
[ ] **4.** The nurse should ask the hospital's attorney about the client's right to refuse treatment.

A nurse prepares to teach a 60-year-old male client who is highly anxious about a heart catheterization that he will undergo next week.

55. Which form of instruction is most beneficial when preparing the anxious client?
[ ] **1.** Provide detailed explanations.
[ ] **2.** Use short, simple sentences.
[ ] **3.** Draw elaborate diagrams.
[ ] **4.** Show a teaching videotape.

56. If the nurse documents all of the following information in the database assessment file, which finding is probably the most significant source of conflict for this client?
[ ] **1.** The client is facing forced retirement.
[ ] **2.** The client has 12 grandchildren.
[ ] **3.** The client is learning to use a computer.
[ ] **4.** The client wants to sell his home.

A 38-year-old woman comes to the clinic to receive information and treatment for her fear of flying.

57. If this client is typical of others with phobias, which coping mechanism has she most likely been using to deal with her fear?
[ ] **1.** Suppression
[ ] **2.** Compensation
[ ] **3.** Avoidance
[ ] **4.** Undoing

58. The nurse performs a physical assessment and collects the woman's health history. Which assessment findings would the nurse expect to note as the woman discusses her phobia related to flying? Select all that apply.
[ ] **1.** Sweating
[ ] **2.** Tachycardia
[ ] **3.** Tremors
[ ] **4.** Shortness of breath
[ ] **5.** Uncontrollable crying
[ ] **6.** Facial tics

The phobic client asks the nurse to explain cognitive therapy, the type of treatment that was recommended by her physician.

59. The nurse accurately explains that cognitive therapy involves which of the following?
[ ] **1.** Changing people's irrational beliefs
[ ] **2.** Exposing people to things they fear
[ ] **3.** Helping people verbalize their feelings
[ ] **4.** Rewarding people's altered behaviors

A nurse volunteers to participate in a support group for military personnel with posttraumatic stress disorder (PTSD).

60. When asked to identify the characteristics of PTSD, the nurse correctly responds that most people with this disorder report which finding?
[ ] **1.** Recurring nightmares
[ ] **2.** Auditory hallucinations
[ ] **3.** Rapidly changing emotions
[ ] **4.** Anger that erupts easily

61. Which therapeutic nursing intervention is most beneficial for a client diagnosed with PTSD?
[ ] **1.** Administering antianxiety medications
[ ] **2.** Monitoring the client's physical symptoms
[ ] **3.** Encouraging the client to express his feelings
[ ] **4.** Investigating the client's current family interactions

62. When the counselor asks the members of the PTSD group to draw pictures of their traumatic experience, the nurse understands that the primary purpose for drawing is to help members work out what problem?
[ ] **1.** Dealing consciously with painful memories
[ ] **2.** Bonding with other group members
[ ] **3.** Receiving approval from group members
[ ] **4.** Justifying their participation in the group

A World War II veteran asks the nurse why he is always startled and fearful whenever he attends Fourth of July fireworks displays.

63. Which explanation by the nurse is most accurate?
[ ] **1.** He was frightened of them as a child.
[ ] **2.** He is fearful he will be injured.
[ ] **3.** He associates the sound with gunfire.
[ ] **4.** He is afraid it will trigger memories.

The veteran's wife asks if anyone other than military personnel can have PTSD.

64. The most accurate statement by the nurse is that PTSD can occur in anyone who meets which of the following criteria?

[ ] **1.** The person experienced multiple failures.
[ ] **2.** The person survived a catastrophic event.
[ ] **3.** The person was abandoned as a child.
[ ] **4.** The person inherited a genetic tendency for PTSD.

A 40-year-old woman has multiple symptoms that do not resemble any specific disease. She is anxious and worried because no definite diagnosis has been made. Diagnostic tests are ordered.

65. When the anxious client summons the nurse and says she feels weak and dizzy, which nursing action is most appropriate at this time?
[ ] **1.** Helping the client to relax
[ ] **2.** Giving the client something to eat
[ ] **3.** Administering oxygen by cannula
[ ] **4.** Taking the client's vital signs

The client shares with the nurse that she regrets that she never went to college or had children. The nurse asks the client to continue with her thoughts and reflect on her statement.

66. The best rationale for having the client reflect on her thoughts is that during the middle years of life, adults tend to do what?
[ ] **1.** Assess their accomplishments
[ ] **2.** Set unreasonable goals
[ ] **3.** Envy others' achievements
[ ] **4.** Doubt their judgment

One day while the client's husband is visiting, the client says to the nurse, "Do you think they'll ever be able to find out what's wrong with me?"

67. Which response by the nurse is best in this situation?
[ ] **1.** "That is something to discuss with your physician."
[ ] **2.** "It sounds like you're feeling discouraged."
[ ] **3.** "Let us worry about your lack of progress."
[ ] **4.** "You need to practice a little more patience."

The client's husband states to the nurse, "She sounds just like a hypochondriac to me."

68. The nurse is aware that such attitudes and statements can have damaging consequences for a mentally ill client. What is the most significant consequence of the remark in this situation?
[ ] **1.** It violates the client's right to treatment.
[ ] **2.** It disregards the client's individuality.
[ ] **3.** It interferes with continuity of client care.
[ ] **4.** It disrupts good staff relationships.

After several diagnostic tests, the physician explains to the client that there are no significant findings and diagnoses the condition as hypochondriasis.

69. The nurse reviews the client's medical history, assessing for possible risk factors leading to hypochondriasis. Which of the following reported findings are considered risk factors for this disorder? Select all that apply.
[ ] **1.** Family history of hypochondria
[ ] **2.** Diagnosed anxiety disorder
[ ] **3.** Physical, sexual, or emotional abuse in childhood
[ ] **4.** Witnessed violence in childhood
[ ] **5.** Stressful experience with a loved one's illness
[ ] **6.** Fear of death or disfigurement

The client's husband asks the nurse about the signs and symptoms of this disorder.

70. Which of the following signs and symptoms are closely associated with hypochondriasis? Select all that apply.
[ ] **1.** Repeatedly researching information about specific illnesses and their symptoms
[ ] **2.** Chronic fear that minor symptoms are signs of a serious illness
[ ] **3.** Multiple physical complaints that often change over time
[ ] **4.** Interference of the disorder with social life or work
[ ] **5.** Numerous physician visits, sometimes in the same day
[ ] **6.** Repeatedly obtaining tests for the same symptoms

The client's pastor visits her in the hospital. He approaches the nurses' station and tells the nurse seated there that the client has given him permission to see her chart.

71. Which action by the nurse is most appropriate at this time?
[ ] **1.** Telling him to ask the physician for permission
[ ] **2.** Asking him if he is a certified hospital chaplain
[ ] **3.** Informing him that he cannot read the chart
[ ] **4.** Checking the policy with the nursing supervisor

The nursing team holds a conference concerning a 38-year-old man who has just been admitted with ulcerative colitis, a psychophysiologic disease.

72. When a nursing assistant asks if *psychophysiologic* means that the client is not really sick, which response by the nurse is most accurate?

[ ] **1.** The client pretends to be sick when he needs a rest.
[ ] **2.** The client thinks he is sick, but the tests are all negative.
[ ] **3.** The client would rather be hospitalized than have to work.
[ ] **4.** The client has an illness that is influenced by his emotions.

During a team conference, the nurses discuss important assessment modifications required in the care of the client with ulcerative colitis.

73. Which of the following identified assessment criteria is the highest priority for this client?
[ ] **1.** The number and characteristics of the client's bowel movements
[ ] **2.** How much the client knows about colostomy care
[ ] **3.** Which coping mechanisms the client uses for handling stress
[ ] **4.** The types of relationships the client has with peers

The discussion turns to exploring ways to maintain the client's self-esteem while providing stool care.

74. Which approach is best for managing this client's care?
[ ] **1.** Use a nonjudgmental manner when cleaning the client of stool.
[ ] **2.** Ask the client's wife to help clean him when possible.
[ ] **3.** Hold the client responsible for all his hygiene.
[ ] **4.** Assign only male nurses to care for the client.

The client is scheduled for further testing to determine whether surgery is needed. The client's wife confides to the nurse that her husband is a chronic alcoholic but has not yet told the physician. Diagnostic testing reveals the need for surgery, which is scheduled for the next day.

75. Which finding noted by the nurse during the postoperative assessment is most indicative of the client's alcoholism?
[ ] **1.** Blood pressure is lower than normal.
[ ] **2.** Pain is unrelieved with usual dosages of analgesics.
[ ] **3.** Bowel sounds are absent in the right upper quadrant.
[ ] **4.** Pulse rates are slow, weak, and irregular.

Approximately 36 hours after his admission, the client becomes restless and shouts that he must kill all the bugs in his room.

76. In this situation, which nursing action is most appropriate?
[ ]   **1.** Placing restraints on the client's arms and legs
[ ]   **2.** Reassuring the client that he is not seeing bugs
[ ]   **3.** Remaining at the client's bedside
[ ]   **4.** Closing the client's door so that others are not alarmed

77. Based on this change in the client's condition, which nursing action is most appropriate to perform next?
[ ]   **1.** Notifying the client's wife
[ ]   **2.** Calling the nursing supervisor
[ ]   **3.** Notifying the physician
[ ]   **4.** Documenting the assessed data in the client's chart

78. While caring for a client who is withdrawing from alcohol, the nurse must assess for what additional complication?
[ ]   **1.** Hypothermia
[ ]   **2.** Seizures
[ ]   **3.** Ascities
[ ]   **4.** Jaundice

At the beginning of the next shift, a team member states, "Don't expect me to take care of that good-for-nothing drunk."

79. The nurse counsels the team member privately about her inappropriate remark. What is the first step in understanding and accepting the behavior of clients?
[ ]   **1.** Understanding one's own behavior
[ ]   **2.** Analyzing what motivates clients' behavior
[ ]   **3.** Becoming more familiar with abnormal behavior
[ ]   **4.** Taking courses in counseling

A home health nurse is scheduled for daily visits to change the abdominal dressing of a 45-year-old woman with a history of bipolar disorder.

80. While reviewing the client's psychiatric history, the nurse would expect to note which major characteristic of bipolar disorder?
[ ]   **1.** Ritualistic behavior
[ ]   **2.** Symbolic aggressiveness
[ ]   **3.** Cyclic mood swings
[ ]   **4.** Periodic amnesia

The nurse reads that the client is taking lithium carbonate (Lithane) to treat her bipolar disorder and suspects that she has not been taking her medication as prescribed.

81. When the nurse reviews information about lithium carbonate (Lithane) with the client, which instructions are most important to stress? Select all that apply.
[ ]   **1.** Restrict salt and fluid intake.
[ ]   **2.** Refrain from sexual activity while taking this medication.
[ ]   **3.** Notify the physician if urine output increases.
[ ]   **4.** Drink 10 to12 glasses of water per day.
[ ]   **5.** Increase salt intake.
[ ]   **6.** Avoid eating aged cheeses.

82. Which finding is most important for the nurse to monitor to help determine whether the client's current dose of lithium carbonate (Lithane) is appropriate?
[ ]   **1.** Vital signs
[ ]   **2.** Urine volume
[ ]   **3.** Drug blood levels
[ ]   **4.** Brain wave scans

83. Which finding strongly suggests that the client is experiencing an exacerbation of her bipolar disorder?
[ ]   **1.** The client has been spending money extravagantly.
[ ]   **2.** The client wants to become a 5-year-old again.
[ ]   **3.** The client has been methodically cleaning her house.
[ ]   **4.** The client has insomnia and has been staying up late to read.

Mental Health Needs During Late Adulthood (Over 65)

A nurse performs a home assessment on a reasonably healthy older adult who chooses to live in a supervised retirement community.

84. If the older adult's sons and daughters are visiting on the day of the scheduled nurse's visit, which action is most appropriate before beginning the assessment?
[ ]   **1.** Encourage the client's children to offer their comments at any time.
[ ]   **2.** Ask the client if there is a more private setting for conducting the assessment.
[ ]   **3.** Identify the names and relationships of those present.
[ ]   **4.** Offer to share the assessment results with the client's children.

85. Which question during the client interview is likely to generate the most information?
[ ]   **1.** "Tell me about your family."
[ ]   **2.** "Are you currently married?"
[ ]   **3.** "Who is your nearest relative?"
[ ]   **4.** "Give me a list of your family."

86. Which question best assesses the client's long-term memory?
[ ] 1. "What is your current age?"
[ ] 2. "What is today's date?"
[ ] 3. "What is your date of birth?"
[ ] 4. "What occurred last January?"

87. Which action by the nurse can best determine if an older client's inappropriate responses to several questions are due to miscommunication or impaired cognition?
[ ] 1. Ask the client to repeat the question before answering it.
[ ] 2. Ask questions that require only a "yes" or "no" response.
[ ] 3. Ask the client's next of kin for answers to the questions.
[ ] 4. Ask questions to which the client is sure to know the answers.

88. Which assessment finding is most atypical of a 65-year-old client?
[ ] 1. Making errors in copying a line drawing
[ ] 2. Forgetting the names of longstanding neighbors
[ ] 3. Recalling information slowly
[ ] 4. Naming only two of the last three presidents

89. If the client is typical of others her age, the nurse can anticipate her having which age-related problem?
[ ] 1. Dealing with losses
[ ] 2. Becoming cynical
[ ] 3. Losing patience
[ ] 4. Developing hostility

A 68-year-old man who is currently being treated for major depression is transferred to a medical unit following an episode of acute abdominal pain.

90. In which room is it best for the nurse to place the depressed client?
[ ] 1. A private room where stimuli are reduced
[ ] 2. A semiprivate room with a cheerful roommate
[ ] 3. An empty room at the end of the hallway
[ ] 4. A room within view of the nurses' station

91. Which of the following assessment data documented by the nurse places the client at highest risk for suicide?
[ ] 1. The client feels hopeless about the future.
[ ] 2. The client has a plan in mind for suicide.
[ ] 3. The client states that he would be better off dead.
[ ] 4. The client says he can't stand the distress anymore.

92. If the physician prescribes imipramine hydrochloride (Tofranil) for the client, the nurse should assess for which therapeutic drug effect first?
[ ] 1. Absence of suicidal ideation
[ ] 2. Improved concentration
[ ] 3. Decreased agitation
[ ] 4. Regulated mood

93. Which of the following instructions are appropriate to include in the teaching plan of a client who is just beginning treatment with imipramine hydrochloride (Tofranil)? Select all that apply.
[ ] 1. Avoid eating cheese, chocolate, and pickled foods.
[ ] 2. Take short naps during the day.
[ ] 3. Rise from the chair or bed slowly.
[ ] 4. Expect to wait about 3 weeks before feeling better.
[ ] 5. Refrain from all sexual activity for 1 month after starting the medication.
[ ] 6. Use a good sunscreen when outdoors.

94. Which nursing action is especially important when administering medications to a depressed client?
[ ] 1. Encouraging the client to drink a full glass of water
[ ] 2. Checking that the client has swallowed all oral medications given
[ ] 3. Giving the medications on an empty stomach before meals
[ ] 4. Having the client take each medication separately

95. When the depressed client is scheduled for a series of electroconvulsive therapy (ECT) treatments, which reaction is he most likely to experience in the immediate recovery period?
[ ] 1. Brief episodes of absence seizures
[ ] 2. Sensitivity to light and double vision
[ ] 3. Short-term memory loss and headaches
[ ] 4. Periods of unexplained fear and anxiety

Another client on the same unit is diagnosed with depression. The physician prescribes doxepin (Sinequan) to be taken at bedtime.

96. What suggestion can the nurse make if the client complains of dizziness on rising after taking the doxepin (Sinequan) at bedtime as prescribed?
[ ] 1. "Place a cool compress on your forehead."
[ ] 2. "Get up slowly from a seated position."
[ ] 3. "Remain in bed with your feet elevated above your heart."
[ ] 4. "Take a hot shower."

A nurse who is employed in a nursing home observes that a romantic relationship is developing between two residents.

97. Which action is most appropriate if the nurse discovers the oriented older couple having consensual sexual intercourse?
[ ] **1.** Report it to their adult children.
[ ] **2.** Restore a measure of privacy.
[ ] **3.** Suggest they become roommates.
[ ] **4.** Censure their sexual activity.

An older adult client with chronic mental illness is transferred from a state psychiatric hospital to a nursing home for custodial care.

98. If the client with chronic mental illness develops the following symptoms after the physician discontinues haloperidol (Haldol), which symptom is most likely a consequence of the drug therapy?
[ ] **1.** Facial tics
[ ] **2.** Depression
[ ] **3.** Patchy hair loss
[ ] **4.** Daytime lethargy

A nurse refers her 66-year-old home care client to a mental health clinic for evaluation of a coexisting depressive disorder.

99. If the home health nurse documented all of the following findings, which one is most suggestive that the client is depressed?
[ ] **1.** The client is irritable after her grandchildren visit.
[ ] **2.** The client has multiple, unrelated physical complaints.
[ ] **3.** The client takes lengthy naps in the late afternoon.
[ ] **4.** The client cries when talking about her dead spouse.

100. If the nurse notes the following symptoms after the client begins taking sertraline (Zoloft), which one is most likely drug-related?
[ ] **1.** Polyuria
[ ] **2.** Diplopia
[ ] **3.** Drooling
[ ] **4.** Insomnia

A client who has had a stroke currently lives in a long-term care facility and struggles to manage his activities of daily living.

101. If the client frequently comes to meals with soap on his face or an unbuttoned shirt, which action by the nurse is most beneficial to the client's emotional state?

[ ] **1.** Send him back to his room to finish.
[ ] **2.** Bathe, shave, and dress him daily.
[ ] **3.** Schedule his hygiene activities after meals.
[ ] **4.** Comment on how self-reliant he is.

A nurse joins a group of older adult clients during reminiscence therapy.

102. Which therapeutic activity is most helpful in facilitating reminiscence therapy among older adult clients?
[ ] **1.** Discussing a current event topic
[ ] **2.** Singing popular songs from the 1940s
[ ] **3.** Reading an article from the newspaper
[ ] **4.** Making decorations for a future holiday

103. When one older adult at reminiscence therapy says, "If I had it to do all over again, I wouldn't change a thing," the nurse is most accurate in interpreting this to mean that the client has acquired which developmental characteristic?
[ ] **1.** Trust
[ ] **2.** Integrity
[ ] **3.** Intimacy
[ ] **4.** Autonomy

A group of nurses in a long-term care facility attends an in-service program about documentation.

104. The nurses critique a chart entry that says, "States, 'I feel unwanted.' Appears to be confused." Which statement best describes why this entry is unsatisfactory?
[ ] **1.** The nurse who made the entry failed to interpret the significance of feeling unwanted.
[ ] **2.** The nurse who made the entry failed to indicate the importance of the client's statement.
[ ] **3.** The nurse who made the entry failed to substantiate that the client made the quote.
[ ] **4.** The nurse who made the entry failed to describe the evidence of the confused behavior.

A nurse is employed on a special unit for clients with dementia.

105. What is the best approach for managing a confused client who wanders into other clients' rooms?
[ ] **1.** Place a large sign with the client's name on her door.
[ ] **2.** Keep the room doors on the unit locked at all times.
[ ] **3.** Restrain her in a wheelchair when unattended.
[ ] **4.** Speak to her about invading other people's privacy.

A 70-year-old woman with dementia removes her clothes and walks naked through the halls of a nursing home.

106. Which action is most appropriate for the nurse to take first?
[ ] **1.** Remind her that others can see her.
[ ] **2.** Tell her to put her clothes back on.
[ ] **3.** Explain to the other residents that she is not in her right mind.
[ ] **4.** Take her to a vacant room nearby.

107. Which technique is most therapeutic for helping clients with dementia remain oriented?
[ ] **1.** Address all clients using their first name.
[ ] **2.** Ask clients to identify their goals for the day.
[ ] **3.** Assign clients to greet visitors each day.
[ ] **4.** Post large calendars with the current date.

108. Which technique is best for reducing confusion among clients with dementia?
[ ] **1.** Wear an employee name tag when caring for clients.
[ ] **2.** Adhere to a consistent routine of unit activities.
[ ] **3.** Provide diversional activities such as field trips.
[ ] **4.** Distribute a list of the day's scheduled events.

At a team conference, the nurses explore ways to help a client with dementia understand verbal communication.

109. Which of the following communication methods is best to use with a client with dementia?
[ ] **1.** Speak loudly to get the client's attention.
[ ] **2.** Use short sentences when speaking to the client.
[ ] **3.** Use written forms of communication.
[ ] **4.** Allow the client to listen to news programs.

110. When a client with dementia says, "I want to go home," which response by the nurse is most appropriate?
[ ] **1.** "You are at home."
[ ] **2.** "You are staying here."
[ ] **3.** "You must not like us."
[ ] **4.** "You need to call your family."

The wife of a client on the dementia unit visits her husband on a daily basis. A nurse who regularly cares for the client notices that the woman is beginning to show signs of exhaustion and self-neglect.

111. Which nursing intervention is most beneficial for the client's wife at this time?

[ ] **1.** Suggesting that she make an appointment for a physical examination
[ ] **2.** Discussing modifying the amount of time she devotes to caretaking
[ ] **3.** Reminding her of the scheduled times for visiting clients on the unit
[ ] **4.** Explaining that many staff are available to care for her husband

A female client who is diagnosed with Alzheimer's disease lives in a long-term care memory center. The client's daughter visits regularly.

112. One day the client's daughter states to the nurse, "I'm not sure Mother knows who I am." Which response by the nurse is most therapeutic?
[ ] **1.** "This is probably the beginning of the end for her."
[ ] **2.** "You're distressed that she doesn't respond to you."
[ ] **3.** "Don't worry. We're taking very good care of her here."
[ ] **4.** "There will be good days and bad days. Today is a bad day."

113. When the older client with Alzheimer's disease is confused about how to use a fork, which nursing action is best for prolonging her ability to maintain self-care?
[ ] **1.** Ask the physician to order a liquid diet.
[ ] **2.** Position her so she can mimic other clients.
[ ] **3.** Serve her first so she has more time to eat.
[ ] **4.** Seat her alone so no one will see her mess.

The daughter of the client with Alzheimer's disease wants to take the client home for a day.

114. Which nursing assessment is critical to ensuring the client's well-being during the home visit?
[ ] **1.** The caregiver's understanding of the symptoms the client manifests
[ ] **2.** The caregiver's understanding of when the client must return
[ ] **3.** The caregiver's understanding of when to administer medications
[ ] **4.** The caregiver's understanding of how to provide hygiene measures

An older adult who is dying of a terminal illness has an advance directive indicating that he does not want any heroic measures used to prolong his life.

115. What is the most appropriate nursing action when the terminally ill client's death is imminent?

[ ] **1.** Sitting quietly and holding the dying client's hand
[ ] **2.** Moving the client into the hall where he can be observed
[ ] **3.** Placing the client in a room alone near the nurses' station
[ ] **4.** Telling the client to use the signal if he needs anything

Following the death of the terminally ill client, a nursing assistant is extremely distraught.

116. What nursing approach is most beneficial for helping the nursing assistant at this time?
[ ] **1.** Sending the nursing assistant home for the rest of the shift
[ ] **2.** Terminating the nursing assistant from this type of work
[ ] **3.** Allowing the nursing assistant to express how she feels
[ ] **4.** Asking the nursing assistant to help with post-mortem care

Family members of the deceased client are referred to a grief support group.

117. When a new member to the group tells the nursing leader that she senses her dead husband's presence in their home, which nursing intervention is most appropriate?
[ ] **1.** Recommending more professional counseling
[ ] **2.** Assuring her that it is wishful thinking
[ ] **3.** Letting her be comforted by the experience
[ ] **4.** Encouraging her to stay with relatives

Correct Answers and Rationales

Mental Health Needs During Young Adulthood

1. 4. Alcoholism is a chronic, progressive, often fatal disease that has genetic, psychosocial, and environmental elements. It is characterized by alcohol craving, impaired control over drinking, a preoccupation with alcohol, and the use of alcohol despite the consequences (loss of a job, problems with a spouse or significant other, or trouble with the law). Alcoholism is a physical dependency, and abrupt deprivation leads to severe withdrawal symptoms. Alcoholics experience distorted thinking and denial.

Although an affirmative answer to all the questions is significant, the most suggestive sign of alcoholism is the occurrence of blackouts. Blackouts are a form of amnesia for actions and events that take place when a person is drinking. Alcoholism is a dependency on alcohol-containing substances; it can occur regardless of the type of alcohol consumed and when the person began drinking. Preferring alcohol over soft drinks is a personal choice; however, choosing to drink alcohol can lead to serious consequences, including the increased risk of developing alcoholism.
Client Needs Category—Psychosocial integrity
Client Needs Subcategory—None

2. 1. Denial is one major barrier to recovery from alcoholism. The first step of Alcoholics Anonymous (AA) and other treatment programs is to help the alcoholic give up his or her denial. Most alcoholics are malnourished, but improving the alcoholic's dietary intake does not necessarily help him stop drinking. AA does emphasize belief in a higher power, but participating in an organized religion is not promoted. Alcoholism is not a consequence of weak willpower.
Client Needs Category—Psychosocial integrity
Client Needs Subcategory—None

3. 3. Al-Anon is an organization specifically for family members of alcoholics who may or may not be involved in recovery. Alcoholics Anonymous is for recovering alcoholics. Recovery Anonymous is a support group for persons with mental disorders. Synanon is a private organization involved in drug rehabilitation.
Client Needs Category—Psychosocial integrity
Client Needs Subcategory—None

4. 2. Inflammation of the eyes is almost always present after smoking marijuana. The pulse rate is likely to be rapid. Other signs include euphoria, drowsiness, light-headedness, and hunger. Shivering accompanies

opiate withdrawal, not marijuana use. Rapid breathing and restlessness are observed in abrupt alcohol withdrawal or with use of a central nervous system stimulant.
Client Needs Category—Psychosocial integrity
Client Needs Subcategory—None

5. 1. The most likely effect of marijuana from among those listed is drowsiness. Other symptoms include impaired motor coordination, inappropriate laughter, impaired judgment and short-term memory, and distortions of time and perception. Central nervous system stimulants, such as cocaine and amphetamines, are abused drugs that are more likely to cause hyperactivity, apprehension, and suspiciousness.
Client Needs Category—Psychosocial integrity
Client Needs Subcategory—None

6. 1. Marijuana is known to produce apathy among those who use it. Consequently, many chronic users become disinterested in school, work, or other social responsibilities. As a result, they fail to reach their potential for success. Marijuana is more likely to be psychologically addicting. Most do not use this drug often enough or long enough to show a statistical relationship with lung cancer. Breathing may be impaired, but the respiratory center in the brain is not usually suppressed as it is in heroin or morphine abuse.
Client Needs Category—Psychosocial integrity
Client Needs Subcategory—None

7. 2. Chronic use of marijuana may cause problems with memory, similar to the effect associated with chronic alcohol abuse. One symptom of marijuana use is drowsiness; therefore, sleeping is not a problem. Marijuana use is not associated with drinking large volume of liquids or having a low tolerance for frustration even though the user's judgment is impaired.
Client Needs Category—Psychosocial integrity
Client Needs Subcategory—None

8. 4. SIDS is the unexpected, unexplained death of an infant who is typically between ages 2 weeks and 1 year old. In most cases, the infant is layed down for a nap or to sleep at night and then, after several hours, is found dead in his crib. Common risk factors include prematurity, low birth weight, and an adolescent or opioid-dependent mother.

Because of the abruptness and finality of the situation, the parents of an infant who died from SIDS have a very difficult time accepting their infant's death. Their most immediate need is to experience the reality of their loss. Facilitating an opportunity to have personal contact with the infant promotes the grieving process. The other nursing actions may be completed at a later time.
Client Needs Category—Psychosocial integrity
Client Needs Subcategory—None

9. 2. Most parents feel guilty immediately after the death of a previously healthy infant, as occurs in SIDS. They need reassurance that they are in no way to blame for the child's death. Later, the parents may benefit from professional or support group help in resolving their anger, fear, and depression.
Client Needs Category—Psychosocial integrity
Client Needs Subcategory—None

10. 3. It is important to relieve parents of any self-blame after the unexpected death of an infant. Unfortunately, many parents are suspected of child abuse in cases like this. Informing them of the staff's efforts and where grief support may be obtained are appropriate nursing actions, but they are secondary to relieving undeserved guilt. Indicating that the child may have had brain damage is little consolation immediately after the infant's death.
Client Needs Category—Psychosocial integrity
Client Needs Subcategory—None

11. 1. Domestic abuse is maltreatment by a family member toward someone else living in the household. If the abused individual comes to the emergency department and is treated for trauma (bruising, burns, broken bones, lacerations, or head injuries), the investigation of potential domestic abuse is a priority. Candidly asking if the person is being abused is the most straightforward way to obtain information. Although many victims of abuse protect their abuser, they are not apt to reveal their abuse unless they sense that someone is concerned enough to ask. It is appropriate to assess the children for signs of abuse, but this would be done secondarily. Checking with relatives or friends may damage the nurse-client relationship or jeopardize the victim's safety if the abusive spouse becomes aware of the inquiry. Asking the client to return for a second visit may arouse suspicions in the abuser, which could cause further abuse for the client. The nurse should obtain as much information as possible during the initial visit.
Client Needs Category—Psychosocial integrity
Client Needs Subcategory—None

12. 2. More than anything else, knowing where there is a safe place to go for help empowers the victim to protect herself when exposed to future violence. Giving out a personal phone number is never appropriate. Many women stay in abusive relationships because they think the abuser will change. Trying to terminate an abusive relationship may also escalate the frequency or severity of violence. Most male batterers are resistant to change and are unlikely to participate in joint counseling.
Client Needs Category—Psychosocial integrity
Client Needs Subcategory—None

13. **3.** Many victims of family violence believe that, if they behave in an ideal way, they can prevent the cycle of abuse. Some persons even blame themselves or believe that they deserve the abuse. Battered individuals feel hopeless and powerless and have a great deal of guilt. Often, abused women have no money and lack the skills and self-esteem to earn it. They need a great deal of support to leave their partners, and extended family members may not be willing to take in the victim because of fear for their own safety. Most know that the abuse is serious or even life-threatening, that they may be murdered if they attempt to terminate the relationship, and that their family most likely will be unsupportive.

Client Needs Category—Psychosocial integrity
Client Needs Subcategory—None

14. **1.** Rape is forced sexual activity involving intercourse and penetration of an orifice by the penis. It is a deviant behavior and a crime of violence. Sexual assault refers to other forced sex acts (such as oral or anal intrusion). To preserve possible evidence, a physical examination should be performed before the victim showers or bathes, brushes her teeth, douches, changes her clothes, or has anything to drink. If there is no report of oral sex, rinsing the mouth and drinking fluids may be permitted. Evidence of pubic hair, semen, skin, and nail samples are some of the data collected from the victim. Although a sketch of the rapist or a written description of the crime may be helpful, rape victims are usually not capable of completing these activities independently. It is inappropriate to recommend calling 911 if the victim is in no immediate danger. However, advising the victim to call a support person is appropriate, but not the most important information to convey.

Client Needs Category—Psychosocial integrity
Client Needs Subcategory—None

15. **4.** The most supportive nursing activity is to remain with a rape victim at all times. Such victims of crime suffer a great deal of stress, especially when they must interact with physicians or police officers who are both strangers and men. The other nursing actions are important to the care of rape victims, but they are not as likely to reduce anxiety as the continuous presence of an empathic nurse.

Client Needs Category—Psychosocial integrity
Client Needs Subcategory—None

16. **2.** Victims of violent crimes are likely to perceive strangers as a threat to their safety. Therefore, a priority for nursing care is to limit the number of client contacts with unfamiliar people, even though the strangers are well-meaning staff. The nurse is responsible for assessing the victim for physical and emotional trauma, whereas the police document the circumstances of the

rape. Sedation is generally avoided if at all possible because it interferes with crisis resolution. The nurse must obtain the victim's permission before contacting anyone. If permission is not obtained, contacting someone on behalf of the client violates the client's right to privacy and confidentiality.

Client Needs Category—Psychosocial integrity
Client Needs Subcategory—None

17. **2.** Providing explanations helps to reduce anxiety. It is especially important for clients who are trying to manage the stress of a traumatic experience. Giving clients opportunities to make choices is a therapeutic method of diminishing feelings of powerlessness. Although giving information does support standards of care established in the emergency department and meets the client's need for teaching, these are not the primary reasons for explaining care measures to a rape victim.

Client Needs Category—Psychosocial integrity
Client Needs Subcategory—None

18. **3.** Competent adult clients always have the right to make decisions regarding their treatment. Although a nurse may not feel that the decision is in the client's best interests, the client's right to refuse must be respected. Coercion in any form is inappropriate.

Client Needs Category—Psychosocial integrity
Client Needs Subcategory—None

19. **1.** Although all the options are possible outcomes of the group process, the most desired outcome for a self-help group is that the group members obtain mutual support from one another. Self-help groups allow members to express their feelings openly and honestly. Individual members have been through similar experiences and serve to validate the feelings and experiences of others in the group.

Client Needs Category—Psychosocial integrity
Client Needs Subcategory—None

20. **3.** Eating out of habit or hardly eating anything is an indication that a rape victim is not recovering readily from the crime. The other behavioral symptoms are more characteristic of a mild reaction to the rape trauma and are likely to be relieved with short-term support.

Client Needs Category—Psychosocial integrity
Client Needs Subcategory—None

21. **2.** Most people are momentarily shocked after receiving bad news. Disbelief or denial typically follows. Later, common emotional responses include anger, bargaining, depression, and acceptance—generally in that order.

Client Needs Category—Psychosocial integrity
Client Needs Subcategory—None

22. 4. Denial is the failure to acknowledge an unbearable condition or the failure to admit the reality of a situation. It is a protective mechanism. The need to deny may be so overwhelming that it interferes with a person's good judgment to implement safer sex practices. Concealing the information and avoiding contact with or confronting others are behaviors more indicative of depression and anger.
  Client Needs Category—Psychosocial integrity
  Client Needs Subcategory—None

23. 2. Having a social network of supportive friends and relatives diminishes a crisis. This promotes subsequent coping. Acceptance by religious leaders, new social acquaintances, and sexual tolerance do not provide the same quality of emotional support.
  Client Needs Category—Psychosocial integrity
  Client Needs Subcategory—None

24. 4. Some people entertain thoughts of suicide as their only means of relieving others and themselves of the hopelessness of living with a terminal disease. Signs of despair indicate that a client should be closely observed to ensure safety. Dreams may be an indication that the client is fearful of dying. The other remarks are more suggestive of someone seeking information.
  Client Needs Category—Psychosocial integrity
  Client Needs Subcategory—None

25. 1. Bingeing and purging take place privately. Staying out of the bathroom following a meal interferes with the client's opportunities to induce vomiting and use laxatives or enemas to stimulate bowel elimination. Having the client take an inventory of foods offered in the dormitory may precipitate an uncontrollable urge to go on an eating binge. The bulimic's food binges are not isolated to fast-food establishments. Recording calories only increases the anxiety that bulimics experience when their eating is out of control.
  Client Needs Category—Psychosocial integrity
  Client Needs Subcategory—None

26. 3. A reduction in bingeing is the best therapeutic effect for this client because it breaks the binge-purge cycle. The problem with bulimics is not that they do not eat nutritious food, but that they eat too much food. Usually, the food they eat is high in carbohydrates and calories. After eating large amounts of these types of foods, bulimics feel guilty and have abdominal discomfort. Purging reduces the guilt and decreases the abdominal pain. Antidepressants work well in controlling the symptoms of bulimics who are not clinically depressed. Usually bulimics do not display signs of suicide; therefore, the physician would not prescribe antidepressants for reducing suidical tendencies.

  Client Needs Category—Physiological integrity
  Client Needs Subcategory—Pharmacological therapies

27. 3. Peer censure is much more therapeutic than disapproval from the group leader. If the therapist or members of the treatment team react positively or negatively to the individuals involved in the conflict, it is likely to divide the group members and jeopardize group work.
  Client Needs Category—Psychosocial integrity
  Client Needs Subcategory—None

28. 2. Being overly talkative is a common sign of use of amphetamines such as dextroamphetamine (Dexedrin). This drug is a stimulant; staring into space and slurring words are side effects typical of depressant types of drugs. Some marijuana users wear sunglasses indoors to disguise their inflamed eyes.
  Client Needs Category—Psychosocial integrity
  Client Needs Subcategory—None

29. 1. Young adults who have not acquired the developmental characteristic of intimacy tend to have superficial relationships that are temporary in nature. Worrying about financial security is more common during the middle years of adulthood. A person's sexual identity is established much earlier in life. Assertiveness is more of a unique personality characteristic than one commonly acquired at a particular stage in life.
  Client Needs Category—Health promotion and maintenance
  Client Needs Subcategory—None

30. 4. Rationalization is a coping mechanism in which a person fails to take responsibility for something by offering some acceptable explanation for it. Indicating health risks from being overweight is an example of intellectualization. The failure to resist ice cream demonstrates that the client has insight into his behavior. Projection is the mechanism of accusing others of one's own feelings that are too painful to acknowledge.
  Client Needs Category—Psychosocial integrity
  Client Needs Subcategory—None

31. 2. Non-English-speaking clients or those who speak very little English feel more comfortable communicating with and through a translator of their own gender. This reduces embarrassment about questions pertaining to genitourinary functions, bowel elimination, reproductive history, and other sensitive issues related to mental health history. Translation cards have key words and phrases in various foreign languages and may be helpful in conveying important words in the foreign language; however, it would be difficult for the nurse to ask all questions included in the admission database using such cards. Having a member of the housekeeping staff translate sensitive history to the nurse is inappropriate. Having a family member translate the information may or may not be a good choice, depending on the nature of the relationship and the level of understanding of medical terminology. Also, the nurse would not be sure that the information is being accurately conveyed.

> **Client Needs Category**—*Psychosocial integrity*
> **Client Needs Subcategory**—*None*

32. 4. As long as a health belief has no detrimental effect, it is best to integrate it in the care plan. Rejecting an otherwise neutral cultural practice interferes with a therapeutic nurse-client relationship. However, the nurse must be mindful of the client's need for safety and the safety needs of the other clients and staff.

> **Client Needs Category**—*Health promotion and maintenance*
> **Client Needs Subcategory**—*None*

33. 2. Snorting cocaine on a routine basis will most likely ulcerate, erode, and perforate the nasal mucosa and septum. Even with routine use of cocaine, the breath sounds should be clear, not congested. Cocaine users have a runny nose due to the irritation of the drug in the nasal passages; they usually do not have frontal sinus pain.

> **Client Needs Category**—*Psychosocial integrity*
> **Client Needs Subcategory**—*None*

34. 1. Cocaine abuse can result in cardiac arrhythmias and death because toxicity may occur anytime and with any dose. Cocaine is a central nervous system stimulant; it increases respirations and raises blood pressure. The client's blood glucose level may decrease, not elevate, due to calorie use during periods of hyperactivity.

> **Client Needs Category**—*Psychosocial integrity*
> **Client Needs Subcategory**—*None*

35. 4. Hallucinations are sensory experiences of which only the client is aware. They may be auditory, visual, olfactory, or tactile. An auditory hallucination involves hearing a voice or sound that no one else perceives. The person rarely volunteers his altered perceptions. The observant nurse draws inferences based on the client's nonverbal cues. The first three examples are not associated with the behavior of a hallucinating client.

> **Client Needs Category**—*Psychosocial integrity*
> **Client Needs Subcategory**—*None*

36. 2. Schizophrenia is a group of mental disorders characterized by a gradual deterioration of mental functioning. As a result of the schizophrenic's disordered thoughts, he may have difficulty putting thoughts into words. The nurse should never pretend to understand the meaning of a client's illogical statement or twist the words to interpret the statement as something logical.

> **Client Needs Category**—*Psychosocial integrity*
> **Client Needs Subcategory**—*None*

37. 1. Hospitalization is indicated when a client poses a danger to himself or others. In this case, the client is neglecting his bodily needs and, therefore, hospitalization is warranted. The other options suggest that the client is having problems with socialization skills, but they are not conditions that improve with hospitalization.

> **Client Needs Category**—*Psychosocial integrity*
> **Client Needs Subcategory**—*None*

38. 2. The most common side effects of risperidone (Risperdal) include insomnia and agitation. Orthostatic hypotension also occurs with reflex tachycardia. Risperidone (Risperdal) does not increase extrapyramidal symptoms. Anticholinergic symptoms such as urine retention are not commonly reported. Weight gain, not loss, may develop.

> **Client Needs Category**—*Physiological integrity*
> **Client Needs Subcategory**—*Pharmacological therapies*

Mental Health Needs During Middle Age (35-65)

39. 2. Regardless of the cause or the client's level of mental functioning, it is important to establish that there are limits for the client's behavior. Leaving the room first is insufficient to establish a relationship between the nurse's response and the unacceptable behavior. Ignoring the behavior is more likely to communicate permission to repeat it. The same is true for trying to avoid being a repeat target.

> **Client Needs Category**—*Psychosocial integrity*
> **Client Needs Subcategory**—*None*

40. 1. One of the best ways to modify behavior is to impose a significant consequence that has been previously communicated to the client. Wearing protective garments will not stop the behavior, although it is appropriate hygienically. It is unrealistic to think that a client with impaired cognition will be persuaded to change his behavior as a result of intellectual reasoning.

> **Client Needs Category**—*Psychosocial integrity*
> **Client Needs Subcategory**—*None*

41. 2. To obtain the most valid results from the mental status assessment of a client who is cognitively impaired, it is best to allow extra time for the client to respond to questions. A certain number of open-ended questions are necessary during a mental status examination, regardless of the client's cognitive ability. Omit-

ting the assessment or deferring the entire assessment to someone else violates standards of care.
Client Needs Category—*Psychosocial integrity*
Client Needs Subcategory—*None*

42. 1. Panic attacks are one type of anxiety disorder. The physical symptoms are generally a consequence of sympathetic nervous system stimulation, as in the release of adrenaline, which causes an increased heart rate. Clients may think that they are having a heart attack or even dying. Sympathetic nervous system stimulation is also associated with hypertension, a dry mouth, and dilated pupils.
Client Needs Category—*Physiological integrity*
Client Needs Subcategory—*Physiological adaptation*

43. 4. Panic attacks are due to the interplay of biological and physiological factors. A person who begins to experience the symptoms typically fears that the symptoms are life-threatening. The combination of symptoms followed by fear followed by intensified symptoms creates a vicious circle. To the client experiencing panic attacks, these symptoms are real and usually have a known cause. The client does not feign the attacks or seek attention through them; such attacks are a source of true distress.
Client Needs Category—*Psychosocial integrity*
Client Needs Subcategory—*None*

44. 4. Most people experience increased anxiety during situations in which they have no prior experience. To a client who is already anxious, this unfamiliarity adds to the anxiety. Providing explanations and instructions helps to diminish the client's insecurity, thereby decreasing the anxiety. Standing within an arm's length invades a client's personal space and heightens anxiety. A nurse wearing a laboratory coat may nonverbally upset a client, depending on what the coat represents from past experiences. Wearing a name tag and introducing yourself are always appropriate, regardless of the client or the occasion. Coffee and tea contain stimulating chemicals and should be avoided in an anxious client.
Client Needs Category—*Psychosocial integrity*
Client Needs Subcategory—*None*

45. 1. Being reassured about safety helps more than the other actions to reduce the client's feelings of fear and loss of control; feeling safe interrupts the vicious cycle of fear and panic. Being believed, trusted, and accepted are integral to establishing a therapeutic relationship.
Client Needs Category—*Psychosocial integrity*
Client Needs Subcategory—*None*

46. 4. Staying with a frightened client communicates genuine concern, and the presence of a caring person tends to reduce anxiety. The first choice is an example of giving advice, which is a nontherapeutic communication technique. It is inappropriate to try to shame the client with the possibility of physician intervention in response to out-of-control behavior. The third nontherapeutic example is one of generalizing, which disregards this client's right to be considered unique.
Client Needs Category—*Psychosocial integrity*
Client Needs Subcategory—*None*

47. 1. Antianxiety drugs such as alprazolam (Xanax) produce a calming effect. Alcohol consumption with this medication is likely to potentiate the drug's action and endanger the client's safety from profound sedation. Drug dependency is related to this drug's dosage and length of administration. Insomnia is unlikely because the drug causes sedation. Blood levels are not commonly monitored when benzodiazepines such as alprazolam (Xanax) are prescribed.
Client Needs Category—*Physiological integrity*
Client Needs Subcategory—*Pharmacological therapies*

48. 2. Many clients who experience panic attacks develop agoraphobia, a fear of being in a place or situation where help may be unavailable. Some clients who experience panic attacks seek psychiatric treatment and some take more than the prescribed amount of medication, but these are not characteristic of the majority of individuals with this anxiety disorder. Persons with panic disorder rarely develop psychotic symptoms.
Client Needs Category—*Psychosocial integrity*
Client Needs Subcategory—*None*

49. 1, 2, 5, 6. Obsessive-compulsive disorder (OCD) is a type of anxiety disorder. Obsessions are irrational thoughts, unwanted ideas, or impulses that occur repeatedly in a person's mind. Obsessions are often intense, frightening, or bizarre and commonly focus on fear of dirt and germs, contamination, and violent or aggressive behavior. Religious thoughts or sexual feelings are also common. Compulsions are the repetitive rituals that individuals perform to lessen anxiety and make them feel temporarily better. Unfortunately, the good feelings do not last, and the ritual begins again. Typical compulsions include excessive washing (particularly of the hands or body), cleaning, checking, counting, arranging, and hoarding. Compulsions commonly occupy a great deal time, which interferes with work performance and normal lifestyle.

Clients with OCD are preoccupied with order and symmetry; they are ashamed of their problem and, therefore, try to hide it. Stress and other psychological factors make the problem worse. The disorder usually begins in adolescence or early adulthood. Of the clients listed, those demonstrating OCD tendencies include the client who repeatedly washes her hands, the one who makes coffee several times per day, the man who cannot throw anything away, and the woman who repeatedly checks and rechecks the locks on her door. Sexual promiscuity is common among those in a manic phase of bipolar disorder. Drinking a fifth of whiskey every day is indicative of alcoholism.

Client Needs Category—Psychosocial integrity
Client Needs Subcategory—None

50. 1, 3. Effective treatment of OCD includes the administration of SSRIs such as fluvoxamine (Luvox). Serotonin is thought to be lacking in clients with OCD; SSRIs replace the missing serotonin in the brain. Cognitive-behavioral therapy is also beneficial because it teaches clients how to confront their thoughts and refuse their rituals. Eventually, anxiety decreases and the clients lessen their preoccupation with thoughts and actions. ECT is used in some circumstances for clients who have severe depression that is unresponsive to other forms of therapy. Clients with OCD do not need a lobotomy, which involves removal of part of the brain. Tranquilizers are also not used for treatment of this disorder.

Client Needs Category—Psychosocial integrity
Client Needs Subcategory—None

51. 4. Displacement is a coping mechanism in which a person transfers his angry feelings for one person onto someone else who is less likely to retaliate with significant consequences. Introjection involves taking on the characteristics of another. Projection is characterized by accusing someone of one's own weaknesses. Compensation is demonstrated by overcoming some inadequacy by excelling at another activity.

Client Needs Category—Psychosocial integrity
Client Needs Subcategory—None

52. 3. By remaining calm, the nurse models the type of behavior that is expected and reduces stimuli that the client may interpret as threatening. Using additional medication relieves the client of responsibility for managing his feelings. Physical activity is a way of dissipating anger, but it should not supersede discussing the client's feelings. Although encouraging the client to discuss what triggered his anger would be beneficial, it would be inappropriate to suggest talking to the client's wife.

Client Needs Category—Psychosocial integrity
Client Needs Subcategory—None

53. 1. Gathering staff is a show of force, which is sometimes all that a client needs to realize that it is best to regain self-control. Asking a physician to intervene implies that nurses are unable to effectively manage a disruptive client's behavior. It is unsafe to go anywhere alone with a client who is beyond anger and in danger of losing self-control. Displaying restraints as a means of controlling the client's behavior is an implied threat, which is unethical.

Client Needs Category—Psychosocial integrity
Client Needs Subcategory—None

54. 2. Administering medications against a client's will when the circumstances indicate a danger to the client or others is legally permissible. To avoid liability, documentation must objectively describe the evidence of danger and the *lack* of success when alternative measures were attempted. In most cases, the nurse should be respectful of the client's right to refuse the medication. However, if the client is demonstrating signs that harm to himself or others is possible, the client's rights are waived. The nurse does not need to get permission from a judge to administer the drug, and the hospital attorney does not need to be notified.

Client Needs Category—Safe, effective care environment
Client Needs Subcategory—Coordinated care

55. 2. Using short, simple sentences is best when teaching anxious clients who have short attention spans and difficulty concentrating. Detailed explanations or elaborate diagrams would overwhelm an anxious client. Videotapes are not as effective as one-on-one instruction in this situation. The nurse needs to periodically assess the client's comprehension and repeat information that is unclear.

Client Needs Category—Health promotion and maintenance
Client Needs Subcategory—None

56. 1. Middle-aged adults forced into early retirement are likely to experience a great deal of stress because adults at this stage in life are very concerned with their future financial security. The other events are challenging but probably not major sources of conflict as adults achieve generativity.

Client Needs Category—Health promotion and maintenance
Client Needs Subcategory—None

57. 3. Phobic people avoid what they perceive as the cause of their discomfort. Suppression is a coping mechanism in which a person chooses to refrain from thinking about something that is a source of conflict. Compensation is characterized by pursuing an activity that ensures success to make up for feeling inadequate. Undoing is a coping mechanism in which one makes amends for having offended someone.

Client Needs Category—Psychosocial integrity
Client Needs Subcategory—None

58. **1, 2, 3, 4.** Phobias are a type of anxiety involving persistent, irrational fears. They can be classified as social (public speaking), agoraphobia (fear of crowds or public places), and simple (fear of certain objects or stimuli, such as animals, insects, heights, enclosed spaces, and flying). Common signs and symptoms include sweating, tachycardia and palpitations, tremors, shortness of breath, nausea, nightmares, and flushing. The client may manifest such signs and symptoms when coming in contact with the fear or by thinking or discussing the fear. Uncontrollable crying is more indicative of depression, and facial tics are commonly associated with Tourette syndrome.

Client Needs Category—Psychosocial integrity
Client Needs Subcategory—None

59. **1.** Cognitive therapy involves confronting irrational thoughts and behaviors. The expected outcome is that the client will recognize the flaws in her thinking and ultimately change her behavior. The remaining options describe desensitization therapy, assertiveness training, and behavioral modification in that order.

Client Needs Category—Psychosocial integrity
Client Needs Subcategory—None

60. **1.** Clients with PTSD generally reexperience their traumatic events in some way, such as through upsetting dreams, nightmares, or flashbacks. Some clients have visual hallucinations, but generally not auditory hallucinations. Most have a numbed or blunted emotional response to others with whom they interact.

Client Needs Category—Psychosocial integrity
Client Needs Subcategory—None

61. **3.** Clients with PTSD who are able to recall the precipitating traumatic event use a tremendous amount of energy to control their feelings or to suppress the memory of it. Giving clients permission to talk about the traumatic event can be very therapeutic. Many clients with this disorder abuse drugs and alcohol to help numb their consciousness; antianxiety drugs are likely to do the same. Improving damaged relationships is a goal of therapy, but it is not the primary focus of treatment. Monitoring the client's physical symptoms is advisable, but it is not as therapeutic as the use of appropriate communication skills.

Client Needs Category—Psychosocial integrity
Client Needs Subcategory—None

62. **1.** Art is used as a therapeutic tool to promote the expression of thoughts or feelings that are too difficult to verbalize. Although the other outcomes in the remaining options may occur, none is the primary purpose underlying the intervention.

Client Needs Category—Psychosocial integrity
Client Needs Subcategory—None

63. **3.** A stimulus that evokes a physiological response similar to that of the original traumatic event can trigger intense anxiety. The stimulus of the fireworks is similar to that of gunfire and can produce the anxiety from that time. If the client had been frightened of fireworks as a child, he probably would have manifested a continued fear response prior to his military experience. In this case, the startle response is not associated with a fear of getting injured from the fireworks or a fear of painful memories.

Client Needs Category—Psychosocial integrity
Client Needs Subcategory—None

64. **2.** PTSD can occur in anyone who is involved in an uncommon event outside the realm of usual human experience. This can involve natural disasters such as earthquakes or situational disasters such as being raped. None of the other situations play a role in development of this disorder.

Client Needs Category—Health promotion and maintenance
Client Needs Subcategory—None

65. **4.** Assessment is the first step in the nursing process. Therefore, the nurse should take the client's vital signs before implementing any further action. After completing the assessment and finding the client in no immediate danger, the nurse can address other nursing interventions.

Client Needs Category—Safe, effective care environment
Client Needs Subcategory—Safety and infection control

66. **1.** Middle adulthood is characterized as a period of either generativity or stagnation. During this stage in the life cycle, it is common for people to assess their accomplishments. In some cases, those who view themselves as not having accomplished much experience what is known as a *midlife crisis*. People usually establish goals at an earlier age. Middle-aged people may regret, but typically do not doubt, their judgment. They may also envy others' achievements but being envious of others is something that happens at all stages of life, not just during middle age.

Client Needs Category—Health promotion and maintenance
Client Needs Subcategory—None

67. **2.** Therapeutic communication requires that the nurse assess hidden meanings within a client's statements or questions, then verbalize the feeling or tone for validation. Deferring discussion to the physician is a form of scapegoating, which conveys to the client that the nurse chooses to remain uninvolved. Telling the client to let the staff worry or to practice more patience is giving advice, which is a nontherapeutic form of communication.

Client Needs Category—Psychosocial integrity
Client Needs Subcategory—None

68. **2.** Emotional care involves a sincere respect, interest, and concern for people. Nurses demonstrate emotional care when they accept a person's individual differences and treat each client as unique. It is important in this situation for the nurse to remain objective in providing emotional care, especially if the nurse shares the husband's opinion about the client's condition. A health care worker's biases and prejudices, if unchallenged, can interfere with objective care. Although all the other outcomes are possible, the most detrimental effect is to the client.

Client Needs Category—Psychosocial integrity
Client Needs Subcategory—None

69. **1, 2, 3, 4, 5.** Hypochondriacs are often preoccupied with vague physical complaints, such as fatigue, headaches, nausea, or dizziness. They fear or believe that they have a major disease, despite constant reassurance that they are healthy. Hypochondriacs may even fixate on specific diseases after reading or hearing about them. Risk factors for hypochondria include a family history of hypochondria; a diagnosed anxiety disorder; physical, sexual, or emotional abuse in childhood; witnessed violence in childhood; a stressful experience with a loved one's illness; and alcoholism. Fear of death is a common symptom of hypochondriacs, but it is not considered a risk factor.

Client Needs Category—Psychosocial integrity
Client Needs Subcategory—None

70. **1, 2, 3, 4, 5, 6.** Hypochondriasis is a psychological disorder characterized by the belief that real or imagined minor physical symptoms are a sign of serious illness. Even when several doctors assure the person otherwise, a hypochondriac is convinced that he has a serious disease. Major signs and symptoms of this disorder include becoming knowledgeable about specific illnesses and their symptoms; a chronic fear that minor symptoms are signs of a serious illness; multiple, vague physical complaints that often change over time (headache, dizziness, backache, stomachache); interference with social life, work, or marriage and the loss of income; multiple doctor visits, sometimes several in the same day; and repeated requests for tests for the same symptoms. In many cases, clients go from physician to physician hoping that they will be diagnosed with a physical disease.

Client Needs Category—Psychosocial integrity
Client Needs Subcategory—None

71. **3.** Only hospital employees who are immediately involved in the care of a client may have access to the client's health record. This is a Health Insurance Portability and Accountability (HIPPA) Act regulation designed to protect the client's health information and treatment. Some examples of a client's protected health history include name, address, phone number, age, Social Security number, and insurance or banking account numbers. A signed, written release from the client must be obtained before confidential information is divulged. The nurse must take all necessary measures to safeguard health information in the client's medical record and to maintain confidentiality.

Client Needs Category—Safe, effective care environment
Client Needs Subcategory—Coordinated care

72. **4.** A client with ulcerative colitis has an inflamed bowel and experiences severe diarrhea with up to 30 stools per day. Endoscopic examinations and X-rays confirm the presence of pathology; therefore, option 2 is inaccurate. In addition, the client does experience physical symptoms, which makes option 1 incorrect. The exact cause of the disease is unknown, but emotional stress is one of many cofactors. Most clients with psychophysiological diseases would rather work than experience their symptoms.

Client Needs Category—Psychosocial integrity
Client Needs Subcategory—None

73. **1.** Meeting physiological needs always takes precedence over other needs, including security, love, and belonging. The most important information needed at this time concerns the client's bowel elimination and its impact on fluid status, nutrition, and electrolyte balance.

Client Needs Category—Physiological integrity
Client Needs Subcategory—Basic care and comfort

74. **1.** Cleaning stool is never pleasant; however, the nurse can avoid making the client feel responsible for his condition or offensive to others by conveying a nonjudgmental attitude when providing care. Treating the client with dignity will help sustain his self-esteem. Having the client's wife or a male nurse clean his stool or making the client responsible for all of his hygiene would not promote his self-esteem; in fact, these measures might have the opposite effect.

Client Needs Category—Psychosocial integrity
Client Needs Subcategory—None

75. **2.** A consequence of alcohol abuse is a tolerance to all sedative drugs. A need for a higher dosage or more frequent administration can indicate that the client abuses alcohol or some other central nervous system depressant drug. An alcoholic's blood pressure and pulse become abnormally high during withdrawal from alcohol. There is no cause-and-effect relationship between the absence of bowel sounds and the abuse of alcohol.

***Client Needs Category**—Psychosocial integrity*
***Client Needs Subcategory**—None*

76. 3. Visual hallucinations occur in advanced withdrawal from alcohol. These are real and terrifying experiences for the alcoholic. To maintain safety and reduce the client's fear and anxiety, it is essential that a nurse remain with the client. Restraints should be used only when all other alternatives for maintaining the safety of the client or others have been exhausted. In the client's mind, the hallucination is real; telling him that he is not seeing bugs would be illogical and untrue. Closing the client's door is unsafe and likely to heighten his fear.

***Client Needs Category**—Psychosocial integrity*
***Client Needs Subcategory**—None*

77. 3. It is always best to notify the physician first whenever there is a sudden change in a client's condition. Usually the nursing supervisor is not called unless the client becomes combative or his condition continues to worsen. Alcohol withdrawal is generally treated with one of the minor tranquilizers, such as lorazepam (Ativan), or a central nervous system depressant such as phenobarbital; however, a physician must prescribe these. Notifying the client's wife may be indicated, but only after the physician has been notified and the client's safety is secured. Documenting the incident is important after the situation is under control.

***Client Needs Category**—Physiological integrity*
***Client Needs Subcategory**—Physiological adaptation*

78. 2. Seizures occur from rebound central nervous system stimulation as the alcohol is metabolized from the client's system. Seizures occur in some clients as early as within the first 24 hours of withdrawal. Of the choices listed, seizures are the most severe. Hypothermia does occur during alcohol withdrawal, but its severity is of much less concern to the nurse than are seizures. Ascities and jaundice result from liver damage caused by chronic alcohol abuse.

***Client Needs Category**—Physiological integrity*
***Client Needs Subcategory**—Physiological adaptation*

79. 1. Staff members are better able to understand client behavior by increasing their own self-awareness. Nurses who are generalists are not academically prepared to analyze a client's motivation or provide psychotherapy. Knowledge of abnormal behavior is important, but it is not the first step in understanding the behavior of others.

***Client Needs Category**—Psychosocial integrity*
***Client Needs Subcategory**—None*

80. 3. Clients with bipolar disorder, formerly called manic-depressive disorder, have cycles in which they display a marked change in mood between mania (abnormal highs) and depression (lows). The disorder is called bipolar because of the swings between the opposing poles in mood. Mania often affects thinking, judgment, and social behavior, causing serious problems. Bipolar disorder is a recurring illness that can be treated with long-term medication. The exaggerated mood is followed or preceded by an interval of normal mood. None of the other behaviors is symptomatic of bipolar disorder.

***Client Needs Category**—Psychosocial integrity*
***Client Needs Subcategory**—None*

81. 4,5. Lithium carbonate (Lithane) is a mood-stabilizing drug approved for the treatment of mania and for preventing the recurrence of manic-depressive cycles. Clients who take this medication should drink 10 to 12 glasses of water each day and increase their salt intake. Sexual activity need not be restricted. Lithium carbonate (Lithane) usually causes polyuria; therefore, notifying the physician about increased urine output is unnecessary. Avoiding aged cheeses or wine is an instruction given to clients who take monoamine oxidase inhibitors (MAOIs), not lithium.

***Client Needs Category**—Physiological integrity*
***Client Needs Subcategory**—Pharmacological therapies*

82. 3. Lithium carbonate (Lithane) has a narrow therapeutic range. Toxic reactions occur when blood levels are more than 1.5 mEq/L. Common side effects include GI discomfort, nausea, muscle weakness, vertigo, and a dazed feeling. Blood levels are usually drawn throughout therapy, and the lithium dosage is adjusted according to the results. The client who takes lithium carbonate (Lithane) may develop polyuria, but the volume of urine eliminated is not used to monitor the lithium level. Close monitoring of kidney, cardiovascular, and thyroid functions is important. Neither vital signs nor brain scans are used to evaluate the client's ability to metabolize her lithium dose.

***Client Needs Category**—Physiological integrity*
***Client Needs Subcategory**—Pharmacological therapies*

83. 1. Spending money extravagantly is a sign that a client with bipolar disorder is having difficulty using good judgment. Wanting to become a 5-year-old again could be interpreted as an example of an altered thought process related to schizophrenia. Methodically cleaning the house could indicate obsessive-compulsive behavior. Staying up late may be a sign of grandiose ideas and hyperactivity that often accompany a manic phase of bipolar disorder. However, such behavior is not as suggestive of loss of control as the client's spending money extravagantly.

> *Client Needs Category—Psychosocial integrity*
> *Client Needs Subcategory—None*

Mental Health Needs During Late Adulthood (Over 65)

84. **2.** Privacy is important whenever the nurse gathers information of a personal nature. Regardless of the environment, clients have the right to expect that what they reveal will be kept private and confidential—even from well-meaning family members. Therefore, asking the family members to give the client privacy is prudent and advisable.

> *Client Needs Category—Safe, effective care environment*
> *Client Needs Subcategory—Coordinated care*

85. **1.** An indirect leading statement or open-ended question is purposely general and nonspecific. It allows the client to give as much information as she wants. Close-ended questions or statements, exemplified in the other three options, provide facts or sometimes one-word replies.

> *Client Needs Category—Psychosocial integrity*
> *Client Needs Subcategory—None*

86. **3.** Asking the client to identify her birth date is a standard technique for assessing long-term memory. To evaluate the client's response, the nurse should know the answer to the question. Asking the client her current age and today's date helps in the assessment of short-term memory and orientation. Asking what occurred last January is too vague a question for a valid assessment.

> *Client Needs Category—Psychosocial integrity*
> *Client Needs Subcategory—None*

87. **1.** Asking a client to repeat the question helps to rule out a hearing deficit or possible dementia. A client has a 50% chance of being right when responding only with a "yes" or "no." Asking the next of kin is appropriate if the client is not a reliable historian. Asking questions only the client can answer does not provide comprehensive objective data.

> *Client Needs Category—Psychosocial integrity*
> *Client Needs Subcategory—None*

88. **2.** Being unable to provide the names of long-standing neighbors is the most significant sign of mental deterioration from among the options provided. In the normal progression of dementia, short-term memory loss is affected followed by long-term memory im-

pairment. The other assessment findings are normal or typical for an adult who is 65 years old.

> *Client Needs Category—Psychosocial integrity*
> *Client Needs Subcategory—None*

89. **1.** Late adulthood is a time when most people deal with multiple losses, including family and friends. The characteristics in the other options reflect myths about aging that many younger people believe are true.

> *Client Needs Category—Health promotion and maintenance*
> *Client Needs Subcategory—None*

90. **4.** In the interest of client safety, it is best to locate a depressed client where he can be frequently and closely observed by the nursing staff. Placing the depressed client alone or at the end of the hallway increases the potential for attempting suicide. Being in a room with a cheerful person and being placed in a non-stimulating environment are not considered therapeutic modalities for relieving depression.

> *Client Needs Category—Psychosocial integrity*
> *Client Needs Subcategory—None*

91. **2.** A plan for suicide indicates that the client has given serious thought to ending his life. A client who has developed a suicide plan is much more likely to act on his feelings. The remaining examples are characteristic of passive suicide ideation, which is not associated with as much lethal risk as an active suicide plan.

> *Client Needs Category—Psychosocial integrity*
> *Client Needs Subcategory—None*

92. **3.** Imipramine hydrochloride (Tofranil) is administered for depression. Client manifestations that occur quickly following initiation of the medication include improvement in sleep, appetite, and psychomotor disturbances (agitation and anxiety). Cognitive symptoms of depression, such as low self-esteem, guilt, suicidal ideation, and lack of concentration, tend to improve more slowly. Mood may be the last symptom to improve.

> *Client Needs Category—Physiological integrity*
> *Client Needs Subcategory—Pharmacological therapies*

93. **3, 4.** Imipramine hydrochloride (Tofranil) is a tricyclic antidepressant that is used to reduce the intensity and frequency of panic attacks and can also be used to reduce depression. Nursing instructions should include rising from the chair slowly because this drug has been associated with cardiac problems and ECG changes. Also, as with any antidepressant, it may take 3 to 4 weeks before the client begins to feel better. Avoiding cheese, chocolate, and pickled foods is related to monoamine oxidase inhibitors (MAOIs), not tricyclic antidepressants. The other choices are not related to tricyclic antidepressants.

> *Client Needs Category*—*Physiological integrity*
> *Client Needs Subcategory*—*Pharmacological therapies*

94. 2. The nurse must check that the depressed client has swallowed his medication. Some clients "cheek" medications, then use them as a method of suicide after accumulating a sufficient quantity. Taking medications with a full glass of water is appropriate for clients who do not have fluid restrictions. Some medications are better absorbed on an empty stomach; some that cause stomach upset are better taken with food. Taking one or all the prescribed drugs at one time is preferred as long as the client does not have difficulty swallowing them.

> *Client Needs Category*—*Physiological integrity*
> *Client Needs Subcategory*—*Pharmacological therapies*

95. 3. Following ECT, it is common for clients to experience headaches and temporary retrograde and antegrade memory loss for events nearest in time to the treatment. Proponents of ECT claim that the capacity to remember information eventually returns to the pretreatment level. The effects identified in the other options may occur, but they are not effects associated with ECT.

> *Client Needs Category*—*Physiological integrity*
> *Client Needs Subcategory*—*Physiological adaptation*

96. 2. Doxepin (Sinequan) and other tricyclic antidepressants may cause orthostatic hypotension, especially in the morning. The nurse should instruct the client to rise slowly and dangle his feet over the side of the bed before standing. This helps him gain his balance before walking. Placing a cool compress on the forehead may help the client initially, but orthostatic hypotension is still a concern when the client rises. Advising the client to take a hot shower may increase the dizziness due to increased vasodilation. Having the client elevate his feet will not decrease dizziness when he rises.

> *Client Needs Category*—*Physiological integrity*
> *Client Needs Subcategory*—*Physiological adaptation*

97. 2. Providing privacy is appropriate for preserving the sexually active couple's self-esteem. Reporting the clients' sexual behavior to their adult children is inappropriate, as long as the clients are competent and consenting adults and are in their right mind. The request to become roommates is better initiated by the residents. Censuring sexuality is inappropriate; even older adults have a need for love and affection.

> *Client Needs Category*—*Psychosocial integrity*
> *Client Needs Subcategory*—*None*

98. 1. Involuntary facial movements and tongue and eye movements indicate the development of tardive dyskinesia, a negative consequence of antipsychotic (neuroleptic) drug therapy. The condition is usually irreversible, even after the drug is discontinued. About 20% of those treated with antipsychotic medications in the long-term develop tardive dyskinesia. None of the other assessment findings is linked to antipsychotic drug withdrawal.

> *Client Needs Category*—*Physiological integrity*
> *Client Needs Subcategory*—*None*

99. 2. Depression in the elderly is often masked under the guise of multiple physical complaints. It is often easier to seek help for physical problems than to verbalize the need for emotional help. Elderly clients with depression are usually very demanding (use the call bell often) and frequently complain about every aspect of their care. Being irritable after a visit from active grandchildren is normal for some older adults. Sleeping a great deal of the time is suggestive of depression, but taking a lengthy nap regularly in the afternoon is not necessarily pathologic. Crying when talking about a dead spouse is normal if the death has been recent. If the crying is brief, it is not interpreted as unresolved grief.

> *Client Needs Category*—*Psychosocial integrity*
> *Client Needs Subcategory*—*None*

100. 4. SSRIs such as sertraline (Zoloft) tend to cause insomnia, nervousness, headache, anxiety, urine retention, blurred vision, and dry mucous membranes.

> *Client Needs Category*—*Physiological integrity*
> *Client Needs Subcategory*—*Pharmacological therapies*

101. 4. Self-worth is maintained by experiencing satisfaction in accomplishments. Giving genuine praise promotes a positive self-concept. The longer a person can maintain independence, the less likely that physical deterioration will occur. All the other choices communicate to the client that he is unable to manage his self-care satisfactorily.

> *Client Needs Category*—*Psychosocial integrity*
> *Client Needs Subcategory*—*None*

102. 2. Techniques that may facilitate reminiscing include singing songs from an earlier period and looking at picture albums, old catalogs, movies, and magazines. Discussing current events and reading a recent newspaper article help clients remain oriented to the present. Making holiday decorations is more likely to provide diversional therapy and help clients remain oriented.

> *Client Needs Category*—*Psychosocial integrity*
> *Client Needs Subcategory*—*None*

103. **2.** During senescence, it is common for people to review their life experiences. If clients believe that their lives have been satisfying and worthwhile, they acquire integrity. If clients have regrets, they close their lives with a feeling of despair. Trust is acquired during infancy. Intimacy is established during young adulthood. The toddler stage in the life cycle is associated with autonomy.

Client Needs Category—Health promotion and maintenance
Client Needs Subcategory—None

104. **4.** Words may not mean the same thing to all people. Reporting what was observed is a much more accurate and objective method for documenting behavior, especially in view of the fact that the nurse's notes are part of the permanent record that can be used as submissible evidence in a court of law. None of the other critiques identify the vague and subjective quality of the nurse's charting.

Client Needs Category—Safe, effective care environment
Client Needs Subcategory—Coordinated care

105. **1.** Labeling rooms with easily identifiable words or pictures promotes environmental awareness. Sensory cues restore the confused client's ability to reorient. Locking the unit deprives all the clients of a certain amount of freedom and privacy. Physical restraint used unnecessarily is considered battery. A confused client is unable to process information about the consequences of her behavior.

Client Needs Category—Psychosocial integrity
Client Needs Subcategory—None

106. **4.** It is essential that the nurse treat a client with cognitive impairment with dignity. Shielding her from public view by taking her to a vacant room is the most appropriate action for the nurse to take in this situation. It would be inappropriate and a violation of confidentiality to tell others about the client's mental impairment. The other options are better suited for a client with a higher level of cognitive function.

Client Needs Category—Psychosocial integrity
Client Needs Subcategory—None

107. **4.** Displaying a large calendar with easy-to-read words and numbers in a prominent place is one way to help older clients remain oriented. All of the other options have therapeutic benefits but are not useful in orienting clients to present reality.

Client Needs Category—Psychosocial integrity
Client Needs Subcategory—None

108. **2.** Consistent repetition in the unit routine helps clients with cognitive impairments stay oriented to activities in which they are expected to participate. Wear-

ing a name tag is a helpful technique, but routinely assigning the same employee to care for the same clients is even better. Altering a set routine of activities with field trips tends to disorient clients, at least temporarily. Clients with dementia are usually incapable of reading and following a written schedule.

Client Needs Category—Psychosocial integrity
Client Needs Subcategory—None

109. **2.** To facilitate attention, concentration, and retention, all verbal communication with a client with dementia should be brief and simple. Directions are given in understandable language with a minimum of distracting stimuli in the environment. Speaking loudly does not improve memory. Writing down some information may help a client to remember oral instructions, but overall it is not the best recommendation of the choices provided. Listening to a news program helps maintain reality orientation, but it does not promote memory.

Client Needs Category—Psychosocial integrity
Client Needs Subcategory—None

110. **2.** It is best to reinforce that the client is in the appropriate place. Trying to convince him that he is at home may provoke the client or agitate him further. Treating his request lightly communicates disrespect. Using the family as a scapegoat avoids responsibility for helping the client understand and cope.

Client Needs Category—Psychosocial integrity
Client Needs Subcategory—None

111. **2.** Nurses need to be alert to signs of burnout and exhaustion among family members. A caring staff member encouraging longer periods of separation can relieve the family's potential for feeling guilty. The client's wife may benefit from a physical examination, but that is not the most therapeutic action in the list of choices. Clients in a long-term health care facility have a right to see visitors at any time within reason. Indicating that the staff is capable of caring for the client's husband may imply that the wife is unappreciated or that her presence is an inconvenience.

Client Needs Category—Psychosocial integrity
Client Needs Subcategory—None

112. **2.** Reflection is a therapeutic communication technique in which the listener reflects the talker's expressed thoughts and related feelings. One of the greatest stressors for family members of clients with Alzheimer's is that those afflicted are physically present but emotionally absent. The remaining responses are clichés. They probably will not encourage the client's daughter to talk more about her feelings.

Client Needs Category—Psychosocial integrity
Client Needs Subcategory—None

113. **2.** Providing a client with environmental cues relieves confusion. Repetitious reminders help the confused person maintain or relearn how to function. A liquid diet is unappetizing and unnecessary as long as the client can chew, swallow, and digest food naturally. Serving this client early will not eliminate her confusion. Seating her alone deprives her of any role models to imitate and shows disregard for her dignity.
   Client Needs Category—*Psychosocial integrity*
   Client Needs Subcategory—*None*

114. **3.** Drugs are potentially unsafe if not administered correctly. The nurse usually takes the time to explain drug administration verbally in such situations; however, it is also helpful to reinforce verbal instructions with written information. Before the client leaves, the nurse needs to determine that the client's daughter has an accurate understanding of the instructions. The family is most likely already familiar with the other types of information.
   Client Needs Category—*Health promotion and maintenance*
   Client Needs Subcategory—*None*

115. **1.** A dying client with an advance directive should not be abandoned even though he does not want heroic measures taken to keep him alive. A nurse in the hall or in a nearby room does not guarantee that the dying client will receive support from the nursing staff. A dying client having access to a signal light does not replace the sustained presence of another human being.
   Client Needs Category—*Psychosocial integrity*
   Client Needs Subcategory—*None*

116. **3.** Expressing feelings to an understanding listener helps facilitate the grieving process. Communication helps people deal openly with their emotions and feelings, which is healthier than suppressing the event's emotional impact. Being sent home or terminated does not help promote grieving. Asking the nursing assistant to perform postmortem care in this emotional state shows a disregard for the trauma she is experiencing.
   Client Needs Category—*Psychosocial integrity*
   Client Needs Subcategory—*None*

117. **3.** Having a paranormal experience, such as sensing a deceased person's presence or seeing or talking to the deceased, can be comforting. As long as there is no potential for being financially, emotionally, or physically disadvantaged, the nurse should not dispute the bereaved person's experience.
   Client Needs Category—*Psychosocial integrity*
   Client Needs Subcategory—*None*

Postreview Tests

Comprehensive Test 1

Directions: With a pencil, blacken the space in front of the option you have chosen for your correct answer.

1. Which assessment finding provides the nurse with the best indication that a client's tracheostomy needs suctioning?
[ ] **1.** The client's pulse rate is decreased.
[ ] **2.** The client's skin is cool and moist.
[ ] **3.** The client's respirations are noisy.
[ ] **4.** The client is coughing up sputum.

2. Before suctioning a client with a tracheostomy, which nursing action should the nurse perform first?
[ ] **1.** Clean the tracheostomy with a sterile, cotton-tipped applicator.
[ ] **2.** Instill 5 mL of saline within the tracheostomy.
[ ] **3.** Administer 100% oxygen for 1 to 2 minutes.
[ ] **4.** Occlude the vent on the catheter for 15 seconds.

3. When changing a sterile abdominal dressing, which nursing action violates the principles of asepsis?
[ ] **1.** The nurse dons clean gloves to remove the soiled dressing.
[ ] **2.** The nurse places the soiled dressing in a moisture-resistant bag.
[ ] **3.** The nurse washes her hands before donning sterile gloves.
[ ] **4.** The nurse cleans the wound from the outer edge toward the center.

4. If a client with a conductive hearing loss asks the nurse how a hearing aid improves hearing, which response by the nurse is most appropriate?
[ ] **1.** "A hearing aid amplifies sounds that are heard."
[ ] **2.** "A hearing aid makes sounds sharper and clearer."
[ ] **3.** "A hearing aid produces more distinct, crisp speech."
[ ] **4.** "A hearing aid eliminates garbled background sounds."

5. The nurse observes a patient care technician assigned to a client who just returned to his room following a bronchoscopy. Which action would prompt the nurse to intervene?

[ ] **1.** The patient care technician takes the client's radial pulse.
[ ] **2.** The patient care technician offers the client some water.
[ ] **3.** The patient care technician raises the head of the bed.
[ ] **4.** The patient care technician takes the client's tympanic temperature.

6. When a client becomes angry and shouts at the nurse when a meal is not to his liking, which response by the nurse is most appropriate?
[ ] **1.** Say something humorous and promise to call the dietitian.
[ ] **2.** Listen attentively, allowing the client to express himself.
[ ] **3.** Leave the room, and allow the client a period of privacy.
[ ] **4.** Explain that, although the meal looks tasteless, it is nutritious.

7. At the time of a retinal detachment, the client will most likely describe which symptom?
[ ] **1.** Seeing flashes of light
[ ] **2.** Being unable to see light
[ ] **3.** Feeling discomfort in light
[ ] **4.** Seeing poorly in daylight

8. Which medication administration technique is best for a 3-month-old infant?
[ ] **1.** Putting the medication in the infant's bottle, and giving it during the next feeding
[ ] **2.** Placing the medication in a needleless syringe, and administering it orally
[ ] **3.** Giving the medication in a medicine cup while pinching the infant's nose shut
[ ] **4.** Mixing the medication with a small amount of cereal, and giving it with a spoon

9. Which assessment finding best indicates that Bryant's traction is applied properly to a small child?
[ ] **1.** The child can sit up without experiencing discomfort.
[ ] **2.** The child can reach the trapeze hanging above the bed.
[ ] **3.** The child's buttocks are raised slightly off the mattress.
[ ] **4.** The child's legs are pulled toward the bottom of the bed.

10. When planning care for a client in sickle cell crisis, what should be the main nursing priority?
[ ] **1.** Promoting self-care
[ ] **2.** Preventing immobility
[ ] **3.** Relieving discomfort
[ ] **4.** Improving self-esteem

11. A client newly diagnosed with cancer receives external radiation therapy. Which of the nurse's instructions regarding bathing is most appropriate?
[ ] **1.** Avoid getting the irradiated skin wet.
[ ] **2.** Use alcohol instead of soap on the irradiated skin.
[ ] **3.** Cover the reddened irradiated area with clear plastic.
[ ] **4.** Use a soft cloth to wash the irradiated skin.

12. If the physician orders "diet as tolerated" for a client postoperatively, which diet is most appropriate initially?
[ ] **1.** Bland diet
[ ] **2.** Soft diet
[ ] **3.** Clear liquid diet
[ ] **4.** Regular diet

13. If a pregnant client in her third trimester tells the nurse that she has had a severe headache for the past 2 days, which nursing action is most appropriate?
[ ] **1.** Informing her to increase her rest and leisure activities
[ ] **2.** Advising her to eliminate coffee or other sources of caffeine
[ ] **3.** Telling her to take two aspirin and lie down for an hour
[ ] **4.** Requesting that she be examined in the physician's office immediately

14. Laboratory data of an adult client diagnosed with *Pneumocystis carninii* pneumonia indicate that he is immunosuppressed. Which admission information is most helpful in determining the client's susceptibility to this infection?
[ ] **1.** The client's immunization history
[ ] **2.** The client's family history
[ ] **3.** The client's hygiene practices
[ ] **4.** The client's sexual practices

15. Which statement made by the parents of a toddler best suggests that the child has cystic fibrosis?
[ ] **1.** "Our child's perspiration is very salty."
[ ] **2.** "Our child vomits immediately after eating."
[ ] **3.** "Our child's stools are soft and bright yellow."
[ ] **4.** "Our child's urine is very light-colored."

16. If a client has been taking corticosteroid medication for a prolonged period, which statement provides the best indication that he understands the danger related to this medication?
[ ] **1.** "I should never suddenly stop taking my medication."
[ ] **2.** "My reaction time will be slowed while taking this drug."
[ ] **3.** "If I forget to take one dose, I should call the physician."
[ ] **4.** "I shouldn't take this drug for more than 6 months."

17. When monitoring the treatment response of a client with diabetes insipidus, which component of the urinalysis is most important for the nurse to assess?
[ ] **1.** Urine pH
[ ] **2.** Urinary casts
[ ] **3.** Specific gravity
[ ] **4.** Microscopic cells

18. While visiting a client who takes a prescribed diuretic, how can a home health care nurse best evaluate the drug's effectiveness?
[ ] **1.** Monitor the client's weight.
[ ] **2.** Palpate the client's peripheral pulses.
[ ] **3.** Assess the client's appetite.
[ ] **4.** Elicit the client's reflexes.

19. When applying nitroglycerin ointment to a client's chest, which nursing technique is most appropriate?
[ ] **1.** Squeezing a ribbon of ointment on paper
[ ] **2.** Rubbing the ointment thoroughly into the skin
[ ] **3.** Reapplying the ointment every 4 hours
[ ] **4.** Spreading the ointment directly over the heart area

20. Which instruction regarding rescue breathing is important to include in the parent-teaching plan when a newborn is at risk for sudden infant death syndrome?
[ ] **1.** Cover the nose and mouth with the rescuer's cheek; blow as much air as is possible.
[ ] **2.** Cover the nose with the rescuer's cheek; blow just enough air to make the chest rise.
[ ] **3.** Cover the nose and mouth with the rescuer's cheek; blow puffs of air from the cheeks.
[ ] **4.** Cover the mouth with the rescuer's cheek and pinch the nose closed; blow puffs of air.

21. When planning the care of a 75-year-old hospitalized client who develops pneumonia, what should be the priority focus?
[ ] **1.** Relieving the cough
[ ] **2.** Maintaining oxygenation
[ ] **3.** Providing nourishment
[ ] **4.** Encouraging independence

22. The nurse caring for a client after a subtotal thyroidectomy places the client in semi-Fowler's position. What is the rationale for this action?
[ ] **1.** It helps the client talk.
[ ] **2.** It reduces incisional edema.
[ ] **3.** It decreases sputum production.
[ ] **4.** It promotes client comfort.

23. When assessing a client who has attempted suicide by taking an overdose of medication, which question is most appropriate to ask initially?
[ ] **1.** "How many pills did you take?"
[ ] **2.** "Why did you take the pills?"
[ ] **3.** "What is the name of the drug?"
[ ] **4.** "Where did you get the pills?"

24. A 6-year-old child has just had placement of bilateral myringotomy tubes. As the parents prepare for discharge, the nurse correctly includes which instruction in the child's discharge plan?
[ ] **1.** Allow the child to eat only soft and liquid foods.
[ ] **2.** Speak in a louder voice when talking to the child.
[ ] **3.** Insert earplugs whenever the child swims or showers.
[ ] **4.** Irrigate the ears daily with tap water while the tubes are in place.

25. In an adult client, the nurse plans to administer 2 mL of medication I.M. Which technique is most accurate?
[ ] **1.** The nurse adds 2 mL of air to the vial before withdrawing the drug.
[ ] **2.** The nurse withdraws the medication using a tuberculin syringe.
[ ] **3.** The nurse selects the deltoid muscle for injecting the medication.
[ ] **4.** The nurse inserts a ⅝" needle into the muscle at a 45-degree angle.

26. Which action by the nurse is most appropriate while assessing the neurologic function of a client who has a freshly applied plaster cast to the lower extremity?
[ ] **1.** Asking the client to wiggle his toes
[ ] **2.** Depressing the nail bed to observe the color
[ ] **3.** Feeling the temperature of the toes
[ ] **4.** Palpating the pedal pulses bilaterally

27. The noon blood glucose level of a client with type 1 diabetes mellitus is 250 mg/dL. The physician orders a sliding scale insulin regimen based on the client's blood glucose level. The order reads, "Give regular insulin using the following scale." How many units of insulin should the nurse plan to give?

0 to 140 mg/dL	None
141 to 200 mg/dL	2 units
201 to 250 mg/dL	4 units
251 to 300 mg/dL	6 units
301 to 350 mg/dL	8 units
351 to 400 mg/dL	10 units
Over 400 mg/dL	Notify physician

[ ] **1.** 2 units
[ ] **2.** 4 units
[ ] **3.** 6 units
[ ] **4.** 8 units

28. A homeless person has an enlarged, tender liver, and a hepatitis B infection is suspected. Which information in the client's history is most likely the etiologic factor for the disease?
[ ] **1.** The client eats food that he finds in garbage cans.
[ ] **2.** The client has open skin sores over his lower extremities.
[ ] **3.** The client smokes cigarettes extinguished on the street.
[ ] **4.** The client occasionally shares needles to inject heroin.

29. Which client poses the greatest risk of developing complications for herself and her fetus during pregnancy?
[ ] **1.** The client who regularly restricts food intake to avoid gaining weight
[ ] **2.** The client who remains sexually active throughout the pregnancy
[ ] **3.** The client who participates regularly in an aerobic exercise program
[ ] **4.** The client who is 32 years old and pregnant for the first time

30. A physician orders 2 mg/kg of a drug. If the client weighs 88 lb, how many milligrams of the medication should the nurse administer?

_____

31. A nurse massages the uterus of a postpartum client. Which assessment finding best indicates that the intended effect of this nursing action has been achieved?
[ ] **1.** Postpartal pain is relieved.
[ ] **2.** The uterus becomes firm.
[ ] **3.** The client passes clots from the vagina.
[ ] **4.** Uterine contractions cease.

32. A client with diabetes comes to the emergency department. The nurse obtains a finger stick blood glucose reading and notes that it is 510 mg/dL. The physician orders I.V. insulin. Which type of insulin can be given I.V. and subcutaneously?
[ ] **1.** Regular
[ ] **2.** NPH
[ ] **3.** Lente
[ ] **4.** 70/30

33. A depressed client states to the nurse, "No one really cares what happens to me." What is the nurse's most appropriate response?
[ ] **1.** "You're exaggerating! Lots of people care about you."
[ ] **2.** "Talking like that will only make you feel worse."
[ ] **3.** "Tell me why you think no one cares what happens to you."
[ ] **4.** "It sounds like you're feeling ignored or abandoned."

34. Which nursing action best determines if a client has a fecal impaction?
[ ] **1.** Auscultating the bowel sounds
[ ] **2.** Measuring the abdominal girth
[ ] **3.** Inserting a finger within the rectum
[ ] **4.** Assessing for diarrhea

35. Following an 8-year-old boy's tonsillectomy, the nurse instructs the parents to avoid giving the child aspirin or aspirin products. What is the best explanation for the nurse's instruction?
[ ] **1.** Aspirin lowers the temperature and, therefore, can mask a fever.
[ ] **2.** Aspirin can cause Reye's syndrome.
[ ] **3.** Aspirin irritates the stomach and could cause an ulcer.
[ ] **4.** Aspirin reduces inflammation and conceals an infection.

36. What is the best evidence that a postpartum client's Kegel exercises are effective?

[ ] **1.** The client can perform deep-knee bends without back discomfort.
[ ] **2.** The client can touch her toes without abdominal discomfort.
[ ] **3.** The client can do several situps without stopping.
[ ] **4.** The client can stop and restart her flow of urine while voiding.

37. A pregnant client with known HIV infection is admitted to the hospital in active labor. Which method of fetal assessment is most appropriate?
[ ] **1.** Fetal scalp sampling
[ ] **2.** Amniocentesis
[ ] **3.** External fetal monitoring
[ ] **4.** Internal fetal monitoring

38. When performing a mental status assessment on an adult client with hypothyroidism, which behavior should the nurse expect?
[ ] **1.** Quick recall of events
[ ] **2.** Rapid response to questions
[ ] **3.** Bizarre thought processes
[ ] **4.** Impaired cognitive function

39. The nurse is caring for a client who has just been diagnosed with sinus bradycardia. Indicate on the illustration the area where the heartbeat's electrical impulse is initiated.

40. When a schizophrenic client claims to see demons in his room, how should the nurse document the finding?
[ ] **1.** "Experiencing hallucinations."
[ ] **2.** "Frightened by hallucinations."
[ ] **3.** "States, 'Seeing demons in my room.'"
[ ] **4.** "Having distorted sensory perceptions."

41. The nurse assists with the delivery of a stillborn infant who is gestationally small with a malformed cranium. To promote the parents' grieving process, which nursing action is most appropriate?

[ ] **1.** Allowing the parents to see and touch their dead infant

[ ] **2.** Covering and shielding the dead infant from parental view

[ ] **3.** Describing the positive characteristics of the dead infant

[ ] **4.** Discharging the mother within 24 hours after delivery

42. Which nursing technique is most accurate for removing an object that completely obstructs the airway of an unconscious adult?

[ ] **1.** Administering up to 5 abdominal thrusts

[ ] **2.** Administering 2 quick ventilations of air

[ ] **3.** Administering 5 chest thrusts and a breath

[ ] **4.** Administering 15 chest compressions

43. Which action provides the best evidence that a client with a colostomy is adjusting to his changed body image?

[ ] **1.** The client wears loose-fitting garments.

[ ] **2.** The client takes a shower each day.

[ ] **3.** The client empties the appliance.

[ ] **4.** The client avoids foods that form gas.

44. After an upper GI X-ray, it is most important for the nurse to monitor which of the following?

[ ] **1.** The client's ability to eat

[ ] **2.** The passage of stool

[ ] **3.** The color of the client's urine

[ ] **4.** The client's swallowing ability

45. A 17-year-old unmarried postpartum client is being discharged from the hospital. Which client factor best indicates the need for referral for community-based assistance after discharge?

[ ] **1.** The client is a primipara.

[ ] **2.** The client lives alone.

[ ] **3.** The client had a previous spontaneous abortion.

[ ] **4.** The client continues to see the newborn's father.

46. A hospitalized client diagnosed with cancer has a sealed source of radiation inserted into her vagina. Which information is most important for the charge nurse to obtain to ensure the safety of the nurse assigned to care for the client?

[ ] **1.** Whether the nurse is sensitive to radiation

[ ] **2.** Whether the nurse is pregnant

[ ] **3.** Whether the nurse has attended the radiation safety in-service

[ ] **4.** Whether the nurse will be reassigned to another unit later in the shift

47. A team conference is scheduled to discuss interventions necessary to resolve the inadequate dietary intake of a client diagnosed with Alzheimer's disease. Which nursing intervention will most likely facilitate the desired outcome?

[ ] **1.** Providing high-calorie finger foods every waking hour

[ ] **2.** Serving foods that are easy to digest

[ ] **3.** Giving the client additional time to eat each meal

[ ] **4.** Asking the client's family for a list of the client's favorite foods

48. Which assessment technique is best for detecting thrombophlebitis in a client's lower extremity?

[ ] **1.** Have the client dorsiflex his feet.

[ ] **2.** Palpate the dorsalis pedis pulses.

[ ] **3.** Observe the client's gait while walking.

[ ] **4.** Monitor the temperature of the client's unaffected leg.

49. Which of the following characteristics are indicative of normal sinus rhythm? Select all that apply.

[ ] **1.** T wave precedes a QRS complex.

[ ] **2.** Heart rate is between 60 and 100 beats/minute.

[ ] **3.** The atrioventricular (AV) node initiates the impulse.

[ ] **4.** Each impulse occurs regularly.

[ ] **5.** Ventricles depolarize and contract.

[ ] **6.** Ventricular rate is slower than the atrial rate.

50. When a hospitalized client diagnosed with Graves' disease is scheduled to undergo a subtotal thyroidectomy, the nurse omits palpating the thyroid gland. How can this action be interpreted?

[ ] **1.** The nurse's action is inappropriate because it eliminates essential information.

[ ] **2.** The nurse's action is inappropriate because the data are needed for comparison.

[ ] **3.** The nurse's action is appropriate because palpation can cause extreme discomfort.

[ ] **4.** The nurse's action is appropriate because palpation can cause thyroid storm.

51. Which statement made by an alcoholic client who takes disulfiram (Antabuse) best indicates the need for further health teaching?

[ ] **1.** "If I miss one dose of the drug, I'll experience nausea, vomiting, and fainting."

[ ] **2.** "I can get very sick if I consume alcohol in any form while taking this drug."

[ ] **3.** "I can have a reaction even 2 weeks after I stop taking this drug."

[ ] **4.** "I shouldn't apply aftershave lotion or cologne to my skin while taking this drug."

52. When discontinuing the administration of I.V. fluid, which nursing action is essential?

[ ] **1.** Monitoring urine specific gravity

[ ] **2.** Putting on clean gloves

[ ] **3.** Checking the client's blood glucose level

[ ] **4.** Assessing the amount of blood loss

53. A few days before a client has a malignant growth removed from his colon, he says to the nurse, "I'm scared that I'll have to have a colostomy. This operation worries me. What if the surgeon can't get all of the cancer?" Which nursing response is most therapeutic?

[ ] **1.** "There is no need to worry or be afraid. Trust me."

[ ] **2.** "Tell me more specifically about your concerns."

[ ] **3.** "You know as well as I that you have an excellent surgeon."

[ ] **4.** "Try to relax. Worrying will only make matters worse."

54. In which circumstance is it essential for the nurse to supply the physician with topical anesthesia?

[ ] **1.** When testing deep tendon reflexes

[ ] **2.** When removing vaginal secretions

[ ] **3.** When measuring intraocular pressure

[ ] **4.** When examining the tympanic membranes

55. If a client with type 1 (insulin-dependent) diabetes mellitus receives 5 units of NPH insulin every morning at 7 a.m., the nurse should closely monitor the client for signs of hypoglycemia at what time?

[ ] **1.** 3:00 p.m.

[ ] **2.** 12:00 a.m.

[ ] **3.** 7:30 a.m.

[ ] **4.** 10:00 p.m.

56. A client with a nasogastric tube has just returned from the recovery room following gastric surgery. Which postoperative assessment finding is essential to report to the physician or charge nurse?

[ ] **1.** The client says that his throat hurts.

[ ] **2.** The client indicates the tape on his nose is coming loose.

[ ] **3.** The client states he feels nauseated.

[ ] **4.** There is bright red, bloody drainage in the tube.

57. The nurse caring for a middle-aged adult would expect which characteristic behavior indicating the developmental task of generativity?

[ ] **1.** The client expresses fear of having further serious illnesses.

[ ] **2.** The client wishes to know the purpose of his medications.

[ ] **3.** The client wants to resume writing a book about his boyhood.

[ ] **4.** The client desires to learn more about using a computer.

58. Which culturally sensitive nursing technique is best for determining whether a male Jewish client follows the strict Orthodox customs of his religion?

[ ] **1.** Ask if he speaks the Hebrew language.

[ ] **2.** Inquire about his dietary preferences.

[ ] **3.** Question whether he wears a yarmulke.

[ ] **4.** Assess whether he has been circumcised.

59. Which nursing action is most appropriate when a chest tube is inadvertently pulled from its insertion site?

[ ] **1.** Quickly covering the opening to keep out air

[ ] **2.** Reinserting the displaced chest tube

[ ] **3.** Checking the client's breath sounds

[ ] **4.** Telling the client to hold his breath

60. When developing the care plan of a client who has a nasogastric (NG) tube for gastric decompression, which nursing order should be modified because it is considered unsafe?

[ ] **1.** Encourage liberal fluid intake every hour.

[ ] **2.** Irrigate the NG tube if drainage stops.

[ ] **3.** Offer throat lozenges every 4 hours, as needed, for discomfort.

[ ] **4.** Provide oral hygiene every 4 hours during the day and as needed.

61. If the nurse is giving an enema to an adult client, how far should the enema tip be inserted into the anal canal?

[ ] **1.** 1″ to 2″ (2.5 to 5 cm)

[ ] **2.** 3″ to 4″ (7.5 to 10 cm)

[ ] **3.** 5″ to 8″ (15 to 20 cm)

[ ] **4.** 9″ to 10″ (22.5 to 25 cm)

62. Which technique should the nurse plan to use when giving perineal care to an uncircumcised male client?

[ ] **1.** Washing the anal area at a separate time

[ ] **2.** Retracting the foreskin, then cleaning the area beneath the foreskin

[ ] **3.** Washing the scrotum before the penis

[ ] **4.** Washing the penis carefully with sterile normal saline solution

63. An adult comes to the clinic with recurring back pain. Which information is most important to obtain prior to developing a teaching plan?
[ ] **1.** The client's age
[ ] **2.** The client's occupation
[ ] **3.** The client's gait
[ ] **4.** The client's medications

64. Which advice is most appropriate for the nurse to give to a young man whose girlfriend has been raped?
[ ] **1.** Always act happy and enthusiastic around her.
[ ] **2.** Prevent her from isolating herself from people.
[ ] **3.** Encourage her to talk about her traumatic experience.
[ ] **4.** Take frequent vacations or engage in pleasurable activities.

65. Which statement by a female client indicates that she understands the correct procedure for performing breast self-examination (BSE) taught by the nurse?
[ ] **1.** "I'll perform the entire examination while laying on my back with my arm down at my side."
[ ] **2.** "I'll examine my breasts while standing in front of a mirror to detect any changes."
[ ] **3.** "I'll lie on my abdomen to detect any breast pain or tenderness."
[ ] **4.** "I'll examine my breasts while lying prone as well as sitting upright."

66. Which finding provides the best indication that a client with nephrotic syndrome (acute glomerulonephritis) has experienced a therapeutic effect from corticosteroid therapy?
[ ] **1.** Increase in body weight
[ ] **2.** Increase in muscle mass
[ ] **3.** Increase in urine output
[ ] **4.** Increase in blood pressure

67. During the night, a client is startled and continues to worry about an alarm that sounded from his electronic I.V. infusion pump. Which nursing intervention is most appropriate to relieve the client's anxiety at this time?
[ ] **1.** Infuse the solution by gravity.
[ ] **2.** Explain why the alarm sounded.
[ ] **3.** Give a prescribed tranquilizer.
[ ] **4.** Stay with the client until he falls back to sleep.

68. An adolescent brings in her 3-month-old infant for a well-baby checkup. The client tells the nurse that she is frustrated because she has gotten little sleep since the baby was born. Which nursing response is most appropriate?

[ ] **1.** Explain that this is a normal feeling, and suggest that the client ask a family member or friend for occasional relief.
[ ] **2.** Explain that parenting is a big responsibility, and suggest that the client place the child for adoption.
[ ] **3.** Explain that this feeling usually precedes abusive behavior, and inform her that this information must be reported.
[ ] **4.** Explain that this feeling is temporary, and encourage the client to be patient until the frustration disappears.

69. One hour after delivery, the nurse notes that a postpartum client has pronounced vaginal bleeding. Which action should the nurse take first?
[ ] **1.** Call the physician.
[ ] **2.** Massage the uterus.
[ ] **3.** Count the pulse.
[ ] **4.** Elevate the legs.

70. A postoperative client asks the nurse why performing leg exercises is important. The best explanation is that leg movement that involves contracting and relaxing leg muscles helps to prevent which condition?
[ ] **1.** Loss of muscle strength
[ ] **2.** Formation of blood clots
[ ] **3.** Swelling of the extremities
[ ] **4.** Development of varicose veins

71. If a child with asthma receives aminophylline (Truphylline) by I.V. infusion, which adverse drug effect is the nurse most likely to observe?
[ ] **1.** Bradycardia
[ ] **2.** Drowsiness
[ ] **3.** Restlessness
[ ] **4.** Hypotension

72. Which behavior best suggests that an older nursing home resident is depressed?
[ ] **1.** The client demands more attention from the staff.
[ ] **2.** The client does not eat the food that is provided.
[ ] **3.** The client sleeps a great deal of the time.
[ ] **4.** The client spends lots of time complaining about her aches and pains.

73. Which prescribed antibiotic should the nurse question before administering it to a child younger than age 8?
[ ] **1.** Cefazolin (Kefzol)
[ ] **2.** Amoxicillin (Amoxil)
[ ] **3.** Tetracycline hydrochloride (Tetracyn)
[ ] **4.** Gentamicin (Garamycin)

74. Which response is most appropriate when an older woman with Alzheimer's disease says she must leave the long-term care facility so that she can be home when her children return from school?
[ ] **1.** "Nonsense! Your children are adults with their own children."
[ ] **2.** "I'm sure a neighbor will take care of them for a while."
[ ] **3.** "I'll call the school and tell them to expect you later."
[ ] **4.** "You're in a nursing home. I'm your nurse."

75. A nurse conducts a "Healthy Heart" class for community leaders and informs them that they should take an aspirin if they feel they are having chest pain related to a heart attack. What is the best rationale for this instruction?
[ ] **1.** Aspirin is administered for its analgesic action.
[ ] **2.** Aspirin is administered for its antipyretic action.
[ ] **3.** Aspirin is administered for its antithrombotic action.
[ ] **4.** Aspirin is administered for its antiplatelet action.

76. When performing cardiopulmonary resuscitation (CPR) on an unresponsive infant, the nurse correctly assesses the pulse at which location?
[ ] **1.** Over the radial artery
[ ] **2.** Over the femoral artery
[ ] **3.** Over the brachial artery
[ ] **4.** Over the carotid artery

77. If the nurse finds a client who has fallen out of the hospital bed, which nursing action is best to perform initially?
[ ] **1.** Reporting the accident to the proper person
[ ] **2.** Helping the person back to bed or a chair
[ ] **3.** Making sure the side rails are raised
[ ] **4.** Checking the client's physical condition

78. Which behavior best indicates healthy parent-newborn attachment?
[ ] **1.** The parents observe the care of their newborn.
[ ] **2.** The parents are satisfied with the baby's gender.
[ ] **3.** The parents watch and listen to their newborn.
[ ] **4.** The parents touch and talk to their newborn.

79. If a postoperative client is on a clear liquid diet, which food item is most appropriate to provide?
[ ] **1.** A glass of milk
[ ] **2.** A bowl of ice cream
[ ] **3.** A dish of gelatin
[ ] **4.** A cup of creamed soup

80. The nursing team evaluates the effectiveness of interventions used to improve a confused client's orientation. Which client action provides the best evidence of progress in accomplishing the goal?
[ ] **1.** The client walks with others to the dining room.
[ ] **2.** The client dresses himself without difficulty.
[ ] **3.** The client locates his room without assistance.
[ ] **4.** The client talks on the telephone to his family.

81. A nurse instructs a client with asthma about how to use a metered-dose aerosol inhaler. The nurse correctly informs the client to take which step after inhaling slowly and deeply when the cartridge is depressed?
[ ] **1.** Immediately exhale the aerosol.
[ ] **2.** Briefly hold the inhaled breath.
[ ] **3.** Quickly swallow the bubble of air.
[ ] **4.** Subsequently cough, then breathe.

82. Which assessment finding best indicates that a 2-year-old girl has symptoms related to otitis media?
[ ] **1.** The child has a runny nose.
[ ] **2.** The child is cutting teeth.
[ ] **3.** The child swallows frequently.
[ ] **4.** The child tugs at her ear.

83. For a client with Ménière's disease, which medication is most appropriate to administer during an acute attack?
[ ] **1.** Acetaminophen (Tylenol)
[ ] **2.** Meclizine (Antivert)
[ ] **3.** Meperidine (Demerol)
[ ] **4.** Triazolam (Halcion)

84. Following a thyroidectomy, it is most appropriate for the nurse to monitor the client for signs of which electrolyte imbalance?
[ ] **1.** Hypokalemia
[ ] **2.** Hyponatremia
[ ] **3.** Hypomagnesemia
[ ] **4.** Hypocalcemia

85. Which nursing action is best for preventing skin breakdown when a client with jaundice complains of severe itching?
[ ] **1.** Bathing the client with very warm water
[ ] **2.** Dusting the client's body with cornstarch
[ ] **3.** Trimming the client's fingernails
[ ] **4.** Using hypoallergenic bed linens

86. A new patient has arrived at the gynecologist's office for an annual examination and Papanicolaou test. Prior to the physical examination, the nurse is conducting a reproductive and sexual assessment. Place in ascending chronological order the nursing actions completed by the nurse. Use all the options.

1.	Ask the client if she would like to use the bathroom.
2.	Introduce yourself and explain the sequence of events.
3.	Help the patient into the stirrups for the physical examination.
4.	Focus on general questions of sexual health and reproduction.
5.	Have the client change into a paper gown and offer a lap gown.
6.	Address detailed sexual history and reproductive questions.

| |
| |
| |
| |
| |
| |

87. A client with hyperparathyroidism is prone to hypercalcemia. Which nursing intervention is most appropriate to include in this client's care plan?
[ ]   **1.** Monitor the client's respirations.
[ ]   **2.** Provide a high fluid intake.
[ ]   **3.** Offer supplemental nourishment.
[ ]   **4.** Administer skin care frequently.

88. Which physical assessment finding best suggests that a client has an abdominal aortic aneurysm?
[ ]   **1.** A pulsating mass felt when palpating the client's abdomen
[ ]   **2.** An extra heart sound heard during chest auscultation
[ ]   **3.** Uneven chest movements noted when observing respirations
[ ]   **4.** A hollow sound heard when percussing the abdomen

89. If a known substance abuser experiences a racing heart, what is the most appropriate question for the nurse to ask?
[ ]   **1.** "When was the last time you used heroin?"
[ ]   **2.** "When was the last time you used cocaine?"
[ ]   **3.** "When was the last time you used barbiturates?"
[ ]   **4.** "When was the last time you used marijuana?"

90. Which assessment finding provides the best evidence that a client remained adequately oxygenated while being suctioned?
[ ]   **1.** The heart rate stayed within 88 to 92 beats/minute.
[ ]   **2.** The client's pulse was bounding.
[ ]   **3.** The client remained alert during suctioning.
[ ]   **4.** The client's capillary refill remained stable at 5 seconds.

91. A friend shares with a nurse that she is engaged to be married. The nurse knows that her friend's fiancé has tested positive for human immunodeficiency virus (HIV). What is the nurse legally obligated to do?
[ ]   **1.** Inform the friend of the fiancé's HIV infectious status.
[ ]   **2.** Recommend that the friend be tested for HIV antibodies.
[ ]   **3.** Advise the friend to postpone the marriage indefinitely.
[ ]   **4.** Safeguard information in the fiancé's health history.

92. During the first stage of a client's labor, the nurse finds that the fetal heart rate decreases during a contraction and returns to normal at the end of the contraction. Which nursing action is most appropriate in response to the assessment finding?
[ ]   **1.** No action is indicated at this time.
[ ]   **2.** Notify the physician immediately.
[ ]   **3.** Turn the client onto her back in bed.
[ ]   **4.** Elevate the head of the client's bed.

93. Which comment made by a client who is taking aspirin is most likely related to the effects of drug therapy?
[ ]   **1.** "My thoughts are racing."
[ ]   **2.** "I'm urinating a lot."
[ ]   **3.** "I've developed diarrhea."
[ ]   **4.** "I hear buzzing in my ears."

94. Which statement provides the best indication that a client understands the nurse's teaching about his newly prescribed medication, alprazolam (Xanax)?
[ ]   **1.** "I should not drink alcohol while taking this drug."
[ ]   **2.** "I will need to continue taking this drug for life."

[ ] **3.** "I might have trouble sleeping because this drug causes insomnia."

[ ] **4.** "I will need a blood test periodically."

95. A 78-year-old man arrives at the hospital and is suspected of having pneumonia. Which laboratory tests should the nurse anticipate the physician ordering to confirm the diagnosis?

[ ] **1.** Complete blood count (CBC) and chest X-ray

[ ] **2.** Hemoglobin and hematocrit

[ ] **3.** Pulmonary function tests and lung biopsy

[ ] **4.** Electrolytes and lung computed tomography

96. A toddler is brought to the emergency department for a broken arm that was a result of a fall from a tree. The nurse instructs the client's mother about cast care. Which instruction given by the nurse is most accurate regarding the drying of the child's cast?

[ ] **1.** Increase the temperature of the room.

[ ] **2.** Turn the child every 1 to 2 hours.

[ ] **3.** Fan the wet cast with folded newspaper.

[ ] **4.** Take the child outside in the sun during the day.

97. Which statement made by a primigravid client at 38 weeks' gestation best indicates that lightening has occurred?

[ ] **1.** "I don't have to urinate as frequently now."

[ ] **2.** "My backaches seem to be relieved."

[ ] **3.** "I can breathe so much easier now."

[ ] **4.** "I've noticed slight contractions lately."

98. A 76-year-old man is found slumped in his chair. The rescuer assesses for a pulse and finds a weak, thready one. The client, however, is not breathing and the rescuer begins rescue breathing. Which of the following provides the best evidence that rescue breathing is being performed appropriately?

[ ] **1.** The chest rises when air is forced in.

[ ] **2.** The pupils of both eyes are dilated.

[ ] **3.** A carotid pulse is palpated at the neck.

[ ] **4.** The rescuer forms a seal over the victim's nose.

99. After having a rectal tube in place for 20 minutes, a client's abdominal distention remains unrelieved. What is the most appropriate action for the nurse to take at this time?

[ ] **1.** Rotate the tube several times within the rectum.

[ ] **2.** Insert the rectal tube farther into the rectum.

[ ] **3.** Remove the tube, and reinsert it in 2 to 3 hours.

[ ] **4.** Replace the tube with one of larger diameter.

100. A client begins taking phenytoin (Dilantin) for seizures, and the nurse provides instructions regarding the medication and its side effects. Which nursing instruction is most accurate?

[ ] **1.** "Drink generous amounts of fluid."

[ ] **2.** "Reduce or control your weight."

[ ] **3.** "Use stress management techniques."

[ ] **4.** "Perform regular oral hygiene."

101. The nurse performs cardiopulmonary resuscitation on a 6-month-old infant. Which technique regarding chest compressions is most accurate?

[ ] **1.** Using both hands

[ ] **2.** Using two fingers

[ ] **3.** Using the heel of one hand

[ ] **4.** Using the palm of one hand

102. When teaching a client the signs and symptoms of a myocardial infarction (MI), the nurse is most correct in instructing that the pain associated with an MI is caused by which condition?

[ ] **1.** Ischemia of the heart muscle

[ ] **2.** Damage to the coronary arteries

[ ] **3.** Impending circulatory collapse

[ ] **4.** Left ventricular muscle fatigue

103. A hospitalized client with congestive heart failure receives furosemide (Lasix) twice per day. As the nurse monitors the client's laboratory test values, which one should be reported to the physician immediately?

[ ] **1.** Potassium: 3.0 mEq/L

[ ] **2.** Sodium: 137 mEq/L

[ ] **3.** Calcium: 9.1 mg/dL

[ ] **4.** Chloride: 102 mEq/L

104. When caring for the newborn of a mother who has heavily consumed alcohol throughout her pregnancy, which assessment finding is most likely to be observed?

[ ] **1.** Lethargy

[ ] **2.** Irritability

[ ] **3.** Flaccidity

[ ] **4.** Jaundice

105. The nurse administers a minor tranquilizer to an anxious client and evaluates its effectiveness 30 minutes later. Which nursing action provides the best indication that the drug is effective?

[ ] **1.** Assessing the client's facial expressions

[ ] **2.** Asking the client to rate the anxiety on a scale of 0 to 10

[ ] **3.** Observing the length of time a client sleeps

[ ] **4.** Monitoring the client's interactions with others

106. One day ago, a client had a below-the-knee amputation. Today the nurse changes the dressing for the first time. During the dressing change, the client says, "I just can't look at it!" Which comment by the nurse is most appropriate at this time?

[ ] **1.** "Look away until you feel ready."

[ ] **2.** "Maybe you should get counseling."

[ ] **3.** "I'd be curious to see how it looks."

[ ] **4.** "Come on! It doesn't look that bad."

107. For a client with a lower respiratory tract infection, when is the best time to plan postural drainage?

[ ] **1.** When the client has an empty stomach

[ ] **2.** When the nurse observes that the client is short of breath

[ ] **3.** When the client experiences coughing

[ ] **4.** When the respiratory therapist orders it

108. Which assessment finding provides the earliest indication that a client is hypoxic?

[ ] **1.** The client is cyanotic.

[ ] **2.** The client is disoriented.

[ ] **3.** The client is restless.

[ ] **4.** The client is hypotensive.

109. A 75-year-old client has a perineal prostatectomy related to cancer of the prostate. After surgery, which nursing action is essential to include in the client's care plan?

[ ] **1.** Instruct the client to perform Valsalva's maneuver during defecation.

[ ] **2.** Place the client in high Fowler's position immediately after surgery.

[ ] **3.** Administer laxatives to promote bowel elimination.

[ ] **4.** Provide perineal care following each bowel movement.

110. Prior to a debilitated older client's discharge from the hospital, a home health nurse performs a home assessment. Which assessment finding presents the greatest safety hazard for the client?

[ ] **1.** The television set is in the bedroom.

[ ] **2.** The client takes showers rather than tub baths.

[ ] **3.** There are throw rugs throughout the house.

[ ] **4.** There are grounded electrical outlets in the kitchen.

111. When a client who tests positive for the human immunodeficiency virus (HIV) is admitted to the hospital, which guidelines must be followed?

[ ] **1.** Strict isolation

[ ] **2.** Standard precautions

[ ] **3.** Droplet precautions

[ ] **4.** Contact isolation

112. When obtaining the health history of a client diagnosed with an inguinal hernia, which information is most likely a contributing factor for the problem?

[ ] **1.** The client had an umbilical hernia as a child.

[ ] **2.** The client does not get much physical exercise except at work.

[ ] **3.** The client lifts heavy mailbags in his job as a postal worker.

[ ] **4.** The client has been underweight most of his adult life.

113. The physician orders an immune assay enzyme test to confirm a diagnosis of acute bronchiolitis secondary to the respiratory syncytial virus (RSV) for a 12-month-old child. Which type of specimen is most appropriate for the nurse to collect?

[ ] **1.** Throat swab

[ ] **2.** Nasal secretions

[ ] **3.** Sputum specimen

[ ] **4.** Blood specimen

114. An obstetric nurse is discharging a mother and newborn. While escorting the family to the car, which of the following observations demonstrate correct car seat placement? Select all that apply.

[ ] **1.** The car seat is facing the rear in the passenger's front seat.

[ ] **2.** The base of the seat is tethered to a hook on the floor.

[ ] **3.** The mother is seated beside the car seat.

[ ] **4.** The car seat is facing forward in the back seat.

[ ] **5.** The car seat is placed between the mother and father in the front seat.

[ ] **6.** The car seat is facing the rear in the back seat.

115. The nurse finds a client with diabetes weak, perspiring, and shaking. After the nurse gives the client a glass of juice, which assessment finding provides the best indication that the nurse has managed the client's symptoms successfully?

[ ] **1.** The client says he feels better.

[ ] **2.** The client's skin is warm.

[ ] **3.** The client's blood glucose level is 80 mg/dL.

[ ] **4.** The client's blood pressure is stable.

116. When obtaining the health history of a young woman with thrombophlebitis, the nurse should ask if she routinely takes which medication?

[ ] **1.** Iron supplement

[ ] **2.** Oral contraceptive

[ ] **3.** Nasal decongestant

[ ] **4.** Stomach antacid

117. Following the physician's explanation of the risks and benefits of a transurethral resection of the prostate (TURP), the best indication that the client understands the effect this surgery will have on his sexual function is which statement?

[ ] **1.** "I won't ejaculate normally anymore."

[ ] **2.** "I won't be able to have an orgasm anymore."

[ ] **3.** "I won't be able to have an erection anymore."

[ ] **4.** "I won't desire to have sex anymore."

118. If a postoperative client received an overdose of heparin, the nurse would anticipate the physician to order which antidote?

[ ] **1.** Protamine sulfate

[ ] **2.** Naloxone hydrochloride (Narcan)

[ ] **3.** Vitamin K
[ ] **4.** Calcium gluconate

119. A non-English-speaking Hispanic client is admitted to the hospital to rule out myocardial infarction. The nurse performs a cultural assessment. Which information should be included in the client's cultural assessment? Select all that apply.
[ ] **1.** The client's food preferences
[ ] **2.** When the client's last bowel movement occurred
[ ] **3.** The client's primary language
[ ] **4.** Whether the client can tell time
[ ] **5.** The client's religion
[ ] **6.** Whether the client is in pain

120. As a preschooler who is recovering from infectious gastroenteritis is advanced to solid foods, the nurse is correct to initially serve which food?
[ ] **1.** Buttered rice
[ ] **2.** Cereal
[ ] **3.** Applesauce
[ ] **4.** Ice cream

121. Which nursing intervention is most appropriate for meeting the needs of an infant with congenital heart disease?
[ ] **1.** Respond quickly to the infant's crying.
[ ] **2.** Place the infant in the prone position.
[ ] **3.** Avoid holding and cuddling the infant.
[ ] **4.** Use a firm, small-hole nipple for feedings.

122. When instructing a postoperative client about the use of enoxaparin (Lovenox), the nurse should include which statement about the drug's therapeutic action?
[ ] **1.** "It promotes wound-tissue healing."
[ ] **2.** "It breaks up clots that have formed."
[ ] **3.** "It decreases postoperative bleeding."
[ ] **4.** "It reduces formation of postoperative blood clots."

123. An 8-year-old boy is sent to the school nurse when his teacher notices recurrent staring episodes with frequent blinking. Shortly after an episode, the student is alert and oriented and responds when his name is called. Which type of seizure is the student most likely experiencing?
[ ] **1.** Myoclonic
[ ] **2.** Absence
[ ] **3.** Partial
[ ] **4.** Clonic

124. A client in her fourth month of pregnancy is scheduled to have an abdominal ultrasound. Which statement by the client indicates a need for additional teaching before the procedure is performed?
[ ] **1.** "A gel will be applied to my abdomen."
[ ] **2.** "I will need to drink a quart of water before the test."
[ ] **3.** "I will need to remain flat for 12 hours after the procedure."
[ ] **4.** "There is no risk of radiation associated with this procedure."

125. The physician orders seizure precautions for a recently admitted client. When the nurse prepares the client's room, which equipment is least likely to be needed if the client has a seizure?
[ ] **1.** A padded tongue blade at the head of the bed
[ ] **2.** An oral airway and oxygen at the bedside
[ ] **3.** Suction equipment at the bedside
[ ] **4.** Padding on the side rails of the bed

126. Which action by the nurse in the nursery will best prevent a newborn from experiencing heat loss secondary to evaporation?
[ ] **1.** Wrapping the infant in warmed blankets
[ ] **2.** Thoroughly drying the child after bathing
[ ] **3.** Positioning the crib away from outside windows
[ ] **4.** Positioning the crib away from air conditioning vents in the nursery

127. A 30-year-old pregnant client has been told by her physician that she has gestational diabetes mellitus. Which statement by the client indicates that she understands the physician's explanation of this disorder?
[ ] **1.** "The disorder was present during my childhood."
[ ] **2.** "The disorder is well controlled with oral hypoglycemics."
[ ] **3.** "The disorder will probably go away after I deliver."
[ ] **4.** "The disorder may cause me to have a small baby."

128. Which finding would the nurse expect in a 7-month-old infant admitted to the hospital with a tentative diagnosis of bacterial meningitis?
[ ] **1.** Elevated white blood cell count
[ ] **2.** Bulging fontanel
[ ] **3.** Low-pitched cry
[ ] **4.** Increased glucose level in cerebrospinal fluid

129. The school nurse plans a discussion with a group of 13-year-olds about seizure disorder. During the teaching session, the nurse correctly identifies which condition as the most common risk factor for the development of seizure disorder?

[ ] **1.** Head trauma that results in long-term brain changes

[ ] **2.** Illegal drug use that results in unconsciousness

[ ] **3.** An underlying psychiatric disorder such as schizophrenia

[ ] **4.** Recent spinal cord damage from a sports accident

130. While assisting with a health screening clinic at a local preschool, the nurse would expect to observe which developmental characteristic among the 6-year-old participants?

[ ] **1.** The children are usually very reserved.

[ ] **2.** The children tend to enjoy pretend play.

[ ] **3.** The children tend to show little or no reaction to criticism.

[ ] **4.** The children almost always finish tasks they have started.

Correct Answers and Rationales

1. 3. Typical signs that a tracheostomy needs suctioning include noisy respirations, dyspnea, sputum color changes, and increased respiratory and pulse rates. Auscultation of the chest helps most to determine when to suction a tracheostomy.

Client Needs Category—*Safe, effective care environment*

Client Needs Subcategory—*Safety and infection control*

2. 3. Before suctioning, the nurse gives the client oxygen to prevent hypoxemia and hypoxia while removing air and debris from the upper airway. Just before inserting the catheter, the nurse may instill saline solution to liquefy thick secretions. After inserting the catheter, the nurse positions the tip at the desired level, usually 6″ to 10″ (15 to 25 cm), occludes the vent, and twists the catheter to remove it. Afterward, the client is reoxygenated a second time. Usually, cleaning the tracheostomy is done last after the sterile procedure is completed, following the general principal of "clean to dirty."

Client Needs Category—*Physiological integrity*

Client Needs Subcategory—*Physiological adaptation*

3. 4. The most appropriate aseptic technique for cleaning wounds is to work in such a way that debris and microorganisms are carried away from the impaired skin. Therefore, wounds should always be cleaned starting at the wound itself and working outward. It is appropriate to use clean gloves to remove a soiled dressing, to place the soiled dressing in a container that acts as a barrier against transmitting microorganisms that may be present, and to perform hand washing before donning sterile gloves.

Client Needs Category—*Safe, effective care environment*

Client Needs Subcategory—*Safety and infection control*

4. 1. A hearing aid amplifies sound waves transmitted by air and bone conduction. Hearing aids do not improve the quality of the sounds by making them crisper, sharper, or less garbled.

Client Needs Category—*Health promotion and maintenance*

Client Needs Subcategory—*None*

5. 2. Food and fluids are withheld temporarily following a bronchoscopy until the gag reflex returns. If the gag reflex is absent, aspiration may occur. Taking vital signs, including radial pulse and tympanic temperature, is an appropriate measure that provides a baseline for further care. Raising the head of the bed is a safe action.

> ***Client Needs Category***—*Safe, effective care environment*
> ***Client Needs Subcategory***—*Safety and infection control*

6. 2. It is therapeutic to allow an angry person to express his feelings within social limits. By remaining neutral, the nurse demonstrates acceptance of the client as an individual and acts as a role model in helping the client regain control. Using humor, leaving the client, or providing an explanation may add to his angry feelings; the client may interpret these actions to mean that the circumstances leading to his anger are unimportant.

> ***Client Needs Category***—*Psychosocial integrity*
> ***Client Needs Subcategory***—*None*

7. 1. Most clients with a retinal detachment describe seeing flashes of light. Only the most profoundly blind cannot see light. Photophobia, or feeling discomfort in light, is associated with many primary and secondary disorders; however, those with retinal detachment do not generally experience it. The client with a retinal detachment generally retains vision in a large portion of the retina. The visual defect is evident only in the area of the tear or separation of the sensory layer from the pigmented layer. Therefore, in the intact retina, vision during daylight is unchanged.

> ***Client Needs Category***—*Physiological integrity*
> ***Client Needs Subcategory***—*Physiological adaptation*

8. 2. Giving an infant medication using a needleless syringe helps reduce the incidence of choking, coughing, and vomiting. Medications are not routinely given in an infant's bottle because the infant may not finish the bottle and may not get the prescribed amount of medication. Pinching a child's nose is not recommended because this action increases the chance of aspiration. Solid (not liquid) forms of medication may be crushed and mixed with jelly, cereal, pudding, or applesauce. However, solid foods should not be given to infants under 4 or 5 months old because they still possess the extrusion reflex; the food will be spit out and not swallowed.

> ***Client Needs Category***—*Safe, effective care environment*
> ***Client Needs Subcategory***—*Safety and infection control*

9. 3. When a child is in Bryant's traction, the buttocks just clear the mattress. The ropes that lead to pulleys above the bed keep the child's legs at a 90-degree angle to his trunk. The child should not sit up or use a trapeze. The legs are pulled toward the ceiling.

> ***Client Needs Category***—*Physiological integrity*
> ***Client Needs Subcategory***—*Reduction of risk potential*

10. 3. Red blood cells are formed in the bone marrow found in long bones and in the sternum. In sickle cell anemia, a genetic disorder affecting the red blood cells, the cells are malformed in a characteristic sickle shape. During sickle cell crisis, the red blood cells clump together and clog the arteries, causing the client much pain, especially in the chest, joints, and abdomen. Consequently, the priority nursing goal is to relieve the client's discomfort. Analgesics are routinely administered and adjusted according to the client's response. Activity, including self-care, is usually limited during sickle cell crisis to prevent hypoxia. Although promoting a chronically ill client's self-esteem is an appropriate nursing goal, it is not a priority during the acute phase of this illness.

> ***Client Needs Category***—*Physiological integrity*
> ***Client Needs Subcategory***—*Physiological adaptation*

11. 4. To avoid additional injury to radiated skin, the client is instructed to use gentle washing with warm water and a soft cloth. Water will not harm the skin, but harsh soaps, lotions, alcohol-based cosmetics, and rubbing the skin are avoided. Covering the reddened area with clear plastic will not serve any therapeutic purpose, and the tape used to hold the plastic may cause further skin breakdown.

> ***Client Needs Category***—*Health promotion and maintenance*
> ***Client Needs Subcategory***—*None*

12. 3. A clear liquid diet is generally offered initially after surgery. This diet moistens the mouth, provides fluid and some energy-supplying calories, and stimulates peristalsis. It is also the least likely diet to contribute to nausea or vomiting. If tolerated well, the client can progress to a full liquid, soft, or regular diet.

> ***Client Needs Category***—*Physiological integrity*
> ***Client Needs Subcategory***—*Basic care and comfort*

13. 4. Any pregnant client in the third trimester with a persistent, severe headache needs to be promptly examined by a physician. A persistent headache may be insignificant, but it is also a sign of pregnancy-induced hypertension, formerly known as *toxemia* or *eclampsia*. The other suggestions are appropriate after the client has been medically assessed.

> ***Client Needs Category***—*Physiological integrity*
> ***Client Needs Subcategory***—*Physiological adaptation*

14. **4.** Acquired immunodeficiency syndrome is suspected when individuals succumb to opportunistic infections. Because homosexual and heterosexual transmissions are the most common modes of acquiring human immunodeficiency virus, assessing a client's sexual practices is important. If the client does not report any high-risk sexual practices, the nurse may assess the possibility of I.V. drug use and a history of having received blood or blood products. A client's immunization history, family history, and hygiene practices are not likely to provide etiologic information about opportunistic infections.

> *Client Needs Category—Health promotion and maintenance*
> *Client Needs Subcategory—None*

15. **1.** Parents of children with cystic fibrosis commonly report that the child's perspiration tastes very salty. This is attributed to the fact that children with cystic fibrosis lose large amounts of salt in their perspiration. Vomiting immediately after eating is not a usual sign of cystic fibrosis, but it is associated with pyloric stenosis. Soft, bright yellow stools are characteristic of a breast-fed infant. In cystic fibrosis, the stools are large, foamy, and foul-smelling. Very light-colored urine usually indicates that the urine is dilute. This characteristic is related to the hydration status and function of the kidneys and is unrelated to cystic fibrosis.

> *Client Needs Category—Physiological integrity*
> *Client Needs Subcategory—Physiological adaptation*

16. **1.** For the person who takes corticosteroids for a prolonged time, abruptly discontinuing the medication can cause life-threatening consequences. Acute adrenal insufficiency (also known as *addisonian* or *adrenal crisis*) can occur, leading to possible death due to fluid volume depletion, hypotension, and shock. Taking a steroid medication does not interfere with a person's reaction time. A missed dose does not warrant consulting the physician. Although long-term corticosteroid therapy causes many side effects, individuals can take the medication for long periods of time.

> *Client Needs Category—Physiological integrity*
> *Client Needs Subcategory—Pharmacological therapies*

17. **3.** Diabetes insipidus is characterized by excessive urine production and elimination as a result of alterations in antidiuretic hormone. The specific gravity is an indication of the ratio of water to dissolved substances. In diabetes insipidus, the specific gravity is 1.002, little more than water. As the client improves, the specific gravity increases as less water is excreted in the urine.

> *Client Needs Category—Physiological integrity*
> *Client Needs Subcategory—Physiological adaptation*

18. **1.** Daily to weekly weight assessments are an appropriate way of monitoring the effectiveness and compliance of a client who takes a diuretic at home. Other valuable assessments include measuring the client's blood pressure, listening to breath sounds, and inspecting the skin and lower extremities for signs of edema. Pulse rate, appetite, and reflexes are not affected by diuretics.

> *Client Needs Category—Physiological integrity*
> *Client Needs Subcategory—Physiological adaptation*

19. **1.** To apply topical nitroglycerin ointment, the nurse squeezes a ribbon of the drug onto calibrated application paper. The paper is then placed on the client's chest, back, or arms, but not directly over the heart area. Applying the ointment over the heart may interfere with the assessment of heart sounds or obtaining an apical pulse rate; it may also be hazardous if the client requires defibrillation. The paper is covered with plastic wrap and taped to hold it in place. The nurse must avoid coming into direct skin contact with the ointment while measuring or applying it; such contact can result in absorption of the medication, causing a severe headache. The drug should not be rubbed into the client's skin. The nurse must follow the physician's orders regarding reapplication of the ointment. Usually, nitroglycerin ointment is left on longer than 4 hours.

> *Client Needs Category—Physiological integrity*
> *Client Needs Subcategory—Pharmacological therapies*

20. **3.** An infant is given controlled, gentle breaths of air from the rescuer. The breaths are sometimes described as puffs of air. The volume is just large enough to make the chest rise. The rate of rescue breaths for an infant is approximately 20 per minute.

> *Client Needs Category—Health promotion and maintenance*
> *Client Needs Subcategory—None*

21. **2.** Maintaining and improving oxygenation is a priority goal when planning the nursing care of a client with an acute respiratory tract infection. In some circumstances, such as when the client's airways contain moist secretions, it is important to promote rather than relieve coughing. Nourishment is important in the care of any client with an infection, but impaired breathing is more life-threatening than a brief reduction in caloric intake. Eventually, the client can begin assuming self-care; however, during the acute phase of illness, the nurse should promote rest and offer assistance to reduce the client's oxygen requirements.

> *Client Needs Category—Physiological integrity*
> *Client Needs Subcategory—Physiological adaptation*

22. **2.** A client with a subtotal thyroidectomy has a neck incision. Therefore, elevating the head, as in semi-Fowler's position, tends to relieve edema and decrease the potential for airway obstruction. Controlling edema will help the client talk and feel more comfortable; however, these are secondary benefits. Elevating the head has little effect on decreasing sputum production.
Client Needs Category—Physiological integrity
Client Needs Subcategory—Reduction of risk potential

23. **3.** The name of the drug is essential in determining the potential effects and the treatment needed. Although determining the approximate number of pills and when they were taken will help to assess the potential lethality of the overdose, this information is not as critical initially. While the client's life is threatened, discussing the reason for the overdose is not a priority. The source of the pills does not affect the client's treatment.
Client Needs Category—Psychosocial integrity
Client Needs Subcategory—None

24. **3.** Custom-made earplugs are used as a barrier against water entering the tubes used to equalize pressure within the middle ear. The introduction of water from such activities as swimming or showering can cause suppurative (pus-producing) otitis media. No dietary restrictions are necessary while myringotomy tubes are in place. The child's hearing should improve as pressure within the middle ear is relieved. Instilling water is contraindicated for the same reasons that water from swimming and showering is prohibited from entering the ears.
Client Needs Category—Health promotion and maintenance
Client Needs Subcategory—None

25. **1.** Adding a volume of air equal to the amount of drug to be withdrawn from a vial increases the pressure within the vial and facilitates filling the syringe. A tuberculin syringe holds a maximum volume of 1 mL; therefore, it will not accommodate the 2-mL volume of medication needed in this situation. The deltoid muscle is not used when the volume of the medication exceeds 1 mL. It is appropriate to select a 1½″ to 2″ needle to reach the depth where muscle is located. The needle is inserted at a 90-degree angle when administering an I.M. injection.
Client Needs Category—Safe, effective care environment
Client Needs Subcategory—Safety and infection control

26. **1.** Observing whether a client can move the fingers or toes of a casted extremity is the best method for assessing neurologic function because muscles cannot move unless the nervous system is intact. Monitoring capillary refill, feeling the skin temperature, and palpating the pedal pulses are appropriate techniques for assessing a client's vascular status.
Client Needs Category—Physiological integrity
Client Needs Subcategory—Physiological adaptation

27. **2.** A sliding scale is a type of insulin regimen used to regulate blood glucose levels throughout the day. The amount of insulin given is based on the client's blood glucose reading. In this case, because the blood glucose level is 250 mg/dL, the nurse should plan to give 4 units of insulin.
Client Needs Category—Safe, effective care environment
Client Needs Subcategory—Safety and infection control

28. **4.** Hepatitis B is transmitted by infected blood, serum, semen, vaginal fluid, and sharing of contaminated needles. Viruses depend on living cells to grow and reproduce. Therefore, it is extremely unlikely that the virus could be transmitted by entering open sores or smoking cigarettes long since extinguished. Hepatitis A is associated with eating unsanitary, contaminated food.
Client Needs Category—Health promotion and maintenance
Client Needs Subcategory—None

29. **1.** Reasonable weight gain is expected during pregnancy. Poor nutrition due to poverty or lack of knowledge is a leading contributor to high-risk pregnancies. To ensure the health of both the mother and her fetus, it is important for the mother to eat a variety of foods. Many physicians do not restrict sexual activity during pregnancy unless complications, such as uterine bleeding or placenta previa, are evident or the membranes rupture. A certain amount of regular exercise is preferable to sporadic activity. The type and amount of exercise depends on the health, habits, and obstetric history of each client. Pregnancy beyond age 35 is considered a risk factor.
Client Needs Category—Health promotion and maintenance
Client Needs Subcategory—None

30. **80.** There are 2.2 lb per kg; therefore, 88 pounds divided by 2.2 equals 40 kg. Because the client should receive 2 mg for every kg, the nurse multiplies; $2 \times 40 = 80$ mg. Using the ratio-and-proportion method, the dosage is calculated as follows:

Step 1 (known ratio to unknown ratio):

$$\frac{2\,mg}{1\,kg} = \frac{X\,mg}{40\,kg}$$

Step 2 (cross-multiply and solve for X):

$$1\,X = 80$$
$$X = 80$$

Client Needs Category—*Safe, effective care environment*
Client Needs Subcategory—*Safety and infection control*

31. **2.** Massaging the uterus causes the myometrium to contract and become firm, occluding the blood vessels and thereby controlling postpartum bleeding. This is more important than assessing for clots that come from the vagina. The client may experience pain when the uterus is massaged. The discomfort is due to uterine contraction, which intensifies (not ceases) as the uterus is massaged.

Client Needs Category—*Physiological integrity*
Client Needs Subcategory—*Physiological adaptation*

32. **1.** Regular insulin, a short-acting type, is the only insulin that can be given I.V. and subcutaneously. If regular insulin is given I.V., the client's blood glucose level should be carefully monitored shortly after infusion. The onset of action and peak effect of regular insulin will be faster if given I.V.

Client Needs Category—*Physiological integrity*
Client Needs Subcategory—*Pharmacological therapies*

33. **4.** Paraphrasing the content of the client's statement is a therapeutic communication technique that helps the client know that the message was heard and how it was interpreted. This technique will likely encourage the client to continue verbalizing. Classifying the statement as an exaggeration is belittling. Telling the client that talking will contribute to sadness is an indirect way of saying that this line of communication should cease. Demanding an explanation by asking "why" is also a block to therapeutic communication. It requires that the client justify a rationale for the statement and puts the client on the defensive.

Client Needs Category—*Psychosocial integrity*
Client Needs Subcategory—*None*

34. **3.** The only reliable method for confirming the presence of hard, dry stool within the rectum is digital examination. Auscultating bowel sounds and measuring abdominal girth are appropriate physical assessment techniques, but they do not aid in determining whether the client has a fecal impaction. Assessing for diarrhea is always important in relation to fluid and electrolyte imbalances, but it may not be an indication of fecal impaction.

Client Needs Category—*Physiological integrity*
Client Needs Subcategory—*Basic care and comfort*

35. **2.** Acetylsalicylic acid, also known as *aspirin,* can cause Reye's syndrome in children. To reduce the potential for developing this disorder, salicylates are avoided both preoperatively and postoperatively.

Client Needs Category—*Physiological integrity*
Client Needs Subcategory—*Pharmacological therapies*

36. **4.** If the pubococcygeal muscles are being contracted and relaxed properly during the performance of Kegel exercises, the client should be able to stop and restart the flow of urine during voiding. Kegel exercises are performed to relieve stress incontinence; they are ineffective in relieving back pain, improving abdominal tone, or performing situps.

Client Needs Category—*Health promotion and maintenance*
Client Needs Subcategory—*None*

37. **3.** External fetal monitoring minimizes the risk of exposing the fetus to the mother's HIV-infected blood. Fetal scalp blood sampling, amniocentesis, and internal fetal monitoring are all invasive techniques that would increase the fetus's risk of exposure to HIV.

Client Needs Category—*Safe effective care environment*
Client Needs Subcategory—*Safety and infection control*

38. **4.** Persons with hypothyroidism (myxedema) are most likely to demonstrate a general slowing of thought processes. Although persons with hypothyroidism are slow in responding, their thought processes are usually based in reality. Quick recall of events, rapid verbal responses, and bizarre thinking are uncharacteristic of clients with this disorder.

Client Needs Category—*Physiological integrity*
Client Needs Subcategory—*Physiological adaptation*

39.

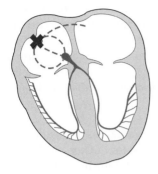

In a sinus rhythm, the sinoatrial (SA) node initiates the electrical impulses. The SA node is located in the upper part of the right atrium.

Client Needs Category—*Physiological integrity*
Client Needs Subcategory—*Physiological adaptation*

40. 3. Charting must be as clear and objective as possible. Quoting the client is always appropriate. Interpreting or labeling what the nurse suspects is occurring is not the best form of documentation.

Client Needs Category—*Safe, effective care environment*
Client Needs Subcategory—*Coordinated care*

41. 1. Having direct contact with a stillborn infant tends to initiate healthy grieving. Although providing a verbal description that focuses on the infant's attributes is therapeutic, it is not as personal as seeing and touching the infant. Preventing any interaction between the parents and infant interferes with the grief process. Many postpartum clients are discharged within 24 to 48 hours after delivery; this would have no bearing on resolving the grief of a perinatal loss.

Client Needs Category—*Psychosocial integrity*
Client Needs Subcategory—*None*

42. 1. To remove an object from the airway of an unconscious, nonpregnant adult, the rescuer administers up to 5 forceful thrusts upward from the abdomen. If the series of abdominal thrusts does not clear the airway, the rescuer performs a finger sweep followed by 2 breaths. The cycle is repeated until respiration is restored. If the adult is conscious, abdominal thrusts are repeated until the object is dislodged or the victim becomes unconscious. Ventilating the client is ineffective as long as the airway is obstructed. Chest compressions are performed when the victim no longer has a pulse.

Client Needs Category—*Physiological integrity*
Client Needs Subcategory—*Physiological adaptation*

43. 3. Performing self-care indicates that a client has progressed from denial and anger to a stage of acceptance. Wearing loose-fitting garments can be viewed as an attempt to hide the change in body image. Although showering daily and avoiding gas-forming foods are ap-

propriate, they may only be an indication that the client is self-conscious about possible fecal odor.

Client Needs Category—*Psychosocial integrity*
Client Needs Subcategory—*None*

44. 2. Following any GI procedure that uses barium as a contrast medium, the nurse should monitor the client's bowel elimination. Retained barium can cause constipation and even bowel obstruction. A laxative or some other method of promoting the passage of the stool is needed if elimination is delayed. The stool color appears white or chalky as barium is eliminated. Assessing the color of the client's urine and the ability to swallow and eat are unrelated to the consequences of the radiographic procedure.

Client Needs Category—*Physiological integrity*
Client Needs Subcategory—*None*

45. 2. An adolescent mother who lives alone is most likely in need of financial assistance and the emotional support that various organizations, including a teen parenting group, can provide. The client's primipara status and previous spontaneous abortion are unrelated to her ability to care for herself and her newborn. The fact that the client continues to see the newborn's father is no guarantee that he will provide the level and type of support this young mother needs.

Client Needs Category—*Health promotion and maintenance*
Client Needs Subcategory—*None*

46. 2. The care of clients with radioactive implants is best assigned to nonpregnant nurses because acute or chronic exposure to ionizing radiation can cause gene mutation and birth defects. All nurses—male and female, pregnant and nonpregnant—are at risk for radiation if precautions of time, distance, and shielding are not followed. Whether the nurse has attended the radiation safety in-service or is being reassigned to another unit later in the shift are topics that the charge nurse may need to know; however, they are not as important as the staff nurse's pregnancy status.

Client Needs Category—*Safe, effective care environment*
Client Needs Subcategory—*Safety and infection control*

47. 1. High-calorie finger foods are best for clients with Alzheimer's disease, who find it almost impossible to sit or stand in one location for more than a few minutes. The problem is not the quantity or variety of food, the time available for eating, the client's personal preferences, or digestibility of food; rather, the underlying problem for these clients is their limited attention span and ability to concentrate on any physical task.

Client Needs Category—*Physiological integrity*
Client Needs Subcategory—*Basic care and comfort*

48. 1. To detect the presence of thrombophlebitis, the nurse has the client dorsiflex each foot separately and notes if the client experiences calf pain. The presence of calf pain is considered a positive Homans' sign and needs to be reported immediately. Although palpating the pedal pulse to assess the client's distal arterial blood flow and observing for evidence of guarding while walking can provide supportive evidence of thrombophlebitis, these are not the primary assessment techniques for detecting the disorder. Monitoring the temperature of the unaffected leg offers no useful comparative value in this situation.

Client Needs Category—*Physiological integrity*
Client Needs Subcategory—*Physiological adaptation*

49. 2, 4, 5. A normal heart rate is between 60 and 100 beats/minute. Each impulse occurs regularly, producing a regular heart rate. The ventricles depolarize and contract to pump blood through the system. The AV node is the gatekeeper, sending impulses to the ventricles. The sinoatrial (SA) node initiates the impulse. P waves, which are the impulse from the SA node, precede the ventricular repolarization of the QRS complex. Ventricular rates, which are slower than atrial rates, are indicative of heart block.

Client Needs Category—*Physiological integrity*
Client Needs Subcategory—*Physiological adaptation*

50. 4. Because the thyroid gland is manipulated preoperatively or during its surgical removal, any postoperative palpation increases the client's risk of developing thyroid crisis or storm, a life-threatening condition. None of the other interpretative analyses is accurate.

Client Needs Category—*Safe effective care environment*
Client Needs Subcategory—*Safety and infection control*

51. 1. Missing a dose of disulfiram (Antabuse) will not cause a drug reaction. The reaction occurs when the client ingests alcohol or applies it to his skin. To ensure that a reaction does not occur, the client must abstain from alcohol for at least 2 weeks or more after discontinuing the drug.

Client Needs Category—*Physiological integrity*
Client Needs Subcategory—*Pharmacological therapies*

52. 2. Standard precautions are followed for every patient, regardless of the potential for direct contact with blood, such as when removing an I.V. device from its site. Normally, blood glucose levels are not checked after the I.V. solution is discontinued, unless the solution contained large amounts of dextrose, such as in total parenteral nutrition. Blood loss should be minimal or nonexistent when the I.V. is discontinued. Urine output should be assessed after the I.V. has been discontinued, but monitoring the specific gravity (the concentration of the urine) is not necessary.

Client Needs Category—*Safe, effective care environment*
Client Needs Subcategory—*Safety and infection control*

53. 2. When a client verbalizes or manifests symptoms of anxiety, it is best for the nurse to help him express his concerns. Belittling his fears by saying "There is no need for fear," using a reassuring cliché such as "trust me" or "you have an excellent surgeon," and giving advice such as "try to relax" are all nontherapeutic ways of communicating.

Client Needs Category—*Psychosocial integrity*
Client Needs Subcategory—*None*

54. 3. Topical anesthesia is needed when a tonometer is used to measure the pressure within a client's eyes. The anesthetic, prepared in liquid eyedrop form, makes it possible to apply the tonometer to the cornea without the client feeling as if something is touching the eye. The other assessment procedures include using a reflex hammer, a vaginal speculum, and an otoscope—none of which requires the application of a topical anesthetic.

Client Needs Category—*Physiological integrity*
Client Needs Subcategory—*Physiological adaptation*

55. 1. NPH is an intermediate-acting type of insulin. The onset of action is 1 to 3 hours, and the peak effect occurs in 6 to 12 hours. Hypoglycemia can occur at the expected onset and again when the insulin level peaks. In this case, the NPH insulin should peak sometime between 1 p.m. and 7 p.m., during which time the nurse should assess for hypoglycemia. Therefore, checking the client's glucose level at 3:00 p.m. would be appropriate. Because the client has breakfast at 7:00 a.m. and eating raises blood glucose levels, the nurse will not detect hypoglycemia at 7:30 a.m. Checking the glucose level at 10:00 p.m. or 12:00 a.m. is well beyond the time for peak action to occur.

Client Needs Category—*Physiological integrity*
Client Needs Subcategory—*Physiological adaptation*

56. 4. Bright red, bloody drainage indicates that the client is hemorrhaging. Preventing life-threatening consequences depends on prompt collaboration with the physician. The nurse can use comfort measures to relieve a sore throat, which is not a life-threatening condition. Loosening of the tape on the client's nose is not a valid reason for notifying the physician. Nausea is common shortly after surgery; most likely the physician will have written an order for an antiemetic.

Client Needs Category—*Physiological integrity*
Client Needs Subcategory—*Physiological adaptation*

57. 3. Eric Erikson describes generativity as a concern for leaving something of worth to society. Adults over age 40 typically seek to identify a positive contribution for which they will be most remembered. For some, their legacy is having been a good parent, an upstanding citizen, or a community volunteer; for others, more tangible activities, such as writing or painting, are their legacy.
Client Needs Category—*Health promotion and maintenance*
Client Needs Subcategory—*None*

58. 2. Asking about dietary practices is the most direct method among the options provided for determining if the client follows Orthodox Jewish lifestyle. Hebrew is commonly spoken by individuals who have emigrated from Israel. Reform, Conservative, and Orthodox Jewish men may wear a yarmulke, or skullcap, especially on the Sabbath or when attending synagogue. Many Christian men, as well as Jews, are circumcised.
Client Needs Category—*Physiological integrity*
Client Needs Subcategory—*Basic care and comfort*

59. 1. To reduce the potential for recollapsing the lung, air is prevented from entering the opening from which a chest tube has been pulled. When the tube comes out, its sterility is compromised. If replaced, a new, sterile tube must be used. Holding the breath may help temporarily, but the client cannot sustain this effort. Breath sounds should be assessed, but only after the chest tube has been reinserted.
Client Needs Category—*Safe, effective care environment*
Client Needs Subcategory—*Safety and infection control*

60. 1. Fluids are restricted to a few ice chips or small sips of water. Because the NG tube is connected to suction, large amounts of fluid will be sucked back into the suction canister. Therefore, the fluid serves no purpose. Irrigating an NG tube is not unsafe; however, the nurse must follow the physician's written order or the facility's standards for care when carrying out this procedure. Relieving throat discomfort and providing oral hygiene are appropriate nursing care measures.
Client Needs Category—*Physiological integrity*
Client Needs Subcategory—*Physiological adaptation*

61. 2. The tip of the enema tubing is inserted approximately 3″ to 4″ (7.5 to 10 cm) when giving an enema to an adult client. This allows the tube to enter the anal canal and pass the internal sphincter, where the solution is instilled. Introducing the tube farther may injure mucous membranes. Introducing it a shorter distance places the solution in the rectum and causes the client to expel the enema before it can be effective.
Client Needs Category—*Physiological integrity*
Client Needs Subcategory—*Physiological adaptation*

62. 2. Retracting the foreskin is necessary to remove secretions and prevent infection. The foreskin is replaced after the area is cleansed. The anal area is washed after the penis and scrotum are cleaned; usually the penis is cleaned before the scrotum. The penis is washed with plain or soapy water; normal saline solution is unnecessary for this procedure.
Client Needs Category—*Physiological integrity*
Client Needs Subcategory—*Basic care and comfort*

63. 2. Knowing a client's occupation and the type of work performed provides valuable information about whether or not to include principles of body mechanics in a teaching plan for a client with recurrent back pain. The client's age and energy level affect the strategies selected for providing the health teaching. Observing the client's gait is more medically diagnostic because a limb that is shorter than another may suggest an alteration in the alignment of spinal vertebrae. Assessing the client's medications may prove helpful when developing a care plan, especially if the medications are used to treat musculoskeletal problems. However, knowledge of medications the client is taking is not as helpful as exploring the occupation of the client and type of work he performs.
Client Needs Category—*Health promotion and maintenance*
Client Needs Subcategory—*None*

64. 3. Talking and dealing with an anxiety-provoking experience is healthier than avoiding or suppressing it. Failing to deal with the terror of an event can also lead to posttraumatic stress disorder. Most victims can detect insincerity when others pretend to be happy in their presence. Although interacting with others who have experienced a similar traumatic event is therapeutic, socializing for the sake of socializing is not. Taking vacations and participating in pleasurable activities are a form of stress management, but they serve as distractions and delay processing the impact of a traumatic event.
Client Needs Category—*Psychosocial integrity*
Client Needs Subcategory—*None*

65. **2.** Standing in front of a mirror helps the client to detect any physical breast changes, such as redness, changes in the nipple, or dimpling of the skin. Performing the entire examination while lying on the back, lying on the abdomen, or sitting when palpating the breast are not recommended methods of BSE.

Client Needs Category—Health promotion and maintenance
Client Needs Subcategory—None

66. **3.** Corticosteroid therapy reduces the immunologic injury to the nephrons. As the nephrons recover, the client's urine output increases. Weight gain is a nontherapeutic effect of steroids due to altered glucose metabolism and sodium retention. Long- and short-term high-dose therapies with corticosteroids are likely to create muscle weakness and atrophy. Blood pressure decreases from previously hypertensive levels as renal function improves.

Client Needs Category—Physiological integrity
Client Needs Subcategory—Pharmacological therapies

67. **2.** One of the best techniques for reducing a hospitalized client's anxiety is to explain procedures before performing them and offer instructions about any equipment involved in the client's care. Many hospitalized clients exaggerate the significance of common procedures and equipment and sometimes overreact to unaccustomed sights and sounds. In this case, the nurse should explain why the alarm sounded to help calm the client. Switching the infusion to gravity flow without explaining why is unlikely to relieve the client's anxiety. A tranquilizer or hypnotic medication should not be given until the results of other nursing interventions are evaluated. Staying with the client until he falls asleep may be time-consuming and keeps the nurse from other nursing duties.

Client Needs Category—Psychosocial integrity
Client Needs Subcategory—None

68. **1.** It is not unusual for any new mother to feel frustrated and overwhelmed by parenting demands. Explaining to the adolescent that this is normal and suggesting coping methods and occasional respite from family or friends are appropriate nursing measures in this case. Suggesting that the client place the newborn for adoption is extreme, given the circumstances. The information as presented does not warrant reporting the situation to child protective services. Telling the mother to be patient until the feeling goes away does not help her deal with the situation at hand.

Client Needs Category—Health promotion and maintenance
Client Needs Subcategory—None

69. **2.** When vaginal bleeding is noted shortly after delivery, the nurse first massages the uterus. This is often sufficient to cause contraction of the uterus, which may have become relaxed and soft. Normally, firming the uterus controls bleeding. If this conservative measure is ineffective, the nurse collects more data, such as the client's current vital signs, and informs the physician. I.V. fluids and drugs (such as oxytocin [Pitocin]) are required if independent nursing measures do not sufficiently control blood loss. Elevating the client's legs is ineffective in controlling the bleeding caused by a boggy uterus.

Client Needs Category—Physiological integrity
Client Needs Subcategory—Physiological adaptation

70. **2.** The main reason for performing leg exercises is to promote venous circulation, thereby preventing the formation of blood clots. Leg exercises are generally used as an alternative when ambulation and activity are less than adequate. Exercise helps to maintain muscle strength, reduces dependent edema, and relieves blood congestion in varicose veins. However, these are the secondary benefits of leg exercises.

Client Needs Category—Health promotion and maintenance
Client Needs Subcategory—None

71. **3.** Aminophylline (Truphylline), a bronchodilator, is most likely to produce stimulating effects, such as restlessness, insomnia, irritability, tachycardia, and hypertension. It is sometimes difficult to differentiate between the effects of the drug therapy and the manifestations of hypoxia. Breath sounds and respiratory effort are monitored frequently along with vital signs. Drug blood levels are monitored to evaluate a person's ability to metabolize the drug; dosages are adjusted based on the response. Bradycardia, drowsiness, and hypotension are all opposite to the stimulating effects associated with aminophylline (Truphylline).

Client Needs Category—Physiological integrity
Client Needs Subcategory—Pharmacological therapies

72. **3.** Excessive sleeping is one method some depressed clients use to withdraw from others. Not eating the food that is provided can have several explanations, not just depression. Complaining about aches and pains may be an activity that draws attention to the client and is not typically associated with depression.

Client Needs Category—Psychosocial integrity
Client Needs Subcategory—None

73. **3.** Tetracycline hydrochloride (Tetracyn) is not recommended for children under age 8 unless its use is absolutely necessary. This family of antibiotics causes permanent yellow, gray, or brown tooth discoloration.

Penicillins, cephalosporins, and aminoglycosides will not discolor a child's teeth.

Client Needs Category—Physiological integrity
Client Needs Subcategory—Pharmacological therapies

74. 4. It is best to first promote reality orientation when any client with dementia becomes confused. Disagreeing may agitate the client, interfering with the effectiveness of any therapy provided. Collaborating in the delusion by offering to call the school or indicating that a neighbor will care for her children contributes to the altered thought processes.

Client Needs Category—Psychosocial integrity
Client Needs Subcategory—None

75. 4. Aspirin is used during the acute stages of a myocardial infarction (MI) primarily for its antiplatelet action. This action helps restore blood flow through the arteries. Aspirin also has analgesic, anti-inflammatory, antipyretic, and antithrombolytic actions, but none of these is the reason for its administration during a possible MI.

Client Needs Category—Physiological integrity
Client Needs Subcategory—Pharmacological therapies

76. 3. The brachial artery is used for assessment during CPR of an infant. The rationale is that an infant's neck is short and fat, which makes assessing the carotid pulse difficult. Also, the airway of an infant is short, soft, and compliant, so palpating for a carotid pulse may close or occlude the infant's airway. The radial and femoral arteries are not routinely used when assessing a client of any age during CPR.

Client Needs Category—Safe, effective care environment
Client Needs Subcategory—Safety and infection control

77. 4. The nurse's first concern is to assess the client's physical condition before attempting any change in the client's position. After examining the client, the nurse should solicit adequate help to move the client to a safer, more comfortable place, usually the bed or chair. If the client is placed back in bed, the side rails should be raised. After all the data are collected and the nurse provides comfort and reassurance to the client, the accident should be reported to the supervisor and physician. A written description of the accident and its outcome is recorded and kept on file in the administration office.

Client Needs Category—Safe, effective care environment
Client Needs Subcategory—Safety and infection control

78. 4. The best evidence of healthy parent-newborn attachment is that the parents hold, touch, and talk to their newborn child. Physical contact tends to stimulate the beginning of parental love and protectiveness. It communicates comfort and security to the infant. Being pleased with the baby's gender is a positive sign, but it is not as indicative of the future relationship between parents and an infant. Observing others caring for the infant or watching from a distance is not as effective as eye-to-eye and direct skin contact in promoting bonding.

Client Needs Category—Health promotion and maintenance
Client Needs Subcategory—None

79. 3. Gelatin is permitted on a clear liquid diet. Clear liquids include fluids and foods that are transparent. Milk and other items containing milk, such as ice cream and creamed soup, are not permitted on a clear liquid diet but may be included on a full-liquid one.

Client Needs Category—Physiological integrity
Client Needs Subcategory—Basic care and comfort

80. 3. A sign that a client is able to orient himself is the ability to find his own room without assistance. Walking with others is not evidence that the client can independently find the dining room. The ability to dress is evidence that the client is able to perform activities of daily living, but does not reflect improvement in orientation. Talking on the telephone indicates that the client has retained the ability to communicate verbally.

Client Needs Category—Psychosocial integrity
Client Needs Subcategory—None

81. 2. It is best to hold aerosolized medication in the lungs for a few seconds to maximally disperse the inhaled drug throughout the lungs. Immediately exhaling causes inadequate distribution and absorption. Swallowing the inhaled medication fails to distribute the drug to the appropriate location for absorption. Coughing causes the aerosolized medication to be displaced into the upper airways.

Client Needs Category—Physiological integrity
Client Needs Subcategory—Pharmacological therapies

82. 4. A young child may not be able to verbally indicate the location of discomfort. Pulling at the infected ear is a common indication of a middle ear infection. A runny nose and swallowing frequently can be signs of many problems; however, they are not specific to an otitis media infection.

Client Needs Category—Physiological integrity
Client Needs Subcategory—Physiological adaptation

83. **2.** Ménière's disease is a disease of the inner ear that results in episodes of dizziness (vertigo), ringing in the ears (tinnitus), and hearing loss. It has no known cause, and the frequency and severity of the attacks vary. Several types of medications may be used during an acute attack. Some include central nervous system depressants, such as diazepam (Valium) or lorazepam (Ativan). Meclizine (Antivert) is an antivertigo-antiemetic drug that is commonly prescribed for motion sickness and vertigo due to vestibular disease. Acetaminophen (Tylenol) has antipyretic and analgesic actions and is not usually used for Ménière's disease. Meperidine (Demerol), an opioid analgesic, is also not used for this disease. Triazolam (Halcion), a benzodiazepine, is commonly prescribed for sleep, not vertigo and tinnitus.

> **Client Needs Category**—*Physiological integrity*
> **Client Needs Subcategory**—*Pharmacological therapies*

84. **4.** Calcium is chiefly regulated in the blood by parathyroid hormone and calcitonin (a hormone released by the thyroid). Following a thyroidectomy, clients are monitored for hypocalcemia because it is possible that the parathyroid glands may have been accidentally removed. Hypocalcemia is manifested by tingling and numbness of the extremities and mouth and muscle contractions of the fingers and hands. The other choices are not related to a thyroidectomy.

> **Client Needs Category**—*Physiological integrity*
> **Client Needs Subcategory**—*Physiological adaptation*

85. **3.** The fingernails are cut short to maintain skin integrity. Some health care professionals also recommend that the client wear cotton gloves to prevent opening the skin in case scratching cannot be controlled. Warm water accentuates the itching sensation. Dry cornstarch absorbs perspiration but does not relieve itching. Because jaundice is not related to an allergic reaction, using special hypoallergenic linens is inappropriate.

> **Client Needs Category**—*Physiological integrity*
> **Client Needs Subcategory**—*Basic care and comfort*

86.

2.	Introduce yourself and explain the sequence of events.
4.	Focus on general questions of sexual health and reproduction.
6.	Address detailed sexual history and reproductive questions.
1.	Ask the client if she would like to use the bathroom.
5.	Have the client change into a paper gown and offer a lap gown.
3.	Help the patient into the stirrups for the physical examination.

Completing a reproductive history and physical examination can be stressful for the client. To ease the client's anxiety and build a trusting relationship, the nurse should begin by introducing herself and explain the sequence of events. Next, the nurse begins collecting the client history, focusing first on general questions about sexual health and reproduction before addressing more detailed concerns. Once the history has been completed, the nurse should allow the client to use the bathroom, especially if the bathroom is in the hall, prior to having her change into a paper gown. Clients typically feel less vulnerable answering questions while fully dressed. Lastly, just before the physician arrives for the physical examination, the nurse helps the client into the stirrups.

> **Client Needs Category**—*Physiological integrity*
> **Client Needs Subcategory**—*Physiological adaptation*

87. **2.** A client with hyperparathyroidism is prone to forming kidney stones. Therefore, keeping the urine dilute and promoting frequent urinary elimination by providing a high fluid intake help reduce the potential for stone formation. Hypercalcemia also increases the risk of hypertension and cardiac arrhythmias; it is not associated with respiratory problems, so there is no need to monitor respirations. The client's diet should be limited in calcium; therefore, offering a supplement is unnecessary. The client is not at increased risk for skin breakdown with this condition, so frequent skin care is also unnecessary.

> **Client Needs Category**—*Physiological integrity*
> **Client Needs Subcategory**—*Physiological adaptation*

88. **1.** An aneurysm is the ballooning or dilation of the blood vessel as a result of a weakness in the vessel wall. The aorta is commonly affected by high blood pressure. Smoking and age are other factors related to an abdominal aortic aneurysm. When the descending aorta develops an aneurysm, an examiner may feel a pulsating abdominal mass. Other signs and symptoms include mild mid-abdominal or back pain, peripheral emboli, and cool, cyanotic extremities. Extra heart sounds are associated with disorders of the conduction system or congestive heart failure, not abdominal aortic aneurysms. Uneven chest movements are more often a sign of a pneumothorax or flail chest. Hollow sounds are normal assessment findings when percussing most areas of the abdomen.

> **Client Needs Category**—*Physiological integrity*
> **Client Needs Subcategory**—*Physiological adaptation*

89. **2.** Cocaine is a central nervous system stimulant that increases blood pressure and heart rate and causes cardiac arrhythmias. Any or all of these cardiovascular side effects can result in chest pain, tachycardia, or palpitations in an otherwise young, healthy person. Opioids, including heroin, barbiturates, and marijuana, are central nervous system depressants that are more likely to cause bradycardia and hypotension.

Client Needs Category—*Physiological integrity*
Client Needs Subcategory—*Physiological adaptation*

90. 1. A heart rate that remains within 60 to 100 beats/minute is within normal limits, indicating that the client is adequately oxygenated and not suffering from hypoxia. Tachycardia, bounding pulses, and arrhythmias are warning signs of oxygen deprivation. Noting the client's alertness and capillary refill time are not the best methods for evaluating the client's oxygenation status during suctioning.

Client Needs Category—*Physiological integrity*
Client Needs Subcategory—*Physiological adaptation*

91. 4. The nurse has an ethical responsibility to protect the confidentiality of the person who is HIV-positive. When persons test positive for HIV, they are provided counseling and education concerning measures for preventing its transmission. Legally, HIV-infected persons are required to divulge their infectious status to any and all potential sexual partners. When safe sex practices and blood and body fluid precautions are followed, it is possible to prevent transmission of HIV from an infected person to a noninfected person. All of the remaining options are inappropriate.

Client Needs Category—*Safe, effective care environment*
Client Needs Subcategory—*Coordinated care*

92. 1. Early decelerations are usually benign and require no intervention. However, the nurse should continue to monitor the client to detect the presence of late decelerations, a more serious condition that requires intervention. If late decelerations occur, the nurse should turn the client onto her side, elevate her legs, and notify the physician.

Client Needs Category—*Health promotion and maintenance*
Client Needs Subcategory—*None*

93. 4. Buzzing, or tinnitus (ringing in the ears), is a common side effect experienced by individuals who take large, frequent doses of aspirin. GI upset and prolonged bleeding are other side effects associated with aspirin. Racing thoughts, polyuria, and diarrhea are not associated with aspirin use.

Client Needs Category—*Physiological integrity*
Client Needs Subcategory—*Pharmacological therapies*

94. 1. The combination of alcohol and a minor tranquilizer can cause central nervous system and respiratory depression. Many people have died accidentally or purposely when these two drugs are mixed. Generally, minor tranquilizers are given in low doses for short periods of time while an individual develops other effective coping techniques. Benzodiazepines such as alprazolam (Xanax) cause drowsiness rather than insomnia. Blood tests are generally unnecessary to monitor the effectiveness of benzodiazepine drug therapy.

Client Needs Category—*Physiological integrity*
Client Needs Subcategory—*Pharmacological therapies*

95. 1. The most common diagnostic tests for pneumonia are a CBC (with white blood cell count) and a chest X-ray. Other diagnostic and laboratory tests used to establish a diagnosis include a sputum culture and Gram stain, arterial blood gas studies, pulse oximetry, blood cultures, and a bronchoscopy. Pulmonary function tests, hemoglobin and hematocrit, electrolyte levels, and lung computed tomography are not used to diagnose pneumonia but may be used to diagnose other pulmonary disorders.

Client Needs Category—*Physiological integrity*
Client Needs Subcategory—*Physiological adaptation*

96. 2. Frequently turning a client with a wet plaster cast helps to dry the complete circumference of the cast. The room would need to be heated to an uncomfortably high temperature to have a significant effect on drying the cast. Manually fanning the cast is tedious and time-consuming. It would be impractical to take a client outside in the sun to dry a plaster cast.

Client Needs Category—*Physiological integrity*
Client Needs Subcategory—*Basic care and comfort*

97. 3. When a pregnant client says that breathing is eased, it is an indication that lightening has occurred. This means that the fetus has settled into the pelvic inlet. Lay persons often remark that the baby has "dropped." Multipara clients may not experience this phenomenon until just before or during true labor. Urination generally increases with lightening because of the pressure exerted by the fetus upon the bladder. Lightening may increase the incidence of backaches due to the descent of the fetus and relaxation of the pelvic joints prior to delivery. Braxton Hicks contractions are irregular, weak uterine contractions. When these contractions become more noticeable, they indicate impending labor.

Client Needs Category—*Health promotion and maintenance*
Client Needs Subcategory—*None*

98. **1.** Seeing the chest rise is the best evidence that rescue breathing is being performed appropriately. A rising chest indicates that the airway is open and no air is leaking from the victim's nose or mouth. It also indicates that the rescuer is administering a sufficient volume of air. Dilated pupils are a sign that the brain is not receiving adequate oxygenation. A pulse indicates that cardiac compressions are unnecessary. The rescuer needs to seal or cover both the nose and the mouth.

Client Needs Category—Physiological integrity
Client Needs Subcategory—Physiological adaptation

99. **3.** If a rectal tube has not brought relief after about 20 minutes, it is best to remove the tube temporarily and reinsert it a few hours later to allow the gas to travel further down the large intestine. Rotating a rectal tube or replacing the tube with a larger one does not increase its effectiveness. If a rectal tube is already inserted correctly beyond the internal rectal sphincter, inserting it further will not improve the potential for relieving intestinal distention.

Client Needs Category—Physiological integrity
Client Needs Subcategory—Physiological adaptation

100. **4.** One of the side effects of phenytoin (Dilantin) is gingival hyperplasia. Therefore, attention to good oral hygiene is required. Phenytoin (Dilantin) does not require additional fluid intake. Weight gain rarely occurs when taking this medication. The need for stress management techniques is not necessary while taking this drug because one of its side effects is drowsiness.

Client Needs Category—Physiological integrity
Client Needs Subcategory—Pharmacological therapies

101. **2.** Because of the disproportionate size of an adult's hand compared with an infant's heart and chest, the rescuer uses just two fingers to perform the chest compressions on an infant who is 1 year old or younger. The rate of compressions for an infant is 100 per minute. The heel of one hand is used on children between ages 1 and 8. The interlocked fingers of both hands are used when performing chest compressions on individuals over the age 8. The palms of the hands are not used during chest compressions regardless of the victim's age.

Client Needs Category—Safe, effective care environment
Client Needs Subcategory—Safety and infection control

102. **1.** An MI results from inadequate blood circulation to the heart muscle, resulting in poor myocardial oxygenation. Diminished oxygenation leads to ischemia or angina pain. Pain that accompanies an MI is not caused by damage to the arteries, impending circulatory collapse, or left ventricular muscle fatigue.

Client Needs Category—Physiological integrity
Client Needs Subcategory—Physiological adaptation

103. **1.** Potassium levels are normally between 3.5 mEq/L and 5.0 mEq/L. Because the potassium level is under 3.5 mEq/L, it is considered hypokalemia. Furosemide (Lasix) is a diuretic that depletes potassium. Therefore, the nurse should monitor the client's potassium daily. All of the other laboratory test values listed are within normal limits.

Client Needs Category—Physiological integrity
Client Needs Subcategory—Physiological adaptation

104. **2.** Infants who are born with fetal alcohol syndrome tend to be extremely irritable at birth. As they mature, they may develop disorders characterized by hyperactivity. Lethargy, flaccidity, and jaundice are not exhibited by infants with fetal alcohol syndrome.

Client Needs Category—Physiological integrity
Client Needs Subcategory—Physiological adaptation

105. **2.** One of the best ways to quantify the client's subjective response to a medication is to use some form of rating scale. The heart rate and blood pressure may be lowered with antianxiety medication, but that does not help evaluate the client's perception. The other assessment techniques are too vague to be significant.

Client Needs Category—Psychosocial integrity
Client Needs Subcategory—None

106. **1.** Although it is therapeutic to involve a client with a change in body image during his care, acceptance of the change in body image cannot be rushed. Therefore, it is best for the nurse to accept the client's behavior and choice without judgment. This shows respect for the individual's unique effort to cope. In the early postoperative period, it is premature to suggest that the client needs professional help to adjust. How the nurse would deal with the same circumstance is immaterial. Saying that the stump does not look that bad is an evaluative statement based on the nurse's standards and experiences.

Client Needs Category—Psychosocial integrity
Client Needs Subcategory—None

107. **1.** Postural drainage is performed before eating or after consumed food has left the stomach. Done on a full stomach, the positioning, coughing, or expectorating may cause the person to feel nauseated and vomit. Postural drainage is performed according to a scheduled routine to mobilize secretions, not just when an individual feels short of breath or is actively coughing. Although the respiratory therapist is consulted when planning postural drainage, this is not the deciding factor in when it takes place.

> *Client Needs Category—Physiological integrity*
> *Client Needs Subcategory—Basic care and comfort*

108. **3.** The earliest signs of hypoxia are manifested by behavioral changes, such as restlessness, apprehension, anxiety, decreased judgment, and drowsiness. As hypoxia progresses, the nurse typically observes dyspnea, tachypnea, and tachycardia. The client's blood pressure may become elevated due to anxiety. Cyanosis is one of the last signs the nurse is likely to observe in a client who is hypoxic.

> *Client Needs Category—Physiological integrity*
> *Client Needs Subcategory—Physiological adaptation*

109. **4.** Maintaining cleanliness is of highest priority following a perineal prostatectomy because the client is at high risk for wound infection from organisms present in stool. Straining during defecation is contraindicated; therefore, performing Valsalva's maneuver (bearing down against a closed glottis) is inappropriate. A high Fowler's position can contribute to discomfort in the perineal incisional area. Laxatives are generally too harsh for prophylactically maintaining comfortable stool elimination.

> *Client Needs Category—Safe, effective care environment*
> *Client Needs Subcategory—Safety and infection control*

110. **3.** Throw rugs are the greatest potential hazard. Due to their instability, individuals tend to slip on throw rugs or fall when tripping on a wrinkled portion of rug or a curled edge. A television in the bedroom is no more unsafe than having one in any other room of the house. Taking a shower is safer than bathing in a tub. Grounded outlets for cords with three prongs are safer than the customary two-pronged plug.

> *Client Needs Category—Safe, effective care environment*
> *Client Needs Subcategory—Safety and infection control*

111. **2.** Standard precautions (formerly known as universal precautions) are followed when caring for all clients, even those already infected with HIV. Transmission of other infectious diseases is prevented by following either airborne, droplet, or contact precautions.

> *Client Needs Category—Safe, effective care environment*
> *Client Needs Subcategory—Safety and infection control*

112. **3.** The most common cause of a hernia is performing an activity that increases intra-abdominal pressure, such as lifting heavy objects. Increasing intra-abdominal pressure causes the intestine to protrude through areas in the abdominal musculature that are structurally weak. There is no correlation between having an umbilical hernia as a child and having an inguinal hernia as an adult. Inactivity plays a role in weakening abdominal muscles; however, in this situation, the client's hernia is most likely due to his heavy lifting. Being underweight is not a factor related to inguinal hernias.

> *Client Needs Category—Physiological integrity*
> *Client Needs Subcategory—Physiological adaptation*

113. **2.** RSV is highly contagious and spread by droplet contamination. It is associated with lower respiratory tract infections (bronchiolitis and pneumonia) in children under age 2. The past medical history reveals that the child has had a previous upper respiratory tract infection or otitis media, which supports the diagnosis. Hospitalization is usually required with RSV, and the main goal is to assist the child to breathe. An immune assay enzyme test to confirm RSV infection requires a specimen of nasal secretions. Throat swabs, sputum specimens, and blood specimens are not used to perform this particular diagnostic test.

> *Client Needs Category—Physiological integrity*
> *Client Needs Subcategory—Physiological adaptation*

114. **2, 6.** The car seat for a newborn should be tethered to a stationary area of the car, such as a hook on the floor. Correct car seat placement includes placing the seat in the rear seat and in a rear-facing position. Even though it is helpful to have the mother seated beside the car seat, this is not required.

> *Client Needs Category—Safe, effective care environment*
> *Client Needs Subcategory—Safety and infection control*

115. **3.** The described symptoms are typical of a hypoglycemic reaction. Therefore, a normal blood glucose level is the best evidence that hypoglycemia has been corrected. The blood pressure is generally within normal limits or increased during hypoglycemia because of anxiety and adrenaline secretion. Assessing the blood pressure or skin temperature is not as valuable in determining the client's response to the nursing intervention. (Clients who perspire during a hypoglycemic reaction usually have skin that is cool and moist; the return to a warm temperature may be an indicator of other things, not just a response to treatment.) Objective data such as a blood glucose levels are more accurate than having the client say he is feeling better.

> *Client Needs Category—Physiological integrity*
> *Client Needs Subcategory—Physiological adaptation*

116. **2.** Oral contraceptives containing estrogen place individuals taking them at risk for thromboembolic disease. The risk of blood clot formation is from 3 to 11 times higher with this form of birth control than with other birth control measures. A history of blood clots is generally a contraindication to taking oral contraceptives. Iron supplements, nasal decongestants, and antacids do not promote the formation of blood clots.

Client Needs Category—*Physiological integrity*
Client Needs Subcategory—*Pharmacological therapies*

117. **1.** Following a TURP, men experience retrograde ejaculation. That is, ejaculation is dry during orgasm. Semen is deposited into the bladder. The first voiding after intercourse is likely to appear cloudy because it contains the seminal fluid and sperm. Because of this change in physiology, men can expect to be unable to impregnate a sexual partner. Despite retrograde ejaculation, following a TURP men experience orgasms, achieve erections during sexual excitement, and maintain normal libidos.

Client Needs Category—*Health promotion and maintenance*
Client Needs Subcategory—*None*

118. **1.** Heparin is an anticoagulant. The antidote for an overdose of heparin is protamine sulfate. Naloxone hydrochloride (Narcan) is used for respiratory depression and opioid overdoses. Vitamin K is the antidote for warfarin (Coumadin) overdose. Calcium gluconate is the antidote for magnesium overdose and is used most often when magnesium levels are toxic related to preeclampsia during pregnancy.

Client Needs Category—*Physiological integrity*
Client Needs Subcategory—*Pharmacological therapies*

119. **1, 3, 5.** Cultural information can be invaluable when providing care for clients who are of a different culture, ethnicity, or religion. Therefore, performing a comprehensive cultural assessment will improve the client's care. Assessment of the client's food preferences is important because eating is important to recovery. Food preferences and diet may also be the cause of the disorder. The client's primary language and his ability to speak and understand treatment goals and discharge instructions are important for the nurse to assess. Assessing language also provides information about whether an interpreter might be needed during the hospitalization. The client's religion is important to assess because of its possible prevalence in the client's daily life and current health practices and beliefs.

Bodily functions, such as bowel movements, urination, and menstruation, are sensitive topics that most clients from a different culture are reluctant to discuss with the nurse during the initial admission assessment. Breast and penis or scrotal diseases as well as reproductive disorders are also topics that may be embarrassing for the client to discuss (especially if the client's language skills are inadequate or his understanding of the language is limited).

Asking the client if he can tell time is an inappropriate question. What the nurse really needs to know is the client's orientation to time because time is a cultural belief. In some cultures, such as in the United States, life is scheduled around a strict time frame; being "on time" is a value. However, in some cultures time is not valued. Personal interactions, human contacts, and official business are more highly valued.

Asking the client whether he is in pain is not part of the cultural assessment. What the nurse really needs to know is how the client expresses the pain based on cultural, ethnic, and religious beliefs and values.

Client Needs Category—*Psychosocial integrity*
Client Needs Subcategory—*None*

120. **3.** Bananas, rice, applesauce, and toast (the BRAT diet) are usually the first solid foods offered to a child who is recovering from gastroenteritis. Butter should not be put on the rice because of the fat content. The diet is advanced gradually, with milk products added last.

Client Needs Category—*Physiological integrity*
Client Needs Subcategory—*Basic care and comfort*

121. **1.** Measures should be taken to minimize crying because excessive crying increases oxygen demand, which increases cardiac workload. The infant should be placed in semi-Fowler's position. Holding is encouraged to decrease the infant's anxiety and cardiac workload. The infant is fed using a soft nipple with a large hole to decrease the effort required to suck.

Client Needs Category—*Physiological integrity*
Client Needs Subcategory—*Basic care and comfort*

122. **4.** Enoxaparin (Lovenox) is a subcutaneously administered anticoagulant that reduces the risk of developing deep vein thrombosis and pulmonary emboli after surgical procedures when the client cannot ambulate as usual. There is no indication that enoxaparin (Lovenox) has any effect on tissue healing or bleeding, and it does not break up clots that have formed.

Client Needs Category—*Physiological integrity*
Client Needs Subcategory—*Pharmacological therapies*

123. **2.** Absence seizures occur most frequently in childhood and adolescence. They involve a lapse of consciousness for 5 to 10 seconds with a blank facial expression and often include frequent repetitive movements. Afterward, the child typically resumes normal activity as if there had never been any seizure activity. Myoclonic and clonic seizures involve motor function disturbances. Partial seizures are common types of seizures that do not result in loss of consciousness, but they are not the most common type for this age-group.

> *Client Needs Category—Physiological integrity*
> *Client Needs Subcategory—Physiological adaptation*

124. **3.** No restrictions are placed on a client's activity when an ultrasound is done. The other statements indicate that the client understands the procedure: The client should drink approximately 1 quart of water 1 to 2 hours before the procedure to facilitate visualization by elevating the uterine contents higher into the abdomen; a gel is applied to the abdomen to reduce friction as the transducer is moved over the abdomen; and radiation is not used with ultrasonography.

> *Client Needs Category—Safe, effective care environment*
> *Client Needs Subcategory—Safety and infection control*

125. **1.** It is no longer justified to use a padded tongue blade during a seizure to keep the tongue from the back of the throat. Many clients have experienced oral problems and choking on snapped tongue blades. An artificial airway may be required to maintain a patent airway during a tonic-clonic seizure. Suctioning equipment is appropriate in seizure precautions. Side-rail padding can protect the client from injury.

> *Client Needs Category—Safe, effective care environment*
> *Client Needs Subcategory—Safety and infection control*

126. **2.** Removing moisture from the infant's body will prevent heat loss by evaporation, which occurs when a liquid is converted to a vapor. Wrapping an infant in a warmed blanket prevents heat loss by conduction, which occurs if the infant's skin comes into direct contact with a cold surface or object. Positioning the crib away from outside windows on cold days prevents heat loss by radiation, which occurs if the infant is placed near cold objects. Positioning the crib away from air conditioning vents prevents heat loss by convection, which occurs if the infant comes into contact with cold moving air.

> *Client Needs Category—Safe, effective care environment*
> *Client Needs Subcategory—Safety and infection control*

127. **3.** Gestational diabetes usually does not persist after delivery of the baby. Some women who have had gestational diabetes develop type 2 (non-insulin-dependent) diabetes mellitus, but this is not usually the case. Gestational diabetes is present only during pregnancy; therefore, it could not be present in the client's childhood. Oral hypoglycemics are not given during pregnancy because they may harm the fetus. Women who have diabetes during pregnancy are more prone to have large-for-gestational-age babies.

> *Client Needs Category—Physiological integrity*
> *Client Needs Subcategory—Physiological adaptation*

128. **2.** One of the manifestations of bacterial meningitis is a bulging fontanel, which occurs secondary to the increased intracranial pressure. The white blood cell count may be elevated with any type of bacterial infection. The infant will usually have a high-pitched, not a low-pitched, cry. The glucose level in cerebrospinal fluid is decreased, not increased, in bacterial meningitis.

> *Client Needs Category—Physiological integrity*
> *Client Needs Subcategory—Physiological adaptation*

129. **1.** Head trauma resulting in long-term brain changes increases the risk of seizure disorder by approximately 50%. No correlation is noted between drug use and seizure disorder, and seizure disorder is not related to mental illness or spinal cord damage.

> *Client Needs Category—Health promotion and maintenance*
> *Client Needs Subcategory—None*

130. **2.** Children at this age are magical thinkers and enjoy pretend play. As they grow older and begin interacting more with other children, their interest in pretend play decreases. Six-year-old children commonly are very busy, boisterous, and bossy; are sensitive to criticism; and usually have short attention spans demonstrated by beginning one or more tasks but rarely completing them.

> *Client Needs Category—Health promotion and maintenance*
> *Client Needs Subcategory—None*

Comprehensive Test 2

Directions: With a pencil, blacken the space in front of the option you have chosen for your correct answer.

1. A client comes to the clinic complaining of epigastric pain. The client reportedly takes several nonprescription drugs on a regular basis. Which drug is most likely related to the client's current complaint?
[ ] **1.** Milk of magnesia, which the client takes for constipation
[ ] **2.** Aspirin, which the client takes for arthritis
[ ] **3.** Nyquil, which the client takes to fall asleep
[ ] **4.** Benadryl, which the client takes for allergy symptoms

2. A client who is 3 months pregnant complains of feeling tired. Which nursing advice is best to give this client?
[ ] **1.** "Do most of your work just after lunch."
[ ] **2.** "Increase your prenatal vitamins to two."
[ ] **3.** "Sleep later in the morning."
[ ] **4.** "Rest whenever you feel tired."

3. Which food is best for the nurse to include in a diet plan for a pregnant client who needs additional iron?
[ ] **1.** Potatoes
[ ] **2.** Legumes
[ ] **3.** Oranges
[ ] **4.** Cheese

4. An unconscious young adult is brought to the emergency department and is suspected of overdosing on heroin. The nurse should anticipate that the physician will order which drug initially?
[ ] **1.** Methadone hydrochloride (Dolophine)
[ ] **2.** Succinylcholine chloride (Anectine)
[ ] **3.** Naloxone hydrochloride (Narcan)
[ ] **4.** Pancuronium bromide (Pavulon)

5. The nurse should collaborate with the physician about which postpartum client before implementing an order for a laxative?
[ ] **1.** A client who has hemorrhoids
[ ] **2.** A client who is breast-feeding
[ ] **3.** A client who has a third-degree perineal tear
[ ] **4.** A client who had a vacuum extraction delivery

6. When a client with gallstones asks about treatment with extracorporeal lithotripsy, the nurse can best explain that the treatment eliminates the stones by which method?
[ ] **1.** Dissolving them with strong chemicals
[ ] **2.** Pulverizing them with shock waves
[ ] **3.** Removing them with a special endoscope
[ ] **4.** Binding them to a sticky resin material

7. A client who is 4 months pregnant states that she lives on a limited income and has a problem purchasing enough meat to supply sufficient protein for her diet. Which food can the nurse recommend to supplement the client's meat source?
[ ] **1.** Broccoli
[ ] **2.** Cauliflower
[ ] **3.** Fortified cereal
[ ] **4.** Dried beans

8. When teaching a postmenopausal client about breast self-examination, which instruction by the nurse is most accurate?
[ ] **1.** "Examine your breasts on awakening."
[ ] **2.** "Examine your breasts on the first day of the month."
[ ] **3.** "Examine your breasts after you finish your shower."
[ ] **4.** "Examine your breasts before your yearly mammogram."

9. The urine of a client who is 6 months pregnant tests positive for albumin. The nurse correctly assumes that the client is probably developing which complication of pregnancy?

[ ] **1.** Preeclampsia
[ ] **2.** Liver failure
[ ] **3.** Amniotic embolism
[ ] **4.** Gestational diabetes

10. A 10-year-old child is admitted to the hospital with endocarditis secondary to rheumatic fever. Which assessment finding in the child's medical history is most consistent with this condition?
[ ] **1.** The child had a congenital heart defect at birth.
[ ] **2.** The child had a recent untreated streptococcal infection.
[ ] **3.** The child has consistently had clubbing of the fingers.
[ ] **4.** The child failed to receive proper immunizations for measles.

11. A pregnant client is admitted to the labor and delivery area with vaginal bleeding. The physician's routine admission orders include the administration of an enema. Which action by the nurse is most appropriate?
[ ] **1.** Administer the enema as ordered.
[ ] **2.** Withhold the enema at this time.
[ ] **3.** Give the enema only if the client reports constipation.
[ ] **4.** Substitute a laxative for the cleansing enema.

12. A client had a hysterectomy 10 hours ago. The nurse assesses the client and finds that her blood pressure has fallen abruptly. Which action by the nurse is most appropriate at this time?
[ ] **1.** Continue to monitor the blood pressure every 15 minutes.
[ ] **2.** Document the information on the client's chart.
[ ] **3.** Inform the surgeon about the client's condition.
[ ] **4.** Change the client to a Fowler's position.

13. A postoperative client who just had a transurethral prostatectomy asks why he must drink so much water. Which response by the nurse is most accurate?
[ ] **1.** "It helps keep the catheter unobstructed."
[ ] **2.** "It promotes excretion of toxic wastes."
[ ] **3.** "It helps increase your bladder capacity."
[ ] **4.** "It promotes postoperative bladder retraining."

14. The physician performs a vaginal examination on a client in labor and states that the client is completely effaced and fully dilated. At this time, the nurse correctly plans to meet the needs of the client who is entering which stage of labor?
[ ] **1.** First
[ ] **2.** Second
[ ] **3.** Third
[ ] **4.** Fourth

15. When a female client requires urinary catheterization, where should the nurse insert the catheter? Indicate the correct location on the diagram.

16. A nursing home resident has a history of repeated falls after attempting to get up from his wheelchair. Which nursing action is most appropriate to prevent further falls?
[ ] **1.** Using a sheet to tie the client to the wheelchair
[ ] **2.** Keeping the client within view of the nurse's station at all times
[ ] **3.** Requesting an order for a restraint alternative
[ ] **4.** Obtaining a physician's order for a sedative

17. Which assessment finding best justifies withholding the I.M. administration of penicillin (Bicillin) until consulting the prescribing physician?
[ ] **1.** The client states that the injection sites are painful.
[ ] **2.** The client shows the nurse a red, itchy rash.
[ ] **3.** The client's body temperature has dropped to 100° F (37.8° C).
[ ] **4.** The client complains of a sore mouth.

18. The admitting nurse documents a client's dietary information. Which information is most likely to contribute to the client's complaint of constipation?
[ ] **1.** The client eats five daily servings of fresh vegetables.
[ ] **2.** The client eats breakfast cereal with skim milk daily.
[ ] **3.** The client drinks an average of four glasses of liquids per day.
[ ] **4.** The client substitutes grains and beans for meat.

19. A physician orders two drops of medication to be administered in the client's right eye b.i.d. How many times a day does the nurse administer the drops?
[ ] **1.** Once
[ ] **2.** Three times
[ ] **3.** Four times
[ ] **4.** Twice

20. A postoperative client asks the nurse to explain the purpose of the Penrose drain positioned in his abdomen. Which statement by the nurse best explains the reason for using a Penrose drain?
[ ] **1.** "Using a Penrose drain decreases scar tissue formation."
[ ] **2.** "Inserting a Penrose drain helps fluid escape from the surgical area."
[ ] **3.** "Instilling a Penrose drain provides a means for irrigating the wound."
[ ] **4.** "Providing a Penrose drain releases accumulating intestinal gas."

21. During a home health visit, the nurse asks the mother of a 7-year-old to describe how she gives the child's medication through a gastrostomy tube. Which response by the mother indicates the need for additional teaching?
[ ] **1.** "I crush the medication finely and mix it with 30 mL of warm water."
[ ] **2.** "Before giving the medication, I flush the tube with 50 mL of water."
[ ] **3.** "I mix the medication into the bag of tube-feeding formula before instilling it."
[ ] **4.** "I flush the tube with 50 mL of water after administering the medication."

22. The nurse knows that a safe pediatric dose of oral cephalexin (Keflex) is 25 mg/kg/day in four equally divided doses. What is the safe single mg dose for a child weighing 44 lb?

_____

23. A physician orders postural drainage for a client with pneumonia. Which nursing action best facilitates a therapeutic outcome for the client?
[ ] **1.** Placing the client in a supine position
[ ] **2.** Encouraging the client to cough deeply
[ ] **3.** Having the client breathe through his mouth
[ ] **4.** Instructing the client to breathe slowly

24. Which assessment finding indicates that a 75-year-old client with diabetes requires additional teaching regarding foot care?
[ ] **1.** The client has placed lamb's wool between his toes.
[ ] **2.** The client states that his wife uses a razor blade to remove his calluses.
[ ] **3.** The client's toenails are short and cut straight across.
[ ] **4.** The client's chart indicates that he notified his physician of a foot injury.

25. When preparing a client for insertion of a nasogastric tube (NG), how should the nurse position the client's neck to facilitate introducing the tube into the nostril?
[ ] **1.** Flexed
[ ] **2.** Extended
[ ] **3.** Rotated to the left
[ ] **4.** Hyperextended

26. When providing discharge instructions to a client receiving warfarin sodium (Coumadin), the nurse teaches the importance of regular monitoring for which laboratory value?
[ ] **1.** Platelet levels in the blood
[ ] **2.** Partial thromboplastin time
[ ] **3.** Circulating blood volume
[ ] **4.** International Normalized Ratio (INR)

27. A previously healthy client comes to the emergency department complaining of severe nausea and vomiting hours after eating in a restaurant. Which assessment question best determines if a food-borne pathogen is the cause of the client's symptoms?
[ ] **1.** "What foods did you eat?"
[ ] **2.** "Did you take something for your nausea?"
[ ] **3.** "Did your food look spoiled?"
[ ] **4.** "Have you ever had food poisoning?"

28. If the care plan of a client receiving internal radiation therapy includes all the following nursing interventions, which intervention requires revision because it is unsafe?
[ ] **1.** Maintain a radiation symbol on the outside wall or door to the client's room.
[ ] **2.** Inform all non-nursing personnel that the client is receiving radiation therapy.
[ ] **3.** Wear a radiation-monitoring badge when providing care to the client.
[ ] **4.** Assign the same personnel to consistently care for the client.

29. Which question is essential for the nurse to ask before a client undergoes an intravenous pyelgram (IVP)?
[ ] **1.** "Are you afraid of needles?"
[ ] **2.** "Have you ever had X-rays taken?"
[ ] **3.** "Do you have any allergies to seafood?"
[ ] **4.** "Have you experienced fear of confined places?"

30. Which diversional activity is best to include in the care plan of a client with recent loss of vision?
[ ] **1.** Listening to a radio or audiotapes
[ ] **2.** Talking with other clients on the unit
[ ] **3.** Listening to television
[ ] **4.** Reading books set in Braille

31. An 8-year-old child is brought to the emergency department after falling from a swing. Which assessment finding provides the nurse with the best evidence that the child has a compound fracture?
[ ] **1.** Complaint of pain at the injury site
[ ] **2.** Abnormal mobility of the injured extremity
[ ] **3.** Grinding sensation over the injury site
[ ] **4.** Bone protruding at the injury site

32. If a client is to receive 1,000 mL of dextrose 5% in normal saline solution over an 8-hour period, the nurse correctly sets the infusion pump to administer which volume?
[ ] **1.** 50 mL
[ ] **2.** 100 mL
[ ] **3.** 125 mL
[ ] **4.** 150 mL

33. Which laboratory test, if elevated, is most indicative that a child has rheumatic fever?
[ ] **1.** Antinuclear antibody test
[ ] **2.** Antistreptolysin O titer
[ ] **3.** Heterophile antibody titer
[ ] **4.** Fluorescent antibody test

34. A 350-lb (159-kg) client with diabetes is hospitalized. The nurse plans to give the client's morning insulin in the abdomen. Which needle angle is most appropriate?
[ ] **1.** 15 degrees
[ ] **2.** 30 degrees
[ ] **3.** 45 degrees
[ ] **4.** 90 degrees

35. When planning discharge instructions for a client who had a prostatectomy, which information is most appropriate for the nurse to include?
[ ] **1.** Avoid eating foods containing roughage.
[ ] **2.** Avoid heavy lifting and strenuous exercise.
[ ] **3.** Use an enema if constipation occurs.
[ ] **4.** Limit fluid intake to eight glasses per day.

36. Which nursing intervention is best to include in the care plan of a client with expressive (motor) aphasia?
[ ] **1.** Use a louder than normal voice when communicating with the client.
[ ] **2.** Write questions and directions for the client to read.
[ ] **3.** Speak in short sentences to promote understanding.
[ ] **4.** Give the client time to respond to questions.

37. A chest tube was placed in a client with a hemothorax 4 hours ago and connected to a closed water-seal drainage system. When the oncoming shift nurse assesses the system, which assessment finding should be reported immediately?
[ ] **1.** Approximately 2 cm of water is in the water-seal chamber.
[ ] **2.** The water-seal chamber is bubbling continuously.
[ ] **3.** Dark, bloody drainage is in the collection chamber.
[ ] **4.** Diminished breath sounds are heard in the lung with the hemothorax.

38. Where should the nurse place her fingers to assess the femoral pulse of a client who has just returned from cardiac catheterization?
[ ] **1.** Behind the knee
[ ] **2.** On the dorsum of the foot
[ ] **3.** Into the inguinal area
[ ] **4.** Over the lower tibia

39. Which assessment finding best indicates that a pregnant client is in the transition phase of labor?
[ ] **1.** The client states that she feels a gush of water coming from her vagina.
[ ] **2.** The client states that she feels as if she needs to have a bowel movement.
[ ] **3.** The client tells her coach not to touch her but also asks not to be left alone.
[ ] **4.** The client asks for blankets and tells the nurse that she cannot stop shivering.

40. The nurse asks a postpartum client to explain how she performs Kegel exercises. Which description provides the best indication that she is performing Kegel exercises correctly?
[ ] **1.** "I tighten, then alternately relax, my perineal muscles."
[ ] **2.** "I lie supine and alternately raise and lower my legs."
[ ] **3.** "I tighten my abdominal muscles for 45 seconds for a total of 10 repetitions."
[ ] **4.** "I roll from side to back to side four to six times an hour."

41. Which nursing action best demonstrates the correct technique for withdrawing a parenteral drug from a multiple-dose vial?
[ ] **1.** Withdrawing the entire volume in a syringe, then discarding the unneeded portion
[ ] **2.** Injecting 1 mL more of air than the amount of the drug to be withdrawn
[ ] **3.** Refrigerating the medication vial for 10 minutes before withdrawing the drug
[ ] **4.** Injecting the same volume of air into the vial as liquid that will be removed

42. When administering an injection, which technique is potentially unsafe?

[ ] **1.** The nurse wears clean gloves when administering the injection.

[ ] **2.** The nurse discards the empty syringe in a biohazard container.

[ ] **3.** The nurse recaps the needle securely before discarding the syringe.

[ ] **4.** The nurse uses an alcohol swab to disinfect the injection site.

43. For a child with hemophilia, the nurse should immediately report which assessment finding to the physician?

[ ] **1.** The child is experiencing anorexia.

[ ] **2.** The child has discomfort from joint pain.

[ ] **3.** The child's mood is somewhat depressed.

[ ] **4.** The child has developed nasal congestion.

44. Before discharging a client with leukemia, which question is most important for the nurse to ask?

[ ] **1.** "Are you glad you're finally going home?"

[ ] **2.** "Is there someone to drive you home?"

[ ] **3.** "Have you decided what you'll do to keep busy?"

[ ] **4.** "Do you have any questions about your home care?"

45. When an unlicensed care technician provides care for a 10-month-old infant, which observation indicates the technician requires additional teaching?

[ ] **1.** The room temperature is set at 75° F (24° C) during the infant's bath.

[ ] **2.** For oral hygiene, the infant's teeth are swabbed with wet gauze.

[ ] **3.** Prior to bathing, the water temperature is checked with an elbow.

[ ] **4.** The infant's chest is sprinkled with baby powder after the bath.

46. In the emergency department, the nurse notes multiple needle punctures on a client's arms. The nurse correctly suspects that the client is abusing which category of drugs?

[ ] **1.** Opiates

[ ] **2.** Barbiturates

[ ] **3.** Amphetamines

[ ] **4.** Hallucinogens

47. An older adult client is comatose and on life support. The family asks that life-support measures be discontinued. Which method is best for determining whether it is appropriate to carry out the family's request?

[ ] **1.** Considering the cost of continued life-support measures

[ ] **2.** Checking if the client's insurance covers life-support measures

[ ] **3.** Validating that all immediate relatives are in total agreement

[ ] **4.** Examining the specifications in the client's advance directive

48. When a client ingests a toxic substance either intentionally or accidentally, which information is most important for the nurse to obtain?

[ ] **1.** The client's age

[ ] **2.** Who found the client

[ ] **3.** The substance involved

[ ] **4.** The client's past medical history

49. A nursing assistant voices concern for her safety when assigned to care for a client with acquired immunodeficiency syndrome (AIDS). Which information is best for allaying the nursing assistant's fears?

[ ] **1.** The life expectancy for AIDS clients is longer than in previous years.

[ ] **2.** AIDS is commonly transmitted by contact with blood and body fluids.

[ ] **3.** Mechanical barriers such as gloves can prevent viral transmission.

[ ] **4.** If the nursing assistant is infected, insurance may assist with her cost of care.

50. Immediately after a pregnant client's membranes rupture, which nursing action is a priority?

[ ] **1.** Monitoring the fetal heart rate

[ ] **2.** Beginning antibiotic administration

[ ] **3.** Putting a waterproof pad beneath the client

[ ] **4.** Placing the client in Trendelenburg's position

51. Which of the following risk factors increases a 75-year-old client's susceptibility to pneumonia?

[ ] **1.** Sudden weight gain

[ ] **2.** Smoking and alcohol intake

[ ] **3.** Anemia and hyperactive gag reflex

[ ] **4.** Dehydration

52. Which position is best for a client with suspected heart failure?

[ ] **1.** Semi-sitting (low Fowler's)

[ ] **2.** Right side-lying (Sims')

[ ] **3.** Sitting upright (high Fowler's)

[ ] **4.** Lying supine with the head lowered (Trendelenburg's)

53. When the client with a slow-bleeding cerebral aneurysm asks for assistance to the toilet for a bowel movement, which nursing response is most appropriate?
[ ]   **1.** The nurse complies with the client's request.
[ ]   **2.** The nurse offers to obtain a bedside commode.
[ ]   **3.** The nurse places the client on a bedpan.
[ ]   **4.** The nurse suggests administering a suppository.

54. If the nurse collects all the following data when performing a newborn's initial assessment, which assessment finding is most important to report?
[ ]   **1.** Blue hands and feet
[ ]   **2.** Flaccid muscle tone
[ ]   **3.** Heart rate over 100 beats/minute
[ ]   **4.** Loud, vigorous cry

55. A maintenance worker in a health agency comes to a nurse after receiving a minor finger burn. Which first-aid measure is correct in this situation?
[ ]   **1.** Apply petroleum jelly to the burn.
[ ]   **2.** Cover the burn with nonallergenic tape.
[ ]   **3.** Immerse the burned area in cool water.
[ ]   **4.** Place the burned area in warm water.

56. Which assessment finding provides the best evidence that a client with acute angle-closure glaucoma is responding to drug therapy?
[ ]   **1.** Swelling of the eyelids is decreased.
[ ]   **2.** Redness of the sclera is reduced.
[ ]   **3.** Eye pain is reduced or eliminated.
[ ]   **4.** Peripheral vision is diminished.

57. Which nursing action is most correct prior to instilling eardrops in a client's ear?
[ ]   **1.** Warm the medication to room temperature.
[ ]   **2.** Refrigerate the medication for 30 minutes.
[ ]   **3.** Clean the outer surface of the dropper.
[ ]   **4.** Fill the dropper with no more than 1 mL of medication.

58. Which teratogenic effect is the best rationale for advising pregnant women to avoid consuming alcohol?
[ ]   **1.** Mental retardation
[ ]   **2.** Congenital cataracts
[ ]   **3.** Seizure disorders
[ ]   **4.** Missing limbs

59. Which initial nursing response is best if a child confides information that indicates sexual abuse?
[ ]   **1.** Persuade the child to provide details.
[ ]   **2.** Examine the child for genital injuries.
[ ]   **3.** Let the child know he is believed.
[ ]   **4.** Look for signs of sexually transmitted diseases.

60. The nurse assesses a client with chronic alcoholism who has been drinking up to the time of admission. During which time frame after admission is the nurse most likely to observe signs of alcohol withdrawal in this client?
[ ]   **1.** 1 to 2 hours
[ ]   **2.** 4 to 6 hours
[ ]   **3.** 12 to 72 hours
[ ]   **4.** 3 to 7 days

61. When caring for a client who has been burned around the face and neck, which assessment finding should the nurse immediately report to the physician?
[ ]   **1.** Fluid overload
[ ]   **2.** Signs of hemorrhage
[ ]   **3.** Signs of infection
[ ]   **4.** Respiratory distress

62. Which nursing measure for preventing contractures is best to include in the care plan of an immobile client?
[ ]   **1.** Encourage the client to perform isometric exercises.
[ ]   **2.** Help the client to perform range-of-motion (ROM) exercises.
[ ]   **3.** Elevate the client's extremities on pillows.
[ ]   **4.** Use a pressure-relieving mattress.

63. When assessing a client with severe burns, which assessment finding provides the best evidence that the wound is infected?
[ ]   **1.** The wound has a foul odor.
[ ]   **2.** The eschar is black.
[ ]   **3.** The white blood cell (WBC) count is 5,000/mm^3.
[ ]   **4.** The heart rate is increased.

64. A 6-year-old child is recovering from acute noninfectious gastroenteritis. The physician leaves orders to advance the child to solid food. Which food is best for the nurse to offer the child initially?
[ ]   **1.** Vanilla pudding
[ ]   **2.** Chicken broth
[ ]   **3.** Oatmeal and milk
[ ]   **4.** Strained applesauce

65. Which activity is most appropriate for a client diagnosed with generalized anxiety disorder?
[ ]   **1.** Playing cards
[ ]   **2.** Assembling models
[ ]   **3.** Using a treadmill
[ ]   **4.** Painting pictures

66. A client who takes furosemide (Lasix) for congestive heart failure comes to the clinic for a routine visit. The client's laboratory report reveals a potassium level of 3.1 mEq/L. Which question elicits the best information to assess whether the client is demonstrating signs and symptoms of hypokalemia?

[ ] **1.** "Have you been having leg cramps or muscle weakness?"
[ ] **2.** "Have you noticed a slowing of your heart rate?"
[ ] **3.** "Have you had a rapid weight gain lately?"
[ ] **4.** "Have you noticed if your speech has become slurred?"

67. When a client with type 1 diabetes comes to the clinic for a routine visit, the nurse should plan to ask which question in relation to possible complications?

[ ] **1.** "Have you had your eyes checked recently?"
[ ] **2.** "What's the color of your urine?"
[ ] **3.** "What's your usual blood pressure?"
[ ] **4.** "Have you had any heart palpitations?"

68. A client with type 2 diabetes takes glyburide (DiaBeta) daily at 7:30 a.m. The nurse correctly advises the client to watch for signs and symptoms of hypoglycemia at what time?

[ ] **1.** 11:00 a.m.
[ ] **2.** 12:00 p.m.
[ ] **3.** 5:00 p.m.
[ ] **4.** 8:30 a.m.

69. When collecting data from the parent of a child who is suspected of having rheumatic fever, the nurse demonstrates an accurate understanding of the etiology by asking if the child has recently had which condition?

[ ] **1.** Chickenpox
[ ] **2.** Sore throat
[ ] **3.** Influenza
[ ] **4.** Roseola

70. Which assessment finding would the nurse expect to find in a child who has rheumatic fever?

[ ] **1.** Urticaria
[ ] **2.** Hypothermia
[ ] **3.** Hypotension
[ ] **4.** Arthralgia

71. A primigravid client at 42 weeks' gestation is having a nonstress test. Which finding provides the best evidence of an unfavorable response to the test?

[ ] **1.** Fetal heart rate accelerations are at least 15 beats/minute above baseline.
[ ] **2.** Fetal movement is detected within 20 minutes of beginning the nonstress test.
[ ] **3.** More than two fetal heartbeat accelerations occur during a 20- to 30-minute period.
[ ] **4.** Each fetal heart rate acceleration lasts less than 15 seconds.

72. The radiologist uses a red pencil to mark a cancer client's skin in preparation for radiation treatments. Which action is essential to this client's nursing care?

[ ] **1.** Removing the marks by using acetone after each treatment
[ ] **2.** Washing the area with mild soap and tepid water when bathing
[ ] **3.** Keeping the irradiated skin exposed at all times
[ ] **4.** Rubbing lotion over the area after each treatment

73. A client with an ulcer has been taking aluminum hydroxide gel (Amphojel) for 3 days. Which symptom reported by the client is most likely a side effect of the antacid?

[ ] **1.** Constipation
[ ] **2.** Itchy skin
[ ] **3.** Dry mouth
[ ] **4.** Fatigue

74. A nursing assistant is assigned to care for a 5-year-old child with acute lymphoblastic leukemia. Which of the nursing assistant's actions best indicates the need for additional teaching when caring for this child?

[ ] **1.** The nursing assistant performs oral care using a sponge-type brush.
[ ] **2.** The nursing assistant assesses the child's temperature rectally.
[ ] **3.** The nursing assistant maintains protective isolation precautions.
[ ] **4.** The nursing assistant places a sheepskin under the bony prominences.

75. The physician prescribes pantoprazole (Protonix) for a client with peptic ulcer disease. When the client asks the nurse to explain the medication's action, which description is most correct?

[ ] **1.** Protonix makes gastric secretions more acidic.
[ ] **2.** Protonix covers the ulcer with a protective barrier.
[ ] **3.** Protonix inhibits gastric acid production.
[ ] **4.** Protonix blocks histamine receptors in the stomach.

76. Which volume of irrigation solution is most appropriate when irrigating a client's colostomy?
[ ] **1.** 50 to 100 mL
[ ] **2.** 100 to 150 mL
[ ] **3.** 250 to 500 mL
[ ] **4.** 500 to 1,000 mL

77. As the nurse gathers data from the medical record of an adolescent tentatively diagnosed with type 1 diabetes mellitus, the nurse would expect to note which history finding?
[ ] **1.** A sudden onset of symptoms
[ ] **2.** A sudden documentation of weight gain
[ ] **3.** A notation of ordered oral hypoglycemics
[ ] **4.** Quoted statements that the signs and symptoms are less severe

78. A client has hemiparalysis from a recent stroke. Which technique should the nurse avoid when changing the client's position in bed?
[ ] **1.** Logrolling the client from side to side
[ ] **2.** Sliding the client to move up in bed
[ ] **3.** Lifting the client using a mechanical lift
[ ] **4.** Having the client use an overhead trapeze

79. When administering eyedrops, in which anatomic location should the nurse begin applying the drops?
[ ] **1.** Inner canthus
[ ] **2.** Outer canthus
[ ] **3.** Upper conjunctival sac
[ ] **4.** Lower conjunctival sac

80. Which laboratory test would the nurse expect the physician to order to determine the infectious status of a 6-month-old infant whose mother tests positive for human immunodeficiency virus (HIV) infection?
[ ] **1.** Enzyme-linked immunosorbent assay (ELISA)
[ ] **2.** Immunoglobulin A (IgA) test
[ ] **3.** Western blot blood test
[ ] **4.** Rapid plasma reagin (RPR)

81. Which physical assessment technique is most appropriate to use to determine whether a 25-year-old substance abuser's unresponsiveness is related to a heroin overdose?
[ ] **1.** Checking the size of the client's pupils
[ ] **2.** Measuring the client's blood pressure
[ ] **3.** Observing the client's response to pain
[ ] **4.** Smelling the odor of the client's breath

82. The nurse is caring for a pregnant client who is in labor and receiving epidural anesthesia. Which position should the nurse avoid when repositioning this client?

[ ] **1.** Supine
[ ] **2.** Semi-Fowler's
[ ] **3.** Right side-lying
[ ] **4.** Left side-lying

83. The nursing team develops a teaching plan for a 10-year-old client with newly diagnosed diabetes who also has attention deficit hyperactivity disorder (ADHD). Which teaching strategy is most appropriate?
[ ] **1.** Providing individualized teaching in a quiet environment
[ ] **2.** Planning group teaching with other children with ADHD
[ ] **3.** Administering consequences for inappropriate behavior
[ ] **4.** Varying the method of instruction for each session

84. A widow whose husband died 1 month earlier tells a nurse that she plans to sell her home and move in with her daughter and son-in-law. Which nursing response is most appropriate?
[ ] **1.** Encourage the client to move on with her life.
[ ] **2.** Congratulate the client on making a hard decision.
[ ] **3.** Caution the client to postpone making major changes.
[ ] **4.** Suggest the client look into renting an apartment.

85. Which nursing action is most therapeutic for helping an older adult resolve grief associated with the death of a spouse?
[ ] **1.** Recommending taking a cruise with other senior citizens
[ ] **2.** Informing the client that grieving takes about 6 months
[ ] **3.** Allowing the client to verbalize feelings about the loss
[ ] **4.** Referring the client to an accountant for financial advice

86. At a routine home health visit, the nurse observes that an elderly client has several bruises on her arms and legs. The nurse reviews the client's history, which reveals that the client moved in with her daughter 1 month ago. Which assessment finding best indicates that the older adult is a victim of elder abuse?
[ ] **1.** The client sleeps on a couch in the living room.
[ ] **2.** There are conflicting explanations for the injury.
[ ] **3.** The home requires cleaning.
[ ] **4.** The client has lost weight in the last month.

87. A client has had a cancerous breast removed and is now preparing for surgery to have her ovaries removed. The client demonstrates understanding of the surgery when she indicates which as a rationale for her surgery?

[ ] **1.** "The surgery will enhance the action of anti-neoplastic drugs."

[ ] **2.** "The surgery will slow tumor growth and metastasis to other sites."

[ ] **3.** "The surgery will prevent adverse reactions of antineoplastic drugs."

[ ] **4.** "The surgery will increase my blood levels of progesterone."

88. Which information regarding estrogen deficiency is most appropriate to include in the discharge teaching of a client who has had her ovaries removed?

[ ] **1.** Hot flashes and a feeling of warmth are common.

[ ] **2.** Menstrual periods are accompanied by heavy flow.

[ ] **3.** Leg cramps may occur during sleep and inactivity.

[ ] **4.** Orgasms may be absent or reduced in the future.

89. The adult children of an older woman consult the nurse about relocating their aging mother from her home to a nursing home. Which nursing suggestion is most therapeutic for facilitating the mother's transition to the nursing home?

[ ] **1.** Identify the costs and services of several facilities.

[ ] **2.** Involve the mother in planning the relocation.

[ ] **3.** Consult the mother's personal physician about the planned move.

[ ] **4.** Label all the client's belongings with her name.

90. When planning the care of a client with an abdominal hysterectomy, which nursing measure is most helpful for preventing postoperative complications and facilitating an early discharge?

[ ] **1.** Reestablishing oral fluids and nutrition

[ ] **2.** Promoting ambulation and movement

[ ] **3.** Maintaining accurate intake and output

[ ] **4.** Exploring feelings about altered image

91. When a nurse discusses hospice care with the family of a terminally ill client, which statement is most therapeutic?

[ ] **1.** "Hospice nurses give better care than hospital nurses."

[ ] **2.** "Hospice nurses give around-the-clock care at home."

[ ] **3.** "Hospice nurses empower personal end-of-life decisions."

[ ] **4.** "Hospice nurses help extend predicted life expectancy."

92. Which characteristic behavior would the nurse expect to note when observing an 8-year-old child with attention deficit hyperactivity disorder (ADHD)?

[ ] **1.** The child has difficulty understanding instructions.

[ ] **2.** The child is uninterested in the surroundings.

[ ] **3.** The child refuses to play with others.

[ ] **4.** The child often fidgets and squirms.

93. The newborn infant of a diabetic mother is admitted to the nursery. Which intervention is most important to perform initially when providing care for this infant?

[ ] **1.** Check the newborn's blood glucose level.

[ ] **2.** Perform a gestational age assessment.

[ ] **3.** Assess for signs of neurologic deficits.

[ ] **4.** Begin phototherapy immediately.

94. The goal for the initial treatment of a client with newly diagnosed myasthenia gravis is to determine an effective maintenance dose of pyridostigmine (Mestinon). Which side effect of the medication is the best evidence that the client is experiencing an overdose?

[ ] **1.** Drooping eyelids

[ ] **2.** Muscle rigidity

[ ] **3.** Labored breathing

[ ] **4.** Extreme weakness

95. A 17-year-old client is seen in the dermatology clinic for treatment of acne vulgaris. Which nursing instruction is essential when teaching about how to avoid secondary infections and scarring?

[ ] **1.** Avoid wearing cosmetics.

[ ] **2.** Apply a drying agent nightly.

[ ] **3.** Avoid squeezing blackheads.

[ ] **4.** Scrub with a mild face soap.

96. A client has undergone an inguinal hernia repair and is preparing for discharge. Which instruction by the nurse is most appropriate?

[ ] **1.** Avoid forceful coughing.

[ ] **2.** Empty the bladder often.

[ ] **3.** Sleep on the operated side.

[ ] **4.** Limit early ambulation.

97. A client requires gastric decompression. Immediately after a Salem sump tube is inserted, which nursing action is correct?
[ ] **1.** The nurse checks the tube for proper placement.
[ ] **2.** The nurse connects the tube to mechanical suction.
[ ] **3.** The nurse irrigates the tube to keep it patent.
[ ] **4.** The nurse offers the client sips of ice water.

98. A client takes ibuprofen (Motrin) for discomfort associated with osteoarthritis. The best evidence that the client understands the hazards of taking this nonsteroidal anti-inflammatory drug (NSAID) is his ability to identify which common side effect?
[ ] **1.** Double vision
[ ] **2.** Transient dizziness
[ ] **3.** Irregular pulse
[ ] **4.** Upset stomach

99. An employee of a chemical plant comes to the emergency department for treatment of severe chemical burns. Which is the most appropriate emergency nursing treatment for this type of burn?
[ ] **1.** Irrigating the area with large amounts of water
[ ] **2.** Using a sterile dressing to cover the wound
[ ] **3.** Applying a thick layer of petroleum jelly to the area
[ ] **4.** Rubbing the burned skin with crushed ice

100. The nurse can best determine if oropharyngeal suctioning is necessary based on which assessment?
[ ] **1.** Type of cough
[ ] **2.** Sputum color
[ ] **3.** Ability to raise sputum
[ ] **4.** Respiratory rate

101. The family of a 78-year-old woman brings her to the hospital after she fell, struck her head, and briefly lost consciousness. Which instruction is most important to convey to the family prior to discharging the client from the emergency department?
[ ] **1.** Give the client extra fluids for the next 72 hours.
[ ] **2.** Keep the client flat in bed for the next several days.
[ ] **3.** Notify the physician if the client is difficult to arouse.
[ ] **4.** Check the client's eyes, ears, and nose for signs of bleeding.

102. Which assessment finding best indicates that there is an infection under a client's cast?
[ ] **1.** A long crack in the cast
[ ] **2.** A foul odor coming from the cast
[ ] **3.** Blood on the cast surface
[ ] **4.** An indentation in the cast

103. To avoid the potential for Reye's syndrome, it is best for the nurse to recommend that parents avoid administering which drug to their children?
[ ] **1.** Acetaminophen (Tylenol)
[ ] **2.** Ibuprofen (Nuprin)
[ ] **3.** Aspirin (Anacin)
[ ] **4.** Naproxen (Naprosyn)

104. When communicating with a client with expressive aphasia, which nursing intervention is most appropriate?
[ ] **1.** Speak about different subjects in one session.
[ ] **2.** Speak with increased volume and tone.
[ ] **3.** Encourage the client to write messages.
[ ] **4.** Make up gestures to communicate ideas.

105. Which nursing observation is the best evidence that a client's traction is maintained correctly?
[ ] **1.** The client's legs are parallel to the bed.
[ ] **2.** The client states that comfort is not compromised.
[ ] **3.** The counter weights are hanging free of the floor.
[ ] **4.** The client's feet are resting against the footboard.

106. Which cluster of assessment findings best indicates that a client is developing pulmonary edema?
[ ] **1.** Bradycardia, transient confusion, mild anxiety
[ ] **2.** Orthopnea, sudden dyspnea, elevated blood pressure
[ ] **3.** Tachycardia, decreased respiratory rate, weak pulse
[ ] **4.** Flushed face, hypotension, thick tenacious sputum

107. A 5-year-old child is scheduled to have a cardiac catheterization at 8:00 a.m. Which of the following provides the best indication that the child has been appropriately prepared for the procedure?
[ ] **1.** The child's chest has been cleansed with an antiseptic solution.
[ ] **2.** The parents state that the child has had nothing by mouth since 6:00 a.m.
[ ] **3.** The child has been shown pictures of the cardiac catheterization laboratory.
[ ] **4.** The parents state that the child will be unconscious during the procedure.

108. Which is the first step in planning a bladder retraining program for an incontinent client?
[ ] **1.** Determine the client's voiding patterns.
[ ] **2.** Limit the client's oral fluid intake.
[ ] **3.** Develop a regular schedule for urination.
[ ] **4.** Requisition a portable bedside commode.

109. Which observation by the nurse offers the best evidence that a paraplegic client understands the correct way to empty the bladder using Credé's maneuver?
[ ] **1.** The client inserts a straight catheter into the urethra using clean technique.
[ ] **2.** The client takes several deep breaths from the diaphragm before trying to void.
[ ] **3.** The client exhales slowly and steadily while tensing the abdominal muscles.
[ ] **4.** The client applies light pressure over the bladder area with the dominant hand.

110. The care plan for a 7-year-old boy with partial-thickness burns indicates that he should be placed in the prone position for 2 hours each shift. If the nursing assistant carries out the care plan correctly, the nurse will observe that the child is positioned in what manner?
[ ] **1.** On his back
[ ] **2.** On his side
[ ] **3.** On his abdomen
[ ] **4.** In a sitting position

111. The nurse assesses a newborn infant who has just been admitted to the nursery from the delivery room. Which assessment finding best indicates that the infant is experiencing respiratory distress?
[ ] **1.** An abdominal breathing pattern
[ ] **2.** A respiratory rate of 40 breaths/minute
[ ] **3.** An irregular breathing pattern
[ ] **4.** Grunting sounds on expiration

112. A male client who has advanced cancer is taking a chemotherapy drug. Which effect is the client most likely to report as a consequence of the drug therapy?
[ ] **1.** Hair loss
[ ] **2.** Breast enlargement
[ ] **3.** Deepening of the voice
[ ] **4.** Significant weight loss

113. A surgical client experiences abdominal incisional discomfort when coughing postoperatively. Which nursing intervention is most appropriate for reducing the client's discomfort?

[ ] **1.** Tell the client to flex both knees while coughing.
[ ] **2.** Have the client lie supine before trying to cough.
[ ] **3.** Teach the client to apply light pressure to the incision site with a pillow while coughing.
[ ] **4.** Administer an analgesic soon after coughing.

114. A liquid nutritional supplement is ordered for an older adult who is not eating adequately. When is the best time for providing the supplement?
[ ] **1.** Just before the noon meal
[ ] **2.** At the noon meal with other food
[ ] **3.** Immediately after eating lunch
[ ] **4.** Between breakfast and lunch

115. Which nursing intervention is most appropriate for preventing urine and stool from soiling the hip spica cast of an 18-month-old child?
[ ] **1.** Insert cotton wadding between the cast and the skin in the perineal area.
[ ] **2.** Cover the edges of the cast around the perineum with a waterproof material.
[ ] **3.** Offer the bedpan at more frequent intervals.
[ ] **4.** Place plastic pants over the perineal area.

116. A patient care technician is assisting the physician in positioning an 11-year-old child for a lumbar puncture. Which of the following indicates that the technician has positioned the client correctly for this procedure?
[ ] **1.** The child is in the prone position with the head turned to the side.
[ ] **2.** The child is in the recumbent position with the feet slightly elevated.
[ ] **3.** The child is in the supine position with the head of the bed elevated 45 degrees.
[ ] **4.** The child is in the side-lying position with the knees drawn up and back flexed.

117. A nurse and a nursing assistant are transferring an adult client from the bed to a wheelchair. Which intervention is best for ensuring the client's safety during the transfer?
[ ] **1.** Putting slippers on the client's feet
[ ] **2.** Locking the wheels on the wheelchair
[ ] **3.** Raising the upper side rails on the bed
[ ] **4.** Showing the client how to use the trapeze

118. Which nurse acts most appropriately to contain a fire?
[ ] **1.** The nurse who closes all the inside doors
[ ] **2.** The nurse who returns to the nursing station
[ ] **3.** The nurse who searches for signs of smoke
[ ] **4.** The nurse who stays with an immobile client

119. If the physician orders the irrigation of a urinary catheter but does not specify the type of solution to use, which solution would be the nurse's first choice?
[ ] **1.** Distilled water
[ ] **2.** Warm tap water
[ ] **3.** Sterile normal saline solution
[ ] **4.** Diluted hydrogen peroxide

120. If a client has obstructive jaundice, which assessment finding is the nurse most likely to observe?
[ ] **1.** Urine that is very dark brown
[ ] **2.** Saliva that is tan and thick
[ ] **3.** Stool that is green and watery
[ ] **4.** Skin that is pale and quite dry

121. After observing a brown discoloration on the washcloth while bathing an African American child, a nursing assistant reports to the nurse that she suspects the child's hygiene has been neglected. Which statement by the nurse provides the best explanation for the discoloration noted by the nursing assistant?
[ ] **1.** "African Americans bathe less to avoid dry skin."
[ ] **2.** "This is a normal finding from shedding skin cells."
[ ] **3.** "Soap tends to remove melanin from epidermal tissue."
[ ] **4.** "The skin of African Americans tends to retain oil."

122. When a nurse performs a mental status examination on an older adult, the previously cooperative client becomes silent when asked to spell "world" backwards. Which response by the nurse is most appropriate at this time?
[ ] **1.** Discontinue assessing the client.
[ ] **2.** Go on to another mental assessment.
[ ] **3.** Assume the client has early signs of dementia.
[ ] **4.** Presume the client is functionally illiterate.

123. Which goal is most appropriate when managing the care of an older adult client who has osteoporosis?
[ ] **1.** The client will consume more dairy products.
[ ] **2.** The client will acquire increased bone density.
[ ] **3.** The client will ambulate without falling.
[ ] **4.** The client will be restrained in a wheelchair.

124. Which assessment finding is most likely associated with the long-term effects of diabetes mellitus?
[ ] **1.** Diminished vision
[ ] **2.** Frequent indigestion
[ ] **3.** Urine retention
[ ] **4.** Tremors at rest

125. A 5-year-old child is being discharged following a tonsillectomy and adenoidectomy. When preparing discharge instructions for the parents, which information is most appropriate to include?
[ ] **1.** "Children commonly will have a great deal of pain for the first 7 days."
[ ] **2.** "Your child will have difficulty swallowing for about 3 weeks."
[ ] **3.** "Your child may expectorate bright red blood for about 1 week."
[ ] **4.** "A transient earache for about 1 to 3 days is a common complaint."

126. The nurse teaches a client how to change his ostomy appliance in preparation for his discharge home. Which suggestion is most helpful for ensuring that the appliance remains attached?
[ ] **1.** Empty the collection bag frequently.
[ ] **2.** Limit fluid intake throughout the day.
[ ] **3.** Change the appliance each morning.
[ ] **4.** Avoid eating gas-forming vegetables.

127. Which assessment finding is considered abnormal when performing the gestational age assessment of a full-term infant?
[ ] **1.** Lanugo over the shoulders, back, and forehead
[ ] **2.** A strong Moro reflex
[ ] **3.** Anterior transverse crease on the soles of the feet
[ ] **4.** Fully flexed posture

128. The emergency department physician prescribes alteplase, a thrombolytic drug, following a client's myocardial infarction. Which statement about the therapeutic action of this medication should the nurse include in the client's discharge instructions?
[ ] **1.** The medication lowers the client's anxiety level.
[ ] **2.** The medication lowers the systolic blood pressure.
[ ] **3.** The medication prevents the risk of arrhythmias.
[ ] **4.** The medication dissolves any clots in the circulation.

129. The nurse is developing a care plan for the residents of an assisted living facility. Which of the following physiological changes are characteristic of aging? Select all that apply.
[ ] **1.** Cardiac output declines.
[ ] **2.** Aspiration risk increases due to a weaker gag reflex.
[ ] **3.** Renal blood flow decreases.
[ ] **4.** Gastric motility increases.
[ ] **5.** Serum albumin level available for binding decreases.
[ ] **6.** The amount of body water increases.

130. The nurse is caring for a client who requires a venipuncture for a complete blood count. After checking the physician's orders and explaining the procedure to the client, the nurse performs all of the following actions in order of priority. Indicate the correct order in which the procedures are performed. Use all the options.

1. Clean the venipuncture site, wiping in a back and forth motion.

2. Wash the hands and then put on gloves.

3. Feel the vein, and note a rebound sensation.

4. Hold the skin taut, and pierce the skin at a 45-degree angle.

5. Assemble all necessary equipment.

6. Release the tourniquet, and withdraw the needle.

Correct Answers and Rationales

1. 2. Aspirin, or acetylsalicylic acid, is used as an anti-inflammatory agent, analgesic, antipyretic, and antiplatelet agent. It is a known gastric irritant. It should be taken with a full glass of water, food, or milk. Enteric-coated or buffered forms of aspirin help prevent gastric irritation and reduce the risk of bleeding. None of the other medications is associated with gastric irritation.

> *Client Needs Category—Physiological integrity*
> *Client Needs Subcategory—Pharmacological therapies*

2. 4. Getting additional rest is the best choice among the options for restoring energy during the demands of pregnancy. Although it is beneficial to modify the work routine to take advantage of times of peak energy, early morning is usually more of a prime energy time than midafternoon. It is inadvisable to take more than the prescribed dose of a medication, including vitamins. Daytime napping is appropriate, even if the naps are short and frequent.

> *Client Needs Category—Health promotion and maintenance*
> *Client Needs Subcategory—None*

3. 2. Good sources of iron include liver, lean meats, legumes, dried fruits, leafy green vegetables, whole grain, and fortified cereals. Potatoes, oranges, and cheese are not good sources of iron. However, citrus fruits in the diet help with iron absorption.

> *Client Needs Category—Health promotion and maintenance*
> *Client Needs Subcategory—None*

4. 3. Heroin is an opioid derived from morphine. Naloxone hydrochloride (Narcan) is an opioid antagonist that reverses the effects of opioids. Methadone hydrochloride (Dolophine) is an opiate-like drug used for detoxification and for clients in treatment programs for opioid abstinence. Both succinylcholine chloride (Anectine) and pancuronium bromide (Pavulon) are powerful neuromuscular junction blocking agents used as adjuncts to anesthetics.

> *Client Needs Category—Physiological integrity*
> *Client Needs Subcategory—Pharmacological therapies*

5. 3. Laxative use is contraindicated for postpartum clients with a third- or fourth-degree laceration because this type of laceration extends into the rectal sphincter. Instead of a laxative, a stool softener is usually prescribed. To avoid constipation, clients are encouraged to increase fluid intake and ambulate. Hemorrhoids, breast-feeding, and vacuum extraction are not reasons for omitting laxatives or enemas.

Client Needs Category*—Physiological integrity*
Client Needs Subcategory*—Physiological
    adaptation*

6. 2. Persons with only a few gallstones and mild symptoms experience relief by the application of shock waves (lithotripsy) that pulverize the stones. The smaller stones then move into the intestinal tract and are excreted in the stool. None of the other explanations is accurate.
Client Needs Category*—Physiological integrity*
Client Needs Subcategory*—Physiological
    adaptation*

7. 4. Dried beans, rice, peanut butter, peanuts, and whole grains are examples of plant proteins that are cheaper than animal proteins, such as meat, chicken, fish, and dairy products. Plant proteins taken in a sufficient amount or combined with a small amount of meat can satisfy the protein needs of a pregnant woman.
Client Needs Category*—Health promotion and
    maintenance*
Client Needs Subcategory*—None*

8. 2. Postmenopausal women generally pick an arbitrary date, such as the first day of the month, and perform breast self-examination on that date each month. If the client is still menstruating, the best time to examine the breasts is 2 to 3 days after the period, when the breasts are not tender. The time of day is not pertinent. It is better to examine the breasts during a shower, when the client's fingers can easily glide over the breast tissue. Breasts should be examined monthly rather than once a year.
Client Needs Category*—Health promotion and
    maintenance*
Client Needs Subcategory*—None*

9. 1. The presence of albumin in the urine is one of the three primary signs of preeclampsia, which is also referred to as *toxemia of pregnancy* and *pregnancy-induced hypertension*. The excretion of albumin in the urine is not a sign of liver failure, amniotic embolism, or gestational diabetes.
Client Needs Category*—Physiological integrity*
Client Needs Subcategory*—Physiological
    adaptation*

10. 2. Endocarditis is an infection or inflammation of heart valves. There is an association between infections with group A hemolytic streptococci and the development of rheumatic fever complicated by endocarditis. To prevent rheumatic heart disease and endocarditis, the American Heart Association recommends that children with streptococcal infections receive antibiotic therapy during their acute illness for at least 10 full days. Poverty and lack of health insurance often deter parents from seeking medical treatment for ill children. Endocarditis is not generally associated with birth defects, clubbing of the fingers, or failure to receive immunizations for the usual childhood infectious diseases.
Client Needs Category*—Physiological integrity*
Client Needs Subcategory*—Physiological
    adaptation*

11. 2. Not all clients admitted to the obstetric department are given an enema, but some physicians include an enema as part of their routine admission orders. It is appropriate to withhold an enema for clients who are experiencing vaginal bleeding and to collaborate with the physician. Enemas given during labor are not used for constipation but to evacuate stool to prevent contamination of the sterile field during delivery or to stimulate uterine contractions. The nurse should consult the physician before substituting a laxative for an enema.
Client Needs Category*—Physiological integrity*
Client Needs Subcategory*—Reduction of risk
    potential*

12. 3. The nurse's ultimate responsibility is for the patient's safety. A change in vital signs is a sign of systemic complications, such as hemorrhage and shock, and should be reported immediately. After notifying the charge nurse and physician, the nurse should then take frequent vital signs to provide a baseline for further treatment. Documenting the information, which is necessary, does not help the client improve. Fowler's position may lower, not raise, the blood pressure.
Client Needs Category*—Physiological integrity*
Client Needs Subcategory*—Physiological
    adaptation*

13. 1. A large oral intake keeps the urine dilute and less likely to obstruct a urinary catheter with blood clots and tissue debris. A large fluid volume does promote the excretion of toxic wastes, but that is not the best answer in this situation. The bladder capacity of a prostatectomy client is unaffected by the surgery. Specific exercises are used to promote bladder retraining.
Client Needs Category*—Physiological integrity*
Client Needs Subcategory*—Reduction of risk
    potential*

14. 2. The second stage of labor begins when the cervix is completely effaced and fully dilated; this stage of labor ends with delivery of the neonate. During the first stage of labor, the client has regular contractions that serve to dilate and thin the cervix. During the third stage of labor, the placenta is delivered. During the fourth stage of labor, the mother is monitored closely for complications such as hemorrhage.
Client Needs Category*—Health promotion and
    maintenance*
Client Needs Subcategory*—None*

15.

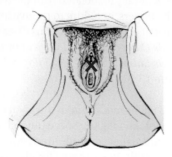

The nurse inserts the urinary catheter in the urinary meatus, which lies just above the vaginal opening and below the clitoris.

    Client Needs Category—Physiological integrity
    Client Needs Subcategory—Reduction of risk potential

16. **3.** The first approach to preventing falls is to assess why the client is trying to get out of the chair. Providing restraint alternatives is a better choice than applying a restraining vest. A restraint alternative is a protective or adaptive device that promotes the client's safety and postural support, which the client can release independently. However, restraining vests are important if restraint alternatives are ineffective and falls are to be avoided. A medical order is required before a restrictive restraint is applied. Tying a person in a chair with a sheet is ineffective for preventing falls because the client can slip under the sheet and onto the floor. Keeping a client within sight at all times is impractical. Sedation should be the last means of keeping the client in the chair.

    Client Needs Category—Safe, effective care environment
    Client Needs Subcategory—Safety and infection control

17. **2.** The presence of a rash is highly suggestive of an allergic reaction, which is common among individuals who are sensitive to penicillins. Before administering subsequent doses, the nurse needs to withhold the dose and notify the physician. The nurse uses alternative I.M. injection sites and rotates each injection site when a site becomes painful. A drop in body temperature indicates that the drug is having some therapeutic effect. A sore mouth can be the result of a superinfection caused by yeast or fungus as a result of antibiotic use. A sore mouth does not warrant withholding the medication; however, it does require further investigation.

    Client Needs Category—Physiological integrity
    Client Needs Subcategory—Pharmacological therapies

18. **3.** Four glasses of fluid per day is an inadequate volume of liquid to ensure moist stool. A healthy daily fluid intake includes 1,200 to 1,500 mL of water and beverages along with an additional 700 to 1,000 mL of water from food sources. Eating five servings of vegetables, eating cereal with skim milk, and substituting plant protein sources for meat are healthy dietary choices, but they do not ensure sufficient fluid intake to prevent constipation. Increasing dietary fiber promotes regular elimination of moist, bulky stools.

    Client Needs Category—Physiological integrity
    Client Needs Subcategory—Reduction of risk potential

19. **4.** The abbreviation b.i.d means twice daily. Therefore, the nurse would not be correct in administering the medication only once a day or more than twice a day.

    Client Needs Category—Safe, effective care environment
    Client Needs Subcategory—Safety and infection control

20. **2.** A Penrose and other types of open drains are placed within an operative site to help drainage escape from a surgical wound. Drains in a wound do not decrease scar formation. A drain is not used to irrigate a wound. A drain may remove air if it is in the area of a wound, but it is not used to release intestinal gas. Nasogastric and nasointestinal tubes are used to remove air and secretions from the stomach or intestine.

    Client Needs Category—Physiological integrity
    Client Needs Subcategory—Physiological adaptation

21. **3.** Medications should never be mixed with the total volume of tube-feeding formula because if the total volume is not ingested, the child will not receive the full amount of medication. Medications should be given separately from the formula. The procedures described in the remaining options are safe and appropriate.

    Client Needs Category—Health promotion and maintenance
    Client Needs Subcategory—None

22. **125.** To solve the calculation, first use the approximate equivalent of 2.2 lb = 1 kg to find the child's weight in kg:

$$\frac{44}{2.2} = 20 \text{ kg}$$

Next, calculate the total daily dose for this child by multiplying the dose by the child's weight in kg:

$$25 \text{ mg} \times 20 \text{ kg/day} = 500 \text{ mg/day}$$

To find the safe amount given in a single dose, divide by 4 (the total number of doses given in 1 day):

$$\frac{500}{4} = 125 \text{ mg/dose}$$

Client Needs Category—*Physiological integrity*
Client Needs Subcategory—*Pharmacological therapies*

23. **2.** Coughing increases intrathoracic pressure, which facilitates raising and expelling secretions from the airways. The client's body position during postural drainage depends on which lobe(s) of the lung needs draining. Lying supine does not encourage drainage from the lungs because it does not capitalize on using gravity. Breathing through the mouth is not related to postural drainage and elimination of secretions. Breathing slowly may increase tidal volume, but it does not promote elimination of pulmonary secretions.

Client Needs Category—*Physiological integrity*
Client Needs Subcategory—*Physiological adaptation*

24. **2.** Because of the changes in circulation in the lower extremities related to the disease process, it is important for the client with diabetes to observe good foot care. Further teaching is needed in this case because the client is at risk for cuts, injury, and infection by having his wife remove his calluses with a razor blade. All the other choices are appropriate when practicing good foot care. Other instructions regarding diabetic foot care include avoiding going barefoot; wearing well-fitting shoes; washing, drying, and covering injuries with sterile gauze; applying lotion to the feet daily; and keeping feet clean and dry and nails short. In addition, the client should carefully examine his feet daily for blisters, cuts, and redness.

Client Needs Category—*Physiological integrity*
Client Needs Subcategory—*Physiological adaptation*

25. **4.** When introducing an NG tube into a nostril, it is best to have the client sit upright with the neck hyperextended. This position helps the nurse to guide and direct the tip of the tube toward the pharynx. After the tube is in the oropharynx, the nurse instructs the client to flex the neck and lower the chin to the chest. Then, the nurse advances the tube into the stomach. Circumduction and rotation of the neck do not facilitate insertion or advancement of an NG tube.

Client Needs Category—*Safe, effective care environment*
Client Needs Subcategory—*Safety and infection control*

26. **4.** The INR is the laboratory test used to assess the effectiveness of warfarin sodium (Coumadin) therapy. Blood levels are obtained on a regular basis to assess the blood's coagulation status. Warfarin sodium (Coumadin) works by interfering with the formation of vitamin K-dependent clotting factors in the liver. Platelet levels are unaffected by warfarin sodium (Coumadin). Partial prothrombin time is used to assess the effectiveness of heparin, not warfarin, therapy. The circulating blood volume remains unchanged with warfarin sodium (Coumadin).

Client Needs Category—*Physiological integrity*
Client Needs Subcategory—*Pharmacological therapies*

27. **1.** Foods of an animal nature are generally involved in outbreaks of food-borne gastroenteritis. Common foods include milk, eggs, and meat. The pathogens tend to grow and reproduce when the food is not refrigerated properly or is undercooked. The appearance, flavor, and odor of contaminated food may be unaffected. Whether a client has previously had a food-borne infection does not necessarily reflect a diagnostic relationship to the present symptoms. Taking something for nausea does not help determine the cause of the problem.

Client Needs Category—*Physiological integrity*
Client Needs Subcategory—*Physiological adaptation*

28. **4.** Care of a client receiving internal radiation therapy is best rotated among all nonpregnant members of the nursing team because rotating care minimizes the time any one individual is exposed to radiation. It is safe and appropriate to warn personnel and visitors of a potential hazard, both verbally and using universal symbols. Radiation badges measure the amount of radiation exposure to the caregiver; therefore, each person involved in the client's care wears a different badge.

Client Needs Category—*Safe, effective care environment*
Client Needs Subcategory—*Safety and infection control*

29. **3.** An IVP is used to evaluate the structures of the urinary system and to assess renal function. An iodine-based dye injected intravenously is commonly used. After injection, the dye passes into the kidneys. X-rays are taken about 30 minutes later. A history of allergies is most important, especially if the client has a history of an allergy to iodine or seafood (which contains iodine). Allergic reactions vary from mild flushing and itching to anaphylactic shock. Delayed response to the dye can occur 2 to 6 hours after the test. If the client is allergic to iodine, the physician is notified before the client has the IVP. Urine output is monitored after the test. The other choices are not essential for the nurse to ask before the IVP.

> ***Client Needs Category***—*Physiological integrity*
> ***Client Needs Subcategory***—*Reduction of risk potential*

30. 1. Of the four options, listening to a radio or audiotapes is the most appropriate diversional activity for a client with a recent loss of vision. The newly blind client may not be ready to interact with others as a means of diversion. Listening to television may create anxiety because the client can only hear, not see, what is happening. Reading books set in Braille requires special education and time to practice the technique.

> ***Client Needs Category***—*Physiological integrity*
> ***Client Needs Subcategory***—*Physiological adaptation*

31. 4. A compound fracture is one in which the bone pierces the skin and the bone is exposed. Pain, impaired mobility, and crepitation (grinding sensation) can be present in closed fractures as well; therefore, these findings do not provide the best evidence of a compound fracture.

> ***Client Needs Category***—*Physiological integrity*
> ***Client Needs Subcategory***—*Physiological adaptation*

32. 3. To determine the number of milliliters of an I.V. solution to infuse in 1 hour, the total quantity (in this example, 1,000 mL) is divided by the total hours of infusion (in this example, 8 hours). Therefore, the hourly volume is 125 mL.

> ***Client Needs Category***—*Safe, effective care environment*
> ***Client Needs Subcategory***—*Safety and infection control*

33. 2. An antistreptolysin O test is useful in the diagnosis of rheumatic fever. This test detects antibodies to the enzymes of the streptococcus group A, which is thought to cause rheumatic fever, glomerulonephritis, bacterial endocarditis, scarlet fever, and other related conditions. The antinuclear antibody test is used to indicate the presence of lupus erythematosus. The heterophile antibody titer is performed to determine if a person has infectious mononucleosis. The fluorescent antibody test is used to diagnose syphilis.

> ***Client Needs Category***—*Physiological integrity*
> ***Client Needs Subcategory***—*Physiological adaptation*

34. 4. Because the client is overweight, inserting the needle at a 90-degree angle is the most appropriate technique. Using a ⅝″ needle rather than a ½″ needle will allow the insulin to reach the subcutaneous tissue. A 15-degree angle is used for intradermal injections, such as in tuberculosis tests. A 30-degree angle is not used with subcutaneous injections. If the client were of normal weight, a 45-degree angle for the injection would be appropriate.

> ***Client Needs Category***—*Safe, effective care environment*
> ***Client Needs Subcategory***—*Safety and infection control*

35. 2. Discharge teaching for a client who has undergone a prostatectomy includes the warning to avoid heavy lifting and strenuous exercise until the physician permits these activities. Constipation is avoided by eating foods high in roughage and enemas are also avoided. A liberal fluid intake is encouraged.

> ***Client Needs Category***—*Health promotion and maintenance*
> ***Client Needs Subcategory***—*None*

36. 4. A client with expressive aphasia hears normally and understands verbal communication but has an impaired ability to provide a clear verbal response. Communication is improved in many instances if the nurse gives the client time to use motions or signs, write an answer (if able), or try to speak. Even though the speech of a client with expressive aphasia is greatly impaired, some affected people can be understood if the listener is patient. It is incorrect to assume that a client with aphasia is also intellectually compromised.

> ***Client Needs Category***—*Physiological integrity*
> ***Client Needs Subcategory***—*Physiological adaptation*

37. 2. Continuous bubbling is abnormal in the water-seal chamber but is normal in the suction-control chamber. Continuous bubbling in the water-seal chamber generally indicates an air leak in the tubing between the client and the water-seal chamber. The source of the air leak needs to be determined, or the therapeutic benefit of the water-seal drainage system will be compromised. The water seal is being maintained by the 2 cm of water. Bloody drainage is normal and a sign that the blood is being evacuated from the thorax. Breath sounds are usually diminished in clients with a hemothorax.

> ***Client Needs Category***—*Physiological integrity*
> ***Client Needs Subcategory***—*Reduction of risk potential*

38. 3. Following cardiac catheterization, the nurse needs to assess the femoral pulse, which is located in the client's groin. The popliteal pulse is felt behind the knee. The pedal pulse is felt on the dorsum of the foot. The posterior tibial pulse is felt in the lower leg.

> ***Client Needs Category***—*Physiological integrity*
> ***Client Needs Subcategory***—*Physiological adaptation*

39. **3.** During the transition phase of active labor, the client may not tolerate touch but fears being left alone. Other signs of transition include nausea and vomiting, trembling of the lower extremities, irritability, and fear of losing control. Rupture of the membranes may occur spontaneously or artificially at any point during labor. The urge to push (the same feeling as the urge to have a bowel movement) occurs during the second stage of labor. Shivering is a normal response that may occur after delivery, during the fourth stage of labor.
> *Client Needs Category*—*Physiological integrity*
> *Client Needs Subcategory*—*Physiological adaptation*

40. **1.** Kegel exercises involve tightening and relaxing the pelvic floor muscles. The exercises are performed four or more times per day and from 5 to 20 times each session. Performed consistently, Kegel exercises prevent or relieve stress incontinence, shorten the second stage of labor, promote healing of perineal and rectal incisions, and increase the potential for sexual orgasm.
> *Client Needs Category*—*Health promotion and maintenance*
> *Client Needs Subcategory*—*None*

41. **4.** The correct procedure is to instill a volume of air equal to the volume that will be removed. Instilling air increases the pressure within the vial and facilitates removal of the drug. Omitting air instillation creates a vacuum in the vial when the drug is withdrawn. Injecting more air than the amount of the drug withdrawn creates excessive pressure in the vial, which may force the plunger out of the syringe. It is generally unnecessary to refrigerate a drug before withdrawing it from a vial unless the manufacturer recommends refrigeration.
> *Client Needs Category*—*Safe, effective care environment*
> *Client Needs Subcategory*—*Safety and infection control*

42. **3.** Recapping needles is a potentially hazardous action that can lead to needle-stick injuries and possible transmission of bloodborne pathogens. Wearing gloves, depositing sharp items in a biohazard container, and swabbing the site are safe and appropriate actions.
> *Client Needs Category*—*Safe, effective care environment*
> *Client Needs Subcategory*—*Safety and infection control*

43. **2.** Mild to severe joint pain indicates bleeding into the joint, which can lead to joint deformities or destruction. Hemophiliacs with symptoms suggestive of bleeding need immediate medical attention. There is no direct connection between hemophilia and anorexia or nasal congestion. Depression may develop as a consequence of coping with a chronic illness. Depression indicates a need for additional nursing assessment for suicidal ideation and continued close observation.
> *Client Needs Category*—*Physiological integrity*
> *Client Needs Subcategory*—*Reduction of risk potential*

44. **4.** The nurse is responsible for determining that the client has sufficient information to manage self-care after discharge. Areas that are unclear, such as the medication schedule and follow-up appointments, are reexplained by the nurse and documented in the client's medical record. Questions about how the client is coping and plans for time management are thoughtful, but they are not more important than the client's ability to manage his or her illness. It is considerate to inquire about home transportation, but the health agency is not responsible for providing transportation unless it is medically necessary.
> *Client Needs Category*—*Health promotion and maintenance*
> *Client Needs Subcategory*—*None*

45. **4.** The use of body powder on an infant is not recommended because of the risk for pneumonitis secondary to aspiration of the talc. A room temperature between 72° and 75° F (22° and 24° C) is appropriate. Wiping the teeth with gauze is appropriate oral care for an infant; as an alternative, having the infant drink water cleans the mouth. It is also appropriate to use the elbow to assess the bath water temperature because the elbow is most sensitive to temperature variations.
> *Client Needs Category*—*Safe, effective care environment*
> *Client Needs Subcategory*—*Coordinated care*

46. **1.** Two abused drugs that may be injected into a vein are cocaine and heroin. Heroin is an opiate. Opiates are any drug containing or derived from opium. Cocaine is a stimulant; it is purified from the leaves of the cocoa plant. Cocaine is also commonly snorted through the nose or inhaled by smoking. Heroin is injected directly into a vein or under the skin, a technique known as skin-popping. Barbiturates, amphetamines, and hallucinogens are more commonly self-administered by the oral route.
> *Client Needs Category*—*Physiological integrity*
> *Client Needs Subcategory*—*Pharmacological therapies*

47. **4.** An advance directive is a legal document that describes how a client wishes to be treated or not treated should the client at some future time be unable to make this decision independently. The client may also select a spokesperson, such as the physician or a spouse, to act on his behalf regarding using or withholding medical treatment. Financial cost or insurance is not considered a priority in arriving at an ethical decision. It is unnecessary for all the client's relatives to agree or disagree on discontinuing life support.

> ***Client Needs Category***—*Safe, effective care environment*
> ***Client Needs Subcategory***—*Coordinated care*

48. 3. Correct treatment of poison ingestion and the possible administration of an antidote depend on identification of the specific substance ingested. The client's age, who discovered the client, and the client's past medical history are relevant but of lesser importance than identifying the substance.

> ***Client Needs Category***—*Physiological integrity*
> ***Client Needs Subcategory***—*Physiological adaptation*

49. 3. Reinforcing the fact that easily implemented techniques (hand washing and wearing gloves) can block the transmission of the virus from client to health care worker is the best information from among the choices. Being told the sources of transmission is not as reassuring as reiterating how the transmission is blocked. Even though many infected people are living longer and some receive medical benefits from insurers, those options hardly give peace of mind.

> ***Client Needs Category***—*Psychosocial integrity*
> ***Client Needs Subcategory***—*None*

50. 1. Immediately after the membranes have ruptured, the nurse monitors the fetal heart rate to detect fetal distress. Natural or artificial rupture of the membranes may result in prolapse of the umbilical cord, which is followed by compression of the cord and interference with fetal oxygenation. Antibiotics are not routinely given when the amniotic membranes rupture. The physician may decide to place the client on antibiotics if the membranes have been ruptured for an extended period of time. Applying pads does not take priority over assessing for fetal distress. In the event of a prolapsed cord, the client is placed in Trendelenburg's position to assist with relieving umbilical cord compression.

> ***Client Needs Category***—*Physiological integrity*
> ***Client Needs Subcategory***—*Reduction of risk potential*

51. 2. Pneumonia occurs most commonly in clients who are in a weak, immunosuppressed state; have chronic disorders, such as AIDS, diabetes, cardiac or pulmonary disorders, cirrhosis, cancer, or renal failure; who are malnourished, smokers, or alcoholics; or have been exposed to toxic airborne substances. Other risk factors for pneumonia include immobility and recent general endotracheal intubation or surgery. Sudden weight gain, anemia, and dehydration are not considered risk factors for pneumonia. Aspiration pneumonia

can occur if the client has a hypoactive, not a hyperactive, gag reflex.

> ***Client Needs Category***—*Physiological integrity*
> ***Client Needs Subcategory***—*Reduction of risk potential*

52. 3. Sitting upright with the feet and legs elevated reduces the myocardial workload. This position also allows for maximum expansion of the thoracic cavity. Low Fowler's position is used if the client cannot tolerate the upright position. Neither lying on the side nor lying with the head lowered would be advisable.

> ***Client Needs Category***—*Safe, effective care environment*
> ***Client Needs Subcategory***—*Safety and infection control*

53. 3. Clients with slow-bleeding cerebral aneurysms are kept quiet to prevent additional or heavy bleeding. Until the physician indicates that it is safe for the client to increase activity, it is best for the nurse to position the client on a bedpan rather than on the bedside commode. A suppository is appropriate if the client is constipated. Clients such as this one who must avoid straining when voiding are generally given a daily stool softener to facilitate ease of elimination.

> ***Client Needs Category***—*Physiological integrity*
> ***Client Needs Subcategory***—*Physiological adaptation*

54. 2. Flaccid muscle tone in a newborn must be reported immediately. A healthy newborn is generally active and displays kicking of the feet and flexion of the arms. The hands and feet may appear blue (acrocyanosis) for a short time after delivery while the rest of the body is pink. As the newborn's respirations improve and the baby is warmed, skin color tends to become pink overall. It is normal for a healthy newborn to have a pulse rate over 100 beats/minute and a loud, vigorous cry

> ***Client Needs Category***—*Physiological integrity*
> ***Client Needs Subcategory***—*Physiological adaptation*

55. 3. Minor burns over a small area are treated first by immersing the affected part in cool water. Cool compresses may also be applied. Ointments or salves are not applied to minor burns. Normally, a dressing is unnecessary for minor burns. However, when a dressing is necessary, sterile gauze is applied over the area and anchored with nonallergenic tape above and below the burn site.

> ***Client Needs Category***—*Physiological integrity*
> ***Client Needs Subcategory***—*Physiological adaptation*

56. 3. Glaucoma is an eye disorder characterized by increased pressure in the eye. There are three types of glaucoma: closed-angle (acute), open-angle (chronic), and congenital. Closed-angle glaucoma is characterized by acute pain. Therefore, a therapeutic response following the treatment of closed-angle glaucoma is a reduction or elimination of pain within the eye. Swollen eyelids are not a manifestation of closed-angle glaucoma. The conjunctiva, not the sclera, is red during an acute attack of closed-angle glaucoma. Loss of peripheral vision is a pathologic consequence of untreated or ineffectively treated glaucoma.

Client Needs Category—*Physiological integrity*
Client Needs Subcategory—*Pharmacological therapies*

57. 1. Liquid and ointment otic (ear) preparations are warmed to room temperature if they have been stored in a cool or cold area. Instilling cold medication into the ear is uncomfortable. Unless the dropper is grossly covered with debris or wax, it is unnecessary to clean it routinely. There are no general limitations on the maximum volume instilled within the ear. The anatomic size of the client's ear canal and the prescribed dose of medication are guidelines for the amount of drug administered.

Client Needs Category—*Physiological integrity*
Client Needs Subcategory—*Pharmacological therapies*

58. 1. Fetal alcohol syndrome may result as a consequence of a mother consuming alcohol during pregnancy. The syndrome leads to mental and physical retardation or structural anomalies involving the head, eyes (widely set), ears, and heart. As children with this syndrome get older, some develop attention deficit hyperactivity disorder. Cataracts, seizures, and missing limbs are not closely associated with fetal alcohol syndrome.

Client Needs Category—*Health promotion and maintenance*
Client Needs Subcategory—*None*

59. 3. When the subject involves sexual abuse, the best initial response is to assume a child is telling the truth. Following that, nursing actions such as those in the alternative options are appropriate.

Client Needs Category—*Psychosocial integrity*
Client Needs Subcategory—*None*

60. 3. On average, signs of alcohol withdrawal are apparent in 12 to 72 hours. However, withdrawal may begin to occur as early as 4 to 6 hours among those who have a pattern of consuming large amounts of alcohol on a routine basis. Initially, clients have a progressive elevation in their vital signs, tremors, and diaphoresis.

If withdrawal is uncontrolled, seizures and hallucinations may also occur.

Client Needs Category—*Physiological integrity*
Client Needs Subcategory—*Physiological adaptation*

61. 4. Burns around the face and neck may compromise breathing as a consequence of inhaling heated air and debris or the swelling of burned tissue. Initially, the burned client will have a fluid volume deficit related to fluid shifts. Hemorrhage does not commonly occur with burns unless there has been an additional injury, such as a wound or fracture. Signs of infection are not evident initially but may occur several days after the injury.

Client Needs Category—*Physiological integrity*
Client Needs Subcategory—*Physiological adaptation*

62. 2. Frequent ROM exercises along with regularly changing a client's position help to prevent contractures. Isometric exercises maintain muscle tone but do not prevent contractures. Elevating extremities on pillows promotes venous circulation and decreases edema formation but does not necessarily prevent contractures. Pressure-relieving devices maintain capillary blood flow, which is necessary for maintaining tissue integrity, not preventing contractures.

Client Needs Category—*Physiological integrity*
Client Needs Subcategory—*Reduction of risk potential*

63. 1. A foul wound odor indicates an infection. The odor of infection is different from the odor associated with burn exudate. Eschar normally turns black after a period of time. A WBC count of $5,000/mm^3$ is normal and, therefore, not an indicator of infection. Tachycardia might occur if an infection is present, but there are other physiological explanations for a rapid heart rate.

Client Needs Category—*Physiological integrity*
Client Needs Subcategory—*Physiological adaptation*

64. 4. For a client recovering from gastroenteritis, solid foods nonirritating to the gastrointestinal tract are added to the diet first. Foods such as bananas, rice, applesauce, toast (BRAT), tea, and yogurt (BRATTY) are provided initially. Milk products are among the last foods reintroduced to the diet because milk and milk products can be hard to digest. Vanilla pudding contains milk, and milk is usually added to oatmeal or cereal. Salty broths such as chicken broth are also avoided. Furthermore, chicken broth is not a solid food.

Client Needs Category—*Physiological integrity*
Client Needs Subcategory—*Physiological adaptation*

65. **3.** Large muscle activities that release nervous energy such as using a treadmill are best for clients with generalized anxiety disorder. Playing cards, assembling models, and painting are too sedentary.

> *Client Needs Category—Psychosocial integrity*
> *Client Needs Subcategory—None*

66. **1.** Normal potassium levels are between 3.5 and 5.0 mEq/L. A value lower than 3.5 mEq/L indicates hypokalemia. Signs of hypokalemia include muscle weakness, leg cramping, shallow respirations, shortness of breath, irregular rapid heart rate, ECG changes, confusion, depression, lethargy, GI symptoms, polyuria, and polydipsia. Rapid weight gain is a sign of hypernatremia (elevated sodium level). Slurred speech is a sign of hypophosphatemia (low phosphate level).

> *Client Needs Category—Physiological integrity*
> *Client Needs Subcategory—Reduction of risk*
> *potential*

67. **1.** Diabetes commonly causes altered blood flow to the retina, resulting in a condition known as *diabetic retinopathy.* Such changes can lead to poor vision and possible blindness. Consequently, clients with diabetes should have their vision checked at least once per year and should be instructed to notify their physician if sudden vision changes occur. Cataracts related to the increased levels of blood glucose may also occur in clients with diabetes. Diabetes is associated with polyuria, but the color of the urine is not typically noted when evaluating for signs and symptoms of diabetes. Neither elevated blood pressure nor heart palpitations are complications of diabetes. Other complications of diabetes include periodontal disease and changes in the circulation of the lower extremities that can result in ulcerations, increased infections, gangrene, and amputations. In addition, changes in the peripheral nerves can cause weakness and pain as well as impaired GI, genitourinary, and vasomotor functioning.

> *Client Needs Category—Physiological integrity*
> *Client Needs Subcategory—Physiological*
> *adaptation*

68. **4.** Oral hypoglycemics are used to treat type 2 diabetes. The onset action of hypoglycemic agents is harder to predict than that of insulin, but the typical time to observe for hypoglycemia is 30 to 60 minutes after ingestion. Peak action occurs in about 1 to 2 hours. Therefore, 8:30 a.m. is the most appropriate time to assess for hypoglycemia.

> *Client Needs Category—Physiological integrity*
> *Client Needs Subcategory—Pharmacological*
> *therapies*

69. **2.** Rheumatic fever may follow a streptococcal infection. Therefore, a history of a recent sore throat, which may have been due to *Streptococcus* microorganisms, is pertinent to the diagnosis. Viral infections, such as influenza, chickenpox, and roseola, are not known to be associated with rheumatic fever.

> *Client Needs Category—Health promotion and*
> *maintenance*
> *Client Needs Subcategory—None*

70. **4.** Joint pain and tenderness (arthralgia) involving one or more joints is noted when assessing a client with rheumatic fever. Urticaria, hypothermia, and hypotension are not typically associated with rheumatic fever.

> *Client Needs Category—Physiological integrity*
> *Client Needs Subcategory—Physiological*
> *adaptation*

71. **4.** When performing a nonstress test, fetal movement must be present. For a nonstress test to be considered favorable, there must also be at least two fetal heart rate accelerations of at least 15 beats/minute within a 20- to 30-minute time frame. Each acceleration must last for at least 15 seconds.

> *Client Needs Category—Physiological integrity*
> *Client Needs Subcategory—Physiological*
> *adaptation*

72. **2.** Because mechanical friction further traumatizes skin affected by radiation, the client's skin should be cleaned with mild soap and tepid water and then patted dry. Vigorous rubbing over the area could cause skin damage. The marks are never removed because they are meant to remain on the skin throughout the interim of radiation therapy. The irradiated skin is protected from direct sunlight. Clothing that covers the area of treatment must fit loosely.

> *Client Needs Category—Physiological integrity*
> *Client Needs Subcategory—Physiological*
> *adaptation*

73. **1.** Constipation is a side effect of antacids containing aluminum and calcium. Antacids containing magnesium cause a laxative effect. None of the other symptoms the client described is associated with antacid drug therapy.

> *Client Needs Category—Physiological integrity*
> *Client Needs Subcategory—Pharmacological*
> *therapies*

74. **2.** Temperature assessment by the rectal route is avoided when a child has leukemia because of the danger of causing injury and bleeding. A sponge or gauze is appropriate to use for mouth care to prevent gums from bleeding. Children with leukemia are maintained in protective isolation because of their compromised immune status. A sheepskin is placed under bony prominences for comfort.

Client Needs Category—*Safe, effective care environment*

Client Needs Subcategory—*Coordinated care*

75. 3. Pantoprazole (Protonix) is a proton pump inhibitor that inhibits the production of gastric secretions, making the gastric contents less acidic. Some antiulcer medications such as sucralfate (Carafate) form a protective coating similar to mucus at the ulcer site. This layer shields the irritated tissue from further irritation by hydrochloric acid and pepsin. Antacids neutralize gastric secretions, raising their pH. Histamine antagonists reduce gastric acid production by blocking histamine-2 receptors.

Client Needs Category—*Physiological integrity*

Client Needs Subcategory—*Pharmacological therapies*

76. 4. The volume used to irrigate a colostomy is the same as the volume used to administer a cleansing enema. Commonly, the volume for a cleansing enema and colostomy irrigation is between 500 and 1,000 mL.

Client Needs Category—*Physiological integrity*

Client Needs Subcategory—*Physiological adaptation*

77. 1. The main difference between juvenile diabetes and adult diabetes is the sudden onset of symptoms. Adult diabetics usually have gradual onset of symptoms. The signs and symptoms are essentially the same and do not vary with age. They include polydipsia, polyuria, polyphagia, nocturia, and weight loss (not weight gain). The onset of diabetic symptoms in children is often associated with ketoacidosis, which is a life-threatening condition. Insulin, not oral hypoglycemics, is used to treat adolescent clients with type 1 diabetes.

Client Needs Category—*Physiological integrity*

Client Needs Subcategory—*Physiological adaptation*

78. 2. Sliding a client up in bed causes friction, which can injure the skin, predisposing it to breakdown and pressure ulcers. It is better to logroll the client or use a mechanical lift or a trapeze to change positions. When rolling a client, the nurse must maintain the correct anatomic position, keeping the limbs supported. A mechanical lift is particularly useful if the client is large or difficult to move. The lift moves and holds the client so that he can be moved in or out of bed. By holding onto the trapeze, the client can assist the nurse in turning and repositioning himself.

Client Needs Category—*Safe, effective care environment*

Client Needs Subcategory—*Safety and infection control*

79. 4. Eyedrops are instilled into the lower conjunctival sac. Before instilling eyedrops, the nurse should first ask the client to look up, then pull the lower lid margin downward by exerting pressure over the bony prominence of the cheek.

Client Needs Category—*Physiological integrity*

Client Needs Subcategory—*Pharmacological therapies*

80. 2. An IgA test is a more reliable test than the ELISA or Western blot test for determining the HIV status of infants and young children. The Western blot test and the ELISA both evaluate the presence of IgG antibodies that can cross the placenta and give a false-positive result if the mother is HIV-positive. IgA antibodies do not cross the placenta; thus, the presence or absence of IgA antibodies is more reliable. The RPR test is a serologic test used to detect syphilis.

Client Needs Category—*Physiological integrity*

Client Needs Subcategory—*Physiological adaptation*

81. 1. Heroin, like morphine, causes the pupils to constrict. Although a person with a heroin overdose might be hypotensive, this finding is not as significant as finding pinpoint pupils. There may be multiple reasons why the client does not respond to pain. Heroin does not produce a characteristic breath odor as occurs with alcohol consumption or medical conditions such as diabetic ketoacidosis.

Client Needs Category—*Physiological integrity*

Client Needs Subcategory—*Pharmacological therapies*

82. 1. The supine position is contraindicated for a client receiving epidural anesthesia because it causes vena cava compression and results in maternal hypotension. Hypotension reduces placental perfusion and fetal oxygenation. Semi-Fowler's and right or left side-lying positions do not compress the vena cava and are, therefore, more appropriate.

Client Needs Category—*Safe, effective care environment*

Client Needs Subcategory—*Safety and infection control*

83. 1. The child who has ADHD requires an environment free of distractions to facilitate processing information. Group teaching creates a greater potential for distraction. Rewarding desirable behavior is considered more therapeutic for effecting change than administering punishment. Having a consistent routine also proves to be more effective than varying the routine.

Client Needs Category—*Psychosocial integrity*

Client Needs Subcategory—*None*

84. 3. After the death of a spouse, it is important to eventually develop a new identity, learn new life skills, engage in new activities, and establish new relationships. Until the acute grief is resolved, however, it is important to delay making major changes. Rushing into decisions too soon often leads to regrets later. Suggesting that the client look into renting an apartment or congratulating her on her decision is inappropriate and nontherapeutic.
   Client Needs Category—*Psychosocial integrity*
   Client Needs Subcategory—*None*

85. 3. Verbalization allows the bereaved to express emotions connected with grief. Many people need to continue processing their grief over and over again, and they may not receive that opportunity from others who feel inadequate to deal with the emotional pain. Grieving is unique to each person, but it may take several years to resolve the loss of a significant person. Giving advice is nontherapeutic; clients may fear losing the nurse's support if they do not take the advice. Recommending a cruise with other senior citizens or referring the client to an accountant for financial advice is unlikely to resolve the client's grief.
   Client Needs Category—*Psychosocial integrity*
   Client Needs Subcategory—*None*

86. 2. Home health care nurses must guard against making assumptions when their clients' environments do not reflect their own values and standards. In this case, although there are obvious health hazards in the home environment such as its lack of cleanliness, the most suspicious finding suggesting elder abuse is the conflicting explanations about the cause of the client's injuries. Although a private bedroom is more desirable than sleeping on a couch, this may be the only option at this time. The cause of the client's weight loss should be investigated, but it is not necessarily the most suspicious finding indicating elder abuse because it may be related to medical causes.
   Client Needs Category—*Psychosocial integrity*
   Client Needs Subcategory—*None*

87. 2. When a malignant breast tumor is hormone-dependent, growth is enhanced by the presence of estrogen, a hormone secreted by the ovaries. Removal of the ovaries eliminates the source of estrogen and thus slows metastasis and growth of any remaining tumor cells. This procedure does not enhance the action of antineoplastic drugs, prevent adverse reactions associated with the administration of antineoplastic drugs, or increase progesterone levels.
   Client Needs Category—*Physiological integrity*
   Client Needs Subcategory—*Physiological adaptation*

88. 1. Symptoms similar to menopause such as hot flashes tend to occur when the ovaries are surgically removed. If there are no contraindications, estrogen replacement therapy can relieve many of the uncomfortable symptoms. Menstrual periods cease when the ovaries are removed. Leg cramps are unrelated to the oophorectomy but are important to report to the physician if they occur. Orgasms are unaffected by removal of the ovaries.
   Client Needs Category—*Physiological integrity*
   Client Needs Subcategory—*Physiological adaptation*

89. 2. Involving the older adult in planning the transition to the nursing home reduces feelings of powerlessness. Feeling that one is part of the solution is better than feeling that one is part of the problem. Obtaining factual information, consulting the physician, and reinforcing positive expected outcomes are helpful but futile if the client feels a loss of control. Labeling the client's clothes is a task that is helpful but does not aid in the client's psychosocial transition.
   Client Needs Category—*Psychosocial integrity*
   Client Needs Subcategory—*None*

90. 2. Ambulation and movement help in preventing thrombi and hypostatic pneumonia. Early ambulation also promotes resumption of peristalsis, which facilitates oral nutrition. Although nutrition and fluids are important, the client's needs can be met temporarily with parenteral therapy. Intake and output are measures for assessing and evaluating whether fluid replacement and output are adequate. The client's emotional adjustment demands the nurse's attention, but physical recovery is primary to the discharge goals.
   Client Needs Category—*Physiological integrity*
   Client Needs Subcategory—*Reduction of risk potential*

91. 3. Hospice nurses are dedicated to facilitating the personal preferences of dying clients and managing how they wish to live and die. Secondarily, they are committed to supporting family members, who tend to be the primary caregivers. Calling hospice nurses "better" nurses is too subjective a statement. Hospice nurses have the same basic education and technical skills as hospital nurses. Hospice nurses make frequent or daily visits to the home, depending on the client needs, but do not provide around-the-clock care. Although some dying clients live longer than expected, that is not an expected outcome of hospice care.
   Client Needs Category—*Psychosocial integrity*
   Client Needs Subcategory—*None*

92. 4. The child with ADHD has such characteristic symptoms as difficulty concentrating, disruptive behavior, failing to complete tasks, constantly moving and fidgeting, and acting in a loud and noisy manner. The child understands but does not follow directions well because he is easily distracted. Lack of interest in surroundings and refusal to play with others are not characteristic of this disorder.

Client Needs Category—*Physiological integrity*
Client Needs Subcategory—*Physiological adaptation*

93. 1. Infants of diabetic mothers are commonly hypoglycemic at birth or shortly thereafter; therefore, the first nursing action is to assess the blood glucose level. If hypoglycemia is not detected and treated with either oral or I.V. glucose, the infant may develop severe, irreversible central nervous system damage and may die. Infants of diabetic mothers are often large for their gestational age, but this assessment does not take priority over determining whether the infant is hypoglycemic. The infant of the diabetic mother is also at risk for respiratory distress and hyperbilirubinemia. However, before receiving oxygen or phototherapy, the infant should be evaluated to determine if there is a need for treatment.

Client Needs Category—*Physiological integrity*
Client Needs Subcategory—*Physiological adaptation*

94. 2. Pyridostigmine (Mestinon) is a drug commonly used to treat myasthenia gravis. It belongs to a group of cholinergic drugs that promote muscle contraction. Muscle weakness and decreased function are common signs of myasthenia gravis; therefore, the goal of drug therapy is to obtain optimal muscle strength. Signs of drug overdose include muscle rigidity and spasm, salivation, and clenching of the jaw. Signs that the drug levels are nontherapeutic (too low) include signs of the disease itself, such as rapid fatigability, drooping eyelids, and difficulty breathing.

Client Needs Category—*Physiological integrity*
Client Needs Subcategory—*Pharmacological therapies*

95. 3. Squeezing blackheads and pimples can cause spread of infection and scarring of the skin. A client with acne vulgaris can wear cosmetics but should avoid those that are oil-based. Makeup should be removed nightly with mild soap. Drying agents should be avoided.

Client Needs Category—*Health promotion and maintenance*
Client Needs Subcategory—*None*

96. 1. To avoid undue strain and tension on the repaired muscle, clients who have undergone a hernia repair must avoid any activity that increases intra-abdominal pressure. Coughing, heavy lifting, sneezing, and straining to have a bowel movement can lead to an incisional hernia until the repaired area has healed. There is no reason for emptying the bladder any more frequently than to maintain comfort. There are no restrictions on turning. Ambulation is not limited unless the client develops a surgical complication.

Client Needs Category—*Physiological integrity*
Client Needs Subcategory—*Physiological adaptation*

97. 1. After inserting the tube, the nurse should check for placement of the tube in the stomach by aspirating stomach contents and injecting air into the stomach while auscultating with a stethoscope. (An X-ray may be ordered to verify placement.) If the client turns blue, has difficulty speaking, or begins to cough or wheeze, the tube is removed immediately because it is either in the client's trachea or occluding the airway. Suction is applied after tube placement has been verified. Irrigation is usually performed when there are large clots or tissue debris occluding the tubing. Irrigation is not done unless tube placement has been verified. Although the client is not allowed to drink or eat, the nurse may offer small sips of water or ice chips sparingly after the tube is connected to suction.

Client Needs Category—*Safe, effective care environment*
Client Needs Subcategory—*Safety and infection control*

98. 4. The most common adverse reactions to NSAIDs include nausea, vomiting, abdominal discomfort, diarrhea, constipation, and gastric or duodenal ulcers. Double vision, transient dizziness, and irregular pulse are not common side effects of NSAIDs.

Client Needs Category—*Physiological integrity*
Client Needs Subcategory—*Pharmacological therapies*

99. 1. Emergency treatment of a chemical burn is directed at diluting and removing the substance as rapidly as possible by flushing the skin with large quantities of water. Applying a sterile dressing may cause tissue to adhere to the skin and pull tissue from the burn area. Specific dressings for burns will be utilized following dilution and removal of the chemical from the skin. Applying a thick layer of petroleum jelly is not appropriate in the emergency department; specific burn ointments are commonly utilized. Rubbing the skin intensifies the burn injury.

Client Needs Category—*Physiological integrity*
Client Needs Subcategory—*Physiological adaptation*

100. 3. Oropharyngeal suctioning is performed when the client is unable to cough and raise sputum. Other indications of the need for suctioning include dyspnea, cyanosis, and moist breath sounds. Identifying the type of cough, sputum characteristics, and respiratory rate are important assessments, but they are not criteria for determining the necessity for suctioning a client.

Client Needs Category—Physiological integrity
Client Needs Subcategory—Physiological adaptation

101. 3. A change in the client's level of consciousness is a clinical indication of intracranial bleeding. If drowsiness or sleepiness occurs and the client cannot be easily aroused, the physician should be notified. Drinking extra fluids or keeping the client in bed is usually unnecessary. Although it is important to observe for signs of bleeding, the most dangerous bleeding occurs within the skull.

Client Needs Category—Physiological integrity
Client Needs Subcategory—Physiological adaptation

102. 2. The presence of a foul or unusual odor from within a cast indicates an infection. A crack or indentation in the cast does not indicate infection but compromises the integrity of the cast. Blood on the cast surface indicates bleeding beneath the cast.

Client Needs Category—Physiological integrity
Client Needs Subcategory—Reduction of risk potential

103. 3. Studies suggest that the use of salicylates, especially aspirin, to relieve a fever or discomfort during a viral illness may lead to Reye's syndrome. Acetaminophen (Tylenol) is safe for the relief of minor symptoms, such as fever and headache. Ibuprofen (Nuprin) and naproxen (Naprosyn) are effective in relieving pain.

Client Needs Category—Health promotion and maintenance
Client Needs Subcategory—None

104. 3. The nurse should encourage the client with expressive aphasia to write messages as a form of communication. Being able to communicate his ideas decreases the client's level of frustration. Many clients with aphasia use communication boards to discuss frequent topics, such as the need to go to the bathroom, the need for a drink, or the need to be handed a book. One topic is discussed at a time to decrease confusion, stimuli, and distractions. Using a normal tone and voice volume is appropriate because the client may not have hearing difficulties. Made-up gestures are not universally known, so accurate communication is not always possible.

Client Needs Category—Physiological integrity
Client Needs Subcategory—Physiological adaptation

105. 3. One of the necessary criteria for maintaining the effectiveness of traction is that the weights must hang free of the floor. The legs may or may not be parallel to the bed, depending on the type of traction applied. Although comfort is a desirable outcome of traction, it is not an indication of the traction's effectiveness. If the feet resist the pull of traction by resting on the footboard, the traction's efficiency is reduced.

Client Needs Category—Physiological integrity
Client Needs Subcategory—Physiological adaptation

106. 2. The symptoms of pulmonary edema include orthopnea (difficulty breathing while lying down), sudden dyspnea, pink frothy sputum, cyanosis, bounding pulse, elevated blood pressure, severe apprehension, and moist or gurgling respirations.

Client Needs Category—Physiological integrity
Client Needs Subcategory—Physiological adaptation

107. 3. If an actual visit to the cardiac catheterization laboratory cannot be arranged, showing the child pictures of the laboratory and equipment will facilitate the teaching process. The site of catheter insertion is the femoral artery or an antecubital vessel; therefore, the chest would not be cleaned with an antiseptic. The child should have nothing by mouth for at least 4 hours prior to the procedure. For this procedure, the child will be lightly sedated but not unconscious.

Client Needs Category—Health promotion and maintenance
Client Needs Subcategory—None

108. 1. The initial step in planning a bladder retraining program is determining the client's voiding pattern. Knowing the voiding pattern helps the nurse develop an individualized voiding schedule. Limiting fluid intake is not recommended; the client needs an adequate fluid intake to keep the urine dilute and prevent a fluid deficit. Requisitioning a commode, if appropriate for the client, is done after collecting data about the voiding pattern.

Client Needs Category—Physiological integrity
Client Needs Subcategory—Physiological adaptation

109. 4. The client performs Credé's maneuver by positioning the hands on the abdomen and applying light pressure over the bladder to initiate voiding. Voiding is achieved without the use of a catheter. The maneuver does not require any special breathing techniques.

Client Needs Category—Physiological integrity
Client Needs Subcategory—Physiological adaptation

110. **3.** The prone position is one in which the client is placed on his abdomen. If a supine position is indicated, the client is placed on his back. A side-lying position is a lateral position. A sitting position is referred to as Fowler's position.
>   ***Client Needs Category***—*Physiological integrity*
>   ***Client Needs Subcategory***—*Physiological adaptation*

111. **4.** Grunting on expiration is a signal of respiratory distress, indicating that effort is needed to move air out of the lungs. Newborn infants normally have a respiratory rate between 30 and 60 breaths/minute. In addition, they normally breathe abdominally and have an irregular breathing pattern.
>   ***Client Needs Category***—*Physiological integrity*
>   ***Client Needs Subcategory***—*Physiological adaptation*

112. **1.** Chemotherapeutic drugs are given to cure cancers, decrease tumor size, or prevent or treat metastases. The side effects of these drugs vary, depending on the length of treatment and the specific drug used. Common side effects of chemotherapy include anorexia, nausea and vomiting, diarrhea, soreness or ulcerations of the mouth, loss of hair (baldness), bone marrow depression, and the inability to fight infection. Voice changes and breast enlargement are not usually associated with chemotherapeutic drugs. Weight loss usually results from the cancer itself, although weight loss can occur due to anorexia, nausea, vomiting, and diarrhea.
>   ***Client Needs Category***—*Physiological integrity*
>   ***Client Needs Subcategory***—*Pharmacological therapies*

113. **3.** Placing a pillow on the abdomen and applying firm, light pressure reduces strain on the incision, which reduces discomfort. Flexing the knees or lying supine are not as likely to promote comfort as applying pressure. It is more advantageous to administer an analgesic shortly before, rather than after, a client coughs or performs other activities that cause discomfort.
>   ***Client Needs Category***—*Physiological integrity*
>   ***Client Needs Subcategory***—*Physiological adaptation*

114. **4.** Liquid nutritional supplements are best offered between meals so that the supplement is not substituted for the meal. If the supplement is given before a meal, the client may not eat an adequate amount of food. If it is given with or soon after a meal, the client may be too full to consume the entire volume.
>   ***Client Needs Category***—*Physiological integrity*
>   ***Client Needs Subcategory***—*Reduction of risk potential*

115. **2.** Covering the edges of the cast with waterproof material such as plastic helps prevent soiling the cast. Cotton wadding should not be inserted unless ordered by the physician. Offering the bedpan at more frequent intervals does not necessarily prevent soiling of the cast, especially if the child is not toilet-trained (which is usual for an 18-month-old child). Plastic pants are contraindicated because they hold moisture and contribute to the disintegration of the cast.
>   ***Client Needs Category***—*Physiological integrity*
>   ***Client Needs Subcategory***—*Reduction of risk potential*

116. **4.** When a lumbar puncture is performed, the client is placed either in a side-lying position, with the knees drawn up and the back flexed, or in a sitting position, with the back flexed. Both of these positions increase the space between the vertebrae to facilitate insertion of the needle within the lumbar interspaces with minimal trauma. Neither the prone position nor the recumbent position is appropriate for increasing the vertebral space. Sitting in the supine position with the head of the bed at a 45-degree angle will not allow access to the vertebral space needed for the procedure.
>   ***Client Needs Category***—*Safe, effective care environment*
>   ***Client Needs Subcategory***—*Safety and infection control*

117. **2.** Locking the wheels ensures that the wheelchair remains in place during the transfer. Although wearing slippers provides warmth and some protection for the client's feet, wearing them is not as important as locking the wheels. Raised side rails and a trapeze can help the client change positions, but they are not the best safety measures during a transfer.
>   ***Client Needs Category***—*Safe, effective care environment*
>   ***Client Needs Subcategory***—*Safety and infection control*

118. **1.** Closing doors helps keep the fire confined to its location of origin and slows or prevents its spread into other areas. It is important to assemble with others at the nursing station to await instructions, but this activity is appropriate only after the environment is secured. Searching for smoke takes valuable time better spent closing doors. Staying with an immobile client is admirable, but nurses have a responsibility to ensure the protection of all clients, not just one who may have difficulty evacuating.
>   ***Client Needs Category***—*Safe, effective care environment*
>   ***Client Needs Subcategory***—*Safety and infection control*

119. 3. Unless the physician orders otherwise, the standard for care is to use sterile normal saline solution when irrigating an indwelling catheter. Normal saline solution is an isotonic solution that will not damage cells. It is incorrect to use an unsterile solution of distilled water or tap water. Hydrogen peroxide is not commonly used when irrigating urinary catheters.

Client Needs Category—Physiological integrity
Client Needs Subcategory—Physiological adaptation

120. 1. A client with obstructive jaundice characteristically has dark brown urine. The change in color is due to the excretion of bilirubin via the kidneys rather than through the intestinal tract. In addition to dark brown urine, clay-colored stools are evident. The other physical assessments have no relationship to obstructive jaundice.

Client Needs Category—Physiological integrity
Client Needs Subcategory—Physiological adaptation

121. 2. All people, regardless of their ethnic background, shed dead skin cells during bathing. In African American clients, the dead skin cells are more obvious because the cells retain their dark pigmentation. This finding is commonly misinterpreted as a disregard for hygiene. Soap cannot physically or chemically remove pigmentation. There is as much ethnic variation in dryness or oiliness of skin among African Americans as in other ethnic groups.

Client Needs Category—Health promotion and maintenance
Client Needs Subcategory—None

122. 2. After allowing sufficient time for a response, moving on to another area of assessment shows respect for the client; however, the nurse must document the lack of response in the client's assessment. Failure to respond to one area of assessment does not justify discontinuing further efforts to assess mental status. With only limited data, it is inaccurate to assume that a client who does not respond is demented or illiterate.

Client Needs Category—Psychosocial integrity
Client Needs Subcategory—None

123. 3. Preventing falls is a major goal when caring for clients with osteoporosis. Even a minor fall can result in a fracture. Consuming dairy products is a healthy behavior, but it is not likely to reverse longstanding osteoporosis. Increasing bone density is a goal of medical therapy. Having osteoporosis does not justify restraining a client in a wheelchair.

Client Needs Category—Physiological integrity
Client Needs Subcategory—Reduction of risk potential

124. 1. Clients with diabetes mellitus are prone to developing visual changes that may result in blindness. Other major diabetic complications include renal failure, coronary artery disease, increased susceptibility to infection, changes in circulation, and peripheral nerve damage. Indigestion, urine retention, and tremors are significant problems, but they are not commonly associated with diabetes mellitus.

Client Needs Category—Physiological integrity
Client Needs Subcategory—Physiological adaptation

125. 4. A transient earache for 1 to 3 days is common following a tonsillectomy and adenoidectomy. The discomfort is due to pain referred from the throat to the ear. When giving discharge instructions, the nurse should advise parents of the possibility of earache. Severe pain for the first 7 days after surgery, difficulty swallowing for 3 weeks, and expectorating bright red blood are not normal and should be brought to the physician's attention.

Client Needs Category—Health promotion and maintenance
Client Needs Subcategory—None

126. 1. Emptying the collection bag decreases the weight and pull on the skin to which the appliance is attached. Fluids are not restricted; restricting fluids concentrates the urine and increases the risk of dehydration, skin irritation, and infection. To avoid skin impairment, an appliance is generally not changed on a daily basis; however, a loose or uncomfortable appliance must be changed. It is unlikely that avoiding gas-forming foods would have any effect on appliance attachment.

Client Needs Category—Health promotion and maintenance
Client Needs Subcategory—None

127. 3. The full-term infant usually has plantar creases over the entire surface of the soles of the feet. The presence of anterior transverse creases is associated with prematurity. Lanugo over the shoulders, back, and forehead is a normal finding in the full-term newborn. A strong Moro reflex and a fully flexed posture are also characteristic of the full-term newborn.

Client Needs Category—Health promotion and maintenance
Client Needs Subcategory—None

128. 2. The mother should be advised to avoid overdressing her infant in warm weather because this reduces perspiration in areas of the body covered with clothes. Applying baby oil may increase, rather than decrease, the problem. Fine cornstarch applied to the affected areas may reduce perspiration, but baby powder (which may contain talc) should be avoided because of the asbestos content of talc. Strong detergents should be avoided because of the risk of atopic dermatitis, but this will not prevent heat rashes.

> *Client Needs Category*—*Health promotion and maintenance*
> *Client Needs Subcategory*—*None*

129. **1, 2, 3, 5.** When developing a care plan for older adults, it is important for nurses to recognize the wide variety of physiological changes that occur with aging and how such changes impact daily life. For example, the efficiency and contractile strength of the heart diminish with aging, resulting in decreased cardiac output. The risk for aspiration increases due to a weaker gag reflex and a delay (not increase) in gastric emptying. Renal blood flow and glomerular filtration rate decrease by 50% between ages 20 and 90. Serum albumin levels also decrease, resulting in less availability of albumin for binding. Older adults have less body water, causing drier mucous membranes.

> *Client Needs Category*—*Physiological integrity*
> *Client Needs Subcategory*—*Physiological adaptation*

130.

5. Assemble all necessary equipment.

2. Wash the hands and then put on gloves.

3. Feel the vein, and note a rebound sensation.

1. Clean the venipuncture site, wiping in a back and forth motion.

4. Hold the skin taut, and pierce the skin at a 45-degree angle.

6. Release the tourniquet, and withdraw the needle.

Prior to any procedure, the nurse needs to review the physician's order for accuracy, and then assemble the needed equipment on a convenient space close to the client. Next, the nurse must wash her hands and put on gloves before touching the client. Assessing the vein status thoroughly is essential to ensuring a successful stick on the initial attempt. After selecting an appropriate vein, the nurse cleans the venipuncture site by wiping in a back and forth motion and allows the site to dry. Holding the skin taut, the nurse pierces the skin with the needle, entering at a 45-degree angle. After obtaining the specimen, the nurse releases the tourniquet and withdraws the needle. Lastly, the nurse applies pressure to the site with gauze or a cotton ball for several minutes.

> *Client Needs Category*—*Physiological integrity*
> *Client Needs Subcategory*—*Reduction of risk potential*

Bibliography

Barry, P.D. *Mental Health and Mental Illness*, 7th ed. Philadelphia: Lippincott Williams & Wilkins, 2002.

Christensen, B.L., and Kockrow, E.O., eds. *Foundations of Nursing*, 4th ed. St. Louis: Mosby–Year Book, 2002.

Cohen, B.J., and Wood, D.L. *Memmler's The Human Body in Health and Disease*, 9th ed. Philadelphia: Lippincott Williams & Wilkins, 2000.

Cohen, B.J., and Wood, D.L. *Memmler's Structure & Function of the Human Body*, 7th ed. Philadelphia: Lippincott Williams & Wilkins, 2000.

Edmunds, M. W. *Introduction to Clinical Pharmacology*, 3rd ed. St. Louis: Mosby–Year Book, 2000.

Fischbach, F.T. *A Manual of Laboratory and Diagnostic Tests*, 7th ed. Philadelphia: Lippincott Williams & Wilkins, 2004.

Harkness, G.A., and Dincher, J. R. *Medical-Surgical Nursing: Total Patient Care*, 10th ed. St. Louis: Mosby–Year Book, 2001.

Kalman, N., and Waughfield, C.G. *Mental Health Concepts*, 5th ed. Albany: Thompson Delmar Learning, 2001.

Keltner, N.L., et al. *Psychiatric Nursing*, 4th ed. St. Louis: Mosby–Year Book, 2002.

Marks, M.G. *Broadribb's Introductory Pediatric Nursing*, 6th ed. Philadelphia: Lippincott Williams & Wilkins, 2003.

Nettina, S.M. *The Lippincott Manual of Nursing Practice*, 8th ed. Philadelphia: Lippincott Williams & Wilkins, 2006.

Reiss, B.S., and Evans, M.E. Pharmacological Aspects of Nursing Care, 6th ed. Albany: Thompson Delmar Learning, 2001.

Roach, S.S., and Scherer, J.C. *Introductory Clinical Pharmacology*, 7th ed. Philadelphia: Lippincott Williams & Wilkins, 2004.

Rosdahl, C B. *Textbook of Basic Nursing*, 8th ed. Philadelphia: Lippincott Williams & Wilkins, 2002.

Scanlon, V.C., and Sanders, T. *Essentials of Anatomy and Physiology*, 4th ed. Philadelphia: F.A. Davis, 2002.

Shives, L.R. *Basic Concepts of Psychiatric-Mental Health Nursing*, 5th ed. Philadelphia: Lippincott Williams & Wilkins, 2001.

Smeltzer, S.C., and Bare, B.G. *Brunner and Suddarth's Textbook of Medical-Surgical Nursing*, 10th ed. Philadelphia: Lippincott Williams & Wilkins, 2003.

Timby, B.K. *Fundamental Nursing Skills and Concepts*, 8th ed. Philadelphia: Lippincott Williams & Wilkins, 2005.

Timby, B.K. *Fundamental Skills and Concepts in Patient Care*, 8th ed. Philadelphia: Lippincott Williams & Wilkins, 2005.

Timby B.K, and Smith, N. *Essentials of Nursing: Care of Adults and Children*. Philadelphia: Lippincott Williams & Wilkins, 2004.

Timby, B.K., et al. *Introductory Medical-Surgical Nursing*, 8th ed. Philadelphia: Lippincott Williams & Wilkins, 2003.

Tucker, S.M., et al. *Patient Care Standards: Collaborative Practice Planning Guides*, 7th ed. St. Louis: Mosby–Year Book, 2000.

2006 Lippincott's Nursing Drug Guide. Philadelphia: Lippincott Williams & Wilkins, 2006.

Wold, G. *Basic Geriatric Nursing*, 3rd ed. St. Louis: Mosby–Year Book, 2003.

About the CD-ROM

This *Lippincott's Review for NCLEX-PN,* Seventh Edition, CD-ROM is just another reason why the book in your hands is so highly regarded by students and faculty. With nearly 2,000 NCLEX©-style questions (multiple-choice and alternate-format), this CD gives you even more options to lead you to exam excellence!

MINIMUM SYSTEM REQUIREMENTS
- Windows 98
- Pentium 166
- 128 MB RAM
- 8 MB of free hard-disk space
- SVGA monitor with high color (16-bit)
- CD-ROM drive

INSTALLATION
Place the CD in your CD-ROM drive. After a few moments, the install process will automatically begin. *Note:* If the install process doesn't automatically begin, click the Start button and select Run. At the command line, type *D:\setup.exe.* (Note: The letter D represents the CD-ROM drive. If your drive is designated by a different letter, use your drive letter instead.) Click OK. Follow the installation instructions.

TECHNICAL SUPPORT
For technical support, call toll-free 1-800-638-3030, Monday through Friday, 8:30 a.m. to 5 p.m. Eastern Time. You may also write to Lippincott Williams & Wilkins Technical Support, 351 W. Camden Street, Baltimore, MD 21201-2436, or e-mail us at techsupp@lww.com.